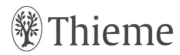

Pathology Q&A

Walter L. Kemp, MD, PhD
Associate Professor
University of North Dakota School of Medicine and Health Sciences
Grand Forks, North Dakota

Travis Brown, MD
Family Physician
Midlothian, Texas

251 illustrations

Thieme
New York • Stuttgart • Delhi • Rio de Janeiro

Acquisitions Editor: Delia DeTurris
Managing Editor: Elizabeth Palumbo
Developmental Editor: Julia Nollen
Director, Editorial Services: Mary Jo Casey
Production Editor: Kenneth L. Chumbley
International Production Director: Andreas Schabert
Editorial Director: Sue Hodgson
International Marketing Director: Fiona Henderson
International Sales Director: Louisa Turrell
Director of Institutional Sales: Adam Bernacki
Senior Vice President and Chief Operating Officer: Sarah Vanderbilt
President: Brian D. Scanlan

Library of Congress Cataloging-in-Publication Data

Names: Kemp, Walter L., author. | Brown, Travis G., author.
Title: Pathology Q&A / Walter Kemp, Travis Brown.
Description: New York : Thieme, [2018]
Identifiers: LCCN 2017023726| ISBN 9781626233805 (softcover : alk. paper) | ISBN 9781626233812 (ebook)
Subjects: | MESH: Pathologic Processes | Examination Questions
Classification: LCC RB119 | NLM QZ 18.2 | DDC 616.07076—dc23
LC record available at https://lccn.loc.gov/2017023726

© 2018 Thieme Medical Publishers, Inc.
Thieme Publishers New York
333 Seventh Avenue, New York, NY 10001 USA
+1 800 782 3488, customerservice@thieme.com

Thieme Publishers Stuttgart
Rüdigerstrasse 14, 70469 Stuttgart, Germany
+49 [0]711 8931 421, customerservice@thieme.de

Thieme Publishers Delhi
A-12, Second Floor, Sector-2, Noida-201301
Uttar Pradesh, India
+91 120 45 566 00, customerservice@thieme.in

Thieme Publishers Rio de Janeiro, Thieme Publicações Ltda.
Edifício Rodolpho de Paoli, 25º andar
Av. Nilo Peçanha, 50 – Sala 2508
Rio de Janeiro 20020-906, Brasil
+55 21 3172 2297

Cover design: Thieme Publishing Group
Typesetting by Prairie Papers

Printed in China by Everbest Printing Co.   5 4 3 2 1

ISBN 978-1-62623-380-5

Also available as an e-book:
eISBN 978-1-62623-381-2

Important note: Medicine is an ever-changing science undergoing continual development. Research and clinical experience are continually expanding our knowledge, in particular our knowledge of proper treatment and drug therapy. Insofar as this book mentions any dosage or application, readers may rest assured that the authors, editors, and publishers have made every effort to ensure that such references are in accordance with **the state of knowledge at the time of production of the book.**

Nevertheless, this does not involve, imply, or express any guarantee or responsibility on the part of the publishers in respect to any dosage instructions and forms of applications stated in the book. **Every user is requested to examine carefully** the manufacturers' leaflets accompanying each drug and to check, if necessary in consultation with a physician or specialist, whether the dosage schedules mentioned therein or the contraindications stated by the manufacturers differ from the statements made in the present book. Such examination is particularly important with drugs that are either rarely used or have been newly released on the market. Every dosage schedule or every form of application used is entirely at the user's own risk and responsibility. The authors and publishers request every user to report to the publishers any discrepancies or inaccuracies noticed. If errors in this work are found after publication, errata will be posted at www.thieme.com on the product description page.

Some of the product names, patents, and registered designs referred to in this book are in fact registered trademarks or proprietary names even though specific reference to this fact is not always made in the text. Therefore, the appearance of a name without designation as proprietary is not to be construed as a representation by the publisher that it is in the public domain.

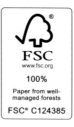

FSC
www.fsc.org
100%
Paper from well-managed forests
FSC® C124385

About this Book

The questions in this book are designed to present a clinical scenario that requires a student to diagnose a pathologic condition. For many questions, the answer to the question is the pathologic diagnosis; however, for other questions, the diagnosed pathologic condition is assumed to be known to the student, and instead, the question stem asks for a specific feature of that condition. The organ-specific sections (e.g., Cardiovascular) can easily be used during the second year of medical school as a review of the material and to study for tests during the year. The mixed question sections would be best for USMLE review; however, the organ-specific sections can also easily be used for USMLE study. The images in the text are chosen to represent common or uncommon but characteristic pathologic findings.

To my wife, Kelly, for her unconditional love and never ending patience for my professional endeavors, including the support of my writing of another book when I had specifically told her not to let me write any more.

To Dr. Gary Dale, for being a good friend and a supportive and collegial mentor during our ten years working together in our home state of Montana, and for showing me the truth to the quote, "Stand up for what you believe in even if it means standing alone."

To my best friend, Brian Kieffer, for always showing me how a person can maintain their dignity and humor even when dealing with adversities in life far greater than anything I myself have ever faced.

Walter Kemp

Dedicated to my wife, to my daughter, Nola, and my son, Abraham, and to the most gifted clinician I have ever known, Dr. Andrey Manov, MD.

Travis Brown

Contents

Preface viii
Acknowledgments.. ix
How to Use This Series x
About the Authors xii

1 Cell Injury, Adaptations, and Death 1

2 Inflammation and Repair 9

3 Hemodynamics 17

4 Diseases of the Immune System 29

5 Neoplasia 45

6 Genetic and Pediatric Diseases 51

7 Environmental and Nutritional Diseases 67

8 Diseases of the Cardiovascular System 77

9 Diseases of the Hematopoietic and Lymphoid Systems 103

10 Diseases of the Respiratory System 125

11 Diseases of the Kidney and Urinary Tract 143

12 Diseases of the Mouth and Gastrointestinal Tract 155

13 Diseases of the Liver, Gallbladder, and Biliary Tract 177

14 Diseases of the Pancreas 197

15 Diseases of the Male and Female Genital Tract 201

16 Diseases of the Breast 213

17 Diseases of the Endocrine System 217

18 Diseases of the Musculoskeletal System 235

19 Diseases of the Peripheral and Central Nervous Systems 241

20 Diseases of the Skin 263

21 Mixed Items 271

22 Images 291

Index 405

Preface

This book is a collection of multiple choice questions (MCQs) to promote the learning of pathology in the framework of preclinical and clinical disciplines. The main features of the book are the following:

The MCQs are all of the type that is used for the Step 1 medical board exams in the United States and are written according to United States Medical Licensing Examination (USMLE) guidelines (i.e., patient-centered vignettes). All questions are "one best answer"; in most cases, there are five answer choices, but in some cases fewer or more choices are given.

Because the MCQs are about pathology, each question is based upon a specific pathologic condition. To correctly answer each question requires a student to use the information given to diagnose the condition, or, the question stem assumes that a student will know the diagnosis, and a question about the disease process is asked instead.

Each MCQ is provided with a level of difficulty, a learning objective, the correct answer, and an explanation.

There are three levels of difficulty: easy, medium, and hard. In general, an easy difficulty question requires only a diagnosis based upon the question stem, whereas a medium difficulty question requires not just the diagnosis of the condition based upon the question stem, but knowledge about that diagnosis so as to answer a question about it (i.e., the student is assumed to know the diagnosis, and a question about the diagnosis is asked), and hard difficulty questions are a combination of medium difficulty questions with less commonly known material about the diagnosis. Question ratings by their nature are subjective; however, every attempt was made to follow the above approach when determining the difficulty of a question. A single question may be easy for one student to answer and hard for another student to answer based upon their knowledge base and test-taking skills.

The learning objective is a brief behavioral statement written using an action verb. If a student can perform the action, then he or she should be able to answer the question correctly. The explanation includes both the reasons why a given answer is correct and why the distractors are wrong.

Many questions are related to the highest levels of Bloom's taxonomy (e.g., interpretation of data and solution of problems) rather than being simple recall questions.

Most MCQs are integrated questions, and a good knowledge of the relevant human physiology, biochemistry, microbiology, and elementary clinical medicine is a necessary prerequisite to determine the right answer to the question. Therefore, the question with its answer explanation can also be used as a powerful tool for reviewing and integrating the medical science disciplines.

The MCQs are grouped in chapters covering most topics presented in standard pathology textbooks. There are 20 to 40 MCQs in each chapter, totaling over 1000 questions.

MCQs are the learning tool most frequently used by medical students. This book is intended as an integrated tool for both course study and board exam preparation. Because the book is organized along clinical rather than strictly pathological lines, it should be useful for Step 1 preparation, but also for Step 2 exam preparation.

Pathology, especially the molecular aspect, is a fast-evolving discipline. The authors have checked sources believed to be reliable, in order to provide information that is in accordance with the currently accepted standards. However, the authors are aware that in several instances the pathology of disease is still controversial. They have tried, as much as possible, to avoid questions addressing controversial issues.

This book is not intended to be a substitute for pathology textbooks. Students are strongly advised to consult their textbooks of pathology for more in-depth coverage of the subject matter.

Walter L. Kemp, MD, PhD
Travis Brown, MD

Acknowledgments

We would like to thank the following members of the University of North Dakota School of Medicine and Health Sciences medical school class of 2018 who assisted in the ranking of questions: Elizabeth Anderson, Joley Beeler, Kacy Benedict, Justin Berger, Whitney Bettenhausen, Jocelyn Fetsch, Brandon Fisher, Jennifer Glatt, Mari Goldade, Jason Greenwood, Mary Jeno, Adria Johnson, Kathryn Johnson, Nolan Kleinjan, Dan Kolm, Anna Kozlowski, Cameron MacInnis, Carrie Mahurin, Megan Schmidt, Nathan Seven, Jared Steinberger, Amber Stola, Vanessa Stumpf, Siri Urquhart, Matt Wagner, and Jill Wieser.

We would also like to thank Delia DeTurris and Julia Nollen for their assistance in writing this question and answer book, as well as Sara D'Emic and all the other individuals at Thieme Publishers who have assisted in its publication.

For their thoughtful and careful review of the proposal and manuscript, thanks to:

Student Reviewers:

Megan Finneran, Chicago College of Osteopathic Medicine

Ramona Mittal, TTUHSC

Megan Cheslock, Oakland University William Beaumont School of Medicine

Amy Leshner, St George's, University of London

Dipak Ramkumar, Dartmouth

Shane Swink, Philadelphia College of Osteopathic Medicine

Jaiye A. Conner, Alabama College of Osteopathic Medicine

Diana Stern, UNECOM

Erin Cummings Scott, Rutgers Robert Wood Johnson Medical School

Amanda Strickland, UT Southwestern Medical School

Instructor Reviewers:

Jenny Libien, SUNY Downstate Medical School

Tipsuda Junsanto-Bahri, Touro College of Osteopathic Medicine–New York

Arben Santo, Edward Via College of Osteopathic Medicine (VCOM)

Pearl Myers, Touro College of Osteopathic Medicine Middletown

Moshe Sadofsky, Albert Einstein COM

Alan Schiller MD, John A. Burns School of Medicine

Robin LeGallo, University of Virginia

Mykhaylo Yakubovskyy, Ross University School of Medicine

Joseph Prahlow, Indiana University School of Medicine

How to Use This Series

Chapter Head

Question Difficulty Key
Green box = Easy question
Yellow box = Medium question
Red box = Hard question

Section Header

1.1 Cellular Adaptations— Questions

| Easy | Medium | Hard |

Question Stem

1. A 50-year-old male dies during a car accident. At autopsy, he is noted to have a moderately stenotic aortic valve. The heart weighs 500 grams. The cause of death from the motor vehicle accident is entirely blunt force injuries of the head and neck, including an atlanto-occipital dislocation. No internal injuries below the neck are identified. There is no history of heart failure. A section of the myocardium from the left ventricle would reveal which of the following processes?

A. Hypertrophy
B. Hyperplasia
C. Atrophy
D. Metaplasia
E. Reversible cell injury
F. Irreversible cell injury

Cardiovascular

2. A 25-year-old male, who is an offensive lineman for the local college football team, dies during a car accident. At autopsy, the injuries, being multiple rib fractures and lacerations of the lungs and heart, with 1500 mL of blood found in the left pleural cavity, are confined to the chest. At autopsy, a biopsy of his left biceps femoris muscle would reveal which of the following?

Answer Options

A. Physiologic hyperplasia
B. Pathologic hyperplasia
C. Physiologic hypertrophy
D. Pathologic hypertrophy
E. Physiologic atrophy
F. Pathologic atrophy

Musculoskeletal

3. A 27-year-old male is in a car accident and sustains a fracture of the 2nd thoracic vertebra, with resultant damage to the spinal cord at the same level, leading to paraplegia, requiring him to be wheelchair bound. Five years following the accident, he develops a neoplasm of the right lower extremity, requiring a wide local excision, which includes a small superficial segment of underlying skeletal muscle. When viewing the microscopic slides, which of the following would the pathologist identify in the skeletal muscle?

A. Physiologic hyperplasia
B. Pathologic hyperplasia
C. Physiologic hypertrophy
D. Pathologic hypertrophy
E. Physiologic atrophy
F. Pathologic atrophy

Musculoskeletal

4. A pathologist is examining the biopsy of an individual's left ventricular myocardium and notices that the cardiac myocytes are enlarged. Of the following conditions, which would best explain this finding?

A. Pulmonary hypertension
B. Systemic hypertension
C. Lambl's excresences on the aortic valve
D. A probe patent fossa ovalis
E. Acute pericardial hemorrhage

Cardiovascular

5. A 2-year-old female aspirates a small coin, unbeknownst to her caregivers. Over the next few days, she develops a cough and becomes less responsive and sleeps longer periods. Her parents also notice that she feels warm to the touch, but do not take her temperature. Six days following the coin being swallowed, her parents find her unresponsive in her bedroom. They call 9-1-1 and she is pronounced dead at the hospital. Autopsy reveals a widespread bronchopneumonia in the right lung and a coin lodged in the right mainstem bronchus, nearly completely blocking it. A microscopic section of the bronchus from where the coin was lodged reveals stratified squamous epithelium, which appears essentially normal, similar to that seen in the inner lining of the esophagus. Which of the following processes has occurred in the bronchus?

A. Hypertrophy
B. Hyperplasia
C. Metaplasia
D. Atrophy
E. Irreversible cellular injury

Respiratory

6. After developing hematuria and flank pain, a 55-year-old male is diagnosed with a renal cell carcinoma in his right kidney. To treat the tumor, the patient's right kidney is resected. Five years later, he dies in a car accident. At autopsy, there is an absence of the right kidney, and the left kidney weighs 300 grams (normal weight is 150-200 grams for an adult male). Of the following processes, which is most likely occurring in the left kidney?

A. Physiologic hypertrophy
B. Pathologic hypertrophy
C. Physiologic hyperplasia, hormonal type
D. Physiologic hyperplasia, compensatory type
E. Pathologic hyperplasia

Genitourinary

Organ System Tag
Organ-specific questions will be tagged as such (in this case: Musculoskeletal) and can be used for review of an isolated system.

Difficulty Level Icon

In general, an easy question requires only a diagnosis based upon the question stem.

A medium question requires not just the diagnosis of the condition based upon the question stem, but knowledge about that diagnosis so as to answer a question about it.

Hard questions are a combination of medium questions with less commonly known material about the diagnosis.

4.   Correct: Systemic hypertension (B).

The pathologist is viewing hypertrophy of the cardiac myocytes. While identification of enlarged cells themselves is a difficulty, enlarged rectangular nuclei (i.e., boxcar nuclei) serve as a marker of cardiac myocyte hypertrophy. Increased blood pressure in the systemic vessels would put strain on the left ventricle and lead to hypertrophy (**B**). Pulmonary hypertension would cause similar changes in the right ventricular myocardium (**A**). Lambl's excrescences are incidental small nodules on the valve leaflets that are of no physiologic consequence (**C**). A probe patent fossa ovalis is usually of no physiologic significance (**D**). However, if a left to right shunt developed, this condition could potentially lead to volume overload in the right atrium and ventricle, with resultant hypertrophy and dilation, but the left ventricle would not be affected. An acute pericardial hemorrhage would not explain hypertrophy, as cardiac myocyte hypertrophy does not develop over such a short period of time, but instead requires a longer exposure to the stimulus (**E**).

5.   Correct: Metaplasia (C).

The bronchus is usually lined by respiratory epithelium (pseudostratified columnar epithelium); however, when the nature of the stimulus to the epithelium changes, which, in this case is trauma caused by the pressure from the coin, the epithelium can change to a different form to better handle the abnormal stimulus. The transition from one epithelium type to another is termed metaplasia (**C**). In the lung, squamous metaplasia most commonly is a result of cigarette smoking, and, in this situation, metaplasia can lead to dysplasia and finally to carcinoma, accounting for the presence of squamous cell carcinomas in the lung. If the coin is removed, the epithelium could transition back to respiratory epithelium; therefore, the change is reversible, and not irreversible cellular injury. (**A-B, D-E**) are incorrect based on the previously discussed information.

6.   Correct: Physiologic hyperplasia, compensatory type (D).

Because of the absence of the right kidney, the left kidney has a higher workload, and in response, the left kidney increases the number of cells in its structure to handle this increased workload and thus, the organ weight has increased. The cells in the kidney are capable of division, and thus hyperplasia can occur (unlike in the cardiac or skeletal muscle). The hyperplasia is physiologic in nature because it is stimulated by an increased workload, and it is to compensate for the loss of the other kidney (**D**). (**A-C, E**) are incorrect based on previously discussed information.

7.   Correct: Ubiquitin-proteasome (E).

The patient has disuse atrophy of the upper and lower extremities. The two primary processes occurring in atrophy are decreased protein synthesis and increased protein degradation. Protein degradation is accomplished by binding of ubiquitin to the substances to be degraded followed by its subsequent destruction by proteasomes (**E**). Cyclooxygenase and thromboxane A2 and 12-lipooxygenase-lipoxin A4 function in inflammation (**A, B**), and plasmin-C3a in the complement cascade (**C**), both of which could be active in the muscle to some degree but are not the main source of protein degradation, and p53-Bax functions in apoptosis (**D**), which might be occurring to some small degree but is not the main cause of the protein degradation.

1.5 Cellular Injury— Answers and Explanations

| Easy | Medium | Hard |

8.   Correct: Karyorrhexis of nuclei (E).

After 1 hour of ischemia, some of the affected myocytes would have irreversible damage, in this case, represented by the subendocardial myocardial infarct. Of the choices, only karyorrhexis of the nuclei is characteristic of irreversible injury, i.e., necrosis (**E**), whereas the other choices are seen with reversible injury (**A-D**). Other microscopic features of irreversible ischemic injury (i.e., necrosis) include increased eosinophilia of the cytoplasm, and other nuclei changes including karyolysis (i.e., fading of the chromatin) and pyknosis (i.e., shrinkage of the nucleus). Karyorrhexis is fragmentation of the nucleus. As the thrombus was lysed relatively early, myocytes closer to the epicardium may have had signs of reversible injury, but not irreversible injury.

9.   Correct: Thrombus of distal branch of left renal artery (E).

The gross description is that of an infarct, which has coagulative necrosis. In coagulative necrosis, the normal organ architecture is preserved in the beginning phases of the development of the infarct. A thrombus of a branch of the renal artery can produce an infarct of the cortex of the kidney (**E**). Infarcts are typically wedge-shaped, essentially exhibiting the downstream effects of a blockage of the arterial system, with the amount of organ affected increasing moving distal from a single point, the tip of the wedge. Preservation of architecture does not occur with liquefactive necrosis (as could be seen with a bacterial pyelonephritis) or caseous necrosis (as could be seen with a tuberculosis infection), and by their nature, tumors do not have preservation of architecture within their boundaries (**A-D**).

6

About the Authors

Walter L. Kemp, MD, PhD, graduated from Creighton University School of Medicine, following which he was a resident in anatomic and clinical pathology at the University of Texas Southwestern Medical Center, and forensic fellow at the Dallas County Medical Examiner's office. After completing his medical training, he was an assistant professor of pathology at the University of Texas Southwestern for two years, being awarded one of the outstanding teacher awards from the second-year medical school class each of those two years. For the next ten years he was the deputy state medical examiner for the state of Montana, during which time he earned his MA and PhD in anthropology from the University of Montana. Beginning in July 2015, he became an associate professor of pathology at the University of North Dakota School of Medicine and Health Sciences, and, in his first year won both the local Golden Apple Award for teaching, and the UNDSMHS's Portrait Award. He has written a pathology review book, a coroner training manual, and has been author or a coauthor for fourteen articles on various topics in medicine.

Travis Brown, MD, graduated from UT Southwestern Medical School in Dallas, Texas. He completed his family medicine residency at John Peter Smith Hospital in Fort Worth, Texas. He is a father of two, medical columnist, and practicing family physician in Midlothian, Texas.

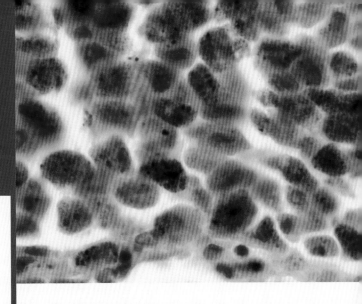

Chapter 1

Cell Injury, Adaptations, and Death

LEARNING OBJECTIVES

1.1 Cellular Adaptations

▶ Discuss examples of the gross and microscopic features produced by hypertrophy, hyperplasia, atrophy, and metaplasia and list disease processes each can result from

▶ Distinguish between physiologic adaptation and pathologic adaptation

▶ List the mediators involved with cellular adaptation

1.2 Cellular Injury

▶ List the morphologic features of reversible and irreversible cellular injury and describe the circumstances and physiologic process under which each occurs

▶ List the reactive oxygen species and describe their effects

▶ Describe the mechanisms of reversible and irreversible cellular injury

▶ Describe the process of apoptosis, including the cellular mediators involved

1.3 Cellular Accumulations, Calcification, and Aging

▶ List and describe the forms of cellular accumulations and list the circumstances or conditions under which they are found

▶ Compare and contrast the different forms of calcification

▶ Describe the function of the telomerase

1.1 Cellular Adaptations— Questions

Easy	Medium	Hard

1. A 50-year-old male dies during a car accident. At autopsy, he is noted to have a moderately stenotic aortic valve. The heart weighs 500 grams. The cause of death from the motor vehicle accident is entirely blunt force injuries of the head and neck, including an atlanto-occipital dislocation. No internal injuries below the neck are identified. There is no history of heart failure. A section of the myocardium from the left ventricle would reveal which of the following processes?

A. Hypertrophy

B. Hyperplasia

C. Atrophy

D. Metaplasia

E. Reversible cell injury

F. Irreversible cell injury

Cardiovascular

2. A 25-year-old male, who is an offensive lineman for the local college football team, dies during a car accident. At autopsy, the injuries, being multiple rib fractures and lacerations of the lungs and heart, with 1500 mL of blood found in the left pleural cavity, are confined to the chest. At autopsy, a biopsy of his left biceps femoris muscle would reveal which of the following?

A. Physiologic hyperplasia

B. Pathologic hyperplasia

C. Physiologic hypertrophy

D. Pathologic hypertrophy

E. Physiologic atrophy

F. Pathologic atrophy

Musculoskeletal

3. A 27-year-old male is in a car accident and sustains a fracture of the 2nd thoracic vertebra, with resultant damage to the spinal cord at the same level, leading to paraplegia, requiring him to be wheelchair bound. Five years following the accident, he develops a neoplasm of the right lower extremity, requiring a wide local excision, which includes a small superficial segment of underlying skeletal muscle. When viewing the microscopic slides, which of the following would the pathologist identify in the skeletal muscle?

A. Physiologic hyperplasia

B. Pathologic hyperplasia

C. Physiologic hypertrophy

D. Pathologic hypertrophy

E. Physiologic atrophy

F. Pathologic atrophy

Musculoskeletal

4. A pathologist is examining the biopsy of an individual's left ventricular myocardium and notices that the cardiac myocytes are enlarged. Of the following conditions, which would best explain this finding?

A. Pulmonary hypertension

B. Systemic hypertension

C. Lambl's excrescences on the aortic valve

D. A probe patent fossa ovalis

E. Acute pericardial hemorrhage

Cardiovascular

5. A 2-year-old female aspirates a small coin, unbeknownst to her caregivers. Over the next few days, she develops a cough and becomes less responsive and sleeps longer periods. Her parents also notice that she feels warm to the touch, but do not take her temperature. Six days following the coin being swallowed, her parents find her unresponsive in her bedroom. They call 9-1-1 and she is pronounced dead at the hospital. Autopsy reveals a widespread bronchopneumonia in the right lung and a coin lodged in the right mainstem bronchus, nearly completely blocking it. A microscopic section of the bronchus from where the coin was lodged reveals stratified squamous epithelium, which appears essentially normal, similar to that seen in the inner lining of the esophagus. Which of the following processes has occurred in the bronchus?

A. Hypertrophy

B. Hyperplasia

C. Metaplasia

D. Atrophy

E. Irreversible cellular injury

Respiratory

6. After developing hematuria and flank pain, a 55-year-old male is diagnosed with a renal cell carcinoma in his right kidney. To treat the tumor, the patient's right kidney is resected. Five years later, he dies in a car accident. At autopsy, there is an absence of the right kidney, and the left kidney weighs 300 grams (normal weight is 150-200 grams for an adult male). Of the following processes, which is most likely occurring in the left kidney?

A. Physiologic hypertrophy

B. Pathologic hypertrophy

C. Physiologic hyperplasia, hormonal type

D. Physiologic hyperplasia, compensatory type

E. Pathologic hyperplasia

Genitourinary

7. A 90-year-old male with severe dementia has been bedridden for 5 years. Physical examination reveals no decubitus ulcers on his back, buttocks, or lower extremities; however, his upper and lower extremities are reduced in circumference, the lower extremities more so than the upper extremities, with apparent significant loss of muscle mass. Which of the following combinations of molecular mediators is most responsible for the decreased size of the skeletal muscles?

A. Cyclooxygenase-Thromboxane A2

B. 12-Lipooxygenase-Lipoxin A4

C. Plasmin-C3a

D. p53-Bax

E. Ubiquitin-proteosome

Musculoskeletal

1.2 Cellular Injury—Questions

Easy	Medium	Hard

8. A 56-year-old male with a history of smoking and hypertension develops an occlusive thrombus in his left anterior descending coronary artery following rupture of an atherosclerotic plaque. He survives the event, but therapeutic lysis of the thrombus is not accomplished until 1 hour after its formation. He is told that he sustained a subendocardial myocardial infarct. If a biopsy of the subendocardial myocytes was performed 24 hours after the occlusion of the vessel, of the following, which intracellular change would be expected to be identified?

A. Swelling of the mitochondria

B. Dilation of the rough endoplasmic reticulum

C. Nuclear clumping of chromatin

D. Lipid vacuoles in the cytoplasm

E. Karyorrhexis of nuclei

Cardiovascular

9. The husband of a 62-year-old female found her unresponsive on the couch in their apartment when he returned home from work. Despite the efforts of emergency responders, she was pronounced dead at the hospital. An autopsy reveals a well-demarcated wedge-shaped yellow lesion in the cortex of the left kidney with preservation of normal gross architecture. Of the following, what is the most likely etiology for this autopsy finding?

A. *Mycobacterium tuberculosis* infection

B. *Klebsiella* bacterial infection

C. Renal cell carcinoma

D. Metastatic colonic adenocarcinoma

E. Thrombus of distal branch of left renal artery

Genitourinary

10. In his autopsy report, a pathologist describes a 5 x 3 cm focus of liquefactive necrosis. The source of the liquefactive necrosis was a thrombus occluding an artery, and the autopsy was performed 2 days following the event that produced the liquefactive necrosis. In which of the following sections of the autopsy report would this lesion most likely be described?

A. Central nervous system

B. Cardiovascular system

C. Respiratory system

D. Hepatobiliary system

E. Genitourinary system

Central nervous system

11. A 37-year-old male with a history of chronic alcohol abuse and gallstones is brought to the emergency room by a friend. The patient has been complaining of severe abdominal pain for 3 days following a bout of increased alcohol consumption. Laboratory testing in the emergency room indicates an elevated amylase and lipase. Despite treatment, the patient dies. An autopsy of the individual most likely will reveal which of the following in the greater omentum?

A. Coagulative necrosis

B. Liquefactive necrosis

C. Gangrenous necrosis

D. Caseous necrosis

E. Fat necrosis

F. Fibrinoid necrosis

Gastrointestinal

12. A pathologist is examining a section of kidney and notes hydropic change in the proximal convoluted tubule epithelial cells. Damage to or decreased function of which of the following cellular structures is most important in directly causing this finding?

A. Rough endoplasmic reticulum

B. Smooth endoplasmic reticulum

C. Sodium-potassium pump

D. Phagocyte oxidase

E. Cytoskeletal proteins

Genitourinary

13. For his research, a scientist exposes cultured cells to certain forms of radiation. Following the exposure, he can examine intracellular proteins for evidence of cross-linking. Of the following, which has the highest propensity for causing such protein changes?

A. Superoxide

B. Hydrogen peroxide

C. Hydroxyl radical

D. Nitric oxide

E. Oxidized glutathione

N/A

3

14. A scientist is studying the effects of an experimental medication, IST-151, on cultured hepatocytes. The medication, unfortunately, results in the death of the hepatocytes and appears to do so predominantly through activation of an intracellular endonuclease, which damages the nucleus of the cell, leading to death. Of the following mechanisms of cellular injury, which one is the most direct in mediating the previously described effects (i.e., activation of the endonuclease)?

A. Mitochondrial damage resulting in decreased production of ATP

B. Mitochondrial damage leading to increased production of reactive oxygen species

C. Calcium influx into the cell

D. Breakdown of lysosomal membranes

E. DNA damage leading to activation of pro-apoptotic proteins

N/A

15. A 46-year-old female receives radiation therapy of the neck for a neoplasm of the thyroid gland. After therapy, it is noted that her thyroid gland has markedly decreased in size, leading to hypothyroidism, and she must be placed on a thyroid replacement therapeutic drug regimen. Of the following, which statement is most characteristic regarding the process by which the thyroid gland decreased in size?

A. The plasma membranes of the thyroid follicular cells lysed

B. Prominent calcium influx led to marked activation of phospholipase

C. Ischemic injury induced by the radiation led to coagulative necrosis

D. Few, if any, inflammatory cells would have been seen histologically

E. Damage to cytoskeletal elements led to dissolution of the cells

Endocrine

16. A scientist is studying apoptosis. By the introduction of a naturally occurring chemical, she wishes to shorten the life span of cultured cells that are derived from a human liver and that have been exposed to radiation. Which of the following effects, if caused by the introduced chemical, would produce her desired outcome?

A. Increased concentration of bcl-2

B. Increased concentration of bcl-xL

C. Increased concentration of BH3 proteins

D. Decreased concentration of Bax

E. Decreased concentration of Bad

N/A

17. A 61-year-old female receives radiation therapy of the neck for a neoplasm of the larynx. After therapy, it is noted that her thyroid gland has markedly decreased in size, leading to hypothyroidism. During the decrease in size of the thyroid gland, biopsies of the parenchyma would have revealed cells with increased eosinophilia, and fragmented nuclei, but essentially no surrounding inflammatory reaction. Of the following cellular components, which one most directly contributed to this lack of an inflammatory reaction?

A. Phospholipase

B. Phagosome oxidase

C. CD95

D. Phosphatidylserine

E. Phosphatidylinositol

Endocrine

1.3 Cellular Accumulations, Calcification, and Aging— Questions

Easy	Medium	Hard

18. A 40-year-old chronic alcoholic with no other medical history died after an alcohol-related seizure, in which he fell down the stairs at his house and fractured his neck. An autopsy is performed that reveals a diffusely golden-yellow discolored liver. Microscopic examination of the liver reveals almost every hepatocyte to be filled with one large vacuole or a few smaller vacuoles. Which of the following mechanisms most likely caused this intracellular inclusion?

A. Abnormal metabolism

B. A defect in protein folding

C. The lack of an enzyme

D. Ingestion of indigestible material

Hepatobiliary

19. A deceased poorly controlled diabetic is found in his messy apartment during a welfare check initiated by concerned friends. At the time of autopsy, his kidneys are noted to be pale. Vitreous electrolyte analysis indicates a vitreous glucose of 576 mg/dL and acetone is detected in the blood. A diagnosis of diabetic ketoacidosis is made. Microscopic examination of the kidneys reveals small clear vacuoles in the renal tubular epithelial cells. Of the following, what is the most likely contents of these vacuoles?

A. Lipofuscin

B. Triglycerides

C. Hemosiderin

D. Glycogen

E. Carbon

Genitourinary

20. A research scientist wants to conduct an experiment using lipofuscin as the substrate to see how it forms and what adverse effects its presence in the cells might create. He collaborates with a medical examiner's office to obtain tissue for his research. All other factors being equal, which of the following might be expected to contain the greatest amount of lipofuscin in each of the parenchymal cells?

A. Liver from a 15-year-old

B. Liver from a 40-year-old

C. Liver from a 75-year old

D. Pancreas from a 15-year-old

E. Pancreas from a 40-year-old

F. Pancreas from a 75-year-old

Hepatobiliary

21. A forensic pathologist is examining a section of skin. Just underneath the dermis is a large collection of macrophages, each containing a stippled, or somewhat chunky-appearing, yellow-brown pigment. The pathologist orders a Prussian blue stain, which causes the pigment to appear blue. Of the following, which is the most likely etiology for the pigment?

A. Abnormal protein accumulation in an alcoholic

B. Previous trauma that resulted in hemorrhage

C. Wear-and-tear pigment in an older individual

D. Cigarette smoking

E. Normal melanin accumulation in a darkly pigmented individual

Integumentary

22. A 36-year-old male crashes while skiing and sustains a large laceration of his thigh, which ultimately heals by secondary intention, leaving a large scar. Six years later, he notices a firm, but ill-defined, mass at the site of the scar. Other than the laceration of the thigh, his past medical history is essentially negative. He consults a surgeon who removes the mass. The mass has a gritty texture to it, and under the microscope appears to be fibrosis with scattered clusters of rounded and globular basophilic material. No cartilage or bone is identified. Which of the following processes is occurring at this site?

A. Metaplastic calcification

B. Dysplastic calcification

C. Dystrophic calcification

D. Metastatic calcification

E. Disuse calcification

Integumentary

23. A researcher is studying a form of lung cancer in which she identifies a gene for a telomerase in the DNA of the tumor cells. Which of the following abilities would this gene provide the cancer cells with?

A. Invade through basement membrane

B. Invade through wall of blood vessel

C. Implant in organs to form a metastasis

D. Increased rate of mitotic activity

E. Ability to divide for an indefinite length of time

N/A

1.4 Cellular Adaptations— Answers and Explanations

Easy	Medium	Hard

1. Correct: Hypertrophy (A)

Because of the stenotic aortic valve, increased pressure is placed on the left ventricular myocardium, which responds by increasing the size of the cells, which is hypertrophy (**A**). The myocardium has adapted to the increased pressure, and since then there has been no heart failure and no reversible or irreversible cell injury (**E, F**). Cardiac myocytes are essentially not capable of division and are increasing in size, not decreasing, so neither hyperplasia nor atrophy is occurring (**B, C**), and there is no switch in type of cell (e.g., cardiac muscle to another form of mesenchymal tissue), so metaplasia is not occurring (**D**).

2. Correct: Physiologic hypertrophy (C)

As the decedent is athletic, there is a stimulus causing enlargement of the biceps femoris muscle, and as athletic activity is a normal activity, the resultant enlargement of the skeletal muscle cells would be considered physiologic and not pathologic. The skeletal muscle cells cannot divide, so they would respond to increased workload by increasing in size (hypertrophy), and not by increasing in number (hyperplasia) (**C**). (**A-B, D-E**) are incorrect based on the previously discussed information.

3. Correct: Pathologic atrophy (F)

Damage to the spinal cord can lead to deinnervation of the lower extremities. Deinnervation is one mechanism causing atrophy, and, as the deinnervation was due to a traumatic injury, the resultant atrophy would be considered pathologic (F) and not physiologic (E). As there is neither an increase in the size of the skeletal muscle cells, nor an increase in their number, the other answers are incorrect (A-D).

4.   Correct: Systemic hypertension (B)

The pathologist is viewing hypertrophy of the cardiac myocytes. While identification of enlarged cells themselves is a difficulty, enlarged rectangular nuclei (i.e., boxcar nuclei) serve as a marker of cardiac myocyte hypertrophy. Increased blood pressure in the systemic vessels would put strain on the left ventricle and lead to hypertrophy (**B**). Pulmonary hypertension would cause similar changes in the right ventricular myocardium (**A**). Lambl's excrescences are incidental small nodules on the valve leaflets that are of no physiologic consequence (**C**). A probe patent fossa ovalis is usually of no physiologic significance (**D**). However, if a left to right shunt developed, this condition could potentially lead to volume overload in the right atrium and ventricle, with resultant hypertrophy and dilation, but the left ventricle would not be affected. An acute pericardial hemorrhage would not explain hypertrophy, as cardiac myocyte hypertrophy does not develop over such a short period of time, but instead requires a longer exposure to the stimulus (**E**).

5.   Correct: Metaplasia (C)

The bronchus is usually lined by respiratory epithelium (pseudostratified columnar epithelium); however, when the nature of the stimulus to the epithelium changes, which, in this case is trauma caused by the pressure from the coin, the epithelium can change to a different form to better handle the abnormal stimulus. The transition from one epithelium type to another is termed metaplasia (**C**). In the lung, squamous metaplasia most commonly is a result of cigarette smoking, and, in this situation, metaplasia can lead to dysplasia and finally to carcinoma, accounting for the presence of squamous cell carcinomas in the lung. If the coin is removed, the epithelium could transition back to respiratory epithelium; therefore, the change is reversible, and not irreversible cellular injury. (**A-B, D-E**) are incorrect based on the previously discussed information.

6.   Correct: Physiologic hyperplasia, compensatory type (D)

Because of the absence of the right kidney, the left kidney has a higher workload, and in response, the left kidney increases the number of cells in its structure to handle this increased workload and thus, the organ weight has increased. The cells in the kidney are capable of division, and thus hyperplasia can occur (unlike in the cardiac or skeletal muscle). The hyperplasia is physiologic in nature because it is stimulated by an increased workload, and it is to compensate for the loss of the other kidney (**D**). (**A-C, E**) are incorrect based on previously discussed information.

7.   Correct: Ubiquitin-proteasome (E)

The patient has disuse atrophy of the upper and lower extremities. The two primary processes occurring in atrophy are decreased protein synthesis and increased protein degradation. Protein degradation is accomplished by binding of ubiquitin to the substances to be degraded followed by its subsequent destruction by proteasomes (**E**). Cyclooxygenase and thromboxane A2 and 12-lipooxygenase-lipoxin A4 function in inflammation (**A, B**), and plasmin-C3a in the complement cascade (**C**), both of which could be active in the muscle to some degree but are not the main source of protein degradation, and p53-Bax functions in apoptosis (**D**), which might be occurring to some small degree but is not the main cause of the protein degradation.

1.5 Cellular Injury— Answers and Explanations

Easy	Medium	Hard

8.   Correct: Karyorrhexis of nuclei (E)

After 1 hour of ischemia, some of the affected myocytes would have irreversible damage, in this case, represented by the subendocardial myocardial infarct. Of the choices, only karyorrhexis of the nuclei is characteristic of irreversible injury, i.e., necrosis (**E**), whereas the other choices are seen with reversible injury (**A-D**). Other microscopic features of irreversible ischemic injury (i.e., necrosis) include increased eosinophilia of the cytoplasm, and other nuclei changes including karyolysis (i.e., fading of the chromatin) and pyknosis (i.e., shrinkage of the nucleus). Karyorrhexis is fragmentation of the nucleus. As the thrombus was lysed relatively early, myocytes closer to the epicardium may have had signs of reversible injury, but not irreversible injury.

9.   Correct: Thrombus of distal branch of left renal artery (E)

The gross description is that of an infarct, which has coagulative necrosis. In coagulative necrosis, the normal organ architecture is preserved in the beginning phases of the development of the infarct. A thrombus of a branch of the renal artery can produce an infarct of the cortex of the kidney (**E**). Infarcts are typically wedge-shaped, essentially exhibiting the downstream effects of a blockage of the arterial system, with the amount of organ affected increasing moving distal from a single point, the tip of the wedge. Preservation of architecture does not occur with liquefactive necrosis (as could be seen with a bacterial pyelonephritis) or caseous necrosis (as could be seen with a tuberculosis infection), and by their nature, tumors do not have preservation of architecture within their boundaries (**A-D**).

10. Correct: Central nervous system (A)

In most organ systems, a thrombus will lead to ischemic injury followed by coagulative necrosis (**B-E**); however, in the brain, a thrombus and the resultant ischemic injury produce liquefactive necrosis (**A**). It should be noted that after an extended period of time, areas of coagulative necrosis in organs other than the brain can become liquefactive necrosis, but this change would not be expected within only 2 days.

11. Correct: Fat necrosis (E)

Based on the clinical history (i.e., abdominal pain with history of gallstones and alcohol abuse) and laboratory testing (elevated amylase and lipase), the individual most likely has acute pancreatitis, with alcohol use and gallstones being two risk factors for this condition, and with the symptomatology and laboratory testing supporting this diagnosis. The release of pancreatic enzymes damages adipose cells in the peritoneal cavity (e.g., the omentum), and the subsequently released fatty acids join with calcium leading to small chalky white patches. This change is termed fat necrosis (**E**). While examination of the pancreas itself could reveal coagulative necrosis or, depending on the time course of the inflammation, liquefactive necrosis (**A, B**), these conditions would not be the main condition identified in the omentum. Gangrenous necrosis is found in the extremities, and caseous necrosis is associated with tuberculosis most commonly (**C, D**). A variety of conditions are associated with fibrinoid necrosis, including some forms of vasculitis, but it would not be present in the omentum in this clinical scenario (**F**).

12. Correct: Sodium-potassium pump (C)

Hydropic change, i.e., cellular swelling, is a sign of reversible cellular injury. The sodium-potassium pump normally pumps sodium out of the cell and potassium into the cell. With ischemia, one cause of reversible cellular injury, the amount of ATP produced is reduced, and without ATP, the sodium-potassium pump will not function, allowing sodium to enter the cell. Water follows sodium into the cell, causing the cell to swell, and producing hydropic change (**C**). (**A-B, D-E**) are incorrect based on the previously discussed information.

13. Correct: Hydroxyl radical (C)

Superoxide, hydrogen peroxide, hydroxyl radical, and nitric oxide are all reactive oxygen species (ROS), which can cause cross-linking of proteins, lipid peroxidation, and DNA damage. Oxidized glutathione is produced in the breakdown of hydrogen peroxide. The most reactive of the four ROS listed is hydroxyl radical (**C**). (**A-B, D-E**) are incorrect based on the previously discussed information.

14. Correct: Calcium influx into the cell (C)

The four main mechanisms by which cellular injury occurs are 1) mitochondrial damage, 2) entry of calcium into the cell, 3) damage to the plasma membrane (causing dissolution of the cell), or 4) DNA damage and/or protein misfolding, which can lead to apoptosis. Calcium influx into the cell can activate a variety of enzymes including phospholipases, proteases, endonucleases, and ATPases (**C**). (**A-B, D-E**) are incorrect based on the previously discussed information.

15. Correct: Few, if any, inflammatory cells would have been seen histologically (D).

Radiation causes damage to DNA, which can trigger the process of apoptosis. During apoptosis, the cells break down into fragments, each with an intact membrane, and little, if, any inflammation is triggered (**D**). (**A-C, E**) are incorrect. See previously discussed information.

16. Correct: Increased concentration of BH3 proteins (C)

BH3 proteins normally detect damaged DNA or misfolded proteins and promote the activation of Bax and Bad, which are pro-apoptotic mediators, leading to the death of the cell. If the chemical that the researcher was using increased the concentration of BH3 proteins, apoptosis would be promoted and the life expectancy of cells previously exposed to radiation would be shorter (**C**). Bcl-2 and Bcl-xL inhibit apoptosis, and therefore, increasing their concentration would lengthen the life span of the cell (**A-B**). Similarly, Bax and Bad promote apoptosis, and decreasing their concentration would inhibit apoptosis and lengthen the life span of the cells (**D-E**).

17. Correct: Phosphatidylserine (D)

With exposure to radiation and subsequent DNA damage, the process of apoptosis can remove the irreversibly injured cells. During apoptosis, which is an organized breakdown of the cell, little if any inflammatory reaction is elicited as the cells are kept intact during the process, preventing cellular components from leaving the cell and triggering inflammation. Phosphatidylserine is expressed on the outside of the cellular fragments and is recognized by phagocytic cells, which promotes uptake of the cellular fragments more quickly, thereby preventing a normal inflammatory response (**D**). Although CD95 is a cellular mediator in apoptosis, being what the Fas ligand binds to, the cellular component most directly involved in the removal of the apoptotic cell without eliciting an inflammatory reaction is phosphatidylserine (**C**). (**A-B, E**) are incorrect based on the previously discussed information.

1.6 Cellular Accumulations, Calcification, and Aging— Answers and Explanations

Easy	Medium	Hard

18. Correct: Abnormal metabolism (A)

The intracellular accumulation described in the question is fat (triglycerides). Accumulation of fat in hepatocytes is caused by abnormal metabolism (**A**). Such fat accumulations can be found most commonly in individuals with alcoholism, diabetes mellitus, or obesity. Hyaline change, resulting from accumulation of proteins associated with alcoholism, does not appear as described (**B**), and is instead more ropy and eosinophilic. The lack of an enzyme could result in fatty accumulation within a cell; however, these defects are frequently hereditary and often produce complications shortly after birth (**C**). Also, compared to fat accumulation associated with alcohol use, they are rare. Fat is not indigestible (**D**). Given time, the fatty accumulations in the hepatocytes would clear.

19. Correct: Glycogen (D)

The description given does not fit for lipofuscin, which is a granular yellow-brown pigment, hemosiderin, which is a more granular or chunky yellow-brown pigment, or anthracotic pigment (carbon), which is finely stippled and black, or green-black (**A, C, E**). Diabetics are described as developing accumulations of glycogen, and not triglycerides, in the kidney, as well as other organs, including the heart (**B, D**).

20. Correct: Liver from a 75-year-old (C)

Lipofuscin is a wear-and-tear pigment that accumulates with age. The older the individual, the more likely their cells will contain the pigment. The heart, liver, and brain are the organs most commonly found to contain the pigment (C). (**A-B, D-F**) are incorrect. See previous discussion.

21. Correct: Previous trauma that resulted in hemorrhage (B)

The pigment being described is hemosiderin. Hemosiderin contains iron and will stain blue with a Prussian stain. Hemosiderin results from the breakdown of red blood cells (**B**). None of the other pigments listed are described in this manner, nor do they stain in this manner (**A, C-E**).

22. Correct: Dystrophic calcification (C)

The description and scenario fit for dystrophic calcification. Deposition of calcium at a site of injury in a person without an elevated calcium concentration in their blood (i.e., normocalcemic) is dystrophic calcification (**C**). If the individual has hypercalcemia, the process is termed metastatic calcification and can occur in otherwise normal tissue (**D**). At this site, if the process progressed, bone could form, which would be a form of metaplasia. Dysplastic calcification and disuse calcification are not terms that are usually used (**A-B, E**).

23. Correct: Ability to divide for an indefinite length of time (E)

A telomerase functions to add nucleotides to the end of a chromosome, maintaining the length of a telomere. When telomeres shorten to a certain point, the end of the DNA is determined by the cell to be damaged, and cell cycles will stop. With maintenance of the telomere length, the cell is able to divide for an indefinite length of time (i.e., is immortal) (**E**). (**A-D**) are incorrect. See previous explanation.

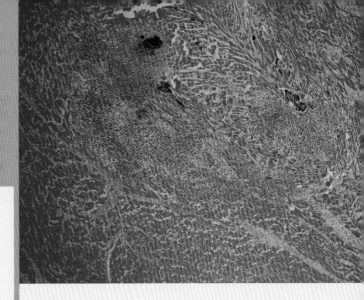

Chapter 2
Inflammation and Repair

LEARNING OBJECTIVES

2.1 Acute and Chronic Inflammation

► List and describe the proteins involved in the process of acute inflammation

► Describe the various morphologic forms of inflammation and list conditions associated with each form

► Describe the process of acute inflammation and the mediators involved with each step

► List the opsonins and the receptor each pairs with

► List diseases resulting from a hereditary deficiency of proteins involved in the process of acute inflammation

► Describe the process of acute inflammation and its outcomes

► Describe the morphologic forms of inflammation and list conditions associated with each

► Describe the process of acute inflammation and list the mediators involved with each step

► Describe the mechanism of formation of reactive oxygen species

► List laboratory tests and physical examination techniques to detect acute inflammatory processes

► Describe the role of cytokines in the development of cachexia in patients with cancer

► Describe mediators responsible for leukocyte rolling, adhesion, and transmigration

► Describe the appearance of caseating granulomas, and list their disease associations

► Describe the morphologic appearance of apoptosis

► Describe the process of apoptosis, including the role of specific mediators, and compare and contrast the extrinsic and intrinsic pathways

► Compare and contrast transudate and exudate

2.1 Acute and Chronic Inflammation—Questions

Easy	Medium	Hard

1. A researcher is studying acute inflammation. Specifically, he has designed an antibody that binds to and blocks the activity of one of the Toll-like receptors. When the antibody is used, which step in acute inflammation would be directly blocked?

A. Identification of the inciting agent

B. Recruitment of white blood cells

C. Removal of the inciting agent

D. Regulatory steps to maintain control of the inflammatory response

E. Resolution of the inflammation

N/A

2. The hospital laboratory receives a specimen from a clinical physician for analysis. The specimen vial contains a watery fluid. Testing indicates a very low concentration of protein, and only a very few red and white blood cells are identified on microscopic examination. Of the following disease types, which is the most likely source of the fluid collection from which this sample was obtained?

A. Acute appendicitis

B. Subdural hematoma

C. Bronchopneumonia

D. Congestive heart failure

E. Acute pancreatitis

F. Sepsis

N/A

3. A 6-year-old boy falls off his bicycle while in the driveway of his house. His mother witnesses him fall and sees that he strikes his knee against the ground but does not hit his head. She feels that he is fine and returns to her work. About 20 minutes later, he comes in the house to get a drink of water. She can see that the skin on his knee where he hit the ground is intact but red. The red discoloration of the skin is not a bruise. Of the following mediators, which played the largest role in producing this visible change in the skin?

A. ICAM-1

B. PECAM-1

C. Histamine

D. Thromboxane A2

E. E-selectin

F. P-selectin

N/A

4. A researcher is studying acute inflammation and has developed an antibody for her research. This antibody, called ILF-2, binds to a receptor on the endothelial cell and blocks it. Binding of the antibody causes impairment of leukocyte rolling, though margination still occurs. Of the following receptors, which is ILF-2 most likely binding to?

A. E-selectin

B. L-selectin

C. ICAM-1

D. PECAM-1

E. Integrin

F. Sialyl-Lewis-X

N/A

5. A medical student is writing a paper on opsonins. In the paper, the student lists the various opsonins and the appropriate receptor that they bind to. In reading the paper, the student's professor identifies one mispairing. Of the following pairings, which represents an opsonin and the wrong receptor for that opsonin?

A. Integrin and ICAM-1

B. IgG and the Fc Receptor

C. CD34 and L-selectin

D. C1q and collectins

E. Complement receptors (1 and 3) and C9

N/A

6. A medical student in a laboratory is studying the effects of a drug that irreversibly binds to and inhibits the function of ICAM-1. When the drug is administered, the student observes that acute inflammation is impaired. Of the following, which protein is also indirectly involved?

A. Sialyl-Lewis-X

B. L-selectin

C. CD11/CD18 integrins

D. VLA-4

E. CD 31

N/A

7. The parents of a young child bring him to a pediatric hospital for evaluation. Their son has frequently sustained middle ear infections and has had two episodes of pneumonia, both requiring hospitalization. Testing indicates that the child has a deficiency in the β subunit of CD18. Which of the following diseases does the child have?

A. Leukocyte adhesion deficiency type 1

B. Leukocyte adhesion deficiency type 2

C. Chronic granulomatous disease

D. Chediak-Higashi

E. Cryopyrin-associated periodic fever syndromes

N/A

8. A 56-year-old male experiences "crushing" substernal chest pain and is taken by private vehicle to the emergency department of the local hospital. A troponin-I test performed in the emergency room indicates a concentration of 0.01 ng/mL, and a 12-lead electrocardiogram (ECG) shows ST elevation in the anterior leads. Streptokinase is administered within 20 minutes of the onset of symptoms and the patient's symptoms resolve. A repeat ECG after administration of the drug is normal. Given that some degree of acute inflammation occurred in this process, of the following, which is the most likely outcome in the myocardium?

A. Resolution
B. Chronic inflammation
C. Scarring
D. Prolonged pericardial effusion
E. Abscess formation

Cardiovascular

9. A 35-year-old female is involved in a motor vehicle accident during which she is thrown against the steering wheel after the airbag fails to deploy, causing her to sustain a laceration of her liver. She is treated nonoperatively and is told at her 6 month check-up that she has had complete resolution of the damage to her liver. Assuming this statement is correct, which of the following could be identified histologically in the region of the liver where the injury occurred?

A. Extensive fibrosis
B. Wavy fibrosis between hepatocytes
C. Increased numbers of blood vessels
D. Multiple foci of neutrophils
E. Hemosiderin-laden macrophages

Hepatobiliary

10. A 12-year-old male with no past medical history is brought to the emergency room by his parents because of flu-like symptoms, including cough, fever, and general malaise, which are associated with the recent development of shortness of breath. During his evaluation, an ultrasound of the chest reveals a large pericardial effusion, which produces right ventricular collapse during diastole. A pericardiocentesis is performed, removing ~ 200 mL of translucent, watery yellow fluid. Of the following, which is the most likely source of the fluid around the heart?

A. A metastatic pediatric neoplasm
B. A parasite
C. A viral infection
D. A bacterial infection
E. A fungal infection

Cardiovascular

11. A 23-year-old female falls off her bike and strikes her thigh against the sidewalk. Bruising occurs at the site of impact, and, within minutes, the tissue expands at this point, creating a noticeable bulge in the skin. Of the following mediators, which most directly and significantly played a role in these changes?

A. Reactive oxygen species
B. Serotonin
C. Thromboxane A2
D. Prostaglandins D2
E. Leukotriene B4

Soft tissue

12. A 24-year-old female develops bacterial meningitis due to *Neisseria meningitidis*. On her initial presentation to the emergency room, being brought in by her family, she is in obvious distress and has a fever of 103°F. Laboratory testing indicates a white blood cell count of 15,000 cells/μL. Of the following mediators, which is least responsible for her symptoms, physical examination, and laboratory findings?

A. IL-1
B. IL-6
C. IL-12
D. TNF
E. CXC chemokines

Central nervous system

13. A 2-year-old boy with recurrent infections is found to improperly synthesize NADPH oxidase, producing a nonworking protein. Of the following, which is most directly responsible for his susceptibility to infections?

A. Elevated concentrations of reactive oxygen species
B. Decreased concentrations of reactive oxygen species
C. Elevated concentrations of activated α1-antitrypsin
D. Decreased concentrations of activated α1-antitrypsin
E. Elevated concentrations of C3a and C5a
F. Decreased concentrations of C3a and C5a

N/A

14. A 17-year-old female is brought to the emergency room by her family because she is acutely short of breath. Despite being given oxygen and epinephrine, her shortness of breath continues and she requires intubation. During the intubation, the emergency room physician notes severe laryngeal edema. This woman has a hereditary condition and commonly develops edema of soft tissue in various locations. Which of the following proteins does she lack?

A. C5

B. C3

C. C3 inhibitor

D. C1 inhibitor

E. Decay-accelerating factor

General

15. A pathologist is examining a slide of the appendix. In the mucosa, submucosa, and muscularis are numerous cells with abundant cytoplasm and multilobed nuclei, with the lobes joined by very thin bridges. Of the following mediators, which was most responsible for attracting these cells to this site?

A. Leukotriene B4

B. Leukotriene C4

C. Leukotriene D4

D. Leukotriene E4

E. Substance P

N/A

16. A pathologist is examining a slide and identifies a lesion that is a roughly circular collection of epithelioid macrophages. There is no central necrosis. Of the following organisms, which is the most likely cause of this lesion?

A. *Staphylococcus aureus*

B. *Streptococcus pneumoniae*

C. *Escherichia coli*

D. *Pseudomonas aeruginosa*

E. *Mycobacterium leprae*

N/A

17. A 56-year-old alcoholic male is admitted to the hospital with a diagnosis of pneumonia. His primary care physician orders a test that identifies an increased speed of sedimentation of red blood cells. Which of the following mediators is responsible for this change?

A. C-reactive protein

B. Serum amyloid A

C. Ceruloplasmin

D. Fibrinogen

E. Creatine kinase

N/A

18. A 68-year-old male with metastatic lung cancer is being evaluated by his oncologist. His chemotherapy regimen was discontinued 3 months ago due to his poor prognosis. His wife is concerned because he has lost 25 lbs. over the past two months. At the present time he is on no medications, and she reports his appetite has been poor. Which of the following polypeptides released by immune cells in response to this patient's cancer is most likely to cause progressive weight loss?

A. TNF-α

B. TGF-β

C. IL-8

D. IL-10

E. IL-13

N/A

19. An immunologist studying the process of leukocyte recruitment in acute inflammation wishes to block the process of transmigration of neutrophils across the endothelial wall. A monoclonal antibody against which of the following adhesion molecules would inhibit transmigration (diapedesis) without interfering with rolling or margination?

A. P-selectin

B. E-selectin

C. Integrin

D. ICAM-1

E. PECAM-1 (CD31)

N/A

20. A 70-year-old male dies of an acute ischemic stroke. During the autopsy an incidental lesion is found in the apex of the right upper lobe of the lung. Microscopy reveals abundant macrophages with indistinct cell boundaries, surrounded by a rim of lymphocytes, and a central zone of necrotic debris. Of the following, which is the most likely cause of this patient's lung lesion?

A. Tissue foreign bodies

B. Tuberculosis

C. Sarcoidosis

D. Crohn's disease

E. Leprosy

Lung

21. A researcher is investigating an experimental drug (F-104), which is known to cause liver failure in mice. Which of the following microscopic findings would suggest that F-104 acted by inducing apoptosis rather than necrosis of the hepatic parenchymal cells?

A. Cytoplasmic blebbing

B. Hepatocyte swelling

C. Chromatin condensation

D. Abundant myelin figures

E. Numerous inflammatory cells

Liver

22. In the previous experiment, which of the following findings would support the hypothesis that F-104-induced apoptosis via the intrinsic pathway?

A. Monoclonal antibody that blocks TNF receptor prevents F-104-induced liver injury

B. Monoclonal antibody that blocks Fas prevents F-104-induced liver injury

C. An experimental drug that inhibits cytochrome c release prevents F-104-induced liver injury

D. An experimental drug that inhibits caspase 8 prevents F-104-induced liver injury

E. An experimental drug that inhibits caspase 10 prevents F-104-induced liver injury

Liver

23. A 56-year-old male presents to an acute care clinic with complaints of shortness of breath and fever. He has no past history of cigarette use. His vital signs are temperature of 101°F, pulse of 107 bpm, and blood pressure of 131/86 mm Hg. A chest X-ray reveals fluid in the left side of the chest and patchy consolidation of the lower lobe of the left lung. He is admitted to the hospital and a thoracentesis is performed. Of the following, what is most likely a characteristic of the fluid?

A. Watery and clear

B. Few cells identified on smear

C. Low specific gravity

D. Elevated protein

E. Numerous neoplastic cells identified on smear

Lung

2.2 Acute and Chronic Inflammation— Answers and Explanations

Easy	Medium	Hard

1. Correct: Identification of the inciting agent (A)

The five possible answers listed are the five general steps of acute inflammation in order from start to finish. The Toll-like receptors are important in allowing immune cells to identify the agent that is precipitating the acute inflammation (**A**). For (**B-E**), see previous discussion.

2. Correct: Congestive heart failure (D)

The fluid described is a transudate, which would produce a serous effusion in a body cavity. A serous effusion is one that is watery, clear, and light yellow in color. Transudates are produced by either high intravascular pressures, such as would occur with congestive heart failure (**D**), or with low oncotic pressure, such as in hypoalbuminemia. With high intravascular pressure, fluid is essentially forced out of the vasculature into the

body cavity or soft tissue, whereas with hypoalbuminemia, the oncotic pressure of the blood, which is the force that draws fluid back into the vasculature from the soft tissue, is low. Hypoalbuminemia can occur in liver failure, because of decreased production of albumin, or in nephrotic syndrome, because of loss of albumin in the urine. The other choices would cause an exudate, which has a high concentration of protein and a prominent cellular component (**A-C, E-F**).

3. Correct: Histamine (C)

Histamine plays a large role in vasodilation, and vasodilation produces the erythema (red discoloration) and heat usually associated with acute inflammation (**C**). Thromboxane A2 causes vasoconstriction (**D**), and the other mediators listed (**A-B, E-F**) participate in the migration of white blood cells through the wall of the blood vessel to the site of the inflammation.

4. Correct: E-selectin (A)

L-selectin and Sialyl-Lewis-X are found on the leukocytes (**B, F**). Integrins (on leukocytes) and ICAM-1 (on endothelial cells) participate in tight adhesion of the white blood cell to the vessel wall (**C, E**), and PECAM-1 participates in transmigration of the white blood cell through the wall of the vessel (**D**). E-selectin is found on endothelial cells and participates in leukocyte rolling and adhesion (**A**).

5. Correct: Complement receptors (1 and 3) and C9 (E)

Opsonin is a general term for a group of molecules that bind to bacteria and dead cells and allow for their recognition by leukocytes as something needing to be ingested and destroyed. The opsonins are IgG, fragments of C3, and collectins. IgG binds to the Fc receptor (**B**), and collectins bind to C1q, (**D**) but fragments of C3 bind to complement receptors (**E**). Integrin and ICAM-1 and CD34 and L-selectin are appropriately paired (**A, C**), but none of these mediators are opsonins.

6. Correct: CD11/CD18 integrins (C)

During the process of firm adhesion and transmigration, CD11/CD18 on the leukocyte binds to ICAM-1 (**C**). Sialyl-Lewis-X binds to P-selectin and E-selectin, L-selectin binds to GlyCam-1 and CD34, VLA-4 binds to VCAM-1, and CD31 on endothelial cells binds to CD31 on white blood cells.

7. Correct: Leukocyte adhesion deficiency type 1 (LAD-1) (A)

LAD-1 is due to a defective production of the β subunit of CD18 (**A**). LAD-2 is due to absence of sialyl-Lewis-X (**B**). Chronic granulomatous disease is due to impaired phagocyte oxidase production (**C**). Chediak-Higashi syndrome is due to a mutation of CHS1, a lysosomal trafficking regulator (**D**). Cryopyrin-associated periodic fever syndromes are due to gain-of-function mutations affecting the inflammasome (**E**).

8. Correct: Resolution (A)

Although the individual was sustaining an acute myocardial infarct, a presumptive diagnosis was made, and restoration of blood flow was made prior to irreversible damage; therefore, resolution of the inflammation is likely (**A**). If the troponin I had been elevated, it would indicate irreversible damage. As the cardiac myocytes are essentially incapable of division, the necrotic cells would have triggered acute inflammation; however, complete resolution is impossible without the potential for division among the surviving cells. In that case, scarring would be the result (**C**). As the underlying etiologic cause is neither infectious nor otherwise likely to linger in the tissue, chronic inflammation, a prolonged effusion, or an abscess would not occur (**B, D-E**).

9. Correct: Hemosiderin-laden macrophages (E)

As a laceration occurred, hemorrhage is expected, and when the red blood cells break down, hemosiderin is deposited (**E**). With complete resolution, all injured cells are replaced, and inflammatory mediators, including inflammatory cells, are no longer present (**D**). During complete resolution, fibrosis would not be deposited (**A-B**). Increased numbers of blood vessels are also indicative of chronic inflammation (**C**).

10. Correct: A viral infection (C)

The effusion as described, being watery, translucent, and yellow, is a serous effusion, which can be found in viral infections (**C**). Given the clinical scenario, the patient most likely has a viral myocarditis or viral pericarditis, both of which are commonly due to Coxsackie virus infection. Bacteria, fungi, and parasites are more likely to produce a fibrinous or suppurative inflammation (**B, D-E**), in which case the effusion would be less watery, and cloudy, not translucent, and a metastatic neoplasm would be more likely to produce a fibrinous or even hemorrhagic effusion (**A**).

11. Correct: Prostaglandin D2 (D)

Prostaglandins D2 and E2 cause increased vasculature permeability and vasodilation, both of which would contribute to fluid leaving the vascular space, entering the tissue, and producing swelling (**D**). Serotonin and thromboxane A2 cause vasoconstriction, which would impede the changes described (**B-C**), and leukotriene B4 is a chemotactic agent (**E**), responsible for helping recruit white blood cells to the site of inflammation. Reactive oxygen species are produced as a tool to destroy invading bacteria (**A**).

12. Correct: IL-12 (C)

The patient has bacterial meningitis, an acute process. IL-1, IL-6, and TNF play a role in acute inflammation, acting on endothelium to increase adhesion molecule expression, activating white blood cells, and promoting systemic effects such as fever, elevation of acute phase proteins, and increasing leuko-

cyte production. Chemokines recruit white blood cells to the site of acute inflammation (**A-B, D-E**). Therefore, in an acute bacterial meningitis, IL-1, IL-6, TNF, and CXC chemokines would all play a role; however, IL-12 functions mostly in chronic inflammation and would not play a role in the acute process (**C**).

13. Correct: Decreased concentrations of reactive oxygen species (B)

NADPH oxidase helps to synthesize reactive oxygen species, which then play a role in killing of infectious agents (**A-B**). α1-antitrypsin is an enzyme that is contained in fluids but is not activated directly by NADPH oxidase, and it plays a role in inhibiting the action of enzymes (**C-D**). C3a and C5a increase vascular permeability and induce vasodilation as well as play a role in recruitment of neutrophils, but they are produced by the action of neutral proteases and not NADPH oxidase (**E-F**).

14. Correct: C1 inhibitor (D)

The patient has hereditary angioedema, which is an inherited defect in C1 inhibitor (**C**), leading to edema of soft tissue, which can involve the larynx. (**A-B, D-E**) are incorrect.

15. Correct: Leukotriene B4 (A)

The cell type described is a neutrophil, which is an acute inflammatory cell. The disease that the patient has is acute appendicitis. Leukotriene B4 is a chemoattractant and plays a role in attracting neutrophils to the site of acute inflammation (**A**). The remainder of the mediators, including substance P, are primarily involved in increasing vascular permeability (**B-E**), so each of these mediators could play a role in the disease process of acute appendicitis; however, that role would not be as a chemoattractant.

16. Correct: *Mycobacterium leprae* (E)

The lesion described is a granuloma. Granulomas are composed of epithelioid macrophages (also referred to as epithelioid histiocytes). While multinucleated giant cells are often found in granulomas, their presence is not necessary for the diagnosis of a granuloma. Granulomatous inflammation is produced by a variety of infectious agents as well as foreign material and other processes. Of the organisms listed, *Mycobacterium leprae* produces granulomatous inflammation (**E**), whereas the other organisms are not associated with granulomatous inflammation (**A-D**).

17. Correct: Fibrinogen (D)

Fibrinogen is an acute phase protein; its concentration is elevated in acute inflammatory processes, such as pneumonia. Fibrinogen binds to red blood cells and thus causes rouleaux, which increases the sedimentation rate (**C**). The test ordered was the erythrocyte sedimentation rate. (**A-B, D-E**) are incorrect.

18. Correct: TNF-α (A)

TNF-α, IL-1, and IL-6 are proinflammatory cytokines that play a critical role in malignancy-related cachexia, and in experimental models, antagonists of these cytokines have been shown to mitigate this effect (**A**). TGF-β is an anti-inflammatory cytokine involved in cellular repair (**B**). IL-8 is a chemokine that recruits neutrophils to the site of infection or inflammation (**C**). IL-10 also plays a critical role in modulating the immune response by down-regulating the expression of Th1 cytokines, MHC class II antigens, and co-stimulatory molecules on macrophages and inhibiting the production of proinflammatory cytokines (**D**). In addition to its anti-inflammatory properties, IL-13 plays an important role in immunity to parasitic infections (**E**).

19. Correct: PECAM-1 (CD31) (E)

PECAM-1 (**E**) plays a critical role in transmigration of the leukocyte across the vessel wall (**E**). The selectins form weak adhesions between leukocytes and endothelial cells, which slows the leukocytes during the process of rolling (**A, B**). Integrins (VLA-4, Mac-1, and LFA-1) on the leukocyte surface bind to ligands on the endothelial surface (ICAM-1, VCAM-1) after the initial process of leukocyte rolling (**C, D**). These interactions result in tight adherence of leukocytes to the vessel wall in preparation for diapedesis into the extravascular site of inflammation.

20. Correct: Tuberculosis (B)

The microscopic description is that of a granuloma with a central area of necrosis (i.e., caseous necrosis). Granulomatous inflammation with caseous necrosis is the classic finding in *Mycobacterium tuberculosis* infection (**B**). This central necrosis has a "cheesy" appearance on gross examination, hence the term "caseous." All the other conditions mentioned are associated with granulomatous inflammation, though not usually with caseous necrosis (**A, C-E**). Crohn's disease would not affect the lung (**D**), and leprosy involves the skin (**E**). Sarcoidosis is a granulomatous disease that most commonly involves the lung, although any other organ can also be involved. Granulomas in sarcoidosis are most commonly non-caseating; however, caseous necrosis has been found in patients with sarcoidosis. The fact that the lesion is in the apex of the lung also supports tuberculosis over sarcoidosis, as *Mycobacterium tuberculosis* is most commonly associated with the upper lobes of the lung because of the organism's aerophilic nature.

21. Correct: Chromatin condensation (C)

Of the choices, chromatin condensation (**C**) is the most characteristic finding in apoptotic cells. Cytoplasmic blebbing could be seen in either apoptosis or necrosis (**A**). Cellular swelling, myelin figures, and abundant inflammatory cells are seen in necrosis, not apoptosis (**B, D-E**).

22. Correct: An experimental drug that inhibits cytochrome c release prevents F-104-induced liver injury (C).

Cytochrome c release from the mitochondria triggers apoptosis via the intrinsic (mitochondrial) pathway. Inhibiting this critical step in activation of the intrinsic pathway would be expected to interfere with F-104 if it acted via the intrinsic pathway (**C**). All the other effects, if observed, would support the hypothesis that F-104 induces apoptosis via the extrinsic (receptor-mediated) pathway (**A-B, D-E**).

23. Correct: Elevated protein (D)

Given the clinical scenario (shortness of breath and fever associated with pulmonary consolidation), the patient most likely has bronchopneumonia, and the infiltrate in the pleural cavity is most likely an empyema, which is a form of exudate (**D**). Exudates are characteristically very cellular, have a high protein and lactate dehydrogenase concentration, and have a high specific gravity. Exudates can occur as a result of infection (e.g., an empyema) or lymphatic obstruction, such as due to a lymphoma. Transudates have low cellularity, low concentration of protein, and low specific gravity (**A-C**). A pleural effusion can be malignant, such as due to primary effusion lymphoma, bronchogenic carcinoma, or metastatic disease (**E**); however, this diagnosis would be much less likely without a contributing history, and the presentation is consistent with pneumonia.

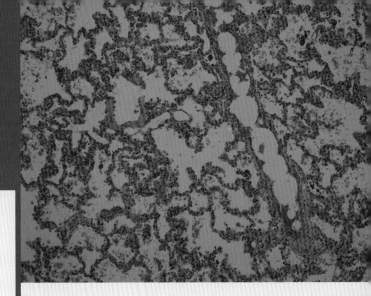

Chapter 3
Hemodynamics

LEARNING OBJECTIVES

3.1 Hemodynamics
▶ List and describe the types of hemorrhage
▶ Describe the morphologic changes associated with acute and chronic congestion
▶ Describe the mechanisms for hyperemia, congestion, and edema
▶ Describe the morphologic features associated with acute and chronic congestion and edema
▶ Describe the risk factors associated with thrombosis
▶ Differentiate amongst the various causes of shock
▶ Identify the underlying cause of shock
▶ Identify the manifestations of vascular congestion
▶ Describe the effect of Starling forces on vascular fluid dynamics
▶ Recognize cerebral edema and its causes

3.2 Coagulation and Thrombolysis
▶ Identify common causes of acquired thrombocytopenia
▶ Describe the regulation of coagulation and thrombolysis
▶ Apply the concepts of hemostasis

3.3 Thrombosis, Embolism, and Infarction
▶ Diagnose fat embolism
▶ Diagnose decompression sickness
▶ Recognize embolic stroke
▶ Identify chronic venous insufficiency
▶ Diagnose mesenteric ischemia
▶ Diagnose renal infarction
▶ Manage superficial thrombophlebitis
▶ Describe the histologic changes in both red and white infarcts; list organs where red and white infarcts commonly occur
▶ Identify common embolic syndromes
▶ Recognize air embolism
▶ Recognize cholesterol embolism syndrome
▶ Recognize causes of cardioembolism

3.4 Hereditary Thrombophilia and Coagulopathy
▶ Identify and discern between the genetic causes of venous thromboembolic disease
▶ Describe the physiologic response to shock
▶ Localize the affected vessel in acute stroke syndromes
▶ Identify common presentations of hereditary thrombophilias

3.1 Hemodynamics—Questions

Easy	Medium	Hard

1. While camping, a 15-year-old boy is bitten by a mosquito. At the site of the mosquito bite, his skin turns red and a small but noticeable bump forms. Which of the following terms best describes the color change in the skin?

A. Lividity

B. Ecchymosis

C. Contusion

D. Congestion

E. Hyperemia

Integumentary

2. A 66-year-old male has a long-standing history of congestive heart failure due to uncontrolled hypertension and has had multiple admissions to the hospital for treatment of pulmonary edema. During his most recent admission, he sustains a fatal cardiac dysrhythmia. Which of the following is likely to be observed in this patient's lungs at autopsy?

A. Dilated alveolar septal capillaries filled with red blood cells

B. Fibrotic and thickened alveolar septal capillaries

C. Loss of alveolar septa, resulting in large airspaces

D. Congestion of centrilobular sinusoids

E. Diffuse macrovesicular steatosis of the liver

Respiratory

3. A 71-year-old male with a history of poorly controlled hypertension due to noncompliance with medications is brought to the emergency room by his family because of increasing shortness of breath. An X-ray of the chest reveals bilateral pleural effusions and enlargement of the heart. Given these features, of the following, which is the most likely causative mechanism for the condition producing his shortness of breath?

A. Increased hydrostatic pressure

B. Increased vascular permeability

C. Decreased colloid osmotic pressure

D. Lymphatic obstruction

E. Sodium retention

Cardiovascular

4. A 68-year-old male with poorly controlled hypertension presents to the emergency room with shortness of breath. A chest X-ray reveals bilateral pleural effusions. An S3 gallop is heard and crackles (rales) are present in both lung fields. Which of the following pigments is most likely to be found within macrophages in his lungs?

A. Bilirubin

B. Hemosiderin

C. Melanin

D. Lipofuscin

E. Calcium

Respiratory

5. A 56-year-old male presents to his physician because of swelling in the right lower extremity distal to the knee. He has a history of mild hypertension, which is well controlled with medication. He also reports no trauma to the extremity, and no skin infections or other known sites of infection. On examination edema is noted, with the circumference of the right calf measuring 3 cm larger than the circumference of the left calf. There is a palpable cord present. Of the following, which aspect of the history, physical, or laboratory testing would be most likely to indicate the cause?

A. AST/ALT levels

B. CK-MB levels

C. BUN/creatinine levels

D. Family history of colon cancer

E. History of recent surgery

Cardiovascular

6. A 40-year-old male is brought to the emergency department by his wife because of his shortness of breath. He reports the onset of a cough two days prior with increasing shortness of breath. On arrival his temperature is 100.5°F (38.0°C), his heart rate is 135/min, and blood pressure is 88/55 mm Hg. Physical examination is unremarkable except for tachycardia. The patient is alert and oriented. His leukocyte count is 18,000/µL, his pCO_2 on arterial blood gas is 30 mm Hg, and serum lactic acid is slightly elevated at 4 mmol/L. A plain chest radiograph shows a right lower lobe infiltrate. What is the most likely diagnosis?

A. Acute pulmonary embolism

B. Septic shock

C. Cardiogenic shock

D. Anaphylactic shock

E. Acute myocardial infarction

Cardiovascular

7. A 76-year-old man is evaluated in the emergency department for hypotension and dyspnea. His temperature is 97.8°F (36.5°C), pulse 125/min, and blood pressure 88/58 mm Hg. Bilateral crackles are present in the lung fields. Pedal edema is noted bilaterally. His extremities are cool, and his urine output is minimal. A plain chest radiograph reveals cardiomegaly and pulmonary edema. What is the pathophysiology of his shock?

A. Septic shock
B. Anaphylactic shock
C. Cardiogenic shock
D. Hypovolemic shock
E. Distributive shock

Cardiovascular

8. In the previous clinical scenario, of the following, which is most likely the underlying cause of this man's shock?

A. Acute pulmonary embolism
B. Acute right ventricular myocardial infarction
C. Pulmonary hypertension
D. Aortic stenosis
E. Pericardial tamponade

Cardiovascular

9. A 67-year-old man is brought to the emergency department with hypotension and tachycardia. He has had no urine output. Which of the following additional findings would suggest hypovolemia rather than sepsis as the underlying cause of this man's low urine output?

A. Low leukocyte count
B. Elevated leukocyte count
C. Hypernatremia
D. Hyperglycemia
E. Elevated serum lactic acid

Cardiovascular

10. A 76-year-old man is found dead at home. Microscopic examination of samples of the liver and lung reveals centrilobular hemorrhagic necrosis of the liver and hemosiderin-laden macrophages in the lungs. Of the following, what additional finding at autopsy would be most likely?

A. Pleural effusion
B. Aortic dissection
C. Deep venous thrombosis
D. Disseminated intravascular coagulation
E. Pericardial tamponade

Cardiovascular

11. A 60-year-old female status post right radical mastectomy and right axillary lymph node dissection develops chronic edema of the right arm. Which of the following is the cause of her edema?

A. Increased plasma oncotic pressure
B. Renal sodium retention
C. Increased interstitial protein
D. Increased vascular permeability
E. Decreased plasma albumin

Cardiovascular

12. A 79-year-old male nursing home resident with dementia is admitted to the hospital for failure to thrive. According to his primary caregiver he has taken very little fluids or food over the preceding three weeks. On admission his serum sodium is 165 mmol/L, and he subsequently receives a large amount of free water in the form of intravenous D5W over a two-hour period. Shortly after finishing the fluids he becomes unresponsive. He dies after a brief attempt at resuscitation. Blood for a chemistry panel is drawn during resuscitation, with laboratory testing revealing the serum sodium to be 124 mmol/L. Examination of the brain at autopsy is most likely to reveal which of the following findings?

A. Liquefactive necrosis
B. Acute thrombosis of the middle cerebral artery
C. Narrowed sulci and distended gyri
D. Passive venous congestion
E. Diffuse axonal injury

Renal

3.2 Coagulation and Thrombolysis—Questions

Easy	Medium	Hard

13. A 58-year-old man with a history of deep venous thrombosis following right total knee replacement is recovering from multiple injuries sustained in a motor vehicle collision. His injuries include fractures to both tibial plateaus. He is on subcutaneous unfractionated heparin for prevention of deep venous thrombosis. On his 6th hospital day his platelet count dropped from 250,000/μL to 110,000/μL. He is otherwise recovering well with no complications, and a lower extremity Doppler is performed, which is negative for deep venous thrombosis. Which of the following additional tests would be most helpful in determining the cause of his thrombocytopenia?

A. PT and PTT
B. Anti-platelet factor 4 antibody
C. Protein C activity
D. Protein S activity
E. Factor Xa level

Hematopoetic

14. A 37-year-old female with a history of deep venous thrombosis during her first pregnancy and two spontaneous abortions is evaluated in the emergency department. Forty minutes prior to arrival she experienced the sudden onset of weakness of the right face, right arm, and right leg. Neurologic examination reveals flaccid paralysis of the right side of the body with expressive aphasia without visual field defect. Magnetic resonance imaging (MRI) of the brain and basic lab work including complete blood count, prothrombin time (PT), and activated thromboplastin time (aPTT) are ordered in the emergency department. The treating physician administers tissue plasminogen activator (t-PA) to the patient according to hospital protocol in the treatment of acute stroke. Which of the following is true regarding the mechanism of t-PA?

A. t-PA prevents platelet activation by inhibiting GpIIb-IIIa complex.

B. t-PA prevents platelet activation by inhibiting GpIb receptors.

C. t-PA increases the degradation of fibrin.

D. t-PA binds anti-thrombin III, leading to thrombin inactivation.

E. t-PA binds and inactivates clotting factors.

Hematopoetic

15. Ristocetin is an antibiotic, which is no longer in use, that causes platelet agglutination by facilitating binding of von Willebrand's factor (vWF) to GpIb. Two tests used in the workup of von Willebrand's disease are the ristocetin cofactor assay and the ristocetin-induced platelet aggregation (RIPA). The ristocetin cofactor assay measures the ability of formalin-fixed (i.e., dead) control platelets to agglutinate in the patient's plasma. The ristocetin-induced platelet aggregation test involves adding ristocetin to a sample of the patient's platelet-rich plasma. Which results on the ristocetin cofactor assay and the RIPA would be consistent with Bernard-Soulier's syndrome?

A. Normal agglutination on ristocetin cofactor assay and normal agglutination on RIPA

B. Normal agglutination on ristocetin cofactor assay and hypoactive agglutination on RIPA

C. Hypoactive agglutination on ristocetin cofactor assay and normal agglutination on RIPA

D. Hypoactive agglutination on ristocetin cofactor assay and hypoactive agglutination on RIPA

E. Hyperactive agglutination on ristocetin cofactor assay and normal agglutination on RIPA

Hematopoetic

3.3 Thrombosis, Embolism, and Infarction—Questions

Easy	Medium	Hard

16. A 17-year-old male sustains a mid-shaft femur fracture after a fall from a horse. The fracture is repaired operatively and the patient is discharged. On the second postoperative day he becomes acutely dyspneic. In the emergency department he is hypoxic and tachypneic, appears confused, and has a petechial rash on his neck and anterior thorax. What is the most likely diagnosis?

A. Aortic dissection

B. Fat embolism

C. Venous thromboembolism

D. Acute myocardial infarction

E. Disseminated intravascular coagulation

Neurologic, hematopoetic, cardiovascular

17. A 23-year-old man is flying home from a 10-day scuba diving vacation. One hour into the flight he develops some mild to moderate pain in his shoulders and knees. Shortly thereafter he reports a substernal burning sensation with inspiration that is associated with low back pain. By the time the flight lands, which is four hours after takeoff, he is unable to move his legs. He is immediately taken to the nearest hospital, but dies of respiratory failure en route. Which of the following would have reduced his risk of developing this illness?

A. Delaying his flight home for 48 hours

B. Wearing insect repellent during his trip

C. Taking a dose of aspirin for a week before and during his trip

D. Walking frequently during his airplane flight

E. Avoiding dental work a month prior to his trip

Cardiovascular

18. A 76-year-old woman is found down at home by a relative and is unresponsive on arrival to the emergency department. A CT scan of the head preformed shortly after arrival shows multiple infarcts of the right and left cerebral hemispheres and an infarct of the cerebellum, which were confirmed with magnetic resonance imaging (MRI) of the brain. Which of the following tests is most likely to reveal the cause of her strokes?

A. A complete blood count

B. Bilateral lower extremity venous Doppler

C. Bilateral lower extremity arterial Doppler

D. Cerebral angiogram

E. Transesophageal echocardiogram

Cardiovascular

19. A 72-year-old man with morbid obesity, hypertension, and diabetes mellitus is evaluated by his primary care physician for progressively worsening edema of the lower extremities over the preceding years. He reports pain in both legs with standing and walking but improvement in the pain and edema with elevation of the legs. His body mass index is 39.5 kg/m². His vital signs are normal. Auscultation of the heart and lungs is normal. He has 3+ pitting edema of the bilateral lower extremities with normal warmth, mild tenderness and numerous varicose veins. Inspection of the skin reveals a reddish-brown hyperpigmented and indurated dermatitis involving the anterior lower legs bilaterally. What is the most likely underlying cause of the patient's symptoms?

A. Damage to valves in the deep venous system of the legs

B. Acute thrombosis of the deep venous system of the legs

C. Atherosclerotic disease of the bilateral iliac arteries

D. Impaired lymphatic drainage of the legs

E. Bacterial soft tissue infection of the legs

Cardiovascular, dermatologic

20. A 78-year-old man with chronic atrial fibrillation presents with abdominal pain. The patient reports the pain started 3 hours ago, is very severe, and is periumbilical. His temperature is 99.0°F (37.0°C), pulse 110/min, and blood pressure 98/58 mm Hg. The patient appears to be in severe pain. Physical examination is remarkable for an irregularly irregular heart rhythm and mild abdominal distension. The abdomen is mildly tender. His leukocyte count is 19.3 × 10³/μL, hemoglobin is 19.0 g/dL, and serum bicarbonate is 18 mmol/L. Five hours after arrival his condition deteriorates, his abdomen becomes grossly distended, his bowel sounds become inaudible, and he dies. Which of the following is the most likely diagnosis?

A. Mesenteric embolic infarction

B. Ruptured abdominal aortic aneurysm

C. Acute appendicitis

D. Acute diverticulitis

E. Small bowel obstruction

Cardiovascular, gastrointestinal

21. A 55-year-old male with well-controlled type 2 diabetes mellitus, hypertension, and paroxysmal atrial fibrillation presents with acute onset of right flank pain with hematuria. His temperature is 98.8°F (37°C), pulse is 90/min, blood pressure is 155/92 mm Hg, respirations are 18/min, and O_2 saturation is 98% on room air. On examination he appears to be in moderate pain, his lungs are clear, he has an irregularly irregular rhythm, and his right flank is tender to palpation. His leukocyte count is 12 × 10³/μL, creatinine is 1.8 mg/dL (from a value of 1.1 mg/dL six months previously), and his aminotransferases are normal. Urinalysis shows numerous red cells with no white cells and no casts. Noncontrast helical CT scan of the kidneys and collection system is unremarkable. Of the following, what is the most likely diagnosis?

A. Acute pyelonephritis

B. Ureterolithiasis

C. Acute appendicitis

D. Glomerulonephritis

E. Renal infarction

Cardiovascular, genitourinary

22. A 32-year-old woman has routine lab work done as part of her annual physical examination. She returns to the clinic 3 days after her blood draw complaining of pain in the left antecubital fossa. On examination there is mild erythema without induration, no palpable fluctuence, and the basilic vein is tender and palpated as a nodular "cord." What is the appropriate management?

A. Anticoagulation with Coumadin

B. Oral antibiotics

C. Warm compresses

D. Topical corticosteroids

E. Incision and drainage

Vascular

23. A pathologist is examining tissue removed from a 57-year-old deceased male. The tissue has preservation of normal architecture; however, there is loss of nuclear and cytoplasmic basophilia. Associated with these changes are abundant extravasated red blood cells in the tissue. The man had no resuscitation performed. Of the following, where did this tissue most likely originate?

A. The heart

B. A kidney

C. The spleen

D. The brain

E. A lung

Lung

24. A 22-year-old female in active labor suddenly develops hypotension and dyspnea. She becomes hypoxic and is intubated for acute respiratory failure. Chest radiograph shows acute pulmonary edema. She dies prior to delivery. Which of the following is most likely to be found at autopsy?

A. Left ventricular hypertrophy

B. Femoral vein deep venous thrombosis

C. Plaque rupture in the left anterior descending coronary artery

D. Disseminated intravascular coagulation

E. Thrombus in the right main pulmonary artery

Cardiovascular, female reproductive

25. A 67-year-old woman has a central venous catheter placed during hospitalization for dehydration. The catheter is placed using guidewire technique and ultrasound guidance, and the tip of the catheter is demonstrated to be in good position in the superior vena cava. On the third hospital day the nurse finds the patient sitting up in bed with the venous catheter partially dislodged. The nurse removes the catheter and holds pressure; however, the patient rapidly becomes tachycardic and hypoxic. Electrocardiogram shows sinus tachycardia and a new right axis deviation. What is the most likely diagnosis?

A. Pulmonary embolism

B. Air embolism

C. Acute myocardial infarction

D. Aortic dissection

E. Sepsis

Cardiovascular

26. A 63-year-old male undergoes left heart catheterization in preparation for possible aortic valve replacement to treat severe aortic regurgitation. The procedure revealed extensive calcification in the thoracic aorta and moderate nonobstructive coronary artery disease. A week after the procedure he presents to his primary care physician complaining that his left big toe has turned blue. In addition to a patchy cyanosis of several toes on both feet, he is noted to have livedo reticularis of the lower extremities and elevation of the serum creatinine. Pulses are brisk in both lower extremities. What is the most likely diagnosis?

A. Granulation tissue in the dermis

B. Excessive collagen deposition in the dermis

C. Foreign body granulomas in the dermis

D. Fibrin thrombi in the arterioles of the dermis

E. Cholesterol deposition in arterioles of the dermis

Cardiovascular

27. A 57-year-old man is evaluated in the emergency room for sudden onset of left hemiparesis, which began 45 minutes prior to his arrival. A CT scan of the head in the emergency department is unremarkable. t-PA is not administered because of his uncontrolled hypertension. He is admitted to a neurologic ICU, and a 2D echocardiogram is performed, which shows a mobile mural thrombus of the left ventricle. Which of the following additional findings are likely to be found on echocardiogram?

A. Atrial fibrillation

B. A large area of poorly contracting left ventricular muscle

C. Hypokinetic right ventricle and dilated pulmonary artery

D. Aortic valve calcification and stenosis

E. Mitral valve vegetation

Cardiovascular

3.4 Hereditary Thrombophilia and Coagulopathy—Questions

Easy	Medium	Hard

28. A 27-year-old male presents with his second unprovoked deep venous thrombosis. He is started on Coumadin and returns in 5 days to check his INR (International Normalized Ratio). Which of the following tests would be least useful to order at his follow-up visit?

A. Homocysteine level

B. Prothrombin Gene Mutation (G20210A)

C. Factor V Leiden

D. Proteins C and S activity

E. Antiphospholipid antibody

Hematopoetic, genetic

29. A 30-year-old man involved in a motor vehicle collision is brought in by EMS for severe bleeding from a laceration of the femoral artery. Shortly after arrival to the emergency department, his systolic pressure has dropped to 65 mm Hg, and his heart rate is 140. He is noted to be confused, and his urine output is low. He is receiving a blood transfusion and is started on Vasopressin. Which of the following physiologic effects would not be expected from Vasopressin?

A. Increase in systolic blood pressure

B. Platelet activation

C. Vasoconstriction

D. Hyponatremia

E. Increased renal tubular sodium absorption

Cardiovascular, renal

30. A 37-year-old female with a history of deep venous thrombosis during her first pregnancy and two spontaneous abortions is being evaluated in the emergency department. Forty minutes prior to arrival she experienced the sudden onset of weakness of the right face, right arm, and right leg. Neurologic examination reveals flaccid paralysis of the right side of the body with expressive aphasia without visual field defect. Magnetic resonance imaging (MRI) of the brain and basic lab work including complete blood count, prothrombin time (PT), and activated thromboplastin time (aPTT) are ordered in the emergency department. Which of the following is most likely to be found on the brain MRI?

A. Acute stroke of the right anterior cerebral artery
B. Acute stroke of the left anterior cerebral artery
C. Acute stroke of the right middle cerebral artery
D. Acute stroke of the left middle cerebral artery
E. Acute stroke of the right posterior cerebral artery
F. Acute stroke of the left posterior cerebral artery

Vascular, neurologic

31. In the previous scenario, which of the following clinical or laboratory findings would suggest a diagnosis other than antiphospholipid antibody syndrome (APS)?

A. Prolonged activated partial thromboplastin time (aPTT)
B. Positive VDRL test
C. Low platelet count
D. Positive antinuclear antibody (ANA)
E. Elevated homocysteine levels

Cardiovascular, neurologic, hematopoetic

3.5 Hemodynamics— Answers and Explanations

Easy	Medium	Hard

1. Correct: Hyperemia (E).

The red discoloration of the skin is a sign of acute inflammation due to the mosquito bite and occurs due to dilation of blood vessels, an active process. The correct term in this situation is hyperemia **(E)**. Congestion is a passive process, which results from impaired venous return **(D)**. Lividity is the postmortem pooling of blood in the skin due to gravity **(A)**. A contusion (i.e., bruise) is due to extravasation of red blood cells into the tissue as a result of trauma **(C)**, and an ecchymosis is also due to extravasation of red blood cells **(B)**, as opposed to hyperemia, where red blood cells should be essentially confined to the blood vessels.

2. Correct: Fibrotic and thickened alveolar septal capillaries (B)

With congestive heart failure, a chronic process, causing multiple episodes of pulmonary edema, chronic pulmonary congestion, characterized by fibrotic and thick alveolar septa and macrophages with hemosiderin would be most characteristic of the clinical scenario **(B)**. For the most recent episode, dilated alveolar septal capillaries filled with red blood cells would be appropriate; however, it would not best describe the overall clinical scenario. For **(C–E)**, see previous information.

3. Correct: Increased hydrostatic pressure (A)

The fluid in the pleural cavities represents pulmonary edema due to heart failure from the uncontrolled hypertension. Although the other mechanisms listed can lead to pulmonary edema, the most likely cause, given the scenario, would be congestive heart failure. Congestive heart failure will increase hydrostatic pressure in the pulmonary vasculature, causing fluid to leak into the surrounding space **(A)**. For **(B–E)**, see previous information.

4. Correct: Hemosiderin (B).

This individual has a clinical scenario consistent with congestive heart failure. In congestive heart failure, a common histologic finding is heart-failure cells, which are macrophages filled with hemosiderin that are found in the alveolar airspaces **(B)**. For **(A, C–E)**, see previous information.

5. Correct: History of recent surgery (E)

This patient has sustained a deep venous thrombosis. Given the unilateral nature, edema due to liver failure, renal failure, or heart failure is less likely **(A–C)**. Unilateral edema of a lower extremity could be due to venous or lymphatic obstruction. A neoplasm would be a rare cause for unilateral swelling of a lower extremity **(D)**. Of the choices, only the history of recent surgery would be expected to reveal a potential cause for this deep venous thrombosis **(E)**.

6. Correct: Septic shock (B)

The patient has multiple diagnostic criteria for sepsis, including fever, a leukocyte count > 12,000/μL, heart rate > 90/min, and CO_2 < 32 mm Hg **(B)**. All of these findings can also be seen in acute pulmonary embolism; however, the finding of an infiltrate on the chest radiograph is consistent with pneumonia and would not be expected in acute pulmonary embolism **(A)**. There is no additional information to suggest cardiogenic shock, anaphylaxis, or acute myocardial infarction **(C–E)**.

7. Correct: Cardiogenic shock (C)

The patient has all the signs and symptoms of cardiogenic shock **(C)**. The presence of signs and symptoms of volume overload such as pedal and pulmonary edema would not be expected in the other types of shock **(A–B, D–E)**.

23

8. Correct: Aortic stenosis (D)

Aortic stenosis can produce cardiogenic shock and left ventricular failure resulting in pulmonary edema **(D)**. The other causes listed are associated with right ventricular failure and would not be expected to cause pulmonary edema **(A–C, E)**.

9. Correct: Hypernatremia (C)

Leukocyte count is frequently low in sepsis, due to bone marrow suppression **(A)**. A high leukocyte count may be seen either in sepsis, due to the response to an infection, or in hypovolemia and dehydration because of the hemoconcentration that occurs **(B)**. Hyperglycemia could be seen in either septic shock or hypovolemic shock, due to cortisol release in the stress response **(D)**. Elevated serum lactic acid levels are a common finding in all forms of shock **(E)**. Hypernatremia occurs when there is severe loss of free water (dehydration), a situation that would be consistent with hypovolemic shock but not septic shock **(C)**.

10. Corect: Pleural effusion (A)

Centrilobular hemorrhagic necrosis of the liver ("nutmeg liver") and hemosiderin-laden macrophages in the lungs are manifestations of chronic passive congestion, which is seen in chronic heart failure. Of the choices, pleural effusions are most characteristic of congestive heart failure **(A)**. The other options **(B–E)** would not be expected as routine autopsy findings in congestive heart failure.

11. Correct: Increased interstitial protein (C)

The lymphatic system returns proteins back to the intravascular space that have been forced out of the arterial capillary system and into interstitial space by hydrostatic pressure. Up to 50% of serum proteins are transported via the lymphatic route each day **(C)**. For **(A–B, D–E)**, see previous information.

12. Correct: Narrowed sulci and distended gyri (C)

This patient sustained cerebral edema due to overcorrection of hypernatremia. The finding of narrowed sulci and distended gyri is the classic description of the edematous brain **(C)**. Liquefactive necrosis would be seen in acute infarction, as would middle coronary artery thrombosis; however, the clinical scenario gives no indication of stroke **(A, B)**. Passive venous congestion would be expected in strangulation or in central venous thrombosis **(D)**. Diffuse axonal injury is seen in trauma **(E)**.

3.6 Coagulation and Thrombolysis— Answers and Explanations

Easy	Medium	Hard

13. Correct: Anti-platelet factor 4 antibody (B)

The > 50% drop in the platelet count is suggestive of heparin-induced thrombocytopenia, and his prior treatment for deep venous thrombosis would likely have meant prior exposure to heparin. Heparin-induced thrombocytopenia is caused by antibodies to heparin-platelet factor-4 complexes **(B)**. Coagulation studies (PT, PTT, Factor Xa level) are unlikely to be helpful as these tests mainly assess coagulation rather than platelet function **(A, E)**. Protein C and S levels would be indicated in the workup for recurrent deep venous thrombosis, or for unprovoked deep venous thrombosis in patients under age 50 **(C, D)**.

14. Correct: t-PA increases the degradation of fibrin. (C)

t-PA converts plasminogen to plasmin, which in turn cleaves fibrin, releasing fibrin degradation products **(C)**. By this mechanism, t-PA prevents further deposition of thrombin and thus clot propagation. GpIb and GpIIb-IIIa are platelet membrane glycoproteins present on the platelet surface that promote platelet aggregation **(A, B)**. Inhibition of GpIIb-IIIa is the mechanism of action of eptifibatide (Intergrilin) **(A)**. There is no drug currently available that inhibits GpIa. Heparin, not t-PA, activates anti-thrombin III **(D)**. **(E)** is incorrect because t-PA acts by promoting fibrinolysis, not by inactivating clotting factors.

15. Correct: Normal agglutination on ristocetin cofactor assay and hypoactive agglutination on RIPA (B)

Ristocetin induces platelet aggregation in a von Willebrand factor (vWF) dependent mechanism by promoting the binding of vWF to GpIb. The ristocetin cofactor assay is an indirect measurement of von Willebrand's factor, which uses control platelets and measures the amount of ristocetin induced platelet agglutination. In von Willebrand's disease, caused by a deficiency of the vWF, platelet agglutination would be hypoactive on both the ristocetin cofactor assay and the RIPA **(D)**. Bernard-Soulier's disease is caused by a genetic deficiency of glycoprotein Ib (GpIb) on platelets. In Bernard-Soulier's disease ristocetin-induced platelet agglutination would be normal on the ristocetin cofactor assay (which uses control platelets) and hypoactive on the RIPA (which uses the patient's own, in this case defective, platelets) **(B)**. For **(A, C, E)**, see previous information.

3.7 Thrombosis, Embolism, and Infarction—Answers and Explanations

Easy	Medium	Hard

16. Correct: Fat embolism (B)

The rapid onset of respiratory failure associated with petechiae and neurologic dysfunction 1 to 3 days after a long bone fracture is classic for fat embolism syndrome (B). The presence of confusion and petechiae make venous thromboembolism less likely (C). There is no history to suggest aortic dissection, acute myocardial infarction, or disseminated intravascular coagulation (A, D, E).

17. Correct: Delaying his flight home for 48 hours (A)

This man's symptoms are characteristic of severe decompression sickness (DCS). Mild cases of DCS usually present with mild joint pains, a mottled appearance of the skin, and pruritus. In severe cases, gas embolism causes damage to the spinal cord resulting in paralysis. Air travel immediately after scuba diving increases the risk of decompression sickness because of the low atmospheric pressure at altitude (A). There is no evidence that aspirin can reduce the risk of DCS (C). For (B, D–E), see previous information.

18. Correct: Transesophageal echocardiogram (E)

The presence of multiple cerebral infarcts suggests embolic stroke. Emboli from thrombi of the left heart or the thoracic aorta would be most likely; thus, a transesophageal echocardiogram is the most appropriate diagnostic test (E). A complete blood count is unlikely to be helpful unless the cause is bacterial endocarditis, which would be much less common in this patient population than cardiac thrombus (A). Deep venous thrombosis would not cause arterial emboli in the absence of a right to left cardiac shunt, making lower extremity venous Doppler unhelpful (B). Arterial Doppler of the lower extremities, being distal, again would not be helpful (C). Finally since in-situ thrombosis is unlikely to happen in multiple vascular territories simultaneously, a cerebral angiogram would not add any additional information (D).

19. Correct: Damage to valves in the deep venous system of the legs (A)

This patient has the classic signs and symptoms of chronic venous insufficiency, including lipodermatosclerosis, varicose veins, and edema. The underlying mechanism is damage to the valves of the deep and perforating system, resulting in venous reflux and venous hypertension (A). A history of prior deep venous thrombosis is common (post-phlebitic syndrome); however, given the bilateral symptoms and gradual onset, an acute DVT in this patient is unlikely (B). Atherosclerotic disease with arterial insufficiency would not cause edema (C), and the presence of characteristic skin changes (lipodermatosclerosis) and varicosities helps distinguish venous insufficiency from lymphedema (D). Mistaking lipodermatosclerosis for cellulitis is a common diagnostic error in the evaluation of chronic venous insufficiency (E).

20. Correct: Mesenteric embolic infarction (A)

This patient presents with abdominal pain out of proportion to physical examination findings and has atrial fibrillation, a risk factor for systemic embolism. This is a classic presentation of mesenteric infarction (A). For (B–E), see previous information.

21. Correct: Renal infarction (E)

This patient has embolic renal infarction from atrial fibrillation (E). In the absence of urine leukocytes, white cell casts, or fever, pyelonephritis is unlikely (A). The absence of a stone on helical CT of the kidneys makes a kidney stone unlikely (B). Appendicitis should be considered; however, appendicitis usually presents with right lower quadrant rather than right flank pain and would not cause hematuria (C). Glomerulonephritis would not cause flank pain (D).

22. Correct: Warm compresses (C)

The management of uncomplicated superficial venous thrombophlebitis is symptomatic. Warm compresses and nonsteroidal anti-inflammatory medication are usually effective (C). In the absence of significant erythema and induration or fever, antibiotics are unnecessary (B). Topical steroids would be indicated for atopic dermatitis but would not help in this case (D). There is no evidence of abscess or septic thrombophlebitis; thus, no indication for incision and drainage (E). Anticoagulation is unnecessary (A).

23. Correct: A lung (E)

The tissue description is that of coagulative necrosis, with preservation of architecture but loss of basophilia. The abundant extravasated red blood cells indicate a red infarct, which most commonly occur in the liver and lungs, organs with dual blood supplies (E). Organs with single blood supplies, such as the heart, kidney, and spleen, have white infarcts unless there has been reperfusion (A–C). The brain can have red infarcts with venous lesions; however, liquefactive and not coagulative necrosis is most common (D).

24. Correct: Disseminated intravascular coagulation (D)

The patient in this scenario dies of an acute catastrophic cardiovascular/pulmonary event (amniotic fluid embolism). Left ventricular hypertrophy is an adaptation to chronic stress (A). (B, E) would be expected if the patient had died of pulmonary embolism; however, pulmonary edema is rare in pulmonary embolism and common in amniotic fluid

25

embolism. Acute myocardial infarction from a ruptured atherosclerotic plaque (**C**) would be extremely rare in a 22-year-old female. Common pathologic findings in amniotic fluid embolism include fetal squamous cells and hair in the arterioles, disseminated intravascular coagulation, pulmonary edema, and diffuse alveolar damage (**D**).

25. Correct: Air embolism (B)

The history of sudden onset of respiratory failure with central venous catheter placement or removal in the upright position is highly suggestive of an air embolism (**B**). The EKG findings of tachycardia and right axis deviation are indicative of right ventricular overload. Pulmonary embolism could present in a similar fashion; however, again, the history of puncture of a large central vein makes air embolism more likely (**A**). For (**C–E**), see previous information.

26. Correct: Cholesterol deposition in arterioles of the dermis (E)

The history of recent angiography in the setting of atherosclerotic disease in the setting of acute kidney injury and livedo reticularis is highly suggestive of cholesterol embolization (**E**). "Blue toe syndrome" is a less common, but classic finding in cholesterol embolization. (**A, B**) describe findings associated with wound healing and scar tissue formation, respectively. Foreign body granulomas are uncommon and inconsistent with the clinical presentation; however, occasionally macrophage granulomas can be seen in cholesterol embolism but would be expected in the arteriole, not the dermis (**C**). (**D**) describes characteristic findings in disseminated intravascular coagulation.

27. Correct: A large area of poorly contracting left ventricular muscle (B)

This patient has developed a ventricular mural thrombus, which most commonly develops after a myocardial infarction. The damaged ventricular wall is highly thrombogenic, and poor contractility of the damaged myocardium creates turbulence that predisposes to thrombus formation. If the infarct results in ventricular wall aneurysm, the risk of thrombus formation is increased further. The infarct should be visible on echocardiogram as an akinetic portion of the ventricular wall (**B**). Thrombi that form as a result of atrial fibrillation are usually visualized in the atria or atrial appendage (**A**). (**C**) describes findings typical of pulmonary embolism. Neither (**D**) nor (**E**) are associated with left ventricular thrombus in the absence of other pathology.

3.8 Hereditary Thrombophilia and Coagulopathy— Answers and Explanations

| Easy | Medium | Hard |

28. Correct: Proteins C and S activity (D)

Proteins C and S are potent inhibitors of several clotting factors. Inherited deficiency of either will lead to a hypercoagulable state. However, Proteins C and S and antithrombin III levels are often low in the setting of acute VTE (venous thromboembolism) due to consumption by the clotting process. Furthermore, both proteins C and S are vitamin K dependent and will be low in the setting of Coumadin therapy (**D**). The remainder of the laboratory studies (**A–C, E**) are all appropriate in the initial workup for possible thrombophilia.

29. Correct: Increased renal tubular sodium absorption (E)

The increase in renal tubular sodium reabsorption (**E**) seen in hypovolemia is due to activation of the renin-angiotensin-aldosterone system, not vasopressin secretion. Vasopressin (antidiuretic hormone) plays a role both in vascular tone and blood pressure control and in water homeostasis. Vasopressin, as its name implies, has vasoconstrictive effects (**C**), which raises blood pressure (**A**) and promotes hemostasis. It also increases water absorption on the distal nephron and thus will cause hyponatremia if its secretion is uncoupled from regulation by plasma osmolality, as is the case in severe hypovolemia (**D**). It also activates platelets (**B**).

30. Correct: Acute stroke of the left middle cerebral artery (D)

A middle cerebral artery (MCA) stroke would be expected to cause neurologic deficits of the contralateral arm, leg, and face (**D**). The presence of aphasia in this case indicates damage of the left posterior inferior frontal gyrus (Broca's area). Anterior cerebral artery (ACA) strokes are less common and would produce contralateral hemiparesis but would not produce hemifacial weakness (**A, B**). The classic finding in posterior cerebral artery (PCA) stroke is homonymous hemianopsia, with larger PCA strokes producing contralateral hemiparesis and hemisensory loss (**E, F**).

31. Correct: Elevated homocysteine levels (E)

Elevated homocysteine levels suggest a diagnosis of hyperhomocysteinemia (E). Inherited deficiency of cystathione β-synthetase or methylene-tetrahydrofolate reductase can cause a familial hypercoagulable state characterized by venous and arterial thrombosis and elevated serum homocysteine levels. Prolongation of aPTT can be seen in antiphospholipid antibody syndromes (APS) with Lupus Anticoagulant (A). Thrombocytopenia is a common manifestation of APS (C). Despite low platelet counts, these patients are prone to thrombosis rather than bleeding. A positive antinuclear antibody is suggestive of systemic lupus, a common cause of secondary APS (D). VDRL (Venereal Disease Research Laboratory) antigen consists of cardiolipin-cholesterol-lecithin mixtures that may produce a false positive syphilis test in patients with APS who have anticardiolipin antibodies (B).

Chapter 4

Diseases of the Immune System

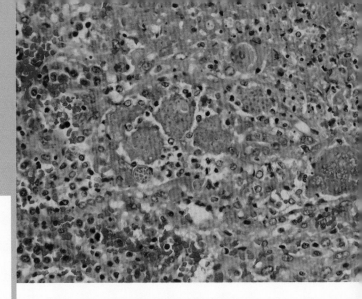

LEARNING OBJECTIVES

4.1 General Concepts and Hypersensitivity Reactions

▶ List the cells of the innate and adaptive immune systems

▶ List locations where a T cell with a γ-δ subunit TCR is located

▶ Describe the mechanism of type 1 hypersensitivity reactions

▶ Describe the mechanism of type 2 hypersensitivity reactions; list some common examples

▶ Given the clinical scenario, identify type 3 hypersensitivity reaction

▶ Given the clinical scenario, identify type 4 hypersensitivity reaction

4.2 Autoimmune Diseases

▶ Diagnose systemic lupus erythematosus

▶ Diagnose drug-induced lupus

▶ Diagnose rheumatoid arthritis

▶ Recognize extra-articular manifestations of rheumatoid arthritis

▶ List the risk factors for rheumatoid arthritis

▶ Recognize common complications of systemic lupus

▶ Identify polymyalgia rheumatica and its complications

▶ Identify systemic sclerosis

▶ Given the clinical scenario, diagnose SLE; describe the mechanism by which SLE damages the kidney

▶ Given the clinical scenario, diagnose Sjögren's syndrome

▶ List the autoantibodies associated with Sjögren's syndrome

▶ Given the clinical scenario, diagnose myasthenia gravis

▶ Describe the pathophysiologic mechanism of myasthenia gravis

▶ Given the clinical scenario, diagnose amyloidosis

4.3 Immunodeficiencies

▶ Describe the mechanism of Chediak-Higashi syndrome

▶ Identify chronic granulomatous disease

▶ Describe the mechanism of hereditary angioedema

▶ Recognize acute retroviral syndrome

▶ Recognize community-acquired pneumonia in patients with AIDS

▶ Describe the features of opportunistic lung infections in patients with HIV/AIDS

▶ Given the clinical scenario, diagnose HIV-associated Kaposi sarcoma; describe causative and epidemiologic features of Kaposi sarcoma

▶ Given the clinical scenario, diagnose hyper-IgM syndrome

▶ Identify severe combined immunodeficiency

▶ Identify X-linked agammaglobulinemia

▶ Identify selective IgA deficiency

▶ List the common causes of CNS infection in HIV/AIDS; given the clinical scenario and laboratory test results, diagnose cryptococcal meningitis

▶ List the common medications used to prevent opportunistic infections in AIDS

▶ Describe the mechanism of Wiskott-Aldrich syndrome.

▶ Describe the mechanism of X-linked lymphoproliferative syndrome

4.1 General Concepts and Hypersensitivity Reactions—Questions

Easy	Medium	Hard

1. A graduate student in an immunology lab is studying a certain cell that plays a role in adaptive immunity. Of the following, which cell type might the student be studying?

A. Macrophage

B. Neutrophil

C. Eosinophil

D. Natural killer cell

E. Lymphocyte

N/A

2. A graduate student has developed a protein that binds to CD3 and blocks its interaction with TCR, which is composed of γ and δ subunits. Of the following, which organ is the student studying?

A. Brain

B. Heart

C. Intestine

D. Liver

E. Kidney

Respiratory

3. A 32-year-old male with a known severe peanut allergy is inadvertently exposed to peanuts by eating a homemade cookie. Within minutes of exposure he develops a widespread rash and difficulty breathing, which resolve with a self-administered epinephrine injection. Which of the following statements is most characteristic regarding this type of allergic reaction?

A. The immediate reaction is triggered by IgM bound to antigen.

B. The immediate allergic reaction is triggered by activation of eosinophils.

C. This type of allergic reaction is caused by excessive a T_H2 response.

D. Prostaglandins do not play a role in this type of reaction.

E. Previous exposure to the antigen is not required for this type of reaction.

Immune

4. A 42-year-old woman presents to her primary care physician complaining of itching and watery eyes, runny nose, and frequent sneezing. She denies fever or cough. She experiences similar symptoms every year in the spring. Which of the following is responsible for her symptoms?

A. Binding of antigen to IgE on mast cell surfaces

B. Recognition of antigen associated with MHC-1

C. Binding of polysaccharide to membrane-bound lectin receptors

D. Destruction of cells coated with IgM

E. Inflammation due to deposition of antigen-antibody complex

Immune

5. A blood type O+ infant is delivered to a multiparous blood type O- mother without prenatal care. The infant is born with severe anemia, jaundice, and severe edema. What is the underlying mechanism of this disease?

A. Crosslinking of IgE on mast cell surfaces

B. IgG binding to cell surfaces

C. Deposition of antigen antibody complexes in the fetal tissue

D. T-cell mediated cytotoxicity

E. Antibody mediated activation of apoptosis

Immune

6. A 32-year-old man hiking in Guatemala is bitten by a rattlesnake. He is treated with equine antivenin. He recovers; however, 2 weeks afterward, he develops rash, fever, and polyarthralgia. Laboratory evaluation reveals a leukocyte count of 3200/μL, a hemoglobin concentration of 16.0 g/dL, a platelet count of 95,000/μL, and a serum creatinine of 1.8 mg/dL. What is the most likely diagnosis?

A. Chikungunya fever

B. Lyme disease

C. Serum sickness

D. Malaria

E. Autoimmune hemolytic anemia

Immune

7. A 32-year-old female immigrant is hired for a food service job at the local cafeteria. As part of her pre-hire physical examination she is given a purified protein derivative (PPD) skin test. She returns to the occupational health clinic 48 hours later with a denuded 22 mm bulla and induration and erythema involving the majority of the volar surface of her right arm. A wound culture is performed; however, there is no growth at 48 hours. A biopsy of the skin lesion would most likely show which of the following?

A. Neutrophil predominant infiltrate

B. Perivascular accumulation of lymphocytes and mononuclear cells

C. Granulomatous inflammation

D. Immune complex deposition in the soft tissue

E. Abundant eosinophils

Immune, dermatologic, infectious disease

8. A 10 year-old girl is stung by a bee while with her family at a school picnic. About 10 minutes later, she becomes nauseated and vomits twice, and shortly thereafter her parents notice that her face begins to swell and she begins to wheeze. Her parents rush her to the hospital, where treatment is administered. Which of the following statements best describes her condition?

A. The reaction is mediated by preformed IgG antibodies.

B. She is having a type II hypersensitivity reaction.

C. The main cellular mediator is macrophages.

D. The most likely cause of her symptoms is foreign body ingestion.

E. A similar reaction can occur in people given penicillin.

Lymphoid

9. Given the previous clinical scenario, of the following, what is the diagnosis?

A. A type I hypersensitivity reaction

B. A type II hypersensitivity reaction

C. A type IIIa hypersensitivity reaction

D. A type IIIb hypersensitivity reaction

E. A type IV hypersensitivity reaction

Lymphoid

10. A 23-year-old male is hit by a bullet during a drive-by shooting at a local store. He is rushed to the emergency room and is determined to have a hemothorax. A chest tube is placed and intravenous fluids and blood are given. Immediately after the transfusion, he develops a temperature of 100.3°F and chills. Shortly thereafter, he develops a blood pressure of 80/50 mm Hg. Of the following, which is most likely occurring?

A. A type I hypersensitivity reaction

B. A type II hypersensitivity reaction

C. A type IIIa hypersensitivity reaction

D. A type IIIb hypersensitivity reaction

E. A type IV hypersensitivity reaction

Lymphoid

11. Given the previous clinical scenario, of the following, which antibody type is responsible for his reaction?

A. IgA

B. IgD

C. IgE

D. IgG

E. IgM

Heme

12. A 47-year-old male with a history of Zollinger-Ellinson's syndrome presents to the emergency room vomiting bright red blood. He has twice before presented to the emergency room vomiting blood. On arrival, a complete blood cell count is performed, revealing a hemoglobin of 5.6 g/dL. A decision to transfuse is made, and he receives 4 units of blood. His blood type is O–. His bleeding is brought under control and he is admitted to the hospital. He is scheduled for surgery the next day. Prior to surgery, a complete blood cell count reveals a hemoglobin of 6.2 g/dL. Of the following, which best explains his low hemoglobin prior to surgery?

A. Bleeding from a second ulcer

B. Insufficient number of units of blood transfused

C. An immediate hemolytic transfusion reaction

D. A delayed hemolytic transfusion reaction

E. Laboratory error

Heme

13. Given the previous clinical scenario, of the following, which antibody type is responsible for the reaction?

A. IgA

B. IgD

C. IgE

D. IgG

E. IgM

Heme

4.2 Autoimmune Diseases— Questions

| Easy | Medium | Hard |

14. A 26-year-old Hispanic female presents to her primary care physician complaining of 2 months of fatigue. She has persistent arthralgias of the distal and proximal interphalangeal joints of both hands and reports that when the weather turns cold her hands frequently change colors. Her physical examination is normal and there is no tenderness or deformity of the joints of the hands. A complete blood count is normal and her antinuclear antibody titer is elevated at 1:90. Which of the following additional tests would confirm the diagnosis of lupus erythematosus?

A. Positive SS-A

B. Positive SS-B

C. Positive anti-cyclic citrullinated peptide (CCP-IgG)

D. Positive rheumatoid factor

E. Positive anti-Smith

Immune, musculoskeletal

15. A 36-year-old African-American with stage 2 hypertension is started on hydralazine for better blood pressure control. Four months after starting the medications, he develops recurring low-grade fevers and pains in the joints of both hands. Examination of both hands is normal; however, there is a slight erythematous dermatitis over both cheeks. Of the following, which test is most likely to be abnormal?

A. Anti-Smith antibody

B. Anti–double-stranded DNA antibody

C. Serum uric acid level

D. Antinuclear antibody (ANA)

E. Low serum complement levels

Immune, musculoskeletal, dermatologic

16. A 55-year-old white female with stable hypertension presents to her primary care physician complaining of fatigue and joint pain. The symptoms started 6 months ago. She reports pain in the metacarpophalangeal (MCP) joints, the proximal interphalangeal (PIP) joints, and both wrists, with the pain worse in the morning, associated with stiffness, and improving somewhat throughout the day. On examination there is tenderness and mild swelling of the MCP joints, the PIP joints, and the wrists, but there is no tenderness or deformity of the distal interphalangeal (DIP) joints. What is the most likely diagnosis?

A. Osteoarthritis

B. Rheumatoid arthritis

C. Lyme disease

D. Systemic lupus

E. Gout

Immune, musculoskeletal

17. Given the patient's most likely diagnosis, of the following tests, which, if positive, would confirm the diagnosis?

A. Rheumatoid factor (RF)

B. Anti-cyclic citrulinated peptide (CCP IgG)

C. *Borrellia* titers

D. Anti–double-stranded DNA (dsDNA)

E. Serum uric acid levels

Immune, musculoskeletal

18. A 45-year-old female immigrant presents with progressive shortness of breath and fatigue that have developed over the past 3 weeks. She also has sores on both legs. She has a long-standing history of joint pain but has not received medical attention for this problem. Her temperature is 98.6°F (37°C), pulse 78 bpm, blood pressure 132/64 mm Hg, respirations 20/min, and oxygen saturation 92% on room air. On examination she has deep cutaneous ulcers around the lateral malleoli of both ankles. Her heart sounds are normal, and there are faint crackles in both lung bases. The abdomen is not tender and the spleen is enlarged. A plain chest radiograph shows bibasilar ground glass opacities. The phalanges demonstrate flexion of the proximal and hyperextension of the distal interphalangeal joints and ulnar deviation. There are several nontender, moveable nodules on the extensor surface of the elbow. What is the most likely diagnosis?

A. HLA-B27-positive spondyloarthropathy

B. ANCA positive vasculitis

C. Psoriatic arthritis

D. Felty's syndrome

E. Systemic lupus erythematosus

Immune, musculoskeletal, dermatologic, vascular

19. In the previous clinical scenario, of the following, what is a risk factor for developing this disease?

A. Multiparity

B. Male sex

C. Breast feeding

D. Haplotype HLA-B27

E. Cigarette smoking

Immune, musculoskeletal, dermatologic, vascular

20. A 40-year-old woman with long-standing lupus erythematosus presents complaining of chest pain. She reports that the pain started 8 hours prior to her arrival, is sharp, is worse with deep breaths and cough, and is improved by sitting up and leaning forward. Her temperature is 100.3°F (37.9°C), pulse 108/min, BP 120/75 mm Hg, respirations 20/min, and oxygen saturation 98% on room air. She looks uncomfortable. On examination her lungs are clear, and her heart rate is regular with no murmurs. A chest radiograph is normal. Her 12-lead ECG shows diffuse ST elevation in all leads. What is the most likely diagnosis?

A. Acute myocardial infarction

B. Pulmonary embolism

C. Aortic dissection

D. Pericarditis

E. Libman-Sacks endocarditis

Immune, cardiovascular

21. A 40-year-old woman is evaluated for eye discomfort. She reports a foreign body sensation in both eyes for the past 3 weeks. Fluorescein examination reveals bilateral corneal ulcers. She has mild cervical lymphadenopathy and bilateral parotid enlargement on examination. Her rheumatoid factor is positive at 75 units/mL. What is the most likely diagnosis?

A. Sjögren's syndrome

B. Rheumatoid arthritis

C. Systemic sclerosis

D. Polymyositis

E. Systemic lupus erythematosus

Immune

22. A 75-year-old male presents complaining of stiffness. He reports a 4-week history of stiffness and pain in both shoulders causing difficulty swinging a golf club. He also has neck stiffness and pain and significant fatigue. The stiffness in his shoulders is worse in the mornings and lasts for at least an hour. The small joints of his hands are not affected. He has lost 10 lbs. over the past month and reports frequent low-grade fevers. On examination his temperature is 98.8°F (37.1°C), pulse 85/min, and blood pressure 135/85 mm Hg. There is moderate tenderness of the shoulder girdle with decreased range of motion with active abduction. The remainder of his musculoskeletal examination is normal. Complete blood count shows a normal leukocyte count and a normochromic normocytic anemia. His rheumatoid factor is negative. His erythrocyte sedimentation rate (ESR) is 109 mm/hr, and his C-reactive protein is 2.3 mg/dL. Of the following, which complication is this patient at risk for?

A. Erosive arthritis

B. Blindness

C. Interstitial lung disease

D. Renal failure

E. Pericarditis

Immune, musculoskeletal

23. A 38-year-old woman presents to her primary care physician complaining of joint pain and fatigue. She reports progressive difficulty over the past two months in grasping objects. Exposure to cold temperatures frequently causes paresthesias and pallor in the fingers, followed by cyanosis, then erythema with rewarming. On examination her vital signs are normal. The heart and lung sounds are normal. There is puffy edema of the fingers with several ulcers of the fingertips and thickening of the skin of both hands. Antinuclear antibody (ANA) is positive. Of the following, what is the most likely diagnosis?

A. Rheumatoid arthritis

B. Systemic lupus erythematosus

C. Polymyositis

D. Subacute endocarditis

E. Systemic sclerosis

Immune, musculoskeletal

24. A 55-year-old woman presents with painless enlargement of the parotid glands, which began 6 months earlier. On examination, ocular dryness and cervical lymphadenopathy are present. Biopsy of the parotid gland is likely to show which of the following?

A. Lymphocytic and plasma cell infiltrate with ductal epithelial hyperplasia

B. Well-demarcated tumor consisting of a mixture of epithelial and myoepithelial cells dispersed within loose myxoid tissue

C. Inflammation with neutrophil predominance and necrosis of salivary ducts

D. Coagulative necrosis of acini with squamous metaplasia of ducts

E. Sheets of small B-cells with infiltration and distortion of epithelial structures and scattered centroblast-like cells

Immune

25. A 34-year-old female is brought to the emergency room by EMS after a seizure during dinner. Her past medical history includes arthritis, which has developed in the last few years. On a recent visit to her family physician for complaints of fatigue, she was found to have a serum leukocyte count of 3.3×10^9/L and a urine dipstick positive for protein, but negative for leukocyte esterase and glucose. Of the following, which is the most likely mechanism for the protein in her urine?

A. An undiagnosed neoplasm

B. A urinary tract infection

C. Antibodies directed against the basement membrane

D. Deposition of antigen-antibody complexes in the glomeruli

E. Accumulation of advanced glycosylation end-products in the glomerulus

Immune

26. A 34-year-old female is evaluated by her family physician for moderate proteinuria, found incidentally on a urinalysis performed to evaluate for a urinary tract infection. A comprehensive metabolic panel shows a serum creatinine of 1.6 mg/dL. A kidney biopsy is performed, revealing an increase in the mesangial matrix. Of the following, which serologic test would be most helpful in confirming her diagnosis?

A. Anti-dsDNA antibodies

B. Anti-SSB antibodies

C. Anti-SSA antibodies

D. Anti-centromere antibodies

E. Anti-scl70 antibodies

Immune

27. A 56-year-old female presents to her family physician. She complains that over the past year she has noticed that her mouth has been much drier, and that she has been using more eyedrops than previously. She has also noticed decreased mobility of the joints in her fingers, a situation which is worse in the morning but improves toward the evening. Of the following, what is the most likely diagnosis?

A. Osteoarthritis

B. Psoriatic arthritis

C. Lyme disease

D. Sjögren's syndrome

E. Osteomyelitis

Immune

28. Given the previous clinical scenario, of the following, what is serologic testing most likely to reveal?

A. Anti-dsDNA

B. Anti-Smith

C. Anti-histone

D. Anti-SSA

E. Anti-centromere

Immune

29. Given the previous clinical scenario, of the following, histologic examination of her submandibular gland would most likely reveal?

A. Granulomas

B. Neutrophilic infiltrate

C. Eosinophilic infiltrate

D. Lymphocytic infiltrate

E. Fibrosis and extensive calcification

Immune

30. A 52-year-old female presents to her internist with neck swelling. On examination there is marked enlargement of the submandibular gland bilaterally. The mucous membranes of the oropharynx are dry, and a small corneal ulceration is present on the right. Given her most likely diagnosis, which of the following complications is she most at risk for?

A. MALToma

B. Thymoma

C. Follicular lymphoma

D. Mantle cell lymphoma

E. Hodgkin's lymphoma

Immune

31. A 38-year-old female presents to the emergency room. She has recently been feeling weak and fatigued, unable to work out at the gym as she normally has in the past. Her trip to the emergency room is because she developed double vision today. Physical examination reveals ptosis. A CT scan of her body reveals a mass in the upper portion of the mediastinum. Of the following, what is the most likely diagnosis?

A. Multiple sclerosis

B. Amyotrophic lateral sclerosis

C. Early onset Parkinson's disease

D. Myasthenia gravis

E. Systemic lupus erythematosus

Immune

32. Given the previous clinical scenario, of the following, what is the most likely mechanism for her symptoms?

A. Antibodies against the acetylcholine receptor

B. Immune-mediated destruction of oligodendroglial cells

C. Elevated T3 hormone concentrations

D. Ischemic injury of the precentral gyrus bilaterally

E. A mass at the optic chiasma

Immune

33. A 73-year-old man with stable hypertension presents to his primary care physician complaining of bruising around the eyes, which occurred after blowing up balloons for his granddaughter's birthday party. He reports no pain and has no other complaints. On examination there are bilateral periorbital purpurae but no other facial trauma. Scalloping of the borders of the tongue caused by the patient's teeth is noted. The lungs are clear, and heart sounds are normal; however, the point of maximal impulse is laterally displaced. Moderate hepatomegaly is noted. What is the most likely diagnosis?

A. T-cell lymphoma

B. Thrombotic thrombocytopenic purpura

C. Leukoclastic vasculitis

D. AL amyloidosis

E. Idiopathic thrombocytopenic purpura

N/A

4.3 Immunodeficiencies— Questions

Easy	Medium	Hard

34. An 18-month-old boy is hospitalized with lobar pneumonia. He has had three ear infections in the past four months. At ages 12 and 14 months he was treated for *Staphylococcus aureus* cellulitis and abscess. He is fair-skinned with silvery-white hair and blue eyes. Angular cheilosis and oral ulcers are present on examination. A complete blood count is remarkable for a leukocyte count of 3.7×10^9/L and a hemoglobin of 8.9 mg/dL. His bleeding time is prolonged. Bone marrow biopsy shows giant azurophilic granules in the myeloid cells. What is the underlying defect?

A. Fusosyl transferase deficiency

B. Phagocyte NADPH oxidase deficiency

C. Myeloperoxidase deficiency

D. Impaired phagosome-lysosome fusion

E. Mutation in the γ-chain subunit of cytokine receptors

Immune

35. A 16-month-old male is admitted with fever and difficulty breathing. He has a history of recurrent *Staphylococcus aureus* skin abscesses and is being treated for pulmonary Aspergillosis. On arrival his temperature is 100.8°F (38.2°C), pulse 118/min, and blood pressure 90/55 mmHg. His weight is below the 10th percentile for age. On examination he has ronchi in both lung fields. There are multiple skin lesions of the face and neck. A plain chest radiograph reveals a small pulmonary abscess in the right middle lobe and left lower lobe pneumonia as well as hilar adenopathy. His leukocyte count is 14.2×10^9/L. Culture of the tracheal aspirate grows out *Burkholderia cepacia*. Biopsy of one of the skin lesions shows aggregates of epithelioid macrophages surrounded by lymphocytes. What additional test results would be expected in this patient?

A. Low gammaglobulin levels

B. Abnormal sweat chloride test

C. Very low IgA levels

D. Abnormal nitroblue tetrazolium test

E. Positive antinuclear antibodies (ANA)

Immune

36. Given the previous clinical scenario, what is the primary defect causing the recurrent infections?

A. Fusosyl transferase deficiency

B. Phagocyte NADPH oxidase deficiency

C. Myeloperoxidase deficiency

D. Impaired phagosome-lysosome fusion

E. Mutation in the γ-chain subunit of cytokine receptors

Immune

37. A 12-year-old girl presents with swelling of the face and lips. The symptoms started gradually 4 hours ago and were preceded by fatigue, nausea, and flu-like symptoms. She has had 3 prior episodes with similar symptoms. Her vital signs are normal. On examination she has diffuse edema of the face and lips. Lungs are clear, without stridor or wheezing, and examination of the skin is normal. Her C1-INH activity is undetectable. Which of the following additional historical or examination findings would be consistent with her illness?

A. Recurrent urticaria

B. Recurrent abdominal pain

C. Elevated serum tryptase

D. Wheezing

E. Resolution of symptoms with epinephrine and glucocorticoids

Immune, pulmonary

38. A 21-year-old male presents to the college health clinic complaining of malaise, fatigue, and sore throat. He denies cough or shortness of breath. The symptoms started abruptly 2 weeks ago and are accompanied by low-grade fever, arthralgia, diarrhea, and a 10 lb. weight loss. His vaccinations are up to date. Temperature is 100.3°F (37.9°C), heart rate is 98/min, and blood pressure is 123/89 mm Hg. On examination there is cervical and axillary lymphadenopathy, pharyngeal erythema without exudates or tonsillar enlargement, and a diffuse maculopapular rash on the face, thorax, and extremities. His heart and lung sounds are normal. A rapid strep test, monospot test, CMV and Lyme titers, and antinuclear antibodies are negative. What test should be ordered next?

A. Anti CCP-IgG

B. Anti-Smith

C. Anti-dsDNA

D. Peripheral blood smear

E. HIV antibodies and viral load

Immune, infectious diseases

39. A 55-year-old man with long-standing HIV disease, recently nonadherent to his antiretroviral therapy, presents complaining of persistent cough. He denies any recent travel or hospitalization. His temperature is 100.4°F (38.0°C), pulse is 106/min, blood pressure is 120/76 mm Hg, and room air oxygen saturation is 93%. On examination he has crackles over the right lower lung field, and a plain chest radiograph shows consolidation of the right lower lobe. Of the following, what is the most likely causative agent?

A. *Pneumocystis jirovecii*

B. *Histoplasma capsulatum*

C. *Streptococcus pneumoniae*

D. *Cryptococcus neoformans*

E. *Mycobacterium tuberculosis*

Immune, infectious diseases, pulmonary

40. A 38-year-old homeless HIV-positive man presents with cough and shortness of breath. His temperature is 101.0°F (38.3°C), pulse is 110/min, blood pressure is 106/60 mm Hg, and room air oxygen saturation is 88%. On examination he is cachectic. He has white pharyngeal exudates. He is tachycardic without murmur. There are fine crackles in both lung fields. His breathing is labored. A plain chest radiograph shows diffuse bilateral interstitial infiltrates. Lactate dehydrogenase level is 530 IU, and the CD 4 count is 173 cells/μL. Of the following, what is the most likely causative agent?

A. *Pneumocystis jirovecii*

B. *Histoplasma capsulatum*

C. *Streptococcus pneumoniae*

D. *Cryptococcus neoformans*

E. *Mycobacterium avium complex*

Immune, infectious diseases, pulmonary

41. A 45-year-old man with known HIV and no prior HAART treatment presents with a rash. His temperature is 99.8°F (37.6°C), pulse is 89/min, and blood pressure is 132/88 mm Hg. Examination of his oropharynx reveals white exudates on the palate and several purple nodular lesions of the gingival mucosa. His lungs are clear, and no murmurs are present. He has several nontender, nonulcerated raised purple lesions on both arms and the anterior chest wall. Biopsy of one of the skin lesions shows whorls of spindle-shaped cells with leukocytic infiltrate and neovascularization. Which of the following is true regarding this skin disease?

A. It is rapidly progressive and fatal if untreated.

B. It is caused by a fastidious gram-negative bacillus.

C. It is uncommon in heterosexual men with HIV.

D. Antibiotic prophylaxis can prevent this disease.

E. Extracutaneous manifestations of this illness are rare.

Immune, dermatologic

42. A 6-year-old boy is brought to his pediatrician with a cough, which started 3 weeks earlier. He has a history of recurrent *Staphylococcus aureus* skin infections. His temperature is 101.4°F, pulse is 110/min, blood pressure is 88/54 mm Hg, oxygen saturation is 89% on room air. On examination he has bilateral crackles. A plain chest radiograph shows bilateral reticulonodular infiltrates. Sputum silver stain reveals *Pneumocystis jirovecii*. He has a younger brother who was also diagnosed with *Pneumocystis* pneumonia. HIV testing is negative; however, serum levels of IgA, IgG, and IgE are low and serum IgM levels are elevated. His condition is a result of which underlying defect?

A. Defective development of the third and fourth pharyngeal pouches

B. Defective CD 40 ligand

C. Mutation in the cytokine receptor common γ-chain

D. Adenosine deaminase deficiency

E. Mutation in Jak3

43. A 7-month-old boy is brought to his pediatrician for a cough, which started 1 week ago. He has also been experiencing diarrhea for the past 3 weeks. His temperature is 99.2°F (37.3°C), pulse is 112/min, blood pressure is 88/48 mm Hg, and room air saturation is 88%. His weight is less than the 10th percentile for age. He is nondysmorphic. There are white plaques on the tongue and oropharynx. No murmur is heard. Bilateral crackles are present on auscultation. Complete blood count shows normal hemoglobin and platelet counts. Serum chemistry is normal. The leukocyte count is 5400 cells/μL, 88% granulocytes and 12% lymphocytes. A plain chest radiograph shows ground-glass infiltrates, and a bronchoalveolar lavage was positive for *Pneumocystis jirovecii*. The cytomegalovirus DNA PCR is positive, and HIV viral load is negative. Serum levels of IgG, IgM, IgA, and IgE are low, and flow cytometry reveals an extremely low T-cell count with a relatively normal B-cell count. Of the following, what is the most likely diagnosis?

A. X-linked agammaglobulinemia

B. Transient hypogammaglobulinemia of the newborn

C. DiGeorge's syndrome

D. Common variable immunodeficiency

E. Severe combined immunodeficiency

44. A 6-month-old boy is brought to his pediatrician for pneumonia. He was treated 2 weeks ago for severe otitis media. On examination, his tonsils and adenoids are absent. Heart sounds are normal, and there are crackles in the left lower lung field. Serum levels of IgG, IgA, and IgM are low, and B-lymphocytes are undetectable. What is the underlying defect responsible for this patient's recurrent infections?

A. Impaired B-cell maturation

B. Impaired cytokine receptor signaling

C. Failure of development of the third and fourth pharyngeal pouches

D. Disruption of the CD40-CD40 ligand interaction

E. Complement deficiency

45. A 33-year-old man is evaluated for recurrent sinusitis. He has had episodes of bacterial sinusitis occurring at least four times a year for the past 3 years. Complete blood count is normal, as is a total hemolytic complement panel (CH50). Serum IgG, IgM, and IgE levels are normal; however, serum IgA levels are undetectable. Which of the following complications is this patient at least risk for?

A. Transfusion reaction

B. Pneumonia

C. Parasitic gastrointestinal infection

D. Crohn's disease

E. Lymphoid malignancy

46. A 32-year-old HIV-positive man presents with fever, headache, and neck stiffness. His temperature is 101.1°F (38.4°C), pulse is 102/min, and blood pressure is 102/58 mm Hg. On examination he appears malnourished. There is oral candidiasis on exam. His heart and lungs are normal to auscultation. Multiple umbilicated papular lesions are noted on the skin. Neurologic examination reveals lethargy and meningismus, but no focal deficits. A CT of the head is preformed and is unremarkable. The opening pressure on lumbar puncture is slightly elevated at 28 cm H$_2$O and fluid analysis reveals a CSF leukocyte count of 38 cells/μL with a mononuclear predominance, as well as elevated protein and low CSF glucose. What is the most likely causative organism of this man's illness?

A. *Toxoplasma gondii*

B. *Mycobacterium tuberculosis*

C. *Streptococcus pneumoniae*

D. *Cryptococcus neoformans*

E. *Molluscum contagiosum*

47. A 57-year-old female immigrant with HIV/AIDS and CD4 count of 53 cells/μL presents with a headache, fever, and confusion. A CT of the head performed on arrival shows multiple enhancing lesions of the frontal and parietal lobe. Which of the following prophylactic treatments could have prevented this complication?

A. Trimethoprim-sulfamethoxazole

B. Itraconazole

C. Fluconazole

D. Azithromycin

E. Acyclovir

Immune, nervous

48. An 8-month-old male is brought to his pediatrician for cough and fever. Past medical history is significant for 3 episodes of otitis media since age 6 months. His brother died at age 11 months of pneumonia. His temperature is 102.4°F (39.1°C), pulse is 120/min, and blood pressure is 88/48 mm Hg. The auscultation of the heart is normal. There are crackles in both lung fields. He has a petechial rash on both lower extremities and a scaly erythematous dermatitis of the extensor surfaces of the arms and legs. His platelet count is 19,000/μL. His serum IgG and IgA levels are normal; however, his IgM levels are very low. What is the underlying cause of this patient's illness?

A. Shiga toxin

B. IgG anti-glycoprotein IIb/IIIa complex

C. Abnormal linking of membrane receptors to cytoskeletal elements

D. Deposition of misfolded fibrillar proteins

E. Mutated cytokine receptor

Immune, pulmonary, dermatologic, hematologic

49. A 33-year-old man develops severe pharyngitis for which he seeks evaluation by his primary care provider. A rapid strep test is negative. He has marked splenomegaly on exam and is noted to be febrile. His monospot test is positive. He dies 3 days later. His brother died at age 18 of Epstein-Barr virus. What is the underlying defect causing this man's disease?

A. Mutation in the gene encoding WASP protein

B. Defect in the receptor for the B-cell activating cytokine

C. Loss of function mutation in CD40

D. Mutation in the gene for SLAM-associated protein

E. Adenosine deaminase deficiency

Immune

4.4 General Concepts and Hypersensitivity Reactions— Answers and Explanations

Easy	Medium	Hard

1. Correct: Lymphocyte (E)

The lymphocyte is a cell type found in adaptive (also referred to as specific, or acquired) immunity (**E**), whereas the other cell types listed play a role in innate (also referred to as native or natural) immunity (**A-D**).

2. Correct: Intestine (C)

The TCR (T-cell receptor) binds to the MHC (major histocompatibility complex) on antigen-presenting cells, with CD4 in helper T cells and CD8 in cytotoxic T cells participating. TCR is normally composed of an α and a β subunit, however, T cells with a TCR composed of a γ and δ subunit are found associated with mucosal surfaces (**C**). For (**A-B, D-E**), see previous information.

3. Correct: This type of allergic reaction is caused by excessive T_H2 response (C)

This patient is experiencing an anaphylactic reaction, a classic type I (immediate) hypersensitivity reaction. Type I hypersensitivity reactions are triggered by crosslinking of membrane-bound IgE on mast cells (**A, B**). Previous antigen exposure is required for the production of this antigen-specific IgE (**E**). This previous exposure results in T_H2 cells secreting IL-4 and IL-5, which promotes B-cell class switching to produce the IgE (**C**). These reactions follow a characteristic pattern of initial reaction (caused by mast cell activation and release of mediators, including prostaglandins) followed 2 to 24 hours later by a late-phase reaction mostly due to activation of eosinophils (**D**).

4. Correct: Binding of antigen to IgE on mast cell surfaces (A)

This woman is presenting with classical symptoms of seasonal allergies, a type 1 hypersensitivity reaction caused by crosslinking of IgE on previously sensitized mast cells (**A**). Recognition of antigen presented on MHC1 activates CD8+ T-cells, which plays an important role in defense against viruses and intracellular pathogens but no role in seasonal allergies (**B**). Recognition of microbial polysaccharides by lectin receptors activates leukocytes in response to extracellular pathogens (**C**). (**D, E**) describe the mechanism of Type 2 and Type 3 hypersensitivity reactions respectively.

5. Correct: IgG binding to cell surfaces (B)

Autoimmune hemolytic disease of the newborn is a type 2 hypersensitivity reaction. In this condition a previously sensitized woman develops IgG antibodies against Rh+ antigens on fetal red cells. These antibodies cross the placenta and lead to lysis of fetal red cells (**B**). For (**A, C-E**), see previous information.

6. Correct: Serum sickness (C)

This patient is suffering from serum sickness, a type 3 (immune complex mediated) hypersensitivity reaction. The history of recent treatment with equine antivenin makes serum sickness much more likely than the other options (**C**). Although Lyme disease, malaria, and Chikungunya fever are present in Central America, again the history suggests another diagnosis (**A-B, D**). The normal hemoglobin concentration makes a hemolytic anemia unlikely (**E**).

7. Correct: Perivascular accumulation of lymphocytes and mononuclear cells (B)

This is a markedly positive PPD test in a patient who probably has latent or active tuberculosis. This type of reaction is a CD4+ T-cell-mediated delayed type hypersensitivity (Type IV hypersensitivity) reaction. Expected findings include dermal edema and perivascular ("cuffing") accumulation of macrophages and lymphocytes (**B**). Granulomatous inflammation would be unlikely in the skin but would likely be seen in the lungs and hilar lymph nodes (**C**). Bacterial infection such as cellulitis would cause a neutrophilic infiltrate, but her wound culture was negative (**A**). Eosinophils would be expected in a drug reaction or parasitic infection (**E**). The mechanism of this type of hypersensitivity reaction does not involve immune complex deposition (**D**).

8. Correct: A similar reaction can occur in people given penicillin (E)

The girl is having a type I hypersensitivity anaphylactic reaction (**B**). After a first exposure to an antigen (**A**), these patients have a heightened T_H2 response that leads to the development of mast cells with IgE that is specific for the antigen. These reactions occur as a result of the binding of antigen to IgE on the surface of mast cells in a previously sensitized individual; however, up to half of all fatal insect sting reactions occur in persons with no prior history of insect stings. Amongst medications, penicillins, aspirin, and nonsteroidal anti-inflammatory drugs are most commonly associated with anaphylaxis. Subsequent exposure to the antigen will cause a release of mediators from the mast cell (**C**), leading to vasodilation and increased vascular permeability, which can clinically cause swelling of the airway. Given her history, foreign body ingestion is not likely, and would be associated with stridor, and not the precipitating bee sting (**D**). In addition to bee stings, other allergens known to cause a type I hypersensitivity reaction are peanuts and penicillin (**E**)

9. Correct: A type I hypersensitivity reaction (A)

See explanation for question #8. The patient is experiencing a type-I hypersensitivity anaphylactic reaction (**A**). These reactions occur as a result of the binding of antigen to IgE on the surface of mast cells in a previously sensitized individual. Type III hypersensitivity reactions are not usually subdivided into types a and b (**C, D**). The reaction is neither type II (**B**) or type IV (**E**).

10. Correct: A type II hypersensitivity reaction (B)

Given that the patient just received blood and immediately afterward developed fever and chills, an immediate transfusion reaction, caused by IgM reacting against AB blood antigens, is the most likely cause. This is a type II hypersensitivity reaction (**B**). The IgM antibodies against the A or B antigen are naturally occurring and do not require previous sensitization to the antigen. Intravascular hemolysis will occur, causing free hemoglobin to be identified in the blood. This type of transfusion reaction can be fatal. For (**A, C-E**), see previous information.

11. Correct: IgM (E)

See explanation for Question #10.

12. Correct: A delayed hemolytic transfusion reaction (D)

Given the fact that the patient has twice before been seen in the emergency room for vomiting blood, he has most likely been transfused. This exposure has caused him to develop antibodies against a blood group antigen that is not A or B (e.g., D, Kell, Duffy, Kidd). When he was exposed to the blood group antigen this time, he had already formed IgG against the antigen, which bound to the antigen and led to extravascular hemolysis, a delayed transfusion reaction (**D**). Because the blood he was given elicited this response, much of it was removed from circulation, and his hemoglobin did not rise much. For (**A-C, E**), see previous information.

13. Correct: IgG (D)

See explanation for question #12.

4.5 Autoimmune Diseases—Answers and Explanations

Easy	Medium	Hard

14. Correct: Positive anti-Smith (E)

Anti-Smith (**E**) is most specific for systemic lupus. Anti-CCP IgG is most specific for rheumatoid arthritis (**C**). SS-A, SS-B, and rheumatoid factor are typically associated with other rheumatologic illnesses but can be seen in patients with lupus, particularly in overlap syndromes, but are not specific for lupus (**A, B, D**).

15.   Correct: Antinuclear antibody (ANA) (D)

This patient has classic hydralazine-induced lupus. Antinuclear antibodies are positive in the majority of patients with drug-induced lupus; however, anti-Smith and anti-dsDNA antibodies are rare in hydralazine-induced lupus (**D, A, B**). An elevated serum uric acid level would suggest gout, which can be provoked in patients treated with hydrochlorothiazide but has not been described as a side effect of hydralazine treatment, and the symmetrical involvement of multiple joints in both hands would be unusual for gout (**C**). Low serum complement levels can be seen in idiopathic systemic lupus but are rare in drug-induced lupus (**E**).

16.   Correct: Rheumatoid arthritis (B)

This patient has rheumatoid arthritis (RA) (**B**). Rheumatoid arthritis, in contrast to osteoarthritis, typically spares the distal interphalangeal joints (**A**). RA is usually polyarticular and symmetric as opposed to gout, which is typically monoarticular and most often affects the metatarsophalangeal joint of the foot (**E**). Including Lyme disease in the differential diagnosis would be appropriate, but Lyme disease is much less common than RA and there is no evidence to suggest she is at risk for Lyme disease (**C**). Similarly, including systemic lupus in the differential diagnosis would be appropriate; however, the clinical history is much more suggestive of RA than lupus (**D**).

17.   Correct: Anti–cyclic citrulinated peptide (CCP IgG) (B)

The most likely diagnosis is rheumatoid arthritis (RA). Of the answers above, only anti-CCP IgG is specific to RA (**B**). For (**A, C-E**), see previous information.

18.   Correct: Felty's syndrome (D)

Physical examination findings include boutonnière deformity and ulnar deviation of the fingers as well as rheumatoid nodules, all of which are highly suggestive of rheumatoid arthritis (RA). The remainder of the extra-articular findings (interstitial lung disease, splenomegaly, and vasculitis) are characteristic of Felty's syndrome, a complication of long standing or poorly controlled RA (**D**). For (**A-C, E**), see previous information.

19.   Correct: Cigarette smoking (E)

Cigarette smoking is strongly associated with the development of rheumatoid arthritis (**E**). Multiparity and breast-feeding both decrease the risk (**A, C**). The HLA-B27 haplotype is associated with several autoimmune diseases including ankylosing spondylitis, Reiter's syndrome (reactive arthritis), and inflammatory bowel disease but is present in patients with RA no more frequently than in the general population (**D**). Male sex is not a risk factor (**B**).

20.   Correct: Pericarditis (D)

Examination: Pleuritic chest pain with diffuse ST elevation on ECG is typical of pericarditis, a common complication of systemic lupus (**D**). The presence of ST elevation in every lead makes acute myocardial infarction and pulmonary embolism unlikely (**A, B**). Patients with systemic lupus do have a 50-fold increased risk for myocardial infarction compared with the general population. Libman-Sacks endocarditis is a classic manifestation of lupus rarely seen in the modern era of disease-modifying therapy and would present as valve vegetations on echocardiogram but would not cause chest pain or ECG abnormalities (**E**). An aortic dissection will often produce a wide mediastinum on chest X-ray (**C**).

21.   Correct: Sjögren's syndrome (A)

Corneal ulcers from keratoconjunctivitis sicca are a common complication of Sjögren's syndrome (**A**). Lymphadenopathy and parotid enlargement are also common in this disease. Rheumatoid factor is positive in 75% of patients, and antinuclear antibodies (ANA) are positive in 50 to 80% of patients with Sjögren's syndrome. Up to 90% of patients are positive for SS-A (Ro) or SS-B (La). For (**B-E**), see previous information.

22.   Correct: Blindness (B)

This patient has polymyalgia rheumatica and is at high risk for giant cell (temporal) arteritis, a condition, which if untreated, commonly causes vision loss and blindness (**B**). Seronegative rheumatoid arthritis is possible; however, the lack of small joint involvement makes this unlikely. Erosive arthritis and interstitial lung disease are complications of rheumatoid arthritis (**A, C**). Renal failure and pericarditis are complications of systemic lupus (**D, E**).

23.   Correct: Systemic sclerosis (E)

The skin changes, digital ischemic ulcerations, and presence of Raynaud phenomenon are highly suggestive of systemic sclerosis (**E**). Up to 95% of patients with systemic sclerosis have positive ANA titers. None of the other choices would be expected to produce the skin changes described in the question, and thus they are unlikely in the absence of an overlap syndrome with other rheumatologic disease (**A-D**).

24.   Correct: Lymphocytic and plasma cell infiltrate with ductal epithelial hyperplasia (A)

Characteristic pathologic findings in Sjögren's syndrome include periductal and perivascular infiltration of lymphocytes. As the disease progresses, extensive lymphocytic infiltration can lead to formation of lymphoid follicles with germinal centers. With time, hyperplasia of the ductal epithelia can progress to atrophy of the acini, fibrosis, and hyalinization (**A**). (**B**) describes pleomorphic adenoma of the parotid gland, not Sjögren's syndrome. Acute inflammatory infiltrate (**C**) or coagulative necrosis (**D**) would not be expected. (**E**) describes lymphoma, which is a complication that can develop in patients with Sjögren's syndrome; however, it would not be expected.

25. Correct: Deposition of antigen-antibody complexes in the glomeruli (D)

Of the choices, the most likely diagnosis is systemic lupus erythematosus, as it can cause fatigue, arthritis, leukopenia, and seizures, whereas none of the other conditions would cause all of these signs and symptoms. The mechanism of glomerular injury in systemic lupus is deposition of immune complexes in the glomerulus (**D**). For (**A-C, E**), see previous information.

26. Correct: Anti-dsDNA antibodies (A)

The presence of proteinuria associated with mesangial proliferation identified on kidney biopsy in a young female patient would most often be associated with underlying systemic lupus. Of the antibodies listed, anti-dsDNA antibodies are most specific to systemic lupus and are present in 40 to 60% of cases (**A**). Anti-SSA and anti-SSB antibodies are common in systemic lupus, but nonspecific (**B, C**). Anti-centromere and anti-SCL 70 antibodies are suggestive of systemic sclerosis (**D, E**).

27. Correct: Sjögren's syndrome (D)

Dry mouth and dry eyes (keratoconjunctivitis sicca) are the hallmark symptoms of Sjögren's disease, an autoimmune disease characterized by lymphocytic infiltration and destruction of the salivary and lacrimal glands (**D**). With osteoarthritis, the pain usually worsens during the day (**A**). While psoriasis and Lyme disease can cause arthritis, they are not usually associated with the dry eyes and mouth (**B, C**). The clinical scenario is not consistent with osteomyelitis (**E**).

28. Correct: Anti-SSA (D)

This patient is suffering from Sjögren's syndrome (SS), characterized by autoimmune destruction of the salivary and/or lacrimal glands. 25% or more of patients with Sjögren's syndrome will experience extra glandular symptoms such as arthritis. Of the antibodies listed in the question, only anti-SSA, present in 70% of patients with Sjögren's syndrome, would be expected (**D**). For (**A-C, E**), see previous information.

29. Correct: Lymphocytic infiltrate (D)

This patient's clinical presentation is consistent with Sjögren's syndrome. Of the answer choices, the most classic histologic finding in a biopsy of a submandibular gland in a patient with Sjögren's syndrome is lymphocytic infiltrate (**D**). For (**A-C, E**), see previous information.

30. Correct: MALToma (A)

This patient presents with physical examination findings consistent with Sjögren's syndrome. Patients with Sjögren's syndrome are at risk for development of lymphoma, which occurs in up to 10% of patient. The majority of Sjögren-associated lymphomas are non-Hodgkin's lymphomas, with MALToma being the most common (**A**). For (**B-E**), see previous information.

31. Correct: Myasthenia gravis (D)

Myasthenia gravis is due to autoantibodies that block the postsynaptic acetylcholine receptors, causing muscle weakness. Ptosis and diplopia are common symptoms and occur due to weakness of extraocular muscles (**D**). The degree of weakness fluctuates, and can become severe very quickly. About one-fifth of patients with myasthenia gravis have a thymoma, which is the mediastinal mass identified on the CT scan. About 50% of thymomas occur in patients with myasthenia gravis. Thymectomy is beneficial to these patients. Although the other conditions could be considered in the differential diagnosis, none are associated with a mediastinal mass (**A-C, E**)

32. Correct: Antibodies against the acetylcholine receptor (A)

See the explanation for question #18. The mechanism by which myasthenia gravis causes disease is blockage of postsynaptic acetylcholine receptors. The other choices (**B-E**) do not apply.

33. Correct: AL amyloidosis (D)

The patient has two characteristic signs of AL amyloidosis: scalloping of the tongue by the teeth due to enlargement of the tongue (macroglossia) and periorbital purpura from trivial injury or Valsalva maneuver (raccoon sign). The displacement of the point of maximal impulse, consistent with cardiac hypertrophy, and the hepatomegaly are also frequently seen in AL amyloidosis (**D**). There is no history of laboratory findings to suggest any of the other diagnoses (**A-C, E**).

4.6 Immunodeficiencies—Answers and Explanations

Easy	Medium	Hard

34. Correct: Impaired phagosome-lysosome fusion (D)

This patient suffers from Chediak-Higashi syndrome. The hallmark of Chediak-Higashi syndrome is impaired phagosome-lysosome fusion, which produces characteristic giant azurophilic granules in neutrophils, eosinophils, and other granulocytes (**D**). The underlying cause is mutations in LYST, a lysosomal membrane trafficking protein. Fucosyl transferase deficiency causes absence of Sialyl-Lewis X and impaired leukocyte adhesion and rolling (leukocyte adhesion deficiency 2) (**A**). The patient's physical appearance and the presence of giant granules are inconsistent with either chronic granulomatous disease (caused by phagocyte oxidase deficiency) or myeloperoxidase deficiency (**B, C**). Mutation in the γ-chain subunit of cytokine receptors is the underlying defect in X-linked SCID (**E**).

35. Correct: Abnormal nitroblue tetrazolium test (D)

This patient suffers from chronic granulomatous disease. The nitroblue tetrazolium test will show absence of superoxide activity (**D**). Cystic fibrosis is high on the differential diagnosis, but this patient has recurrent extrapulmonary infections and cutaneous granulomatous disease, neither of which would be expected in cystic fibrosis. His sweat chloride test therefore would be normal (**B**). The primary defect in chronic granulomatous disease is with the phagocyte; thus immunoglobulin levels are normal or increased (due to persistent and recurrent infection) (**A, C**). (**E**) is incorrect, as this patient has signs and symptoms of immunodeficiency rather that autoimmunity.

36. Correct: Phagocyte NADPH oxidase deficiency (B)

The primary defect in chronic granulomatous disease is deficiency of phagocyte NADPH oxidase, which can be inherited in either an autosomal recessive or an X-linked pattern (**B**). The resultant impairment in superoxide production renders the phagocyte impaired in microbial killing. The clinical picture is that of a much more severe illness than is usually seen with myeloperoxidase deficiency (**C**), which is asymptomatic in 95% of patients and when symptomatic generally causes recurrent *Candida* infections. For (**A, D-E**), see previous information.

37. Correct: Recurrent abdominal pain (B)

In addition to angioedema, recurrent, often severe abdominal pain and skin edema are common manifestations of hereditary angioedema (HA) (**B**). Wheezing, stridor, urticaria, and elevated serum tryptase levels are manifestations of anaphylaxis (Type I hypersensitivity reaction) and are not seen in attacks of hereditary angioedema (**A, C-D**). Likewise, anaphylaxis is usually responsive to epinephrine and glucocorticoids, whereas these agents have no effect on attacks of HA (**E**).

38. Correct: HIV antibodies and viral load (E)

This patient is suffering from acute retroviral syndrome. The main differential diagnosis is pharyngitis from Group A *Streptococcus* and infectious mononu-

cleosis (**D**), which have been excluded. With a negative ANA, acute HIV infection (**E**) should be excluded prior to further workup for autoimmune disease (**A-C**). A Lyme titer (not given as an option in this question) would also be appropriate.

39. Correct: *Streptococcus pneumoniae* (C)

This patient has community-acquired lobar pneumonia (**C**). Despite the emphasis placed on the many opportunistic pathogens that HIV-positive patients are at risk for, the most common causes of community-acquired pneumonia are the same pathogens prevalent in the general population (**C**). For (**A-B, D-E**), previous information.

40. Correct: Pneumocystis jirovecii (A)

The presence of fever, hypoxia, and bilateral diffuse infiltrates with elevated serum LDH is consistent with pneumonia due to *Pneumocystis jirovecii* (**A**). Pneumococcal pneumonia would not be expected to produce bilateral interstitial infiltrates (**C**). All of the other agents listed should be in the differential; however, infection with *Histoplasma* and *Cryptococcus* are less common in patients with CD4 count > 100 cells/μL (**B, D**), and *Mycobacterium avium* complex infections are unusual in patients with CD 4 count > 50 cells/μL (**E**).

41. Correct: It is uncommon in heterosexual men with HIV (C)

This patient's clinical presentation and biopsy findings are consistent with Kaposi sarcoma. Infection with human herpes virus-8 (HHV-8), a sexually transmitted infection, is required to develop this disease. HHV-8 seropositivity is much more common in men who have sex with men than in women or heterosexual men (**C**). The primary differential diagnosis of Kaposi sarcoma (KS) is bacillary angiomatosis, caused by *Bartonella*; however, there is no mention of bacterial organisms on the biopsy (**B**). Antibiotic prophylaxis cannot prevent development of KS, and extraintestinal manifestations are common (**D, E**). Most cases of KS have an indolent course (**A**).

42. Correct: Defective CD 40 ligand (B)

This patient suffers from hyper-IgM syndrome, which, given the presence of a similar illness in his brother, is likely the X-linked form, resulting from a defect in CD40 ligand (**B**). The autosomal recessive form is due to a defect in CD40 itself. Defective development of the third and fourth pharyngeal pouches causes DiGeorge's syndrome (**A**). Adenosine deaminase deficiency and mutations in the cytokine receptor common γ-chain and Jak3 cause severe combined immunodeficiency (SCID) (**C-E**). A child with SCID would not be expected to survive to age 6 years without a stem cell transplant.

43. Correct: Severe combined immunodeficiency (E)

This patient presents with combined defects of both humoral and cellular immunity, consistent with severe combined immunodeficiency (SCID) (E). The presence of relatively normal levels of B-lymphocytes makes X-linked agammaglobulinemia less likely (A). DiGeorge is important in the differential diagnosis of SCID; however, in the absence of cardiac defect or hypocalcemia there is no indication of DiGeorge's syndrome (C). Neither transient hypogammaglobulinemia nor common variable immunodeficiency (CVID) would be expected to produce such severe disease in a 7-month-old, and CVID typically presents with recurrent infections later in childhood or in early adolescence (B, D).

44. Correct: Impaired B-cell maturation (A)

This patient has X-linked agammaglobulinemia. The underlying defect is a mutation in a tyrosine kinase that blocks signal transduction by the pre-B cell receptor required for B-cell maturation (A). For (B-E), see previous information.

45. Correct: Lymphoid malignancy (E)

This patient has selective IgA deficiency, which when symptomatic, causes recurrent sinopulmonary infection. This condition is associated with increased risk for transfusion reactions, pneumonia, *Giardia lamblia* intestinal infections, and, rarely, with Crohn's disease (A-D). Unlike common variable immunodeficiency, selective IgA deficiency has not been associated with an increased risk of malignancy (E).

46. Correct: *Cryptococcus neoformans* (D)

Cryptococcus is the most common cause of central nervous system (CNS) infection in patients with AIDS. In this case, the presence of umbilical papules (molluscum-like rash) is classic for disseminated cryptococcal infection (D). The normal brain imaging, the absence of radiologic signs, and the presence of meningeal signs make *Toxoplasma* less likely (A). The historical and clinical findings in tuberculous meningitis are frequently very similar; however, the molluscum-like rash is a clue to making the right diagnosis (B). *Streptococcus* is excluded based on the CNS fluid analysis (C), and Molluscum does not infect the CNS (E).

47. Correct: Trimethoprim-Sulfamethoxazole (A)

This patient has central nervous system toxoplasmosis with characteristic signs, symptoms, and imaging findings. In addition to preventing *Pneumocystis* infection, trimethoprim-sulfamethoxazole is indicated for the prevention of toxoplasmosis in AIDS (A). For (B-E), see previous information.

48. Correct: Abnormal linking of membrane receptors to cytoskeletal elements (C)

This patient has Wiskott-Aldrich syndrome, characterized by recurrent infections, eczema, and thrombocytopenia. Usually inherited in an X-linked recessive pattern, Wiskott-Aldrich syndrome is caused by mutations in Wiskott-Aldrich syndrome protein (WASP), thought to be involved in linking membrane receptors to cytoskeletal elements (C). For (A-B, D-E), see previous information.

49. Correct: Mutation in the gene for SLAM-associated protein (D)

The history of fatal Epstein-Barr virus (EBV) infections in male siblings is most consistent with X-linked lymphoproliferative disorder, caused in most cases by mutations in the gene coding for SLAM-associated protein (SAP) (D). Patients with this disorder have impaired NK cell function and are susceptible to fulminant infection with EBV. For (A-C, E), see previous information.

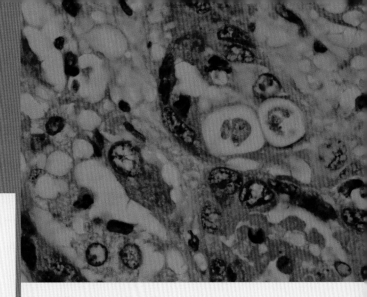

Chapter 5

Neoplasia

LEARNING OBJECTIVES

5.1 Neoplasia

- ▶ Compare grade and stage of tumors
- ▶ List the normal activity of common oncogenes
- ▶ List the tumors associated with tuberous sclerosis
- ▶ Diagnose and list the conditions associated with acanthosis nigricans
- ▶ List common tumor suppressor genes associated with neoplasms, and their chromosome location
- ▶ Describe the association between CNS lymphoma and HIV
- ▶ Given the constellation of neoplasms present in a patient, diagnose the familial neoplasia syndrome that they possess
- ▶ Describe the activity of the APC gene

5.1 Neoplasia—Questions

Easy	Medium	Hard

1. A clinician is reviewing the pathology report of a patient with adenocarcinoma of the colon. Of the following, which helps determine the grade of the tumor?

A. Number of positive lymph nodes

B. Size of the tumor

C. Metastatic spread to another organ

D. Depth of invasion of wall of colon

E. Number of mitotic figures per high-power field

Colon

2. A 60-year-old male presents to his family physician because of complaints of blood in his stool and intermittent constipation. Fecal occult blood testing is positive. A colonoscopy is performed, revealing a large adenocarcinoma of the sigmoid colon. As the tumor was removed at a teaching hospital, a researcher tests the tumor and identifies a mutation of *ras*. Of the following, what was one mechanism by which the tumor developed?

A. Inhibition of apoptosis

B. Abnormal GTPase activity

C. Abnormal tyrosine kinase activity

D. Up-regulation of cytokine receptor

E. Down-regulation of cytokine receptor

Colon

3. The parents of a 17-year-old female bring her to the emergency room after she had a brief seizure at home from which she recovered. A CT scan is performed in the emergency room, identifying a cortical nodule in the left cerebral hemisphere. A CT scan of the body is also performed, identifying a 3.0 cm mass in the left kidney, which is subsequently biopsied and diagnosed as an angiomyolipoma. Of the following, which other tumor is this patient at increased risk for?

A. Medulloblastoma

B. Hepatic neuroblastoma

C. Ewing sarcoma

D. Cardiac rhabdomyoma

E. Retinoblastoma

Kidney, brain

4. A 63-year-old female is being evaluated by her family physician. Over the past 3 months she has developed a velvety hyperpigmentation of the skin of the posterior neck and bilateral axilla. She has lost 15 lbs. since her last visit four months ago and has a body mass index of 23 kg/m^2. Routine blood work is normal except for a hemoglobin level of 8.6 g/dL. Her HbA1c is 5.4%, and a plain chest radiograph is normal. What is the next step in the evaluation?

A. Bone scan

B. CT chest with contrast

C. Skin biopsy

D. Upper and lower endoscopy

E. Bone marrow aspirate

Lung

5. A 46-year-old female presents to her family physician because she palpated a nodule in her left breast during a breast self-examination. She subsequently undergoes a partial mastectomy. The mass is examined by a pathologist who makes a diagnosis of invasive ductal carcinoma. Subsequent genetic testing reveals a mutation of the *BRCA2* gene. Of the following, what is the location for this mutation?

A. 17p

B. 17q

C. 13q

D. 13p

E. 18q

F. 18p

Breast

6. A 4-year-old boy is evaluated by his pediatrician for 1 week of intermittent hematuria. On examination he appears well developed and well nourished, except a right flank mass is palpable. A biopsy of the mass is performed, which reveals primitive looking small blue cells with glomeruloid and tubuloid structures. What is the diagnosis?

A. Medulloblastoma

B. Polycystic kidney disease

C. Clear cell sarcoma

D. Rhabdoid tumor

E. Wilms tumor

Kidney

7. A 46-year-old male presents to his family physician with complaints of a headache. While being evaluated, he has a seizure and is subsequently taken to radiology for a CT scan, which identifies a mass in his corpus callosum. Subsequent biopsy determines the mass to be composed of malignant lymphocytes. Of the following, what other condition does this patient most likely have?

A. Hepatitis C infection associated with cirrhosis of the liver

B. Hashimoto's thyroiditis

C. HIV infection

D. HSV encephalitis

E. Remote head trauma

Brain

8. A 31-year-old female has fecal blood identified during a physical examination. A colonoscopy reveals an ulcerated mass in her proximal rectum. In the past, she has had a ductal carcinoma of her left breast and a malignant thyroid tumor, both excised and treated. Of the following, what is the most likely mutation if she is diagnosed with Cowden's syndrome?

A. Mutation of the *PTEN* gene

B. Mutation of the *CDKN2* gene

C. Mutation of *RB* gene

D. Mutation of the *WT* gene

E. Mutation of the *TP53* gene

Large intestine

9. In the same family, four individuals are diagnosed with malignant melanoma. Of the following, which mutation is most likely?

A. Mutation of the *RET* gene

B. Mutation of the *CDKN2* gene

C. Mutation of *APC* gene

D. Mutation of the *WT* gene

E. Mutation of the *PTEN* gene

Genetic

10. A 35-year-old male presents to his family care physician because of balance problems. A CT scan of his head reveals a mass near the pontomedullary junction. The mass is excised and diagnosed as a schwannoma. Four years later, he presents with headaches and is found to have two meningiomas. Of the following, what is the most likely mutation that he possesses?

A. Mutation of the *PTEN*

B. Mutation of the *CDKN2* gene

C. Mutation of the *NF2* gene

D. Mutation of the *WT*

E. Mutation of the *TP53*

Genetic

11. A 5-year-old male is brought to his pediatrician by his parents for an annual examination. Palpation of his abdomen reveals a mass, which is subsequently resected. The pathologist examining the mass identifies three components: blastemal, stromal, and epithelial. His sister had the same type of tumor. Of the following, what gene mutation do the siblings most likely have?

A. Mutation of the *RB* gene

B. Mutation of the *CDKN2* gene

C. Mutation of the *VHL* gene

D. Mutation of the *WT* gene

E. Mutation of the *APC* gene

Genetic

12. A 41-year-old female has had an invasive ductal carcinoma, a low grade astrocytoma, a leiomyosarcoma, and a rhabdomyosarcoma. She is diagnosed with a facial neoplasia syndrome. Of the following, which gene mutation is most likely present?

A. Mutation of the *MET* gene

B. Mutation of the *CDKN2* gene

C. Mutation of the *ATM* gene

D. Mutation of the *TP53* gene

E. Mutation of the *TSC1* gene

Genetic

13. A 42-year-old male undergoes a colectomy. The pathologist identifies more than 100 polyps in the resected specimen as well as a focus of invasive adenocarcinoma. Of the following, what is the functional mechanism for the gene mutation causing his disease process?

A. Decreased breakdown of β-catenin

B. Increased breakdown of β-catenin

C. Increased activity of β-catenin

D. Decreased activity of β-catenin

E. Lack of production of β-catenin

Large intestine

5.2 Neoplasia—Answers and Explanations

Easy	Medium	Hard

1. Correct: Number of mitotic figures per high-power field (E)

The grade of a tumor is its degree of histologic differentiation (e.g., well, moderate, or poorly differentiated) and represents a subjective determination by the pathologist as to how closely the tumor resembles the tissue type from which it arose (e.g., in colonic adenocarcinoma, whether the tumor cells appear like normal glandular epithelium). In determining the grade of the tumor, the histologic appearance of the tumor is important, including the number of mitotic figures per high-power field (E). The other features listed are used to determine the stage of a neoplasm (A-D). The exact determination of stage depends on the tumor type and characteristics specific to that tumor.

2. Correct: Abnormal GTPase activity (B)

The *ras* oncogene is associated with colonic adenocarcinoma, and the gene product of the ras gene is a GTPase. For (A, C-E), see previous information.

3. Correct: Cardiac rhabdomyoma (D)

The cortical mass is a tuber, and, when combined with an angiomyolipoma in a young patient, the diagnosis is most likely tuberous sclerosis. The tumors associated with tuberous sclerosis also include cardiac rhabdomyomas (D). The other tumors listed are not commonly associated with tuberous sclerosis (A-C, E).

4. Correct: Upper and lower endoscopy (D)

The changes noted on physical examination are consistent with acanthosis nigricans. In the absence of obesity or diabetes, the presence of acanthosis nigricans in adult patients often indicates underlying malignancy, warranting the upper and lower endoscopy (D). Gastrointestinal malignancies, particularly gastric adenocarcinoma, are most commonly associated with acanthosis. The other choices (A-C, E) would not be as useful.

5. Correct: 13q (C)

The *BRCA2* gene is located on the long arm of chromosome 13 (13q) (C). The *BRCA1* gene is located on the long arm of chromosome 17 (17q) (B). The gene for the p53 protein, which is mutated in many types of cancer, is located on the short arm of chromosome 17 (17p) (A). 18q is the site of the *DPC* gene, which can be mutated in pancreatic carcinoma (E). For (D, F), see previous information.

6. Correct: Wilms tumor (E)

Wilms tumor (E), the most common renal malignancy in children, usually presents with a palpable mass or hematuria. This tumor, most often caused by a mutation of the *WT1* tumor suppressor gene on 11p13, is characterized histologically by a mixture of blastemal (small blue cell), stromal, and epithelial (primitive glomeruloid and tubuloid) cell types. The other choices are not correct (A-D).

7. Correct: HIV infection (C)

Of the listed conditions, primary lymphomas of the central nervous system in patients under the age of 70 are most commonly associated with HIV infection (C). Although Hashimoto's thyroiditis and other autoimmune disorders are associated with lymphoma, the lymphoma they are most commonly associated with is mucosa-associated lymphoid tissue (or, MALTomas), of which the brain has none (B). Cirrhosis of the liver is a risk factor for hepatocellular carcinoma (A), and HSV encephalitis and remote head trauma are not commonly associated with an increased incidence of malignancy (D-E).

8. Correct: A

Patients with Cowden's syndrome develop colorectal, thyroid, and breast neoplasms. The underlying mutation is that of *PTEN* (A). Mutations of *CDKN2* are associated with malignant melanoma (B), *RB* with retinoblastoma (C), *WT* with Wilms tumor (D), and *TP53* with breast cancer, brain tumors, and leukemia (E).

9. Correct: B

Familial malignant melanoma is associated with mutations of *CDKN2* (p16) (B). Mutations of *RET* are associated with thyroid medullary carcinoma and pheochromocytomas (A), mutations of *APC* are associated with colonic adenocarcinoma (C), mutations of *WT* are associated with Wilms tumor (D), and mutations of the *PTEN* gene are associated with colonic adenocarcinoma, breast cancer, and thyroid cancer.

10. Correct: C

Multiple meningiomas and schwannomas are characteristic of neurofibromatosis type II, so the patient most likely has a mutation of the *NF2* gene (C). Mutations of *PTEN* are associated with colonic adenocarcinoma and breast and thyroid tumors (A), mutations of *CDKN2* are associated with familial melanoma (B), mutations of *WT* are associated with Wilms tumor (D), and mutations of *TP53* are associated with a variety of tumors including breast cancer, soft tissue sarcomas, leukemia, and brain tumors (E).

11. Correct: D

The tumor description fits that of a Wilms tumor. Wilms tumors are associated with mutations of the *WT* gene (**D**). Mutations of the *RB* gene are associated with retinoblastoma (**A**), mutations of the *CDKN2* gene are associated with familial melanoma (**B**), mutations of the *VHL* gene are associated with renal cell carcinoma (**C**), and mutations of the *APC* gene are associated with colonic adenocarcinoma.

12. Correct: D

The constellation of breast cancer, brain tumors, and soft tissue sarcomas is consistent with Li-Fraumeni's syndrome, which is caused by a mutation of the *TP53* gene (**D**). Mutations of the *MET* gene are associated with papillary renal cell carcinoma (**A**), mutations of the *CDKN2* gene are associated with malignant melanoma (**B**), mutations of the *ATM* gene are associated with leukemia and lymphoma (**C**), and mutations of the *TSC1* gene are associated with tuberous sclerosis and a variety of tumors including renal cell carcinoma, angiomyolipomas, and astrocytomas.

13. Correct: Decreased breakdown of β-catenin (A)

This patient suffers from familial adenomatous polyposis, one of the genetic colon cancer syndromes. In this disorder, patients have a germline loss of function mutation in the *APC* tumor suppressor gene, which usually functions to break down β-catenin, a protein involved in the signal cascade of APC (**A**). The subsequent increased amount of β-catenin appears to prevent cell differentiation and apoptosis. (**B-E**) are incorrect, see previous information.

Chapter 6
Genetic and Pediatric Diseases

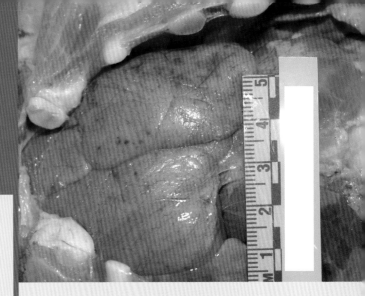

LEARNING OBJECTIVES

6.1 General Genetic Disorders
▶ Given the clinical scenario, diagnose neurofibromatosis; describe the gross and microscopic features of the disease
▶ Given the clinical scenario, diagnose neurofibromatosis type II; describe the gross and microscopic features of the disease
▶ List the tumors associated with von Hippel-Lindau
▶ Given the clinical scenario, diagnose tuberous sclerosis; list the conditions associated with tuberous sclerosis

6.2 Enzyme Deficiencies and Inborn Errors of Metabolism
▶ Recognize galactosemia
▶ Describe the molecular basis and complications of α-1-antitrypsin deficiency
▶ Identify Friedreich Ataxia
▶ Describe and identify the phenomena of incomplete penetrance and variable expressivity
▶ Recognize phenylketonuria

6.3 Genetic Diseases of Structural Proteins
▶ Describe the molecular basis and complications of Marfan's syndrome
▶ Describe the molecular basis and complications of Ehlers-Danlos syndrome
▶ Given the clinical scenario, diagnose Marfan's syndrome; describe the gross and microscopic characteristics of Marfan's syndrome

6.4 Lysosomal and Storage Disorders
▶ Identify Tay-Sachs disease
▶ Identify mucopolysaccharidoses and list the underlying genetic defects
▶ Distinguish Niemann-Pick disease from Tay-Sachs disease
▶ Identify McArdle's disease
▶ Identify von Gierke's disease
▶ Identify Pompe's disease

6.5 Chromosomal Disorders
▶ Describe the processes that can cause trisomy
▶ Identify Edward's and Patau's syndromes
▶ Identify DiGeorge's syndrome
▶ Identify fragile X syndrome and describe the underlying mechanism
▶ Describe the common complications of Klinefelter's syndrome
▶ Describe the common complications of Turner's syndrome

6.6 Pediatric Diseases
▶ Identify fetal alcohol syndrome
▶ Identify 5p- syndrome
▶ Diagnose intussusception
▶ Describe the classic presentation and histologic appearance of neuroblastoma
▶ Recognize Meckel diverticulum and list the "rule of 2's"
▶ List the risk factors for congenital hypertrophic pyloric stenosis
▶ Recognize the common childhood infections
▶ Diagnose congenital adrenal hyperplasia
▶ Recognize common congenital malformation syndromes associated with Wilms' tumor
▶ List the common fetal complications of maternal diabetes
▶ List the risk factors for sudden infant death syndrome
▶ Diagnose cystic fibrosis
▶ Diagnose meconium ileus
▶ Identify necrotizing enterocolitis
▶ Describe the pathogenesis, risk factors, and complications of neonatal respiratory distress syndrome
▶ Describe the complications of prematurity
▶ List the congenital birth defects associated with multifactorial inheritance and the risk of recurrence
▶ Distinguish the different types of congenital abnormalities of morphogenesis

6.1 General Genetic Disorders—Questions

Easy	Medium	Hard

1. A pathologist is performing an autopsy on an individual who died as the result of a motor vehicle accident. During the external examination, the pathologist notes that there are about 20 brown macules on the skin with multiple soft dermal nodules of the same color as the skin. A biopsy of the nodules would reveal?

A. Malignant melanocytes

B. Schwann cells and fibroblasts

C. Entrapped sebaceous fluid

D. Pus

E. Adipose cells and macrophages

Skin

2. A 45-year-old man is referred to dermatology for skin lesions found incidentally on examination. The dermatologist notes that there are about 30 brown macules on the skin with multiple soft nodules on the extensor forearms, neck, and back. Of the following, which organ could the clinician also examine to find characteristic lesions of the disease process?

A. Liver

B. Lung

C. Heart

D. Adrenal gland

E. Eye

Skin

3. A 33-year-old female presents to her family physician complaining of ringing in the ears and balance problems. After a complete physical examination, a CT scan of the head is performed revealing bilateral lesions at the pontomedullary junction. The lesions are removed by a neurosurgeon, and the neuropathologist examining the masses makes the diagnosis of schwannomas. Of the following, which other lesion might the CT scan have identified?

A. A glioblastoma multiforme

B. Metastatic colonic adenocarcinoma

C. A lipoma of the septum pellucidum

D. Meningiomas

E. Hyperostosis frontalis

Central nervous system

4. A 32-year-old male has a seizure at work. During his evaluation in the emergency room, a CT scan of the head reveals a tumor in the left cerebral hemisphere. The biopsy diagnosis is hemangioblastoma. The patient's 30-year-old brother died one week ago in a motor vehicle accident and at autopsy the pathologist found a 2.5 cm yellow and red cortical mass in the left kidney. In addition to the hemangioblastoma, of the following, what other tumor type might the patient have?

A. Rhabdomyoma

B. Retinoblastoma

C. Pheochromocytoma

D. Osteosarcoma

E. Colonic adenocarcinoma

Central nervous system, renal

5. A 21-year-old female has a seizure while playing basketball with her friends. She is taken to the emergency room and a CT scan of the head is performed, revealing a lesion in the right cerebellar hemisphere. A neurosurgeon excises the mass, and a pathologist confirms a diagnosis of subependymal giant cell astrocytoma. When the patient was younger, she had a mass excised from her heart. Of the following, what is her most likely diagnosis?

A. Neurofibromatosis type I

B. Neurofibromatosis type II

C. Tuberous sclerosis

D. α-1 antitrypsin deficiency

E. Osler-Weber-Rendu syndrome

Central nervous system

6.2 Enzyme Deficiencies and Inborn Errors of Metabolism—Questions

Easy	Medium	Hard

6. A 2-week-old infant is evaluated in the emergency department for failure to thrive. The parents report persistent diarrhea, which started at 3 days old. The child's temperature is 103.2°F (39.5°C), pulse is 145/min, and blood pressure is 66/44. On examination bilateral corneal opacities are noted. There is mild hepatomegaly. The heart and lungs are clear. Moderate jaundice is observed. The child's blood glucose is 125 mg/dL, and the urine is positive for reducing substance. What is the most likely underlying condition?

A. Congenital type 1 diabetes

B. Phenylketonuria

C. Homocystinuria

D. Galactosemia

E. Alkaptonuria

Genetics

7. The child in the previous question is diagnosed with sepsis. Blood cultures are most likely to grow which organism?

A. *Escherichia coli*

B. Group B streptococci

C. *Listeria monocytogenes*

D. *Streptococcus pneumoniae*

E. *Klebsiella oxcytoca*

Genetics

8. A 36-year-old male is seen by his primary care physician for a physical exam. On examination the liver edge is nodular. A hepatitis panel is negative. Though the patient smokes, he does not consume alcohol. A liver biopsy is performed that shows numerous eosinophilic, diastase-resistant, PAS-positive cytoplasmic droplets within the hepatocytes. Which of the following is true of this patient's disease?

A. The underlying cause is a mutation in the gene for elastase.

B. His son has a 50% chance of inheriting this disease.

C. Apical bullous emphysema is a classic finding on chest radiograph.

D. Cessation of smoking will not reduce the risk of lung disease in this patient.

E. He is at increased risk for necrotizing panniculitis.

Genetics, pulmonary, gastrointestinal

9. A 19-year-old man is evaluated by neurology for increasing difficulty walking. On examination he has moderate motor weakness of the lower extremities with normal strength in the hands and arms, impaired two-point discrimination and vibration sense in the hands and feet with normal pain and temperature sensation, absent deep tendon reflexes throughout, marked ataxia, and mild dysarthria. Magnetic resonance imaging (MRI) of the brain and spinal cord shows atrophy of the spinal cord and medulla. The patient dies at age 35. What additional findings are likely to be seen at autopsy?

A. Telangiectasias in the brain, conjunctiva, and skin

B. Degeneration of the anterior roots of the spinal cord

C. Aβ plaques and neurofibrillary tangles

D. Axonal loss and gliosis of the posterior columns, spinocerebellar tracts, and distal corticospinal tracts

E. Aggregation of enlarged globoid macrophages in the brain parenchyma and around blood vessels

Central nervous system

10. In the previous patient, what is the underlying abnormality causing this patient's disease?

A. Trinucleotide repeat expansion

B. Single gene deletion

C. Deficiency of an enzyme involved in galactocerebroside catabolism

D. Viral infection

Central nervous system

11. A researcher is studying the genetic basis of a disease known to be familial. The disease is rare outside of affected families. The pedigree of one such family is shown below. Affected individuals are shaded. What is the best explanation for the inheritance pattern of this disease?

A. Mitochondrial inheritance

B. X-linked recessive trait

C. Incomplete penetrance

D. X-linked dominant inheritance

E. Autosomal recessive inheritance

Genetics

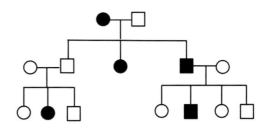

12. A 3-year-old girl, recently adopted from India by relatives, is brought to her pediatrician to establish care for a seizure disorder. The child is fair in complexion compared to her relatives, with light brown hair and brown eyes. Her height and weight are near the 50th percentile for her age. She has a vocabulary of 6 words. Though clean and well dressed, she has a peculiar musty odor, which her relatives say is persistent. What is the most likely diagnosis?

A. Isovaleric acidemia

B. Maple syrup urine disease

C. Phenylketonuria

D. Galactosemia

E. Multiple carboxylase deficiency

Pediatric, genetic, skin, eyes

6.3 Genetic Diseases of Structural Proteins—Questions

Easy	Medium	Hard

13. A 38-year-old male is referred to ophthalmology by his primary care physician for diminished visual acuity in the right eye. On examination his visual acuity is 20/20 in the left eye and 20/45 in the right eye, pupils are equal and reactive, ocular motility is normal, and the posterior segment is normal. Superotemporal dislocation of the lens of the right eye is observed. His skull is somewhat elongated with rather prominent frontal eminences but otherwise the remainder of his physical examination is normal. He denies any recent trauma. Which of the following tests should the patient undergo prior to surgery?

A. Plain chest radiograph

B. Complete blood count

C. 2D echocardiogram

D. Fasting glucose

E. Computed tomograph of the head

Genetics, eyes, central nervous system

14. A 12-year-old boy is evaluated in the emergency department for an elbow dislocation that occurred at home after a fall. He has a history of prior dislocation of both knees and severe myopia requiring glasses at age 4. On examination his skin is hyperextensible and he has multiple atrophic scars on the arms and legs. What is the most likely underlying defect?

A. Defect in fibrillin

B. Defect in dystrophin

C. Defect in collagen

D. Defect in elastase

E. Defect in TGF-b

Genetics

15. A 29-year-old tall male with no past medical history collapses while playing baseball with friends. An autopsy is performed, which identifies a ruptured thoracic aortic aneurysm. Microscopic examination of the aorta at the area of the dissection reveals cystic medial degeneration. Of the following, what is his most likely diagnosis?

A. Syphilitic aortitis

B. Takayasu's arteritis

C. Giant cell arteritis

D. Marfan's syndrome

E. Essential hypertension

Cardiovascular

16. Given the previous scenario, of the following, what other condition related to his disease process may be identified at autopsy?

A. Coarctation of the aorta

B. Ventricular septal defect

C. Myxomatous mitral valve

D. Extralobar pulmonary sequestration

E. Bronchogenic cyst

Cardiovascular

6.4 Lysosomal and Storage Disorders—Questions

Easy	Medium	Hard

17. An 11-month-old male is admitted to the hospital for failure to thrive. He has experienced recurring infections and regression of neurologic milestones starting at age 7 months. Two other siblings have died of a similar illness. On examination he is below the 5th percentile for weight. His heart and lung sounds are normal and hepatosplenomegaly is absent. Moro and rooting reflexes are present. On ophthalmoscopic exam there is a relative paleness of the retina compared with the central macula. Despite heroic care, the infant dies at age 15 months. At autopsy, lipid vacuolation of neurons is observed, with prominent lysosomes filled with whorled membranes being identified by electron microscopy. What is the most likely diagnosis?

A. Niemann-Pick disease

B. Tay-Sachs disease

C. Gaucher's disease

D. Hurler's syndrome

E. Hunter's syndrome

Genetics

18. A 24-month-old male is evaluated in the ER for an upper respiratory tract infection. It is his third such illness in the past 6 weeks. The child is dysmorphic with wide-set eyes (i.e., hypertelorism), marked bulging of the frontal eminence of the skull, and a depressed nasal bridge. Both corneas are opacified. He is unable to crawl and his joints are stiff and relatively immobile. What is the underlying defect?

A. Inability to degrade heparan sulfate and dermatan sulfate

B. Accumulation of glucocerebrosides in phagocytes and cells of the central nervous system

C. Sphingomyelinase deficiency

D. Defective collagen synthesis

E. Trinucleotide repeat expansion in the nontranslated region of a gene on the X chromosome

Genetics

19. A 5-month-old boy is hospitalized for failure to thrive. His weight is less than the 5th percentile for age. On examination he has hepatosplenomegaly, generalized lymphadenopathy, and a persistent Moro reflex. A liver biopsy is performed, which shows a foamy, vacuolated appearance of the Kuppfer cells and hepatocytes with enlarged dilated lysosomes containing concentric lamellated myelin figures on electron microscopy. What is the underlying defect?

A. Deficiency of hexosaminidase A

B. Deficiency of sphingomyelinase

C. Deficiency of glucocerebrosidase

D. Deficiency of α-L-iduronase

E. Deficiency of glucose-6-phosphatase

Genetics

20. A 26-year-old man is brought to the ER by his concerned wife after his urine turned dark after exercise. His brother was recently diagnosed with a genetic muscle disorder. The patient reports doing only very light weight training. He has been experiencing significant fatigue and muscle swelling and cramps with minimal activity. His urine is noted to be tea-colored, his urine myoglobin is elevated, and a serum creatine kinase level is 46,000 mg/dL (normal 50-175 mg/dL). Which of the following additional findings is likely in this patient?

A. Cardiomegaly

B. Hepatomegaly

C. Normal blood lactate levels after exercise

D. Elevated blood cholesterol levels

E. Hypoglycemia

Genetics, musculoskeletal

21. A 5-month-old female is hospitalized for lethargy. She is at the 4th percentile for weight. On examination there is prominent hepatomegaly with a protuberant abdomen, and "doll-like" facies. Her serum glucose is low (39 mg/dL) and is difficult to correct even with adequate enteral feeds. Her triglyceride and lactic acid levels are both elevated. What is the most likely diagnosis?

A. Galactosemia

B. Tay-Sachs disease

C. Gaucher's disease

D. von Gierke's disease

E. Pompe's disease

Genetics

22. A 2-month-old male infant is brought to the emergency room for respiratory distress. There is generalized hypotonia and moderate macroglossia identified on examination, and the liver is palpated 4 cm below the costal margin. A plain chest radiograph shows severe cardiomegaly, with the left ventricle obscuring most of the left hemithorax, and pulmonary edema. Blood glucose levels are normal, but the serum creatine kinase levels are elevated. What is the inheritance pattern of this disease?

A. Mitochondrial

B. Autosomal dominant

C. Autosomal recessive

D. X-linked recessive

E. X-linked dominant

Genetics

6.5 Chromosomal Disorders—Questions

Easy	Medium	Hard

23. A newborn female is examined by her pediatrician shortly after an uncomplicated vaginal delivery at 38 weeks gestational age. The child has epicanthal folds, flattened nasal bridge, macroglossia, and a transverse palmar crease. A karyotype is performed which shows 46 chromosomes in all cells examined. What is the likely underlying cause of this patient's disease?

A. Meiotic nondisjunction of chromosome 21

B. Mitotic nondisjunction of chromosome 21

C. Robertsonian translocation of chromosome 21

D. Trinucleotide repeat expansion

E. Uniparental disomy

Genetics

24. A 3-month-old male infant is examined at his pediatrician's office. The child was born at 40 weeks by uncomplicated vaginal delivery. He has low-set ears, a small mouth, and overlapping fingers. There is a mid-systolic flow murmur with a fixed split S2 heard best over the second left intercostal space. The extremity examination is remarkable for a prominent calcaneus with convex rounded deformity of the foot. What is the most likely diagnosis?

A. Down's syndrome

B. Patau's syndrome

C. Edward's syndrome

D. Velocardiofacial syndrome

E. Fragile X syndrome

Genetics

25. An 11-month-old male infant is brought to his pediatrician's office for evaluation of fever. His medical history is significant for neonatal tetany, which required calcium infusion, and for a cleft palate that was repaired surgically at age 3 months. On examination the child has a high broad nasal bridge with elongated facies. What is the underlying cause of this patient's condition?

A. Trisomy of chromosome 13

B. Mutation of tyrosine kinase on the X chromosome

C. Deletion of part of chromosome 22

D. Trinucleotide repeat expansion on the X chromosome

E. Mutation of a mitochondrial gene

Genetics

26. A 15-year-old boy is brought to his pediatrician for a routine checkup. He has an IQ of 69 and the intellectual capacity of a 10-year-old child. He has an 8-year-old brother with similar intellectual deficits. Both parents have normal IQ and intellectual capacity. On examination he has large everted ears, a large mandible, and prominent, enlarged testes. Which of the following is true regarding this patient's condition?

A. His father is likely a silent carrier of the mutation.

B. The boy could not pass the mutation to his offspring.

C. The disease is caused by trinucleotide repeat expansions, which induce fractures in the X chromosome.

D. The patient's children are likely to be more severely affected than the patient.

E. If the child's parents have a daughter, she has a 50% chance of being affected.

Genetics

27. A 16-year-old boy is brought to his pediatrician by his parents who are concerned about a lack of development of secondary sex characteristics. On examination he has long legs, is taller than average, and has much smaller testes than expected for his age. A chromosomal analysis performed on circulating leukocytes showed a 47 XXY karyotype. Which of the following complications is this patient at increased risk for?

A. Bladder cancer

B. Hodgkin lymphoma

C. Prostate cancer

D. Breast cancer

E. Gastric cancer

Genetics

28. A 32-year-old female presents to her family physician for routine physical. Her height is 63 inches (134 cm) and weight is 138 lbs (62 kg). She has never had a menstrual period. Her vital signs are temperature 99.8°F (37.6°C), pulse 78/min, and blood pressure 176/92 mm Hg. On examination she has multiple pigmented nevi of the skin, and when standing with her arms to her side, her hands end up much farther from her legs than usual. What test should be ordered next?

A. LH and FSH level

B. Serum cortisol level

C. 2D echocardiogram

D. MRI of pituitary

E. Transvaginal ultrasound

Genetics

29. A 17-year-old female is brought to her family physician because she has not had her first menstrual period. The patient is short of stature and on examination there are folds of extra skin on both sides of the neck. Cytogenetic analysis reveals a 45 X karyotype. Which of the following is true regarding this patient's underlying disorder?

A. This is a rare cause of secondary amenorrhea.

B. Most cases like this one are caused by abnormal oogenesis.

C. Most fetuses with this disorder are viable.

D. Half of patients with this condition develop hypothyroidism.

E. Congenital heart disease is uncommon in patients with this condition.

Genetics

6.6 Pediatric Diseases—Questions

| Easy | Medium | Hard |

30. A boy is brought to the pediatrician for evaluation of developmental delay. The child is 7 years old and was placed in the second grade for the second year in a row. His teachers note him to be hyperactive and impulsive. On examination his head circumference is below the 10th percentile for sex and age. He has short palpebral fissures, and a thin vermilion border, and his philtrum is smooth. Which of the following is most likely to account for this child's clinical presentation?

A. Congenital infection with *Treponema pallidum*

B. Fetal anoxia during delivery

C. Trinucleotide repeat expansion of a noncoding region of a gene on the X chromosome

D. Trisomy of chromosome 18

E. Maternal alcohol use

Central nervous system

31. A 2-hour-old boy is examined by the pediatrician in the newborn nursery. The child was born at 39 weeks gestational age by uncomplicated vaginal delivery. The child weighed 2300 grams at birth. On examination the child has microcephaly with rounded facies and prominent cheeks, and there is a holosystolic murmur along the left sternal border. The infant feeds poorly during his hospital stay and exhibits a bizarre high-pitched cry. What is the underlying cause of this child's condition?

A. Maternal alcohol use

B. Partial deletion of the short arm of chromosome 5

C. Deletion of band 12 in the long arm of chromosome 15

D. Trisomy of chromosome 13

E. Hexosaminidase deficiency

Central nervous system

32. An 18-month-old male is brought to the emergency department by his parents for severe abdominal pain that began two hours prior to arrival. The pain is intermittent with episodes occurring every 15 minutes accompanied by inconsolable crying with the child drawing his legs up toward his abdomen. Plain abdominal radiograph shows two concentric radiolucent circles in the right upper quadrant as well as dilation of the bowel with air-fluid levels. Which of the following additional signs or symptoms is this patient likely to have at the time of examination?

A. Fever

B. Absent cremasteric reflex

C. Diarrhea

D. Bloody stools

E. Absent bowel sounds

Pediatric, gastrointestinal

33. An 11-month-old male child is brought to the pediatrician because his mother noticed that his eyes have begun to "dance around." She has noticed rhythmic jerking motions of the extremities and worsening of head and limb control. The child has lost weight since his last visit. On examination there are bilateral periobital ecchymoses and a palpable abdominal mass. A biopsy of the mass is likely to reveal which of the following?

A. Diffused densely packed small blue cells with scanty cytoplasm with fibroblast-like stroma and epithelial elements resembling glomeruli and tubules

B. Sheets of primitive-appearing small cells with dark nuclei in a background of eosinophilic fibrillary material with cells concentrically arranged around a central space

C. Intersecting sharply marginated spindle cells with areas of necrosis

D. Sheets of anaplastic lymphoblasts positive for T-cell markers

E. Neoplastic cells with clear-appearing cytoplasm arranged in "nests" between blood vessels

Pediatric, neurologic

34. A 6-year-old female is brought to the pediatrician for evaluation of bloody stools. The patient's mother noticed bloody stools on two occasions a week apart. The child is without complaint and denies any fever, abdominal pain, vomiting, or myalgias. There are no sick contacts at home or at school. Physical examination including external and digital examination of the rectum is normal. An abdominal ultrasound is normal. Nuclear scintigraphy suggests gastric mucosa present within the small bowel. Which of the following is true regarding this disease?

A. It occurs most frequently in the jejunum.

B. It occurs more frequently in females than in males.

C. This disease occurs in 10% of the population.

D. Peptic ulceration at these sites may occur.

E. The abnormality will contain two layers of the bowel wall on microscopic examination.

Pediatric, gastrointestinal

35. A female infant is brought to the pediatrician for evaluation of vomiting. The parents report forceful vomiting immediately after feedings followed by the desire to feed again. The mother says the child is constantly hungry. On examination the child is normal, except for a 1 cm palpable mass in the right upper quadrant at the edge of the rectus abdominis muscle. Which of the following is a known risk factor for development of this disorder?

A. Female sex

B. Age < 3 weeks

C. Recent quinolone antibiotic use

D. Trisomy 18

E. Galactosemia

Pediatric, gastrointestinal

36. A 6-year-old boy is brought to his pediatrician because of pain and swelling in the neck. His temperature is 101.5°F (38.6°C). On examination there is marked swelling of the parotid and submandibular salivary glands and the testicles. What complications is this patient ultimately at risk for?

A. Deafness

B. Blindness

C. Sepsis and shock

D. Mental retardation

E. Renal failure

Pediatric, infectious diseases

37. An infant born at 39 weeks from an uncomplicated vaginal delivery is being evaluated for ambiguous genitalia. On examination the genitalia cannot be determined to be either male or female. A karyotype of peripheral blood leukocytes is 46 XX. A serum chemistry is remarkable for a serum sodium of 130 mEq/L, a serum potassium of 6.0 mEq/L and a serum glucose of 55 mg/dL. What is the next test to order in the workup for the cause of this patient's genital abnormality?

A. Abdominal and pelvic ultrasound

B. 17-OH progesterone level

C. Estradiol level

D. Free and total testosterone level

E. Thyrotropin-stimulating hormone level

Renal, pediatric

38. A 2-year-old child with mental retardation, born with congenital absence of the iris, and cryptorchidism (repaired surgically at age 14 months) is brought to his pediatrician because his mother feels a "lump in his side" while bathing him. On examination, his heart and lung sounds are normal, testes are normal, and there is a palpable mass in the right flank. An ultrasound is ordered, and afterwards a biopsy is performed. Which of the following findings is likely to be found?

A. Monomorphic cells with prominent eosinophilic nucleoli and filamentous intracytoplasmic inclusions

B. A lace-like reticular network of medium-sized cuboidal cells, which stain positive for α-fetoprotein

C. A mixture of ectodermal, mesodermal, and endodermal structures

D. Solid sheets of small primitive cells concentrically arranged around a central space of eosinophilic material

E. Tightly packed blue cells with both blastemal and epithelial components

Renal, pediatric

39. A 12-week pregnant 24-year-old woman with poorly controlled type 2 diabetes mellitus is seen by her obstetrician for routine prenatal care. She wants to know what effect the diabetes may have on her fetus. She should be informed that uncontrolled diabetes places her fetus at risk for which of the following complications?

A. Congenital infection

B. Mental retardation

C. Spina bifida

D. Infantile leukemia

E. Phocomelia

Endocrine, pediatric

40. An 18-year-old woman brings her 15-month-old daughter and her 2-week-old son to the pediatrician. The woman's 15-month-old daughter has a mild upper respiratory tract infection, but otherwise both children are healthy. The mother is concerned about sudden infant death syndrome because a neighbor's child recently died unexpectedly at age 3 months. She wants to know whether her children are at risk and what steps she can take to reduce the risk of sudden infant death syndrome. Which of the following statements regarding her children's risk for sudden death syndrome (SIDS) is true?

A. Female children are at higher risk than male children.

B. Upper respiratory tract infections do not increase the risk of SIDS.

C. Supine sleeping position increases the risk of SIDS.

D. Bed-sharing with parents is safe after age 4 weeks.

E. Her son is at low risk for SIDS at his present age.

Pediatric

41. A 29-year-old man and his 26-year-old wife are evaluated by their family physician for infertility. Past medical, social, and family history are unremarkable. The man's wife has normal regular menstrual periods. A sperm count is obtained that shows no sperm in his semen. The vas deferens cannot be identified on either side on scrotal and transrectal ultrasonography. What is the next step in the management of this patient?

A. Obtain LH, FSH, and serum testosterone levels

B. Genetic counseling

C. Genetic testing

D. Computed tomography of the kidneys and collection system with IV contrast

E. Testicular sperm extraction and in vitro fertilization

Genetic, male reproductive

42. A 2-day-old, 7.4 lb male infant born at 38 weeks by uneventful spontaneous vaginal delivery is evaluated for persistent vomiting. The child has not passed any meconium since delivery. On examination the abdomen is distended and the infant appears uncomfortable. Plain radiographs demonstrate a low, small bowel obstruction. A contrast enema is performed which reveals microcolon and numerous filling defects in the cecum and terminal ileum. The child voids after contrast enema and improves clinically. What additional investigation should be performed at this time?

A. Diagnostic colonoscopy

B. Dilated eye examination by ophthalmology

C. 2D echocardiogram

D. Genetic testing

E. CT abdomen and pelvis with IV and oral contrast

Pediatric, genetic, gastrointestinal

43. A 3-week-old female infant born at 29 weeks gestational age with birth weight of 980 g is evaluated in the neonatal intensive care unit for abdominal distention and worsening respiratory failure. On examination, the patient is afebrile and tachycardic with crackles present in both lung fields. The abdomen is distended and tender, and bowel sounds are absent. Plain abdominal radiographs reveal dilated loops of small bowel with gas bubbles in the small bowel wall and air present in the distal colon. The child is taken to the operating room for emergency surgery. Which of the following is likely to be seen in the surgical specimen?

A. Acute inflammation with neutrophilic infiltrate in the appendix

B. Transmural coagulative necrosis of the small bowel

C. Acute colitis with pseudomembrane formation

D. Acute small bowel obstruction

E. Embolism of the superior mesenteric artery

Gastrointestinal

44. A female infant is born by emergency caesarian section at 27 weeks. The infant requires a brief resuscitation in the delivery room and then is transferred to neonatal ICU. On examination in the NICU, the child is cyanotic, in respiratory distress with tachypnea, and has nasal flaring and retractions, with crackles identified in both lung fields. A plain chest radiograph shows bilateral reticulonodular "ground glass" opacities. After a 1-week NICU course the patient dies. What is the most likely finding in the lungs on autopsy?

A. Honeycombing

B. Interstitial fibrosis

C. Thick eosinophilic membranes lining the alveoli

D. Numerous macrophages containing dusty brown pigment

E. Interstitial pneumonitis with numerous lymphocytes and plasma cells

Pulmonary

45. Had the child in the previous question survived, which additional complications would she have been at risk for?

A. Intraventricular hemorrhage

B. Ventricular septal defect

C. Pyloric stenosis

D. Peripheral neuropathy

E. Diabetes

Pulmonary

46. A couple visits with their family physician for prenatal counseling. The couple has one child, a boy born at 40 weeks by spontaneous vaginal delivery after an uneventful prenatal course. The child was born with a unilateral cleft lip. There is no family history of congenital birth defects. The parents should be counseled that the risk of their second child having cleft lip or palate is . . .

A. Less than 5%

B. 10%

C. 25%

D. 30%

E. Greater than 30%

Genetics, head and neck

47. An infant born at 39 weeks gestation age via uncomplicated vaginal delivery is noted to have a ring-like constriction of the 3rd digit of the right hand and distal amputation of the 4th digit of the right hand at birth. The child is otherwise normal. What type of morphologic anomaly are these findings an example of?

A. Mutation

B. Disruption

C. Malformation

D. Deformation

E. Sequence

Musculoskeletal

6.7 General Genetic Disorders—Answers and Explanations

Easy	Medium	Hard

1.   Correct: Schwann cells and fibroblasts (B)

This patient has the characteristic features of neurofibromatosis type I: neurofibromas and café-au-lait spots. The neurofibromas are benign tumors composed of Schwann cells, fibroblasts, and collagen **(B)**. For **(A, C-E)**, see explanation.

2.   Correct: Eye (E)

The patient in question has neurofibromatosis. Common clinical findings include multiple hyperpigmented maculae (café au lait spots), multiple soft tissue nodules (neurofibromas), and hamartomas on the iris (Lisch nodules) **(E)**. For **(A-D)**, see previous information.

3.   Correct: Meningiomas (D)

The finding of bilateral schwannomas of the acoustic nerve is essentially diagnostic of neurofibromatosis type 2. Other common findings with neurofibromatosis type 2 include meningiomas (which occur in 50% of patients), spinal cord tumors, and soft tissue tumors **(D)**. For **(A-C, E)**, see previous information. These other conditions listed are not commonly associated with NF2.

4.   Correct: Pheochromocytoma (C)

The patient's brother's renal mass is consistent with a renal cell carcinoma. With the presence of a hemangioblastoma the clinical picture is suspicious for von Hippel-Lindau disease. In addition to these tumors, patients with von Hippel-Lindau disease can have pheochromocytomas as well as tumors of the pancreas **(C)**. The other tumors listed are not routinely associated with von Hippel-Lindau's **(A-B, D-E)**.

5.   Correct: Tuberous sclerosis (C)

The history of cardiac tumor in the presence of a subependymal giant cell tumor is consistent with tuberous sclerosis, an autosomal dominant syndrome characterized by multiple hamartomas and benign tumors of the central nervous system (CNS) and other organs **(C)**. Common CNS lesions include cortical tubers and subependymal nodules as well as subependymal giant cell astrocytomas. Subependymal giant cell astrocytomas and rhabdomyomas, the lesion in the heart, are not routinely found in the other conditions listed **(A-B, D-E)**.

6.8 Enzyme Deficiencies and Inborn Errors of Metabolism—Answers and Explanations

Easy	Medium	Hard

6.   Correct: Galactosemia (D)

The constellation of hepatomegaly, infantile cataracts, and a positive urinary reducing substance is highly suggestive of galactosemia **(D)**. Galactose, fructose and glucose are the most important urinary reducing substances and of the three, glucose is most common. However, there are several additional findings in this patient that suggest another diagnosis. For **(A-C, E)**, see previous information.

7.   Correct: *Escherichia coli* (A)

The most common cause of sepsis in infants with galactosemia is *Escherichia coli* (up to to 80% of cases). **(B-E)** are incorrect.

8. Correct: He is at increased risk for necrotizing panniculitis. (E)

This patient suffers from α-1-antitrypsin deficiency, an autosomal recessive disorder caused by misfolding of a protein, which inactivates neutrophil elastase **(A)**. His son's risk of inheritance is low, barring parental consanguinity **(B)**. Lung disease in α-1-antitrypsin deficiency is characterized by panacinar emphysema, which unlike most other types of pulmonary emphysema, characteristically involves the lower rather than upper lung lobes **(C)**. Smoking increases the risk of development of emphysema in these patients, as with other causes of emphysema **(D)**. Development of necrotizing panniculitis is a well described though less common extra-pulmonary manifestation of this disease.

9. Correct: Axonal loss and gliosis of the posterior columns, spinocerebellar tracts, and distal corticospinal tracts (D)

This patient suffers from Friedreich ataxia, an autosomal recessive disorder and the most common hereditary ataxia. The disease is characterized by loss of axons and gliosis in the posterior columns, distal corticospinal tracts, and spinocerebellar tracts as well as neuronal degeneration in the brainstem, cerebellum, and motor cortex **(E)**. Ataxia-telangiectasia **(A)** presents at a much earlier age and is associated with immunodeficiency. Degeneration of the anterior spinal roots **(B)** would be seen in amyotrophic lateral sclerosis, consistent with this disease's primary involvement of the motor neurons and sparing of sensory roots. Neurofibrillary tangles **(C)** are seen in Alzheimer's disease. **(E)** describes the characteristic feature of Krabbe's disease.

10. Correct: Trinucleotide repeat expansion (A)

Most cases of Friedreich ataxia are caused by trinucleotide repeat expansion in the frataxin gene resulting in diminished or absent production of the gene product **(A)**. For **(B-D)**, see previous information.

11. Correct: Incomplete penetrance (C)

This trait clearly demonstrates the ability to be passed along both maternal and paternal lines, making mitochondrial inheritance **(A)** incorrect. The trait is passed by an unaffected male to his offspring, a phenomenon that would contradict X-linked recessive inheritance **(B)**. The daughters of an affected man are unaffected, making X-linked dominant inheritance **(D)** incorrect. The disease does not appear to skip generations, making autosomal recessive inheritance **(E)** unlikely. The inheritance pattern shown is characteristic of autosomal dominant inheritance with incomplete penetrance, meaning that some individuals with the trait do not manifest the disease.

12. Correct: Phenylketonuria (C)

This patient exhibits several features of classic phenylketonuria, including mental retardation, seizures, fair hair and skin, and a peculiar musty or "mousy" odor **(C)**. Many of the inborn errors of metabolism are characterized by particular odors. Children with maple syrup urine disease may have a sweet odor to the urine or an odor said to be similar to curry **(B)**. Isovaleric acidemia causes an odor similar to valerian root or sweaty feet **(A)**, and multiple carboxylase deficiency causes an odor similar to cat urine **(E)**. The clinical presentation is inconsistent with galactosemia **(D)**.

6.9 Genetic Diseases of Structural Proteins— Answers and Explanations

Easy	Medium	Hard

13. Correct: 2D echocardiogram (C)

The presence of lens dislocation (ectopia lentis) and dolichocephaly is suggestive of Marfan's syndrome. The patient should be evaluated with electrocardiography and echocardiography **(C)** prior to surgery to exclude significant dilation of the aortic root, valvular disease, and aortic dissection (which causes up to 45% of deaths in patients with Marfan's syndrome). For **(A-B, D-E)**, previous information.

14. Correct: Defect in collagen (C)

This patient's constellation of findings is consistent with classic Ehlers-Danlos syndrome, caused by a mutation in the gene for Type IV collagen **(C)**. Marfan's syndrome is caused by a mutation in fibrillin **(A)**. A mutation in dystrophin is the cause of muscular dystrophy **(B)**. Defects in TGF-β and elastase have not been described to cause these symptoms **(D-E)**.

15. Correct: Marfan's syndrome (D)

The history of sudden death due to a ruptured thoracic aortic aneurysm in a tall young patient is suggestive of Marfan's syndrome. The presence of cystic medial degeneration, the classic histologic finding of Marfan's syndrome, is consistent with the diagnosis. Takayasu's arteritis, syphilitic aortitis, and giant cell arteritis can cause a thoracic aortic aneurysm, but the histologic appearance is different **(A-C)**. Essential hypertension is not commonly associated with thoracic aortic aneurysms, especially at such a young age **(E)**.

16.   Correct: Myxomatous mitral valve (C)

This patient has a clinical history suggestive of Marfan's syndrome combined with a characteristic histologic finding for that disorder. Cardiac complications of Marfan's syndrome include aortic dissection, valvular incompetence, and heart failure. Patients can have a myxomatous mitral valve (**C**). The other conditions (**A-B, D-E**) are not associated with Marfan's syndrome.

6.10 Lysosomal and Storage Disorders—Answers and Explanations

Easy	Medium	Hard

17.   Correct: Tay-Sachs disease (B)

This patient suffers from Tay-Sachs disease, an autosomal recessive disorder caused by mutations that prevent degradation of GM2 gangliosides (**B**). The clinical picture can be difficult to discern from severe Neiman-Pick disease, which can also cause the "cherry-red" spot described in the disease; however, the finding of whorled membranes in lysosomes combined with the absence of hepatosplenomegaly makes Tay-Sachs more likely (**A**). For (**C-E**), see previous information.

18.   Correct: Inability to degrade heparan sulfate and dermatan sulfate (A)

This patient suffers from Hurler's syndrome, characterized by coarsening of the facial features, mental retardation, hepatomegaly, joint stiffness, and corneal clouding. Hurler's syndrome is an autosomal recessive disease cause by deficiency of α-L-iduronase, an enzyme which degrades heparan and dermatan sulfate (**A**). For (**B-E**), see previous information.

19.   Correct: Deficiency of sphingomyelinase (B)

This patient has Niemann-Pick disease, an autosomal recessive disease caused by a deficiency of sphingomyelinase (**B**). The classic histologic finding is the "zebra body," a concentric lamellated figure found within the dilated lysosomes. Niemann-Pick disease can be difficult to distinguish from Tay-Sachs disease clinically; however, hepatomegaly is not present in Tay-Sachs disease (**A**). Gaucher's disease (**C**) does not commonly affect the central nervous system. The clinical features and pathologic findings in this patient do not support the diagnosis of Hurler's syndrome (**D**) or von Gierke's disease (**E**).

20.   Correct: Normal blood lactate levels after exercise (C)

This patient suffers from McArdle's disease, an autosomal recessive glycogen storage disease caused by mutation in the muscle isoform of the enzyme phosphorylase. This disease affects skeletal muscle only, unlike other glycogen storage diseases. The classic finding is a failure of exercise to elevate blood lactate levels (**C**). The disease is rare, and the majority of patients report a family history. For (**A-B, D-E**), see previous information.

21.   Correct: von Gierke's disease (D)

Von Gierke's disease, a glycogen storage disease caused by deficiency of glucose-6-phosphatase, should be suspected in any infant with hypoglycemia, hepatomegaly, and elevated triglyceride and lactic acid levels (**D**). Galactosemia usually presents shortly after birth (**A**). Tay-Sachs disease does not ordinarily cause hepatomegaly (**B**). The clinical presentation is inconsistent with Gaucher's or Pompe's disease (**C, E**).

22.   Correct: Autosomal recessive (C)

The child in this case suffers from Pompe's disease, an autosomal recessive disease (**C**) caused by mutation in the gene for lysosomal glucosidase (acid maltase). The finding of hypotonia with massive cardiomegaly and normal blood glucose levels is classic for Pompe's disease. For (**A-B, D-E**), see previous information.

6.11 Chromosomal Disorders—Answers and Explanations

Easy	Medium	Hard

23.   Correct: Robertsonian translocation of chromosome 21 (C)

This patient has classic features of Down's syndrome. In the case of a Robertsonian translocation, chromosome 21 can be translocated onto another acrocentric chromosome, causing the resultant gamete to carry two copies of chromosome 21 and a normal number of chromosomes (**C**). Nondisjunction of chromosome 21 during maternal meiosis is the most common cause of Down's syndrome, and karyotypes of these patients will show 47 chromosomes with three copies of chromosome 21 (**A**). Less commonly, some patients have a mixture of trisomic and normal cells and a blended phenotype. In that circumstance, nondisjunction has occurred in the embryo early in development, rather than in parental meiosis and gametogenesis. For (**B, D-E**), see previous information.

24. Correct: Edward's syndrome (C)

This patient has trisomy 18 (Edward's syndrome) (**C**). There is no mention of epicanthal folds or a flattened nasal bridge to suggest Down's syndrome, and rocker bottom feet, as described in the question, are not typical features of Down's syndrome, velocardiofacial syndrome, or fragile X syndrome (**A, D, E**). The absence of cleft palate, polydactyly, or micropthalmia make Patau's syndrome (**B**) incorrect.

25. Correct: Deletion of part of chromosome 22 (C)

The patient presents with characteristic findings of DiGeorge's syndrome, caused by a deletion of band 11.2q on chromosome 22 (22q11.2) (**C**). The history of neonatal tetanus and cleft palate repair is inconsistent with Patau's syndrome (trisomy 13), Bruton agammaglobulinemia, fragile X syndrome, or a mitochondrial disease (**A-B, D-E**).

26. Correct: If the child's parents have a daughter, she has a 50% chance of being affected (E)

The patient suffers from fragile X syndrome. This disease is caused by amplification of CGG trinucleotide repeats in an untranslated region of the *FMR1* gene on the X chromosome, which leads to abnormal methylation of the gene, leading to dysfunction in the promoter region and transcriptional suppression of the *FMR1* gene. Because this patient is male, the abnormality would have to have been transmitted by his mother (his father would not have transmitted an X chromosome to a male child), making (**A**) incorrect. The child is capable of passing the mutation on to his offspring (**B**). The name "fragile X" is a misnomer caused by weak staining of the expanded region of the chromosome, giving the appearance of a "break" in the chromosome (**C**). In this case the patient's children are not likely to be more severely affected than the patient, as the trinucleotide expansion occurs during oogenesis, not spermatogenesis (**D**). Carrier females have a 50% chance of being affected for reasons that are not understood (**E**).

27. Correct: Breast cancer (D)

Patients with Klinefelter's syndrome are at much higher risk to develop breast cancer than the general male population (**D**). There is some evidence that patients with Klinefelter's syndrome may be at increased risk of non-Hodgkin's lymphoma, but these patients appear to be at average or lower risk for Hodgkin's lymphoma and the other cancers listed as answer choices (**A-C, E**).

28. Correct: 2D echocardiogram (C)

This patient suffers from Turner's syndrome (45 X). The incidence of coarctation of the aorta in this patient population is roughly 30%. All patients with Turner's syndrome should be screened for this poten-tially reversible cause of hypertension and heart failure, especially in the setting of hypertension (**C**). For (**A-B, D-E**), see previous information.

29. Correct: Half of patients with this condition develop hypothyroidism (D)

Up to half of patients with Turner's syndrome develop autoimmune hypothyroidism (**D**). Turner's syndrome is the most common cause of secondary amenorrhea (**A**). In 75% of cases of Turner's syndrome, the X chromosome is maternally derived, indicating that most cases are associated with abnormalities in paternal gametogenesis (**B**). Up to 99% of 45X fetuses are nonviable and are spontaneously aborted (**C**). 30 to 50% of patients have some form of congenital heart disease (aortic coarctation, bicuspid aortic valve, etc.) (**E**).

6.12 Pediatric Diseases—Answers and Explanations

Easy	Medium	Hard

30. Correct: Maternal alcohol use (E)

The patient exhibits classic physical characteristics associated with fetal alcohol syndrome (**E**). Congenital syphilis is characterized by notched incisors, persistent mucopurulent nasal discharge, and outward curvature of the anterior tibia, among other findings (**A**). Fetal anoxia during delivery would not be expected to produce physical malformations (**B**). The description of the patient is inconsistent with either fragile X syndrome (**C**) or Edward's syndrome (**D**).

31. Correct: Partial deletion of the short arm of chromosome 5 (B)

The high-pitched bizarre "cat-like cry" of 5p- deletion syndrome gives rise to its other name, cri du chat (cry of the cat). The child lacks other features of fetal alcohol syndrome (**A**) such as smooth philtrum and thin vermilion border. The child lacks any other features to suggest either Angelman's or Prader-Willi syndromes (**C**) or Patau's syndrome (**D**). Tay-Sachs disease (**E**) typically is asymptomatic at birth with progressive neurologic decline after age 6 months.

32. Correct: Bloody stools (D)

This child has a classic history for intussusception with evidence of bowel obstruction on imaging as well as a "target sign." The classic triad of signs and symptoms of intussusception include colicky abdominal pain, currant jelly bloody stools, and a sausage-shaped abdominal mass palpated in the right upper quadrant (**D**). Intussusception may be mistaken for acute gastroenteritis, though fever and diarrhea are not present in intussusception (**A, C**).

An absent cremasteric reflex would be expected in testicular torsion, a condition which does not cause bowel obstruction (**B**). Likewise in bowel obstruction, bowel sounds are present, though usually high-pitched (**E**).

33. Correct: Sheets of primitive-appearing small cells with dark nuclei in a background of eosinophilic fibrillary material with cells concentrically arranged around a central space (B)

This child has two clinical signs of neuroblastoma, opsoclonus myoclonus syndrome and periorbital ecchymoses ("raccoon eyes"). (**B**) describes the typical appearance of neuroblastoma as well as classic Homer-Wright pseudorosettes. For (**A, C-E**), see previous information.

34. Correct: Peptic ulceration at these sites may occur. (D)

This child has a Meckel diverticulum causing gastrointestinal bleeding. The "rule of 2's" is typically used to remember the features of Meckel diverticulum. The diverticulum occurs within 2 feet of the ileocecal valve, is usually 2 inches long, occurs in 2% of the population, and is 2 times more likely in males than in females. Meckel diverticula are usually composed of normal bowel wall with three bowel wall layers; however, ectopic gastric tissue is not uncommon, is more common in patients with gastrointestinal bleeding, and can lead to peptic ulceration and perforation (**D**). For (**A-C, E**), see previous information.

35. Correct: Trisomy 18 (D)

Congenital hypertrophic pyloric stenosis is more common in males (**A**), usually presents between ages 3 and 5 weeks of age (**B**), and is associated with macrolide antibiotic exposure (azithromycin or erythromycin) (**C**). Galactosemia may be mistaken for pyloric stenosis, but there is no described association (**E**). The condition is more common in patients with trisomy 18, trisomy 21, and Turner's syndrome (**D**). The condition has a multifactorial pattern of inheritance.

36. Correct: Deafness (A)

In the pre-vaccine era, mumps was a common cause of sensorineural deafness in children (**A**). The acute illness causes swelling of the salivary glands and testes. Other common complications include reduced fertility in males and aseptic meningitis. Blindness, renal failure, mental retardation, and sepsis are not a feature of this disease (**B-E**).

37. Correct: 17-OH progesterone level (B)

This infant has laboratory evidence of mineralocorticoid deficiency with genital virilization, both consistent with congenital adrenal hyperplasia (CAH). Classic congenital hyperplasia due to 21-hydroxylase deficiency accounts for 90% of cases of CAH and is characterized by very high levels of 17-hydroxyprogesterone (**B**). For (**A, C-E**), see previous explanation.

38. Correct: Tightly packed blue cells with both blastemal and epithelial components (E)

This patient suffers from WAGR syndrome, caused by deletion of 11p13. This disorder is characterized by Wilms tumor, Aniridia, Genital abnormalities, and mental Retardation (WAGR). The histologic findings in Wilms tumor are described in (**E**). Up to 50% of these patients will develop Wilms tumor. (**A**) describes a rare and deadly renal malignancy (rhabdoid tumor) seen almost exclusively in children under the age of 2 years. Yolk sac tumor (**B**) is the most common testicular tumor in children, however, this patient's mass is intra-abdominal and his testicular examination is unremarkable. Teratomas (**C**) are tumors consisting of components resembling normal derivatives of more than one germ layer. (**D**) describes the classic Homer-Wright rosettes characteristic of neuroblastoma.

39. Correct: Spina bifida (C)

Maternal diabetes increases the risk of several birth defects, including neural tube defects and congenital heart disease as well as both macrosomia and intrauterine growth retardation, polyhydramnios, and macrosomia-related birth injuries such as shoulder dystocia (**C**). For (**A-B, D-E**), see previous information.

40. Correct: Her son is at low risk for SIDS at his present age (E)

Male children are at higher risk for SIDS than female children (**A**). A preceding upper respiratory tract infection is common in infants who later die of SIDS (**B**). The supine sleeping position is associated with a lower risk of SIDS (**C**). Bed-sharing with parents increases the risk of infant death (**D**). Infants are at highest risk for SIDS between the ages of 2 and 4 months (**E**).

41. Correct: Genetic counseling (B)

Mutation in the *CFTR* gene is found in up to 50% of men with congenital bilateral absence of vas deferens (CBAVD). 98% of men with cystic fibrosis have this condition, which almost always causes infertility in these patients. If imaging of the kidneys is necessary, an ultrasound would allow for screening of renal malformations or anomalies without the risks associated with radiation and contrast dye (**D**). Genetic testing would be inappropriate if done before genetic counseling (**C**). Genetic counseling should always be performed before genetic testing to inform the patient of the risks, benefits, limitations, and consequences of testing (**B**). Likewise, given the association of this condition with a serious genetic disease, assisted reproduction would be inappropriate prior to genetic counseling (**E**). LH, FSH, and testosterone testing would not be useful (**A**).

42. Correct: Genetic testing (D)

The patient suffers from meconium ileus, a bowel obstruction characterized by failure to pass meconium within the first 24 hours of life caused by thick tenacious meconium. The finding of microcolon with meconium filling defects in the ileum and cecum is characteristic of this condition. The condition is strongly associated with cystic fibrosis, and patients with this condition should undergo genetic testing for mutations in the *CFTR* gene (**D**). For (**A-C, E**), see previous information.

43. Correct: Transmural coagulative necrosis of the small bowel (B)

The presence of gas bubbles in the small bowel wall is pathognomonic of necrotizing enterocolitis. The dilated loops of small bowel with gas present in the colon is suggestive of ileus rather than obstruction (**D**). Neonatal appendicitis is difficult to distinguish from necrotizing enterocolitis except by laparotomy; however, neonatal appendicitis is a much rarer condition (**A**). Colitis with pseudomembrane formation is the hallmark of *Clostridium difficile* infection; however, the radiologic studies demonstrate gas in the small bowel (**C**). An embolism of the superior mesenteric artery would be rare in infants (**E**).

44. Correct: Thick eosinophilic membranes lining the alveoli (C)

This is a classic presentation of neonatal respiratory distress syndrome, also known as hyaline disease of the newborn, thus named because of the characteristic eosinophilic (hyaline) membranes lining the alveoli (**C**). For (**A-B, D-E**), see previous information.

45. Correct: Intraventricular hemorrhage (A)

Preterm infants are at risk for many complications, including intraventricular hemorrhage, retinopathy of prematurity, patent ductus arteriosus, and necrotizing enterocolitis (**A**), but not the remainder of the conditions listed (**B-E**).

46. Correct: Less than 5% (A)

Cleft lip is a birth defect that is multifactorial with both genetic and environmental factors playing a role. The recurrence risk for most multifactorial birth defects is 2 to 5% for parents with one affected child (**A**). Other birth defects with multifactorial inheritance include spina bifida, congenital hip dysplasia, and pyloric stenosis. (**B-E**) are incorrect.

47. Correct: Disruption (B)

Band-like constrictions and amputations of fingers are typical of amniotic bands, an example of a disruption (secondary destruction of an organ or body region previously normal in development) (**B**). These types of abnormalities are not usually indicative of genetic damage (**A**) and carry no risk of recurrence in subsequent pregnancies. Malformations are primary defects in organogenesis due to inherent abnormalities in development and are frequently genetic in origin (**C**). A deformation consists of abnormal development of a body part or organ system due to extrinsic mechanical factors such as uterine constraint (**D**). Sequences are cascades of anomalies caused by a single primary aberration (such as oligohydramnios and Potter sequence) (**E**).

Chapter 7

Environmental and Nutritional Diseases

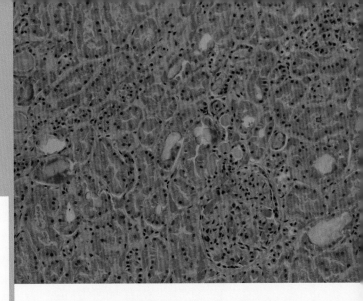

LEARNING OBJECTIVES

7.1 Environmental Toxins

► Identify carbon monoxide poisoning and understand the physiologic effects of carbon monoxide

► Identify asbestosis

► Recognize common symptoms and hematologic findings in lead toxicity

► Recognize arsenic poisoning

► Recognize silicosis and know the common complications of silicosis

► Describe the association between liver angiosarcoma and polyvinyl chloride exposure

7.2 Injury by Therapeutic Drugs

► Recognize methemoglobinemia and list the common causes

► Know the common side effects of oral contraceptive pills (OCPs)

► Recognize warfarin-induced skin necrosis and its association with protein C deficiency

► Recognize salicylate intoxication

► Describe the pathologic findings of an acetaminophen-induced liver injury

► Describe the long-term complications of radiotherapy and chemotherapeutic agents

► Given the clinical scenario, diagnose cobalt toxicity

7.3 Drugs of Abuse

► Recognize levamisole-induced skin necrosis as a complication of cocaine abuse

► Recognize common complications of cocaine abuse

► Recognize signs and symptoms of MDMA (ecstasy) abuse

► Recognize cannabis-induced cyclic vomiting syndrome

7.4 Malnutrition and Dietary Deficiencies

► Identify Wernicke-Korsakoff syndrome and describe the typical pathologic findings

► Recognize refeeding syndrome and describe the role of phosphorus in this disorder

► Describe the pathologic changes associated with vitamin A deficiency

► Describe the pathologic changes associated with vitamin B2 deficiency

► describe the pathologic changes associated with folic acid deficiency

► Describe the complications of morbid obesity

► Given the clinical scenario, diagnose B12 deficiency; describe the association between nitrous oxide and B12 deficiency

► Given the clinical scenario and laboratory testing, diagnose copper deficiency

7.1 Environmental Toxins— Questions

Easy	Medium	Hard

1. A 55-year-old man presents at the start of flu season with headache, malaise, and confusion. His vital signs are temperature 98.7°F (38° C), pulse 110/min, respiratory rate 24/min, and blood pressure 155/92 mm Hg. On examination his lungs are clear, heart sounds are normal, and he has a rosy appearance of his lips and skin. He is slightly confused and oriented only to person. Influenza A and B antigen tests are negative, a complete blood count is normal, and plain chest radiograph is unremarkable. Which additional test is likely to reveal his diagnosis?

A. Pulse oximetry

B. Electrocardiogram

C. CT of the head without contrast

D. Complete blood count

E. Arterial blood gas

Respiratory

2. A 64-year-old retired mechanic presents to his primary care physician for shortness of breath. He has mild hypertension and has never smoked. The symptoms began gradually 6 months ago and have worsened to the point that the patient cannot mow his lawn without resting. His vital signs are temperature 98.6°F (37°C), pulse 61/min, blood pressure 140/92 mmHg, and respiratory rate 18/min. Examination is normal except for fine bibasilar crackles. Plain chest radiograph shows bibasilar fibrosis and pleural plaques. A CT-guided biopsy of the lungs would most likely show which of the following?

A. Macrophages containing hemosiderin

B. Ferruginous bodies

C. Macrophages containing black pigment

D. Abundant silica

E. Widespread granulomas

Respiratory

3. A 56-year-old man presents to his primary care physician for depression. His symptoms began 6 months previously and are accompanied by fatigue, myalgias, and insomnia. His medical history is significant only for mild dyslipidemia, controlled by diet. His vital signs are normal, and his physical examination reveals weakness for the right foot to dorsiflexion and a bluish discoloration at the gum-tooth line. His serum thyroid-stimulating hormone level is normal. Complete blood count is remarkable for a hemoglobin level of 9.2 g/dL and MCV of 72 fL. His blood urea nitrogen level is 42 mg/dL and serum creatinine is 1.7 mg/dL. An examination of his peripheral blood smear would most likely show which of the following?

A. Rouleaux formation

B. Myeloid blasts with Auer rods

C. Basophilic stippling of the red cells

D. Multilobated neutrophils

E. Leukocytosis with basophil predominance

Neurologic, hematologic

4. A 38-year-old factory worker is brought to the emergency department by coworkers after developing severe cramping abdominal pain with diarrhea and vomiting. He is admitted and placed on intravenous fluids. Twelve hours after admission he becomes confused, and his serum creatinine increases from 0.5 mg/dL to 3.8 mg/dL. With supportive care, he improves and is discharged from the hospital five days after admission. Two weeks after the initial illness, the man returns to the hospital complaining of numbness and tingling in the hands and feet. At the time of his second admission, his laboratory studies are remarkable for a serum creatinine of 2.1 mg/dL, a leukocyte count of 2700 cells/μL, a serum hemoglobin of 9.3 mg/dL, platelet count of 54,000 cells/μL, ALT of 502 units/L, and serum total bilirubin of 6.3 mg/dL. Occupational exposure to which of the following would explain this man's constellation of signs and symptoms?

A. Mercury

B. Cadmium

C. Lead

D. Arsenic

E. Hydrocarbon fumes

Neurologic, hematologic, renal, gastrointestinal

5. A 55-year-old man presents to his primary care physician complaining of progressively worsening shortness of breath. The patient has smoked one pack of cigarettes daily for the past 30 years and worked in the demolition industry from age 24 until age 41. Physical examination is normal except for bilateral crackles. Plain chest radiograph shows numerous nodules less than 5 mm in diameter mainly in the upper lobes. Which complications of this illness is this patient at risk for?

A. Lymphoma

B. Tuberculosis

C. Mesothelioma

D. Liver failure

E. Meningitis

Respiratory

6. A 67-year-old man is sent for liver biopsy by his internist after a workup for jaundice revealed a liver mass. The biopsy shows angiosarcoma. Exposure to which of the following agents is a risk factor for this malignancy?

A. Naphthalene

B. Aldehydes

C. Benzene

D. Aflatoxin

E. Vinyl chloride

Gastrointestinal

7.2 Injury by Therapeutic Drugs—Questions

Easy	Medium	Hard

7. A 37-year-old woman undergoes upper endoscopy for workup of possible peptic ulcer disease. She receives topical anesthesia of the upper airway with 20% benzocaine spray, an intravenous injection of midazolam and fentanyl for sedation, and intravenous ondansetron for nausea. During the procedure a large nonbleeding peptic ulcer is observed, and the patient is given a dose of intravenous esomeprazole. While in the recovery room, she becomes hypoxic. On examination her skin and nail beds are blue; she is tachycardic and breathing at 26 breaths/min. An arterial blood gas is immediately drawn, and the respiratory therapist notes a blue-brown color of the arterial blood. Which of the following is the most likely cause of this patient's hypoxia?

A. Benzocaine

B. Fentanyl

C. Midazolam

D. Ondansetron

E. Esomeprazole

Respiratory, hematologic

8. A 42-year-old G2P2 female smoker with a history of well-controlled hypertension presents to her gynecologist for a refill on her estrogen-only oral contraceptive. Her last cervical cancer screening at age 40 was normal. She has no family history of breast or ovarian cancer. Which of the following counseling should she be provided?

A. The medication increases her risk of ovarian cancer

B. The medication increases her risk of endometrial cancer

C. The medication increases her risk of thromboembolism

D. The medication lowers her risk of heart disease

E. The medication lowers her risk of cervical cancer

Reproductive

9. A 56-year-old woman was started on anticoagulation with Coumadin for venous thromboembolism and presents to the emergency department a week later with purple-black discoloration of both breasts. She is admitted, the Coumadin is discontinued, and she is started on subcutaneous low-molecular-weight heparin. By the third hospital day large bullae from sloughing of the skin are present. Which of the following is most likely to have contributed to this condition?

A. Lupus anticoagulant

B. Protein C deficiency

C. Factor V Leiden

D. Concomitant aspirin therapy

E. Subtherapeutic doses of Coumadin

Dermatologic, hematologic

10. A 17-year-old female is brought to the emergency department by police after she was witnessed to ingest an unmarked bottle of liquid in an apparent suicide attempt. On evaluation the patient expresses remorse, but states that she does not know what substance she ingested. Her vital signs are temperature 99.9°F (37.7°C), pulse is 110/min, blood pressure 148/90 mm Hg, and respiratory rate 27/min. The patient is somewhat confused; however, she reports a "ringing" in her ears. Arterial blood gas reveals a pH of 7.5, pCO_2 of 31 mm Hg, and HCO_3 of 22 mEq/L. What substance is the most likely cause of her intoxication?

A. Methanol

B. Acetaminophen

C. Salicylate

D. Hydrocarbon

E. Ammonia

Respiratory

11. A 26-year-old woman ingests a large quantity of acetaminophen at home in a suicide attempt. She experiences nausea and vomiting that resolves, and she does not seek medical attention. She is brought to the emergency department 36 hours after the ingestion by relatives after they discovered she was suicidal. Despite appropriate medical care, the woman dies of multiorgan failure 9 days after admission. What is most likely to be seen at autopsy?

A. Centrilobular necrosis of the liver

B. Infarction of the liver

C. Portal vein thrombosis

D. Cirrhosis of the liver

E. Periportal fibrosis

Gastrointestinal

12. A 40-year old male, long-term survivor of Hodgkin lymphoma, presents for routine follow-up. His treatment included chest radiotherapy and chemotherapy with doxorubicin and bleomycin. He wishes to know the long-term effects of his prior treatment. He should be counseled that he is at increased risk for all of the following except?

A. Coronary artery disease

B. Pulmonary fibrosis

C. Cardiomyopathy

D. Thyroid disease

E. Prostate cancer

Heme

13. A 59-year-old male, former professional football player with a history of dyslipidemia that is well-controlled with simvastatin, bilateral total knee arthroplasty, and left total hip arthroplasty presents with shortness of breath. On examination he has crackles in both lung fields and an audible S3. A 2D echocardiogram shows an ejection fraction of 30%. The patient had a normal nuclear stress one year ago with an ejection fraction at that time of 55%. On further questioning the patient reports progressive memory loss and worsening in both his visual acuity and hearing over the preceding 6 months as well as a burning pain in both feet which started 3 months ago. What is the most likely diagnosis?

A. Chronic traumatic encephalopathy

B. Cobalmin (vitamin B12) deficiency

C. Adverse effect of statin therapy

D. Amyotrophic lateral sclerosis

E. Cobalt toxicity

Lungs, central nervous system

7.3 Drugs of Abuse— Questions

Easy	Medium	Hard

14. An 18-year-old male cocaine abuser presents to his primary care physician with purpuric, necrotic lesions of the face including both malar eminences and necrosis of the distal third of the nose and both ears as well as purpura on both arms and legs. Complete blood count is significant for a leukocyte count of 2,800 cells/μL and a platelet count of 89,000 cells/μL. Antineutrophil cytoplasmic antibodies and lupus anticoagulant are both positive. Which of the following is most likely to have caused this patient's condition?

A. Systemic lupus erythematosus

B. Cotton fever

C. Exposure to an antihelminthic drug

D. Frostbite

E. A blood-borne pathogen

Dermatologic, vascular

15. A 42-year-old man presents to the emergency room with substernal chest pain which started 3 hours prior to arrival. He describes the pain as severe, radiating to the back between the shoulder blades. His temperature is 99.9°F (37.7°C), pulse is 115/min, respirations are 22/min, and blood pressure is 195/110 mm Hg. On examination he is diaphoretic and tachycardic. There is a grade 2/6 diastolic murmur heard best in the right sternal border. His lungs are clear. An electrocardiogram shows sinus tachycardia with left ventricular hypertrophy. A plain chest radiograph shows widened mediastinum. Which of the following recreational drugs is most commonly associated with this condition?

A. Methadone

B. MDMA ("ecstasy")

C. Cocaine

D. Phencyclidine

E. Ketamine

Vascular

16. A 17-year-old female is brought to the emergency department after three seizures at home. Her parents report that she was out late at a party with friends. She has no past medical history. On arrival she is encephalopathic. Her temperature is 104.4°F (40.2°C), pulse is 125/min, respirations are 28/min, and blood pressure is 180/105 mm Hg. A serum sodium drawn in the emergency department is 108 mEq/L. Computed tomography of the head shows cerebral edema. Which of the following recreational drugs is the most likely cause of the patient's symptoms?

A. Methamphetamine

B. MDMA ("ecstasy")

C. Cocaine

D. Phencyclidine

E. Ketamine

Neurologic

17. A 24-year-old male is seen in the emergency department for nausea and vomiting for the fifth time in nine months. He reports severe intractable vomiting that began two days ago, is associated with severe nausea, and is improved by lying in a hot bath. The patient denies headache, vertigo, fever, or diarrhea. Typically these episodes of vomiting last for three days and resolve spontaneously. Prior workup includes a CT of the abdomen and an MRI of the brain, both of which are normal. His neurologic and abdominal exam is normal and lab work including complete blood count, liver enzymes, chemistry, amylase, and lipase are normal except for a slight metabolic alkalosis. Which recreational drug is most likely to be associated with this patient's symptoms?

A. Cocaine

B. Methamphetamine

C. Cannabis

D. Ecstasy (MDMA)

E. Bath salts

Neurologic

7.4 Malnutrition and Dietary Deficiencies—Questions

Easy	Medium	Hard

18. A 63-year-old man is brought to the hospital by neighbors because of confusion. They report that the man has become increasingly disoriented over the preceding three weeks. According to his neighbors he is widowed, lives in dilapidated conditions, and has drunk alcohol very heavily for the entire ten years they have known him. On examination he is disheveled, oriented only to self, his gait is slow, wide-based, and ataxic, and there is nystagmus to lateral gaze on both sides. Strength in the upper and lower extremities is 4/5 throughout, with no focal weakness. There is diminished sensation to light touch in the bilateral feet. Patellar tendon reflexes are diminished and ankle jerk reflexes are absent. Of the following, which part of the brain is most likely to demonstrate characteristic pathology of this man's disease?

A. Cerebellum

B. Brainstem

C. Cerebrum

D. Mammillary bodies

E. Hypothalamus

Neurologic

19. A severely malnourished man from a small village in Africa is taken under the care of a missionary family. The patient's body mass is 15.5 kg/m². He is aggressively fed with nutritious high-calorie and high-protein foods. After a week the patient worsens dramatically. He is taken to an aid station in a nearby village. On examination his temperature is 95.9°F (35.5°C), heart rate is 90/min, and blood pressure is 86/52 mm Hg. On examination he is lethargic and jugular venous pressure is measured at 10 cm H_2O. An S3 is audible and there are crackles in both lung fields. Which of the following is most likely to have caused this patient's condition?

A. Hyperglycemia

B. Hypophosphatemia

C. Polycythemia

D. Thyrotoxicosis

E. Myocardial infarction

Gastrointestinal, cardiovascular

20. A 12-year-old boy is evaluated in a local hospital for malnutrition. On examination he is noted to have dry conjunctiva with softening of the corneas and areas of abnormal keratinized patches on the conjunctiva. Adequate dietary intake of which of the following foods would likely have prevented this condition?

A. Black beans

B. Animal fat

C. Barley

D. Squash

E. Wheat bread

Eye

21. A 36-year-old female with celiac disease is brought to her internist for evaluation of nonresolving sores at the corners of the mouth bilaterally. On examination, her physician notices a smooth reddened appearance to the tongue with several sores on the oral mucosa and lips. Dietary deficiency of which of the following would most likely produce these symptoms?

A. Vitamin B1

B. Vitamin B2

C. Vitamin B3

D. Vitamin C

E. Vitamin E

Gastrointestinal

22. A 36-year-old female has laboratory testing during a routine physical examination. A complete blood count reveals a hemoglobin of 9.9 g/dL with a mean corpuscular volume of 108 fL and a normal leukocyte and platelet count. She denies alcohol use. A follow-up methylmalonic acid level is normal at 155 nmol/L and homocysteine level is elevated at 4.3 mg/L. Which finding would be expected on the patient's peripheral blood smear?

A. Hypersegmented neutrophils

B. Spiculated red cells

C. Bite cells

D. Teardrop-shaped red cells

E. Smudge cells

Heme

23. A 42-year-old man with well-controlled hypertension and morbid obesity (BMI 42 kg/m²) presents to his family physician complaining of fatigue. He states that he began to notice excessive daytime tiredness 6 months ago. He denies any chest pain or dyspnea. On examination his temperature is 98.8°F (32°C), pulse is 65/min, and blood pressure is 144/78 mm Hg. On examination heart and lung sounds are normal and his neurologic exam is unremarkable. A 12-lead EKG shows normal sinus rhythm. A complete blood count shows a hemoglobin level of 18.2 g/dL with normal leukocytes and platelets. Serum thyroid stimulating hormone is 4.2 mU/mmol. His basic metabolic profile is normal except for a serum bicarbonate of 35 mEq/L. What additional testing is likely to reveal the cause of his fatigue?

A. Computed tomography of the chest

B. Nuclear stress testing

C. Serum testosterone level

D. Polysomnogram

E. Magnetic resonance imaging of the brain

Lung

24. A 46-year-old male presents complaining of 3 months of difficulty walking. On examination the patient appears his stated age; however, his hair is prematurely gray. He has a slight yellow color to the skin and sclerae as well as a shiny red appearance to the tongue with lack of obvious filiform papillae. His gait is shuffling and broad-based, and cognition is slow. Strength in the legs is 4/5 bilaterally and hyperreflexia is present. On examination and with his neck placed in flexion the patient experiences an intensely uncomfortable "electric" sensation, which runs down the back and into the arms and legs. When the patient is standing, he loses his balance only when his eyes are closed. Abuse of which of the following drugs can cause this patient's condition?

A. Heroin

B. Cocaine

C. Nitrous oxide

D. Cannabis

E. Amyl nitrite

Central nervous system

25. A 46-year-old woman with a history of gastric bypass surgery is referred to neurology for numbness and tingling in both feet. Past medical history is unremarkable except for bariatric surgery. The patient denies any alcohol use. On examination her gait is ataxic, Rhomberg test is positive, and strength is 4/5 in the upper and lower extremities bilaterally. Deep tendon reflexes in the upper and lower extremities are brisk. A complete blood count is remarkable for a leukocyte count of 3.5×10^9 cells/L and a hematocrit of 33% with a mean corpuscular volume of 109/fL. Cobalamin, folic acid, homocysteine, methylmalonic acid, and glycated hemoglobin levels are all within normal range. Magnetic resonance imaging of the cervical spine shows increased signal intensity in the posterior columns. Which of the following is most likely responsible for this patient's symptoms?

A. Vitamin B12 deficiency

B. Folic acid deficiency

C. Selenium deficiency

D. Copper deficiency

E. Thiamine deficiency

Central nervous system

7.5 Environmental Toxins— Answers and Explanations

Easy	Medium	Hard

1. Correct: Arterial blood gas (E)

The rosy or cherry red appearance of this patient is highly suggestive of carbon monoxide poisoning, a condition seen more frequently during winter months due to the use of gas furnaces. An arterial blood gas with carboxyhemoglobin level will confirm the diagnosis **(E)**. An electrocardiogram (ECG) should be performed on patients with confirmed carbon monoxide poisoning due to increased risk of myocardial ischemia; however, ECG will not assist in diagnosing this condition **(B)**. Pulse oximetry is of no benefit, since it cannot distinguish between oxyhemoglobin and carboxyhemoglobin **(A)**. For **(C, D)**, see previous information.

2. Correct: Ferruginous bodies (B)

This patient has clinical findings consistent with interstitial fibrosis, which, with pleural plaques, is a finding almost synonymous with pulmonary asbestosis. The finding of ferruginous bodies with a thin transparent core (the asbestosis fiber) would be expected **(B)**. **(A, C-E)** are not characteristic of asbestos exposure.

3. Correct: Basophilic stippling of the red cells (C)

This patient has several signs and symptoms of lead poisoning, including abnormal renal function, microcytic anemia, lead lines at his gum line, and foot drop. Of the findings listed as possible answers, basophilic stippling of the red blood cells is the only one expected in lead toxicity **(C)**. For **(A-B, D-E)**, see previous information.

4. Correct: Arsenic (D)

Of the possible answer choices, this patient's symptoms are most consistent with arsenic poisoning. Abdominal pain, vomiting, mental status changes, acute kidney injury, and cardiac arrhythmias are common early manifestations of arsenic poisoning, with dermatitis, peripheral neuropathy, pancytopenia, and acute hepatitis developing 2 to 8 weeks after the initial exposure **(D)**. The clinical scenario is not consistent with exposure to the other chemicals **(A-C, E)**.

5. Correct: Tuberculosis (B)

This patient's occupational history and radiographic findings are consistent with chronic silicosis. Up to 25% of patients with silicosis will develop tuberculosis **(B)**. Mesothelioma would be expected in asbestosis, but not silicosis **(C)**. The other conditions listed **(A, D-E)** are not commonly associated with silicosis.

6. Correct: Vinyl chloride (E)

Vinyl chloride as well as arsenic, anabolic steroids, and Thorotrast (thorium dioxide) have all been associated with development of angiosarcoma **(E)**. Aflatoxin, produced by *Aspergillus* species, is a common contaminant of grain and is one of the most carcinogenic substances known; however, aflatoxin usually produces hepatocellular carcinoma **(D)**. The other answer choices are not associated with angiosarcoma of the liver **(A-C)**.

7.6 Injury by Therapeutic Drugs—Answers and Explanations

Easy	Medium	Hard

7. Correct: Benzocaine (A)

This patient is suffering from methemoglobinemia. Several drugs are known to cause methemoglobinemia, including dapsone and nitric oxide; however, the most severe cases have been associated with 20% topical benzocaine spray **(A)**. For **(B-E)**, see previous information.

8.   Correct: The medication increases her risk of thromboembolism (C)

Oral contraceptives, particularly in smokers over the age of 35 years, raise the risk of heart disease (**D**). These medications also increase the risk of thromboembolism and possibly cervical cancer (**C, E**). On the other hand, women on oral contraceptive medications have a lower risk of ovarian and endometrial cancer (**A, B**).

9.   Correct: Protein C deficiency (B)

This patient is suffering from warfarin (Coumadin)-induced skin necrosis. This complication is seen more frequently in patients who receive large loading doses, and up to 30% of patients have underlying protein C deficiency (**B**). Warfarin-induced skin necrosis is thought to be triggered by a transient hypercoagulable state due to a more pronounced effect of the drug at inhibiting protein C and factor VII early in treatment due to the shorter half-life of these vitamin K-dependent factors. For (**A, C-E**), see previous information.

10.   Correct: Salicylate (C)

Salicylates stimulate the respiratory center producing a respiratory alkalosis early in intoxication, followed by a metabolic acidosis with increased anion gap. Tinnitus is a characteristic symptom of salicylate intoxication not seen in other intoxications (**C**). (**A-B, D-E**) would not cause this clinical scenario.

11.   Correct: Centrilobular necrosis of the liver (A)

The pathophysiology of an acetaminophen overdose is acute centrilobular hepatic necrosis (**A**). Patients who survive can expect a full recovery except in cases of other organ involvement such as renal failure. Liver infarcts and portal vein thrombosis are not seen, and cirrhosis and fibrosis are chronic processes (**B-E**).

12.   Correct: Prostate cancer (E)

Secondary cancers and cardiovascular disease are the most important causes of mortality in patients who survive treatment for Hodgkin lymphoma. Chest radiation increased the risk of coronary artery disease fivefold (**A**). The patient is at risk for pulmonary fibrosis due to the bleomycin and chest irradiation as well as cardiomyopathy from the doxorubicin (**B, C**). Chest and neck radiation also leads to a very high rate of thyroid dysfunction in this population (**D**). Survivors of Hodgkin lymphoma are at increased risk for skin, colon, and breast cancer; however, there is no evidence that prostate cancer rates in long-term survivors are higher than the general population (**E**).

13.   Correct: Cobalt toxicity (E)

Chromium and cobalt toxicity are increasingly recognized as a serious and even life-threatening complication of hip arthroplasty (**E**). Cobalt poisoning occurs as the metal prosthesis wears and releases cobalt into the bloodstream. Symptoms include pain at the site of the prosthesis, cognitive dysfunction, nerve deafness, optic nerve damage and retinopathy, peripheral neuropathy, hypothyroidism, and heart and kidney failure. (**A-D**) do not adequately explain the clinical scenario.

7.7 Drugs of Abuse— Answers and Explanations

Easy	Medium	Hard

14.   Correct: Exposure to an antihelminthic drug (C)

This patient has a classic presentation for levamisole-induced skin necrosis (**C**). Levamisole is a veterinary anthelminthic previously used as an adjunct to fluorouracil in the treatment of colon cancer in humans. Levamisole is a common adulterant in cocaine, thought to enhance the euphoria of the drug by inhibiting both monoamine oxidase and catechol-O-methyltransferase. Levamisole is known to stimulate production of antinuclear and anti-neutrophil cytoplasmic antibodies and cause a necrotizing vasculitis, which particularly affects the ears, nose, and extremities. (**A-B, D-E**) would not adequately explain the clinical scenario.

15.   Correct: Cocaine (C)

The signs, symptoms and radiographic findings in this patient are all consistent with an acute aortic dissection, a condition known to be associated with cocaine use (**C**). Cocaine abuse also causes cardiac arrhythmias, coronary artery thrombosis and myocardial infarction, heart failure, and probably premature coronary artery disease. The other drugs listed are not commonly associated with an aortic dissection (**A-B, D-E**).

16.   Correct: MDMA ("ecstasy") (B)

The presence of hyponatremia and hyperthermia are highly suggestive of ecstasy (MDMA) intoxication (**B**). Users of ecstasy frequently consume large amounts of water during intoxication and the drug itself causes secretion of antidiuretic hormone (ADH). This combination frequently leads to acute hyponatremia, cerebral edema, and seizure. (**A, C-E**) do not adequately explain the clinical scenario.

17. Correct: Cannabis (C)

This patient's symptoms and absence of other organic causes are suggestive of cyclic vomiting syndrome. Heavy cannabis appears to be responsible for some cases (C). Patients with cannabis-related cyclic vomiting syndrome frequently report symptoms improved with hot baths and may spend hours each day in the bathtub during attacks. Cessation of cannabis use appears to resolve most cases in which the drug is related. (A-B, D-E) do not adequately explain the clinical scenario.

7.8 Malnutrition and Dietary Deficiencies— Answers and Explanations

| Easy | Medium | Hard |

18. Correct: Mammillary bodies (D)

The patient suffers from Wernicke-Korsakoff syndrome, a neurologic disorder caused by thiamine (B1) deficiency, not uncommonly seen in alcoholic patients. The hallmarks of this disease are the broad-based ataxic gait, encephalopathy, and eye abnormalities (paralysis of conjugate gaze, nystagmus, and oculomotor palsies). Up to 75% of these patients will also demonstrate a peripheral neuropathy. All cases will have involvement of the mammillary bodies (D). Lesions of the hypothalamus, brainstem nuclei, and the floor of the fourth ventricle and cerebellar atrophy are variably present (A-C, E).

19. Correct: Hypophosphatemia (B)

This patient is suffering from refeeding syndrome. In patients with severe malnutrition, electrolyte shifts and vitamin deficiencies precipitated by aggressive refeeding can cause serious and fatal complications. Hypophosphatemia in refeeding is well-described and appears to be due to an underlying deficiency of total body phosphate stores exacerbated by insulin-mediated shift of phosphate to the intracellular compartment triggered by large carbohydrate loads during refeeding (B). Additionally, insulin increased the activity of many metabolic pathways that consume phosphates including adenosine triphosphate production and hexokinase activity. Severe hypophosphatemia leads to myocardial dysfunction, respiratory failure, and circulatory collapse in these patients. (A, C-E) do not best explain the clinical scenario.

20. Correct: Squash (D)

The patient suffers from xerophthalmia and has classic Bitot's spots, superficial accumulations of keratin on the conjunctiva consistent with Vitamin A deficiency. β-carotene is the most important precursor for Vitamin A production. Sweet potatoes, squash, carrots, and dark leafy vegetables have the highest β-carotene content (D). The other answer choices are poor dietary sources of Vitamin A (A-C, E).

21. Correct: Vitamin B2 (B)

The patient has cheilitis, glossitis, and stomatitis, all signs of vitamin B2 (riboflavin) deficiency (B). Riboflavin is present in abundance in fish, eggs, milk, and green vegetables. This water-soluble vitamin plays a critical role in the electron transport chain in the form of flavin adenine dinucleotide (FAD). (A, C-E) do not best explain the clinical scenario.

22. Correct: Hypersegmented neutrophils (A)

This patient has a macrocytic anemia with an elevated homocysteine level and normal methylmalonic acid level, consistent with folic acid deficiency. One would expect to see neutrophils with more than five nuclear lobules (hypersegmented neutrophils) (A). (B-E) are not features of a macrocytic anemia.

23. Correct: Polysomnogram (D)

This patent is morbidly obese, complaining of daytime fatigue with two lab findings concerning for severe sleep apnea. The presence of an elevated hematocrit and serum bicarbonate are concerning for nocturnal hypoxia and chronic respiratory acidosis. A chest radiograph, arterial blood gas, and echocardiogram to evaluate for pulmonary hypertension would all be reasonable in this patient; however, a polysomnogram is most likely to confirm the diagnosis (D). For (A-C, E), see previous information.

24. Correct: Nitrous oxide (C)

This patient suffers from subacute combined degeneration, caused by vitamin B12 deficiency. He has a yellow discoloration of the skin due to a combination of mild jaundice and anemia associated with glossitis, weakness with upper motor neuron signs, and a true positive Rhomberg test, indicating that impaired proprioception rather than cerebellar dysfunction is the cause of his ataxia. Finally, the Lhermitte's sign is positive. Of the drugs listed as possible answers, only nitrous oxide is known to be associated with vitamin B12 deficiency (C). (A-B, D-E) are incorrect.

25.   Correct: Copper deficiency (D)

This patient presents with a myeloneuropathy with several features suggestive of vitamin B12 (cobalamin) deficiency including a macrocytic anemia, polyneuropathy, and myelopathy with degeneration of the dorsal columns. However, the cobalamin levels as well as the methylmalonic acid and homocysteine levels are normal, which essentially excludes the diagnosis of vitamin B12 deficiency (**A**). Copper deficiency causes clinical symptoms very similar to vitamin B12 deficiency and, though rare, should be considered in the differential diagnosis of a megaloblastic anemia with peripheral neuropathy (**D**). (**B-C, E**) do not explain the clinical scenario.

Chapter 8

Diseases of the Cardiovascular System

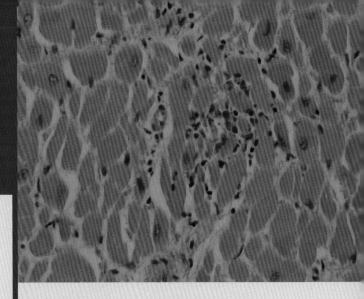

LEARNING OBJECTIVES

8.1 Aneurysms

- ▶ Describe the etiology and complications of thoracic aortic aneurysms
- ▶ Describe the etiology and complication of and the clinical evaluation for abdominal aortic aneurysms
- ▶ Describe a pseudoaneurysm
- ▶ Describe the complications of an aortic dissection
- ▶ Describe the association between size of aneurysm and risk of rupture
- ▶ Identify a mycotic aneurysm
- ▶ Identify a ruptured abdominal aortic aneurysm
- ▶ Identify, diagnose, list the pathologic conditions of, and list the genetic defect in Marfan's syndrome

8.2 Atherosclerosis and Hypertension

- ▶ Diagnose hypercholesterolemia
- ▶ Diagnose acute myocardial infarction; describe the process of atherosclerosis
- ▶ Diagnose and describe the morphologic changes producing stable angina
- ▶ Describe the appearance and clinical importance of fatty streak
- ▶ Diagnose peripheral vascular disease
- ▶ Diagnose a stroke; describe the underlying cause of a cerebral infarct
- ▶ Diagnose hypertension; describe the organs damaged by hypertension and laboratory testing to identify this damage
- ▶ Diagnosis and describe the histologic changes associated with a hypertensive crisis
- ▶ Describe the histologic changes caused by systemic hypertension
- ▶ Describe the causes of secondary hypertension and how to identify them clinically
- ▶ Describe the pathologic and clinical features of renal artery stenosis
- ▶ Diagnose a pheochromocytoma
- ▶ Describe the laboratory testing for a pheochromocytoma
- ▶ Describe the clinical features of Cushing's disease and Cushing's syndrome
- ▶ Diagnose aortic dissection and describe the gross and microscopic appearance of an aortic dissection

- ▶ Describe the association between ruptured berry aneurysms and systemic hypertension
- ▶ Describe the gross and microscopic features of changes induced by hypertension
- ▶ List blood vessels affected by Monckeberg medial calcification
- ▶ Describe the effects of lipoprotein(a)
- ▶ Identify hyaline arteriolosclerosis and describe its relationship to hypertension
- ▶ Identify aortic dissection

8.3 Vasculitis

- ▶ Given the clinical scenario and pathologic findings, diagnose Takayasu's arteritis
- ▶ Diagnose polyarteritis nodosa and describe the appearance of the lesions
- ▶ Given the clinical scenario, diagnose coarctation of the aorta
- ▶ Discuss how to diagnose a coarctation of the aorta by physical examination

8.4 Congenital Heart Disease

- ▶ Diagnose coarctation of the aorta
- ▶ Discuss how to diagnose a coarctation of the aorta by physical examination
- ▶ List the cyanotic congenital heart defects
- ▶ List the most common of the cyanotic congenital heart defects
- ▶ Describe Eisenmenger's syndrome
- ▶ Describe the epidemiology and clinical presentation of a ventricular septal defect
- ▶ Describe the features of tetralogy of Fallot
- ▶ Describe the morphologic features of the congenital heart conditions causing early cyanosis

8.5 Ischemic Heart Disease

- ▶ Diagnose acute myocardial infarct and describe the underlying pathologic changes associated with unstable angina and acute myocardial infarction
- ▶ Describe a vulnerable plaque
- ▶ Describe the role of T lymphocytes in the development of a thin fibrous cap

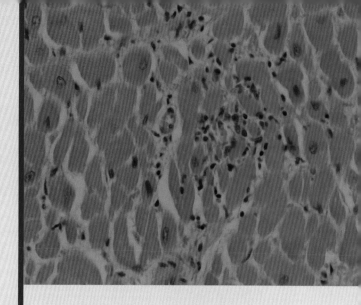

- ▶ Diagnose a coronary artery dissection
- ▶ Describe the use of laboratory testing in the diagnosis of atherosclerosis and angina syndromes
- ▶ Describe the different forms of acute plaque change
- ▶ Describe the most common cause of ischemic heart disease
- ▶ Describe the morphologic changes of atherosclerotic plaques associated with stable angina, unstable angina, and acute myocardial infarction
- ▶ Describe the coronary arterial distribution
- ▶ Describe situations in which a circumferential subendocardial infarct of the entire left ventricle could occur
- ▶ List and describe the complications of a myocardial infarct
- ▶ Describe the gross and morphologic changes of the myocardium following a myocardial infarct
- ▶ List and describe the complications of an acute myocardial infarct

8.6 Cardiomyopathies
- ▶ Diagnose arrhythmogenic right ventricular dysplasia-cardiomyopathy
- ▶ Describe the morphologic features of hypertrophic cardiomyopathy
- ▶ Describe the genetic mutations associated with hypertrophic cardiomyopathy
- ▶ Describe the clinical and morphologic features of hypersensitivity myocarditis
- ▶ Describe the morphologic appearance and list the causes of a dilated cardiomyopathy
- ▶ Describe the gross and microscopic features of hypertrophic cardiomyopathy

8.7 Miscellaneous Cardiovascular Disease
- ▶ Describe the complications of varicose veins
- ▶ Diagnose a pulmonary thromboembolus and describe physical examination findings associated with the condition
- ▶ Describe the association between pancreatic tumors and thrombosis
- ▶ Describe a paradoxical embolus
- ▶ Diagnose and describe complications of a deep venous thrombus
- ▶ Describe the relationship between pulmonary thromboembolus and recent immobility
- ▶ Describe the laboratory evaluation for pulmonary thromboembolus
- ▶ Diagnosis superior vena cava syndrome
- ▶ Describe the association between lymphedema and angiosarcoma
- ▶ Diagnose acute lymphangiitis
- ▶ List tumors of the skin that can be painful
- ▶ Diagnose Kaposi sarcoma and the association between Kaposi sarcoma and HHV8
- ▶ List the tumors associated with tuberous sclerosis
- ▶ Diagnose cardiac myxoma
- ▶ Describe causes of eccentric hypertrophy
- ▶ Describe the pathologic changes on the heart associated with pulmonary fibrosis
- ▶ Describe the pathologic features of left-sided congestive heart failure
- ▶ Describe the complications of pulmonary disease on the heart

8.1 Aneurysms—Questions

Easy	Medium	Hard

1. A 67-year-old male presents to his family physician complaining of a persistent cough and occasional dyspnea, which have developed over the last several weeks. Also, within the last few days, the cough has become productive. His temperature is 100.2°F. Auscultation of the chest reveals decreased breath sounds on the left side and a diastolic murmur. An X-ray confirms an infiltrate in the left lung. His past medical history includes hypertension, and he recalls a rash affecting the palms of his hands while he was in college. Of the following, which is the most likely diagnosis?

A. Granulomatosis with polyangiitis

B. Churg-Strauss syndrome

C. Thoracic aortic aneurysm

D. Chronic rheumatic aortic valvulitis

E. Aortic dissection

Lung, aorta

2. A 65-year-old male with a past medical history of hypertension and hypercholesterolemia, and who has a 50-pack-per-year smoking history presents to the emergency room complaining of abdominal pain. A physical examination reveals a pulsatile mass in the abdomen. Of the following, which played the greatest role in the development of his pathologic condition?

A. C-reactive protein

B. Oxidized LDL

C. Troponin I

D. Matrix metalloproteinases

E. p-ANCA

Aorta

3. A 56 year-old male sustains an acute myocardial infarction. Three days later, the infarct ruptures; however, because of fibrosis in the pericardial sac related to a previous episode of acute pericarditis, the hemorrhage is contained, and he survives the rupture. An echocardiogram obtained five days after the infarct reveals a bulge in the wall of the left ventricle. The left ventricular wall thickness is normal. What is the diagnosis?

A. A left ventricular true aneurysm

B. A pseudoaneurysm

C. Infarct extension

D. Infarct expansion

E. Lobular capillary hemangioma

Heart

4. A 50-year-old male with a history of hypertension complains to his wife of sharp back pain, and shortly thereafter collapses. Emergency medical services responds, but, despite resuscitation, he cannot be revived. They identify pulseless electrical activity on the monitor during the resuscitation attempts. Which of the following best explains the findings by the EMTs?

A. A left-sided hemothorax

B. A hemopericardium

C. An intraluminal thrombus in the abdominal aorta

D. A retroperitoneal hemorrhage

E. Blood in the media of the aorta

Aorta

5. A 66-year-old male with a history of hypertension and hypercholesterolemia, and with a 75-pack-per-year smoking history, presents to his family physician because the big toe of his left foot has developed a blackened tip over the course of several days. Of the following, which is the physician most likely to identify on physical examination and which represents the underlying pathologic cause of the change in the toe?

A. A pulsatile mass in the abdomen

B. Bilateral decreased pulses in the lower extremities compared to the upper

C. A harsh crescendo-decrescendo systolic murmur

D. A bruit in the carotid artery

E. Bilateral jugular venous distension

Aorta

6. A 68-year-old male presents to his family physician for a routine examination. He has not seen a doctor in 10 years. His blood pressure is 155/91 mm Hg. His glucose is 245 mg/dL. Palpation of the abdomen reveals a pulsatile mass, and an ultrasound confirms an abdominal aortic aneurysm of 7 cm in size. The physician schedules the patient with a vascular surgeon. Of the following, which most prompted the quick consultation with the surgeon?

A. The age of the patient

B. The patient's blood pressure

C. The patient's glucose concentration

D. The size of the aneurysm

E. The sex of the patient

Aorta

7. A 36-year-old male complains to his wife of abdominal pain for 1 hour before he collapses. EMTs and the emergency room physician are unable to revive him. An autopsy reveals an aneurysm in his abdominal aorta, which, microscopically, is found to have multiple neutrophils in the wall and bacterial organisms. Which of the following is the most specific name for this aneurysm?

A. True aneurysm

B. False aneurysm

C. Saccular aneurysm

D. Mycotic aneurysm

E. Fusiform aneurysm

Aorta

8. A 67-year-old male with a history of hypertension and a 30-pack-per-year smoking history develops abdominal pain and collapses in front of his wife. At autopsy, he is found to have 2500 mL of blood in his peritoneal cavity. If he had not died, which of the following would this same disease have made him at risk for?

A. Ischemic necrosis of the left big toe

B. An acute myocardial infarct

C. A hemopericardium

D. A sudden lethal ventricular dysrhythmia

E. Intracerebral hemorrhage

Aorta

Consider the following case for questions 9 to 10

A 37-year-old male was found dead in bed by his wife when she awoke in the morning. He had complained of chest pain the night before. He had a brother who died when he was 32 years old of a heart-related condition. At autopsy he was found to have a hemopericardium. There was no atherosclerosis in the coronary arteries.

9. Which of the following enzymes/proteins does he have a deficiency/defect of?

A. Matrix metalloproteinases

B. Lipoprotein(a)

C. Fibrillin

D. C-reactive protein

E. PR3

Aorta

10. Given the previous clinical scenario, of the following, what other condition might be present?

A. A bicuspid aortic valve

B. Myxomatous mitral valve

C. Quadricuspid pulmonary valve

D. Abdominal aortic aneurysm

E. Coarctation of the aorta

Aorta

8.2 Atherosclerosis and Hypertension—Questions

Easy	Medium	Hard

11. A 24-year-old male presents to the emergency room with complaints of crushing chest pain, which radiates into his left arm and jaw. The symptoms have been occurring for 2 hours. Laboratory testing reveals an elevated troponin I. He has no past medical history; however, his father died suddenly in his early 30s while shoveling snow. The patient has no history of tobacco use, diabetes mellitus, or hypertension. On examination, a cloudy ring surrounding the cornea is noted, and nodules are present on both heels. Of the following, which is the most likely source of his disease process?

A. Factor V Leiden mutation

B. Prothrombin gene mutation

C. LDL receptor mutation

D. β-myosin heavy chain gene mutation

E. Plakoglobin gene mutation

Heart

12. A 66-year-old man presents to the emergency room complaining of a squeezing discomfort in his chest that radiates to the left arm. He is noted to be diaphoretic. Laboratory testing indicates a troponin I concentration of 2.63 ng/mL. A 12-lead electrocardiogram shows ST depression and T-wave inversions in the lateral leads. His past medical history includes hypercholesterolemia and tobacco use (3 packs per day for 40 years). Of the following, which was the initiating step in the disease process producing his symptoms?

A. Tearing of the intima

B. Migration of smooth muscle cells from the media into the intima

C. Accumulation of oxidized LDL in intimal macrophages

D. Dysfunction of endothelial cells

E. Dilation of the aortic root

Heart

13. A 62-year-old male presents to his family physician, with a complaint of chest pain. He describes the chest pain as a pressure sensation that occurs consistently after he walks from his house to his mailbox. When he stops walking the pain goes away. He relates that this has been happening for the last 6 months. Of the following, which best explains the scenario?

A. Atherosclerotic plaque producing 10% stenosis of the lumen of the vessel

B. Atherosclerotic plaque producing 25% stenosis of the lumen of the vessel

C. Atherosclerotic plaque producing 40% stenosis of the lumen of the vessel

D. Atherosclerotic plaque producing 60% stenosis of the lumen of the vessel

E. Atherosclerotic plaque producing 80% stenosis of the lumen of the vessel

Heart

14. During the autopsy of a 14-year-old adolescent who died in a motor vehicle accident, the pathologist identifies linear yellow discolorations in the intima of the thoracic aorta. Which of the following statements bests describes the lesion?

A. It is considered a precursor for atherosclerosis.

B. The cells are most likely lipid-laden smooth muscle cells.

C. Given the age of the patient, the lesions are due to a mutation in the LDL receptor.

D. Granulomas will be identified microscopically.

E. Laboratory testing would reveal a p-ANCA.

Aorta

15. A 67-year-old male with a history of essential hypertension, diabetes mellitus, and a 60-pack-per-year smoking history presents to his family physician complaining of pain in his lower extremities when he walks. When he stops walking, the pain goes away. Palpation and auscultation of the abdomen reveal a soft, nontender abdomen, and normal bowel sounds. The symptoms have been occurring for 6 months. Of the following, which is the most likely cause of the symptoms?

A. A thoracic aortic aneurysm

B. An abdominal aortic aneurysm

C. An aortic dissection

D. Giant cell arteritis of the femoral arteries

E. Atherosclerosis of the femoral arteries

Aorta and branches

16. A 72-year-old female is playing cards with friends when she suddenly develops a weakness in her left arm and drops her cards. Her friends call 9-1-1, and she is rushed to the emergency room. A CT scan reveals an infarct in her right cerebral hemisphere. Of the following, which process in the cerebral vasculature most likely led to this pathologic change?

A. Infection

B. Embolism

C. Vasculitis

D. Dissection

E. Aneurysm

Central nervous system

17. A 54-year-old male presents to a family physician for his first doctor visit in 35 years. He has no specific complaints, but is simply coming to the doctor at his wife's insistence. Auscultation of the heart reveals no murmurs, palpation reveals a laterally and inferiorly displaced point of maximum impulse, and retinal examination reveals arteriovenous nicking. Of the following, which laboratory test might reveal more signs of organ injury produced by his underlying disease process?

A. C-reactive protein

B. Test for β-myosin heavy chain gene mutation

C. Test for Factor V Leiden mutation

D. p-ANCA

E. Blood urea nitrogen (BUN)

Heart, kidney

18. A 56-year-old male with a 10-year history of hypertension treated with an ACE inhibitor is brought to the emergency department by his wife. He had been complaining of a headache and had become confused. Ophthalmic examination revealed retinal hemorrhages, and auscultation of the chest revealed rales. If obtained, a biopsy of his kidney would reveal which of the following conditions that best represents his presentation?

A. Fibrinoid necrosis of arterioles

B. Hyaline arteriolosclerosis

C. Cystic medial degeneration of arterioles

D. Necrotizing inflammation of arterioles

E. Medial calcification of arterioles

Heart

19. An autopsy is performed on a 67-year-old male who died as the result of an aortic dissection. His heart weight was 500 grams. The cortical surface of the kidneys was not smooth and instead had a granular appearance. Microscopic examination of the kidneys would most likely reveal which of the following?

A. Glomerulonephritis

B. Hyperplastic arteriolosclerosis

C. Hyaline arteriolosclerosis

D. Fibromuscular dysplasia of the renal arteries

E. Necrotizing transmural inflammation of the renal artery

Heart, kidney

20. A 46-year-old male presents to his family physician with complaints of generalized weakness and muscle cramps. He is afebrile and denies any recent cough, congestion, or difficulty breathing. His blood pressure is 160/95 mm Hg. Laboratory testing reveals a normal concentration of hemoglobin but an elevated sodium concentration and decreased potassium concentration. Of the following, what is his most likely diagnosis?

A. Essential hypertension

B. Pulmonary hypertension

C. Fibromuscular dysplasia of a renal artery

D. Bilateral adrenal hyperplasia

E. Cushing's syndrome

Kidney, heart

21. At the autopsy of a 40-year-old female who died in a motor vehicle accident, the pathologist notes that one kidney is smaller than the other kidney and has a smooth cortical surface. Also, the larger kidney has a more granular cortical surface. Of the following, which physical examination finding would have been present and would directly represent the underlying pathologic condition causing the differences in her two kidneys?

A. An S4

B. An S3

C. A systolic murmur

D. An abdominal bruit

E. A palpable and pulsatile abdominal mass

Kidney

Consider the following case for questions 22 to 23

A 47-year-old male presents to the emergency room. He is diaphoretic and complaining of a headache. Physical examination reveals him to be afebrile and with a heart rate of 113 beats per minute, and a respiratory rate of 18 breaths per minute. His blood pressure is 156/97 mm Hg. He tells the doctor that he has episodes like this every once in a while. His blood pressure is usually about 110/70 mm Hg when he visits his family physician and he has no medical diagnoses.

22. Of the following, which is his most likely diagnosis?

A. Acute myocardial infarction

B. Coarctation of the aorta

C. Primary aldosteronism

D. Pheochromocytoma

E. Polyarteritis nodosa

Kidney, heart

23. Given the previous clinical scenario, of the following laboratory tests, which substance will best assist in making the diagnosis?

A. Troponin I

B. Creatine kinase

C. Metanephrines

D. p-ANCA

E. Aldosterone

Kidney, heart

24. A 51-year-old female presents to her family physician. Over the past 4 years, she has gained about 50 lbs. and she complains that when she is working in her garden, she often cuts her skin with very minor trauma. She is afebrile, with a heart rate of 92 beats per minute, and a blood pressure of 145/95 mm Hg. Her physician notes that she has distinct hair on her upper lip, and her face appears more rounded. Of the following, which is the most likely source of her condition?

A. A pituitary adenoma

B. A thyroid adenoma

C. Fibromuscular dysplasia of the renal artery

D. Tumor of the adrenal medulla

E. Poor diet

Pituitary gland

25. A 53-year-old male presents to the emergency room because of sharp chest pain that started 15 minutes prior to arrival. His only past medical history is hypertension. Physical examination reveals that he is afebrile, with a heart rate of 110 beats per minute and a blood pressure of 170/100 mm Hg. While being admitted, he goes into shock, becomes unresponsive, and is unable to be resuscitated. Of the following, which is the autopsy most likely to reveal?

A. Hyperplastic arteriolosclerosis

B. Blood in the aortic media

C. Coarctation of the aorta

D. A ruptured myocardial infarct

E. Fibrinoid necrosis of the left anterior descending coronary artery

Aorta

26. A 53-year-old male complains to his wife of an excruciatingly painful headache that just developed, and says he is going to lie down for a little while. Several minutes later she goes in to check on him and finds him unresponsive. An autopsy reveals a subarachnoid hemorrhage, but no other hemorrhage in the cranial cavity, including within the brain. Of the following, which medical condition did he most likely have?

A. Pulmonary hypertension

B. Systemic hypertension

C. Takayasu's arteritis

D. Polyarteritis nodosa

E. A ruptured hemangioma of the brain

Cardiovascular

27. A 50-year-old male with a history of hypertension complains to his wife of sharp back pain and shortly thereafter collapses. Emergency medical services responds, but, despite resuscitation, he cannot be revived. An autopsy reveals blood in the pericardial sac. Microscopic examination of the aorta would most likely reveal?

A. Cystic medial degeneration

B. Giant cells and fibrosis

C. Transmural necrotizing inflammation

D. Foamy macrophages in the intima

E. Eosinophilic infiltrate in the media

Aorta

28. A vascular biopsy of a 67-year-old man reveals calcification of the media. The lumen of the vessel is nonstenotic. Which of the following vessels was the likely source of the biopsy?

A. Left anterior descending coronary artery

B. Left renal artery

C. Pulmonary artery

D. Internal carotid artery

E. Right radial artery

Aorta

29. A 53-year-old sustains an acute myocardial infarct. He is found to have a high level of a competitive inhibitor for the activation of plasmin. Which of the following is this inhibitor?

A. C-reactive protein

B. Oxidized LDL

C. Matrix metalloproteinases

D. Lipoprotein (a)

E. Homocysteine

Blood vessel

30. A 63-year-old male died in the hospital and was autopsied. Under the microscope, the pathologist identified arterioles with thick acellular eosinophilic walls, which are related to the underlying cause of death. Of the following conditions, which was the cause of death of the patient?

A. Polyarteritis nodosa

B. Giant cell arteritis

C. Aortic dissection

D. Angiosarcoma of the liver

E. Monckeberg medial calcification

Blood vessels

31. A 57-year-old male with a history of hypertension was found dead in bed by his wife when she awoke in the morning. He had complained of chest pain the night before. At autopsy he was found to have a hemopericardium. The source of the hemorrhage was the aorta. Which of the following was most likely to have been found on microscopic examination of the aorta?

A. Giant cells

B. Hemosiderin

C. Cystic medial degeneration

D. Foam cells

E. Bacterial organisms and a neutrophilic infiltrate

Aorta

8.3 Vasculitis—Questions

| Easy | Medium | Hard |

32. A 37-year-old female is playing softball with her co-workers. While running the bases, she becomes short of breath, and on return to the dugout, sits down, and shortly thereafter passes out and becomes unresponsive. Despite resuscitation, she is pronounced dead. An autopsy reveals a thoracic aortic aneurysm. Histologic examination of the aorta reveals giant cells and fibrosis. Her family has no history of sudden death. Of the following, which is her most likely diagnosis?

A. Marfan's syndrome
B. Takayasu's arteritis
C. Giant cell arteritis
D. Ehlers-Danlos syndrome
E. Kawasaki's disease

Aorta

33. A 32-year-old male has had several episodes of various symptoms requiring medical evaluation, including abdominal pain and muscle aches. He has also occasionally had an unexplained fever. His blood pressure has not been elevated. Immune testing revealed no p-ANCA or c-ANCA. His past medical history includes hepatitis B infection. He is diagnosed with a vasculitis. An echocardiogram reveals no abnormalities of the heart or aorta. Which of the following will a biopsy of the disease process reveal?

A. Temporally dissimilar lesions with giant cells
B. Temporally similar lesions with giant cells
C. Temporally dissimilar lesions without giant cells
D. Temporally similar lesions without giant cells
E. Widespread granulomatous inflammation

Blood vessels

34. A 61-year-old female presents to an acute care clinic with complaints of a headache and double vision. Her erythrocyte sedimentation rate is 73 mm/hr.

A. Leukocytoclastic vasculitis
B. Thromboangiitis obliterans
C. Microscopic polyarteritis
D. Giant cell arteritis
E. Polyarteritis nodosa

Aorta

35. A 35-year-old female with a history of pain and weakness in her joints and muscles is found dead in bed. An autopsy reveals a thoracic aortic aneurysm.

A. Takayasu's arteritis
B. Kawasaki's disease
C. Leukocytoclastic vasculitis
D. Granulomatosis with polyangiitis
E. Eosinophilic granulomatosis with polyangiitis

Aorta

36. A 44-year-old male with a history of chronic sinusitis presents to the emergency room with complaints of blood in his urine. His blood pressure is 181/98 mm Hg and a chest X-ray reveals pulmonary infiltrates.

A. Granulomatosis with polyangiitis
B. Polyarteritis nodosa
C. Thromboangiitis obliterans
D. Giant cell arteritis
E. Microscopic polyarteritis

Heart

37. A 12-year-old male is found dead in bed by his parents. Autopsy reveals a hemopericardium due to rupture of an aneurysm of the left anterior descending coronary artery.

A. Leukocytoclastic vasculitis
B. Thromboangiitis obliterans
C. Eosinophilic granulomatosis with polyangiitis
D. Takayasu's arteritis
E. Kawasaki's disease

Heart

38. A 53-year-old with a 60-pack-per-year smoking history presents to an acute care clinic with ulcers of his fingers.

A. Microscopic polyarteritis
B. Thromboangiitis obliterans
C. Polyarteritis nodosa
D. Giant cell arteritis
E. Leukocytoclastic vasculitis

Heart

8.4 Congenital Heart Disease—Questions

| Easy | Medium | Hard |

39. A 33-year-old male presents to a family physician for a routine visit. It is his first visit since high school. His heart rate is 85 beats per minute. His respiratory rate is 14 breaths per minute. He is afebrile. His blood pressure is 167/103 mm Hg. On auscultation of the chest, a mid-systolic murmur is heard. A chest X-ray reveals an enlarged cardiac silhouette. Of the following, what is his most likely diagnosis?

A. Aortic stenosis due to a bicuspid aortic valve
B. Aortic stenosis due to a calcified tricuspid valve
C. A ventricular septal defect
D. Coarctation of the aorta
E. Thoracic aortic aneurysm

Heart

40. Given the previous clinical scenario, of the following, which physical examination technique is most useful in making the correct diagnosis?

A. Assessment of jugular venous distention

B. Measurement of blood pressure in both the upper and lower extremities

C. Auscultation of the abdomen

D. Palpation of the liver and spleen

E. Ophthalmic examination

Heart

41. A newborn child is noticed by his parents, ten days after they left the hospital, to be breathing fast and to be very irritable. They schedule a visit with their pediatrician the next day, and, during the physical examination, the doctor notices that the baby has blue fingernail beds and that with strenuous crying, his lips become more blue. Of the following, what is the most likely diagnosis?

A. A large atrial septal defect

B. A large ventricular septal defect

C. Tricuspid atresia

D. A patent ductus arteriosus

E. Tetralogy of Fallot

Heart

42. Given the previous clinical scenario, of the following, what structural abnormality is this child most likely to possess?

A. Stenosis of the aorta at the level of the ligamentum arteriosum

B. A connection between the aorta and pulmonary artery

C. Anomalous origin of the left coronary artery from the right sinus of Valsalva

D. Right ventricular hypertrophy

E. Incomplete closure of the foramen ovale

Heart

43. A 46-year-old female with an unrepaired ventricular septal defect develops dyspnea and cyanosis. An echocardiogram reveals dilation and hypertrophy of the right ventricle. Of the following, which condition has she developed?

A. Eisenmenger's syndrome

B. Trousseau's syndrome

C. Osler-Weber-Rendu syndrome

D. Superior vena cava syndrome

E. Inferior vena cava syndrome

Heart

44. A 21-year-old male presents to his family physician for a yearly physical prior to starting medical school. His family physician hears a loud and harsh holosystolic murmur. Of the following, which is the most likely location for the defect producing this murmur?

A. The interatrial septum at the fossa ovalis

B. The interatrial septum in the inferior portion

C. The ductus arteriosus

D. The membranous portion of the interventricular septum

E. The muscular portion of the interventricular septum

Heart

45. A newborn child is noticed by his parents, ten days after they left the hospital, to be breathing fast, and to be very irritable. They schedule a visit with their pediatrician the next day, and, during the physical examination, the doctor notices that the baby has blue fingernail beds, and, with strenuous crying, his lips become more blue. Of the following, which condition does this child most likely have in his heart?

A. Atrial septal defect

B. Ventricular septal defect

C. Severe congenital aortic stenosis

D. Coarctation of the aorta

E. Tricuspid atresia

Heart

46. A newborn child is being evaluated by echocardiography for a suspected congenital heart defect. During the procedure the technologist identifies flow between the left atrium and the right atrium. Of the following forms of congenital heart disease, which is the infant most likely to have?

A. Tetralogy of Fallot

B. Ductus arteriosus

C. Totally anomalous pulmonary venous return

D. Ebstein anomaly

E. Membranous ventricular septal defect

Heart

47. A newborn child is being evaluated by echocardiography for a suspected congenital heart defect. During the procedure the technologist identifies flow from one atrium into the other and flow from one ventricle into the other, in both cases, at separate sites. Of the following forms of congenital heart disease, which is the infant most likely to have?

A. Tetralogy of Fallot

B. Totally anomalous pulmonary venous return

C. Transposition of the great arteries

D. Tricuspid atresia

E. Persistent truncus arteriosus

Heart

8.5 Ischemic Heart Disease— Questions

Easy	Medium	Hard

48. A 55-year-old male with a history of systemic hypertension (for 15 years treated with an ACE-inhibitor) and hypercholesterolemia presents to the emergency room with complaints of crushing chest pain radiating to his jaw and arm. He is noted to be diaphoretic. He has a troponin I concentration of 3.5 ng/mL. He sustains a cardiac arrest while being evaluated. Of the following, which lesion would most likely be identified as a cause of the symptoms?

A. Atherosclerotic plaque in the left anterior descending coronary artery, producing 75% stenosis

B. Hemorrhage in the media of the right coronary artery, with compression of the lumen

C. Occlusion of the circumflex coronary artery, with evidence of bone formation in the plaque

D. Thrombus overlying a ruptured atherosclerotic plaque resulting in occlusion of the vessel

E. A ruptured aneurysm of the left anterior descending coronary artery

Heart

49. An autopsy report on a 53-year-old male who died in a motor vehicle accident describes a lesion in the left anterior descending coronary artery as a vulnerable plaque. Of the following, which was this individual most at risk for if the motor vehicle accident had not claimed his life?

A. Release of foamy macrophages into the lumen of the vessel leading to thrombus formation

B. Extensive calcification of the plaque, leading to occlusion of the vessel

C. Intraplaque thrombosis, leading to occlusion of the vessel

D. Hemorrhage into the media, leading to compression of the lumen

E. Neutrophilic infiltration of the wall and resultant fibrinoid necrosis

Heart

50. A pathologist is examining a cross section of a coronary artery atherosclerotic plaque obtained at autopsy. A change in the plaque was directly responsible for the individual's death. Within the plaque are numerous lymphocytes, with immunohistochemical staining indicating they are T-lymphocytes. Of the following changes in the plaque, which is most directly related to these cells?

A. Extensive calcification of the atherosclerotic core

B. Extensive hemorrhage into the plaque

C. Intraluminal thrombosis

D. A thin fibrous cap

E. Multiple granulomas in the intima

Heart

51. A 27-year-old female in her third trimester of pregnancy suddenly develops crushing chest pain, with radiation of the pain to her jaw, while walking with her husband. She becomes diaphoretic and nauseated. She does not smoke or have hypertension, diabetes mellitus, or high cholesterol, and there is no history of sudden death in her family. She was very healthy as a child, never missing a day of school. Of the following, which is the most likely cause of her symptoms?

A. Occlusive thrombus of the right coronary artery, in a background of multifocal severe atherosclerosis

B. A nonocclusive thrombus of the right coronary artery, in a background of multifocal severe atherosclerosis

C. A coronary artery aneurysm

D. A coronary artery dissection

E. Polyarteritis nodosa

Heart

52. A 57-year-old male with a history of hypertension, diabetes mellitus type 2, and a 50-pack-per-year smoking history presents to his family physician complaining of a squeezing-type chest pain whenever he climbs more than three flights of stairs. He has no other associated symptoms, and the chest pain only lasts for about 3 minutes and goes away when he stops exerting himself. The last time he had chest pain was three weeks ago. Of the following, which laboratory test could be expected to be elevated?

A. Troponin I

B. CK-MB

C. D-dimer

D. C-reactive protein

E. c-ANCA

Heart

53. A 48-year-old male with a history of diabetes mellitus type 2 and hypertension collapses in front of his wife, who performs CPR and revives him. In the hospital, he undergoes a cardiac catheterization to evaluate his coronary arteries. A thrombus, which has an underlying atherosclerotic plaque, is found in his left anterior descending coronary artery. Of the following, what is the likely composition of that plaque?

A. Thin fibrous cap with a large necrotic core

B. Thick fibrous cap with a small necrotic core

C. Fibrous intimal hyperplasia with minimal foam cells or extracellular lipid

D. Thick fibrous cap with prominent calcification

E. Thick fibrous cap with medium necrotic core with abundant cholesterol crystals

Heart

54. A 67-year-old male collapses at work. He is autopsied by the medical examiner, who identifies ischemic heart disease. Of the following, what is the most likely cause of this disease process in the heart?

A. Coronary artery dissection of the right coronary artery

B. Embolism (from endocarditis) to the left anterior descending coronary artery

C. Polyarteritis nodosa

D. Sarcoidosis of the heart

E. Coronary artery atherosclerosis

Heart

55. A 35-year-old pregnant female with no family history of sudden cardiac deaths and no personal history of smoking, hypertension, or diabetes mellitus becomes unresponsive while dancing with her husband. Resuscitation is unsuccessful. Of the following, which is an autopsy most likely to find?

A. An occlusive thrombus overlying a ruptured thin cap atheroma

B. An aortic dissection

C. A coronary artery dissection

D. A nonocclusive thrombus overlying an erosion of an atheroma

E. A thickened interventricular septum

Heart

56. A 51-year-old male with hypertension and a 35 pack per year history of smoking is golfing with friends when he starts complaining of crushing chest pain, collapsing 5 minutes later. Resuscitation is unsuccessful. He has never before complained of chest pain. He does not have diabetes mellitus. His father died at the age of 52 from a myocardial infarct, and one of his brothers had cardiac bypass surgery at the age of 49 years. At autopsy, which of the following lesions is most likely to be found?

A. A nonocclusive thrombus superimposed on a 50% stenotic atherosclerotic plaque

B. A nonocclusive thrombus superimposed on an 85% stenotic atherosclerotic plaque

C. An occlusive thrombus superimposed on a 50% stenotic atherosclerotic plaque

D. An occlusive thrombus superimposed on an 85% stenotic atherosclerotic plaque

E. A thickened interventricular septum

Heart

57. A pathology resident is reviewing organs from an autopsy with the director of the autopsy service. A cross section of the heart reveals changes consistent with ischemic injury throughout all the subendocardial region of the left ventricle (i.e., anterior, lateral, and inferior walls and interventricular septum). Which of the following lesions would explain this finding?

A. A nonocclusive thrombus in the left main coronary artery in an individual who is right dominant with survival for three days in the hospital

B. A nonocclusive thrombus in the right main coronary artery in an individual who is right dominant with survival for three days in the hospital

C. A dissection of the left anterior descending coronary artery with survival for three days in the hospital

D. An aortic dissection with hemorrhage into the retroperitoneal soft tissue with survival for three days in the hospital

E. A hemangioma compressing the left anterior descending coronary artery

Heart

58. A 63-year-old male with a 50-pack-per-year smoking history and hypertension complains to his wife of a sudden crushing sensation in his chest, with the pain radiating into his jaw and left arm. He also started sweating. She wants to drive him to a hospital, but he refuses. One hour later, while they are walking, he suddenly collapses, becomes unresponsive, and cannot be resuscitated. Which of the following is his most likely immediate cause of death?

A. A lethal ventricular dysrhythmia

B. A hemopericardium due to rupture of the anterior wall of the left ventricle

C. Mitral insufficiency due to a ruptured papillary muscle

D. Constrictive pericarditis

E. Rupture of a left ventricular aneurysm

Heart

59. Given the previous clinical scenario, of the following microscopic features, which would examination of the myocardium at the time of the autopsy most likely reveal?

A. Apparently normal cardiac myocytes

B. Prominent coagulative necrosis with a neutrophilic infiltrate

C. Prominent coagulative necrosis with a pronounced neutrophilic infiltrate and a few macrophages

D. Sheets of macrophages in the area of nonviable myocardium

E. Large patches of fibrosis

Heart

60. A 68-year-old female with a 50-pack-per-year smoking history and a history of hypertension sustains an acute myocardial infarct. She is admitted to the hospital, and 10 days later, as she is talking to family, her left arm and leg suddenly weaken. She is diagnosed with a cerebral infarct. After two more weeks in the hospital, she leaves and enters rehabilitation. Which of the following complications of her acute myocardial infarct is the cause of this cerebral infarct?

A. Rupture of the anterior wall of the left ventricle

B. A ventricular aneurysm

C. A mural thrombus

D. Pericarditis

E. A ventricular arrhythmia

Heart

61. A 73-year-old male with a history of high cholesterol and hypertension sustains an acute myocardial infarct while fishing with his friends at a lake. In the emergency room, he is found to have a new systolic murmur. Which of the following complications of his acute myocardial infarct is the cause of this murmur?

A. Pericarditis

B. Rupture of the interventricular septum

C. A mural thrombus

D. Rupture of one of the mitral valve papillary muscles

E. Contractile dysfunction of one of the mitral valve papillary muscles

Heart

8.6 Cardiomyopathies—Questions

Easy	Medium	Hard

62. A 24-year-old male is playing softball with friends when he collapses while running the bases after hitting the ball. He is unable to be resuscitated. Autopsy reveals dilation of the right ventricle, and microscopically, there is fatty infiltration and fibrosis of the thinned wall. Gross and histologic examination of his lungs reveals no pathologic condition. What was his cause of death?

A. Acute cor pulmonale

B. Chronic cor pulmonale

C. Right ventricular infarct

D. Arrhythmogenic right ventricular dysplasia-cardiomyopathy

E. Hypertrophic cardiomyopathy

Heart

63. A 24-year-old female collapses while running with her boyfriend. Although emergency services are called immediately, she is unable to be resuscitated. She has a family history of sudden cardiac death. At autopsy, a patch of fibrosis is identified on the outflow tract of the left ventricle. Which of the following other features is present?

A. Dilation of all four cardiac chambers

B. A thickened interventricular septum

C. Dilation of the right ventricle with fatty infiltration and fibrosis of the posterior wall

D. An intraluminal coronary artery thrombus

E. A bicuspid aortic valve with severe dystrophic calcification

Heart

64. Given the previous scenario, a mutation of which of the following genes is most likely responsible for her condition?

A. One of the enzymes for collagen synthesis

B. β-myosin heavy chain gene

C. Dystrophin

D. Fibrillin

E. Lamin A

Heart

65. A 36-year-old male is found dead in his apartment. His cause of death was a suicidal gunshot wound of the head. Microscopic examination of the heart reveals several areas where there are perivascular infiltrates of eosinophils. The subendocardium is histologically normal. What is the most likely cause of this microscopic finding?

A. Recent switch from paroxetine to buproprion for his depression

B. An ongoing coxsackievirus B infection

C. A mutation of the β-myosin heavy chain gene

D. Release of major basic protein

E. Heavy recent alcohol use

Heart

66. A 43-year-old female with no history of alcoholism or family history of sudden death collapses while grocery shopping. She had been complaining of increased shortness of breath lately to her husband, but refused to see a doctor. Autopsy revealed four-chamber dilation of the heart. Which of the following conditions is the cause of her disease process?

A. A past coxsackievirus B infection

B. A past *Streptococcus pneumoniae* infection

C. A past Group A streptococcus infection

D. A mutation of the fibrillin gene

E. A mutation of the myosin-binding protein C

Heart

67. A 47-year-old chronic alcoholic is found dead in his apartment on a welfare check by police, initiated by neighbors who had not seen him in 3 days. At autopsy, he is found to have dilation of all four chambers of the heart. The wall of the left ventricle is thin, but microscopically, there is myocyte hypertrophy and fibrosis. Of the following, which of these other features might be seen at autopsy and are directly related to the described condition?

A. Fusion, thickening, and shortening of the chordae tendineae of the mitral valve

B. A mural thrombus in the left ventricle

C. Thick interventricular septum

D. Severe coronary artery atherosclerosis of the left anterior descending coronary artery

E. Multiple large clusters of lymphocytes in the wall of the left ventricle

Heart

68. A 35-year-old male with a family history of sudden death collapses while playing football with old college friends. Despite aggressive resuscitation efforts, he dies. An autopsy reveals a thick interventricular septum. Which of the following findings would be identified microscopically?

A. Patchy fibrosis, with myocytes having a normal orientation to each other

B. Clusters of lymphocytes and associated necrosis of cardiac myocytes

C. Fatty infiltration and fibrosis

D. Patches of fibrosis associated with granulomas and giant cells

E. Myocyte disarray

Heart

8.7 Miscellaneous Cardiovascular Disease— Questions

Easy	Medium	Hard

69. A 35-year-old obese and pregnant female develops varicose veins. She asks her obstetrician whether she is at risk of developing any severe consequences as a result of those varicose veins. Of the following, which could be a complication that varicose veins might cause by themselves without the assistance of another morphologic abnormality?

A. Ischemic necrosis of a toe

B. A pulmonary thromboembolus

C. Rupture with bleeding

D. Pressure necrosis of the surrounding skeletal muscle

E. Cerebral infarct

Veins

70. A 37-year-old male is in a motor vehicle accident and sustains a femoral fracture requiring surgical repair. Several days following the accident, he develops shortness of breath and a sharp pain in his chest. His symptoms resolve. Ten days later, he is released from the hospital, and while walking into his house, he suddenly collapses and cannot be revived. He has no past medical history. Of the following, what is his most likely cause of death?

A. A ruptured acute myocardial infarct

B. A ruptured ventricular aneurysm

C. An aortic dissection

D. A pulmonary thromboembolus

E. A ruptured coronary artery aneurysm

Lung

71. A 67-year-old male collapses while having dinner with his wife. An autopsy reveals a pulmonary thromboembolus. Of the following, which pathologic finding is most indicative of a risk factor for his cause of death?

A. A granular renal cortical surface

B. A calcified aortic valve

C. A tumor in the pancreas

D. Pitting edema of the lower extremities

E. Cirrhosis of the liver

Pancreas, lungs

72. A 63-year-old male fractures his ankle while hunting when he steps in a gopher hole. Because of the fracture he has difficulty caring for himself, being mostly bed-ridden, and his daughter comes to take care of him. About 15 days after the accident, she finds him unresponsive on the bathroom floor. An autopsy reveals an acute right-sided cerebral infarct and deep venous thrombi in the lower extremities. Which of the following autopsy findings would allow the pathologist to indicate that DVTs caused the stroke?

A. Thrombosis of the right carotid artery

B. A patent foramen ovale

C. Endocarditis of the aortic valve

D. A mural thrombus in the left ventricle of the heart

E. A papillary fibroelastoma of the aortic valve

Heart, brain

73. An obese 43-year-old female with no significant past medical history presents to her family physician complaining of swelling of her right lower extremity. Physical examination confirms the swelling and identifies a generalized red discoloration of the skin. Palpation identifies a cord-like lesion in the calf. Of the following, which is she most at risk for?

A. Embolic occlusion of a pulmonary artery

B. Embolic occlusion of a coronary artery

C. Embolic occlusion of a cerebral artery

D. Aortic dissection

E. Coronary artery dissection

Veins

74. A 37-year-old male presents to the emergency room complaining of dyspnea, a sharp chest pain on the left side, and a cough, with occasional blood being produced. During the history and physical examination, which of the following is important history to obtain in formulating the diagnosis?

A. History of sudden cardiac death in the family

B. History of easy bleeding with trauma

C. History of a heart murmur previously diagnosed

D. History of recent long-distance travel by car

E. History of a febrile illness as a child resulting in oral erythema

Veins, lung

75. A 37-year-old male presents to the emergency room complaining of dyspnea, a sharp chest pain on the left side, and a cough, with occasional blood being produced. He recently severely sprained his right ankle and has been off work and at home since that time. During the history and physical examination, of the following, which is a likely finding?

A. Pitting edema of the lower extremities

B. A harsh crescendo-decrescendo systolic murmur

C. Accentuation of the pulmonic component of the second heart sound

D. Retinal hemorrhages

E. Slow respiratory rate

Veins, lung

76. Given the previous scenario, of the following, which laboratory test would best help determine the diagnosis?

A. p-ANCA

B. Factor V Leiden gene mutation

C. D-dimer

D. Cholesterol profile

E. C-reactive protein

Veins, lung

77. A 64-year-old female with an 80-pack-per-year smoking history has had a chronic cough and occasionally coughs up blood. Over the course of several days, she develops profound congestion of her head, neck, and upper extremities, and her fingernail beds are blue. Which of the following is the most likely cause?

A. A thoracic aortic aneurysm

B. Acute aortic insufficiency secondary to endocarditis

C. A lung tumor

D. Giant cell arteritis, with near occlusion of the subclavian arteries

E. Congestive heart failure secondary to long-standing hypertension

Lung

78. A 78-year-old woman has a right mastectomy and lymph node dissection for invasive ductal breast carcinoma. Following the surgery, she slowly develops swelling of the right upper extremity. Of the following, which is she at risk for developing because of these changes?

A. Congestive heart failure

B. Aortic insufficiency due to left ventricular overload

C. Hepatocellular carcinoma

D. Angiosarcoma

E. Kaposi sarcoma

Lymph nodes

79. A 25-year-old scratches his right forearm while hiking. Over the next four days, he develops redness, swelling, and notable warmness to the touch at the site. When he awakes on the 5th day, he notices that he has developed red streaks on his right forearm, and that they are painful. What is his diagnosis?

A. Lobular capillary hemangioma

B. Acute rheumatic fever

C. Acute lymphangiitis

D. Thrombophlebitis

E. Osler-Weber-Rendu syndrome

Lymph nodes

80. A 35-year-old male goes to a dermatologist and reports that he has developed a painful red mass underneath the fingernail of his left index finger. He is otherwise healthy, with no other medical diagnoses. What is the most likely diagnosis?

A. Capillary hemangioma

B. Pyogenic granuloma

C. Glomus tumor

D. Bacillary angiomatosis

E. Angiosarcoma

Blood vessels

81. A 46-year-old homosexual male presents to his physician because of the appearance of several brown patches on the skin of his trunk. A biopsy reveals small capillary-like spaces lined with endothelial-like cells with some pleomorphism of the nuclei. Within the tissue section are many red blood cells, not all of which are contained within the vascular spaces. Of the following, which is the most likely etiologic agent directly responsible for this skin change?

A. HIV

B. HSV

C. HHV-6

D. HHV-8

E. CMV

Blood vessels

82. Echocardiography of a 25-year-old male with the diagnosis of tuberous sclerosis reveals a nodule in the myocardium of the left ventricle. Of the following, which is the nodule most likely to be?

A. Myxoma

B. Fibroma

C. Rhabdomyoma

D. Metastatic melanoma

E. Angiosarcoma

Blood vessels

83. A pathologist is performing an autopsy on a 67-year-old female who died in a motor vehicle accident. On opening the left atrium, the pathologist identifies a soft, gelatinous-like mass adherent to the wall of the interatrial septum near the fossa ovalis. Of the following, what is the most likely diagnosis?

A. Papillary fibroelastoma

B. Myxoma

C. Angiosarcoma

D. Lipoma

E. Endocarditis

Blood vessels

84. At autopsy, a patient is found to have eccentric hypertrophy of the left ventricle of the heart. Of the following additional findings, which is the source of the hypertrophy in the heart?

A. An aldosterone-secreting adrenal adenoma

B. Coarctation of the aorta

C. Calcification of a bicuspid aortic valve, producing aortic stenosis without significant regurgitation

D. Healed endocarditis of the aortic valve, with a gaping defect in one leaflet

E. Chronic rheumatic mitral valvulitis, causing mitral stenosis

Heart

91

85. At autopsy, a 73-year-old male is found to have an enlarged liver and spleen (with microscopic evidence of chronic congestion), and pressure on his legs leaves lasting depressions. There is no fluid in the pleural cavities. Of the following, which is the most likely underlying source of the pathologic changes?

A. Coronary artery atherosclerosis

B. Systemic hypertension

C. A calcified bicuspid aortic valve

D. Pulmonary fibrosis

E. Hypertrophic cardiomyopathy

Heart

86. At autopsy, a 72-year-old male is found to have some fibrosis of his pulmonary septa combined with numerous alveolar macrophages filled with small granules of hemosiderin. Which of these other findings is also most likely to be identified at autopsy?

A. Enlarged liver

B. Enlarged spleen

C. Pitting edema

D. Nutmeg appearance to the cut surface of the liver

E. Pleural effusions

Lungs, heart

87. A 62-year-old female with a 65-pack-per-year history of smoking and a diagnosis of chronic obstructive pulmonary disease is on oxygen and dies while visiting her son for Thanksgiving. He requests an autopsy at the local hospital. Which of the following findings in the heart would be most consistent with her disease process?

A. Left ventricular hypertrophy

B. Left ventricular dilation

C. Coronary artery atherosclerosis

D. Right ventricular hypertrophy

E. Fibromuscular dysplasia of the right coronary artery

Heart

8.8 Aneurysms—Answers and Explanations

Easy	Medium	Hard

1. Correct: Thoracic aortic aneurysm (C)

The rash on the palm of the hand during college is most consistent with syphilis, which is a cause of thoracic aortic aneurysms (**C**). A thoracic aortic aneurysm can cause aortic insufficiency and thus the diastolic murmur, and the aneurysm can press on the bronchus, causing retention of secretions and increase the chance for pneumonia, which is the patient's presenting feature. The other conditions listed do not, in total, fully explain the clinical scenario (**A-B, D-E**).

2. Correct: Matrix metalloproteinases (D)

The patient has risk factors for an abdominal aortic aneurysm: hypertension, smoking, and high cholesterol. The physical examination is consistent with this diagnosis as well. Although atherosclerosis is associated with aneurysms, the main factor leading to the development of an abdominal aortic aneurysm is believed to be dysfunctional regulation of matrix metalloproteinases (**D**). The other choices (**A-C, E**) are incorrect.

3. Correct: A pseudoaneurysm (B)

The tear in the wall of the heart allowed blood to leak outside, which was then contained. On imaging, this pathologic change will appear as a bulge in the wall of the heart, when in reality it is not (**B**). As the left ventricular wall thickness is normal, this is not a true left ventricular aneurysm, which results from a transmural myocardial infarct, with subsequent thinning of the wall, which bulges outward (**A**). Infarct expansion would also produce an outward bulge; however, the wall thickness would be thin (**D**). Neither (**C**) or (**E**) would produce similar findings as those described.

4. Correct: Hemopericardium (B)

The clinical history of sharp back pain in the background of hypertension is consistent with an aortic dissection. If the dissection ruptures into the pericardial sac, pulseless electrical activity can occur as the heart attempts to beat but cannot generate a pulse, because, although it can contract, it cannot dilate to fill with blood (**B**). As the patient has an aortic dissection, blood in the media of the aorta would occur, but this answer would not best explain the EMTs' findings (**E**); also, the patient could develop a left-sided hemothorax or retroperitoneal hemorrhage, but neither would explain the PEA as well as a hemopericardium (**A, D**). An intraluminal thrombus would not explain the clinical findings (**C**).

5. Correct: A pulsatile mass in the abdomen (A)

Given the history, the patient is at risk for an abdominal aortic aneurysm, and, the changes in the toe are consistent with plaque or thrombus in the aneurysm embolizing to small vessels in the feet and causing ischemic injury. An abdominal aortic aneurysm could be identified as a pulsatile mass in the abdomen (**A**). None of the other symptoms are characteristic of an abdominal aortic aneurysm (**B-E**).

6. Correct: The size of the aneurysm (D)

At the size of 6 cm and above, abdominal aortic aneurysms have a significant increase in the likelihood of rupture and are thus candidates for repair (**D**). The other choices would not have played a major factor in the decision to pursue repair (**A-C, E**).

7. Correct: Mycotic aneurysm (D)

Although the aneurysm is most likely both saccular and a true aneurysm (**A, C**), based on the description, the most specific name is mycotic aneurysm (**D**). The aneurysm is neither a false aneurysm (**B**) nor a fusiform aneurysm (**E**).

8. Correct: Ischemic necrosis of the left great toe (A)

With the history of hypertension and smoking, the patient is at risk for an abdominal aortic aneurysm. The clinical scenario of abdominal pain, followed by death and the identification of a hemoperitoneum, is consistent with an abdominal aortic aneurysm. The plaque and thrombi within an abdominal aortic aneurysm can break loose, embolize, and lead to ischemic injury of the digits (**A**). The other conditions, while related to hypertension and atherosclerosis, are not directly complications of an abdominal aortic aneurysm (**B-E**).

9. Correct: Fibrillin (C)

Given the family history, Marfan's syndrome, which causes aortic root dilation, and thoracic aortic aneurysms and can contribute to aortic dissections, is the most likely cause. The underlying defect in Marfan's syndrome is in fibrillin (**C**). The other choices are incorrect (**A-B, D-E**).

10. Correct: Myxomatous mitral valve (B)

See previous explanation in question 9. Of the conditions listed, myxomatous mitral valves are commonly found in Marfan's syndrome, affecting around 25% of patients (**B**). The remainder of the conditions listed are not commonly associated with Marfan's syndrome (**A, C-E**).

8.9 Atherosclerosis and Hypertension—Answers and Explanations

Easy	Medium	Hard

11. Correct: LDL receptor mutation (C)

Familial hypercholesterolemia, an autosomal dominant disorder caused by mutation of the LDL receptor, results in severe dyslipidemia (**C**). Typical clinical features include a corneal arcus, tendon xanthomas, and premature heart disease. (**A, B**) would cause thrombosis, (**D**) is associated with hypertrophic cardiomyopathy, and (**E**) is associated with arrhythmogenic right ventricular dysplasia-cardiomyopathy.

12. Correct: Dysfunction of endothelial cells (D)

The clinical scenario is consistent with an acute myocardial infarct, which would be due to atherosclerosis of the coronary arteries. The initiating step in atherogenesis is endothelial injury and endothelial dysfunction (**D**). The majority of early atheromatous lesions have morphologically intact endothelium, and intimal tearing is associated with dissection rather than atherogenesis (**A**). (**B, C**) occur following endothelial dysfunction, and the clinical scenario is not most consistent with an aortic aneurysm or aortic insufficiency (**E**).

13. Correct: Atherosclerotic plaque producing 80% stenosis of the lumen of the vessel (E)

This man's symptoms are consistent with stable angina. The oxygen extraction ratio of cardiac muscle in the resting patient is extremely high compared to other organs (around 75% vol). In a normal patient, during exercise, coronary blood flow increases proportional to the increase in myocardial oxygen demand. In the setting of significant coronary artery stenosis, however, coronary blood flow cannot increase to meet the increase in myocardial oxygen demand, and ischemic symptoms develop, which resolve when the myocardial oxygen demand returns to resting levels. Vascular lesions producing 75% or greater narrowing of the vessel lumen are generally required to produce angina symptoms (**E**). (**A-D**) are incorrect.

14. Correct: It is considered a precursor for atherosclerosis. (A)

The description is that of a "fatty streak." These lesions, composed of foamy macrophages, are precursor lesions to atheromas (**A**). However, not all fatty streaks will progress to atherosclerotic plaques. The cells are lipid-laden macrophages (**B**). Fatty streaks are commonly identified in young individuals and do not represent a familial hypercholesterolemia (**C**). Neither granulomas nor a p-ANCA would be found (**D, E**).

15. Correct: Atherosclerosis of the femoral arteries (E)

The patient has numerous risk factors for atherosclerosis. Atherosclerosis can affect the major vessels supplying the lower extremities, and with activity and increased oxygen demand, ischemia and resultant pain can occur (i.e., claudication). The pain goes away when the activity ceases. Given the chronic nature of the symptoms and the negative abdominal examination, (**B, C**) are unlikely. A thoracic aortic aneurysm would not present with these symptoms (**A**), and giant cell arteritis does not commonly involve the femoral arteries and would be very rare compared to atherosclerosis (**E**).

93

16. Correct: Embolism (B)

The patient had a sudden focal neurological change, which is consistent with a stroke. Strokes can be due to cerebral infarcts, which are most commonly due to plaque fragments that embolize from the carotid arteries to the cerebral arteries (**B**). Although the other conditions listed could cause a stroke, each would be a rare cause compared to atherosclerosis (**A, C-E**).

17. Correct: Blood urea nitrogen (BUN) (E)

The laterally displaced point of maximal impulse is suggestive of cardiomegaly. Arteriovenous nicking is a classic manifestation of hypertension caused by focal compression of a venule of the eye by a thickened arteriole. Both findings are suggestive of systemic hypertension. Of the tests listed, the blood urea nitrogen is most likely to reveal further end organ damage, as in the case of hypertensive nephropathy (**E**). For (**A-D**), see previous information.

18. Correct: Fibrinoid necrosis of arterioles (A)

The patient is presenting acutely with hypertension, and given his clinical findings of confusion and retinal hemorrhages, he most likely is having a hypertensive crisis. Although hyaline arteriolosclerosis is found in hypertension, given his acute presentation, he most likely would have fibrinoid necrosis of arterioles and could develop hyperplastic arteriolosclerosis (**A**). (**C-E**) are not associated with a hypertensive crisis.

19. Correct: Hyaline arteriolosclerosis (C)

Given that the patient died from an aortic dissection and has an enlarged heart, he most likely has systemic hypertension. The changes on the kidney surface are arteriolar nephrosclerosis, which is found in hypertensive patients, and the microscopic correlate is hyaline arteriolosclerosis (**C**). Glomerulonephritis can cause a similar gross appearance in the kidney, but would be much rarer than hypertension (**A**). Given the lack of a hypertensive crisis, (**B**) is not likely. Both (**D, E**) could cause hypertension, but it would be uncommon compared to essential hypertension.

20. Correct: Bilateral adrenal hyperplasia (D)

The hypernatremia, hypokalemia, and clinical symptoms are consistent with hyperaldosteronism. Of the possible answers, only adrenal hyperplasia is likely (**D**). Fibromuscular dysplasia is rare in men (**C**), and, other than the hypertension, there are no clinical signs or symptoms consistent with Cushing's syndrome (**E**). As there is an underlying cause of the hypertension, it is not essential hypertension (**A**), and the pulmonary circulation is not involved (**B**).

21. Correct: An abdominal bruit (D)

The patient has unilateral renal artery stenosis, which, given her age, is most likely due to fibromuscular dysplasia. The kidney that is on the side of the stenosis would be atrophic; however, the other kidney would feel the effects of the hypertension induced by the atrophic kidney and thus has arteriolar nephrosclerosis. Of the possible answers of listed findings, only an abdominal bruit is most characteristic of renal artery stenosis (**D**). For (**A-C, E**), see previous information.

22. Correct: Pheochromocytoma (D)

See the explanation in question 23.

23. Correct: Metanephrines (C)

The patient is having episodic hypertension, which is characteristic for a pheochromocytoma. Laboratory testing for metanephrines will help confirm the diagnosis of a pheochromocytoma (**C**). None of the other laboratory tests listed will directly assist in the diagnosis of a pheochromocytoma (**A-B, D-E**).

24. Correct: Pituitary adenoma (A)

The patient has features of Cushing's disease and Cushing's syndrome, with weight gain, easily damaged skin, and hirsutism. Cushing's disease and Cushing's syndrome are also causes of hypertension. Cushing's disease is due to an ACTH-secreting pituitary adenoma (**A**), while Cushing's syndrome is due to disease of the adrenal glands. Given the clinical scenario, (**B-E**) are not correct.

25. Correct: Blood in the aortic media (B)

The clinical scenario is consistent with an aortic dissection, which, pathologically would be characterized by blood in the aortic media (**B**). Although malignant hypertension can lead to dissection, in most cases of aortic dissection there is not necessarily a precursor hypertensive crisis, and hyperplastic arteriolosclerosis is not often identified (**A**). A coarctation of the aorta is rare compared to an aortic dissection (**C**). As the chest pain is sharp and since the chest pain only began a few minutes prior to his death, a ruptured myocardial infarct is not likely (**D**). Fibrinoid necrosis of a coronary artery would be rare and would present like a myocardial infarct (see previous) (**E**).

26. Correct: Systemic hypertension (B)

The patient most likely had the rupture of a berry aneurysm. While berry aneurysms most commonly develop from a congenital weakness in the wall, systemic hypertension will cause the aneurysm to grow and can trigger rupture (**B**). A ruptured hemangioma could cause a subarachnoid hemorrhage and resultant headache, but this would be rare compared to a ruptured berry aneurysm (**E**). The other conditions (**A, C-D**) are not commonly associated with subarachnoid hemorrhage.

27. Correct: Cystic medial degeneration (A)

Given the clinical scenario, the patient most likely had an aortic dissection due to his underlying hypertension. The characteristic histologic change is cystic medial degeneration (**A**). Although some of the other changes can be found in the aorta under various conditions, such as vasculitis (**B**) and fatty streaks (**D**), none are consistent with the clinical history. Transmural necrotizing inflammation of the aorta would be rare, as would eosinophilic infiltrates (**C, E**).

28. Correct: Right radial artery (E)

Calcification of the media of an artery is found in Monckeberg medial calcification, which most commonly involves the vessels of the forearm (e.g., the radial and ulnar arteries) (**E**). The other vessels listed do not routinely have medial calcification (**A-D**).

29. Correct: Lipoprotein (a) (D)

Lipoprotein(a) is a competitive inhibitor for the activation of plasmin (**D**). If plasmin is not activated, thrombosis is promoted, which can lead to the development of an acute myocardial infarct. The other choices are incorrect (**A-C, E**).

30. Correct: Aortic dissection (C)

The description of thick acellular eosinophilic walls affecting arterioles is consistent with hyaline arteriolosclerosis, which is a feature of hypertension. Of the choices, hypertension is most likely to cause an aortic dissection, and an aortic dissection has a high mortality rate (**C**). In polyarteritis nodosa (PAN), the arterioles, if affected, would have transmural inflammation (**A**); however, PAN does not normally involve arterioles. Giant cell arteritis essentially does not involve arterioles (**B**). Neither angiosarcoma or Monckeberg medial calcification is related to hypertension (**D, E**).

31. Correct: Cystic medial degeneration (C)

Given the history of hypertension and chest pain, if the source of the hemorrhage in the pericardial sac was the aorta, it is most likely from a dissection that ruptured down to the pericardial sac. Microscopic examination of the aorta would reveal cystic medial degeneration (**C**). Although giant cell arteritis could lead to a thoracic aortic aneurysm and potential rupture with a hemopericardium, it would be much rarer than hypertension (**A**). Hemosiderin would indicate an older dissection that was healed (**B**). Neither foam cells or bacterial organisms and a neutrophilic infiltrate are specific to the clinical scenario (**D, E**).

8.10 Vasculitis—Answers and Explanations

Easy	Medium	Hard

32. Correct: Takayasu's arteritis (B)

Causes of thoracic aortic aneurysms include bicuspid aortic valve, syphilis, and vasculitis. Both Takayasu's arteritis and giant cell arteritis can involve the aorta; however, Takayasu's arteritis occurs in patients under the age of 50 years (**B**), and giant cell arteritis occurs above the age of 50 years (**C**). Kawasaki's disease involves the coronary arteries (**E**); Marfan's syndrome, which also causes thoracic aortic aneurysms, would not have giant cells and fibrosis (**A**); and Ehlers-Danlos syndrome also would not have giant cells and fibrosis (**D**).

33. Correct: Temporally dissimilar lesions without giant cells (C)

Given that the diagnosis is a vasculitis, the variation in symptoms, including abdominal pain, and lack of p-ANCA or c-ANCA, and no abnormalities of the aorta, polyarteritis nodosa is a distinct possibility. In this disease process, there are temporally dissimilar lesions, and giant cells are not a component (**C**). The other descriptions are not consistent with polyarteritis nodosa (**A-B, D-E**).

34. Correct: Giant cell arteritis (D)

Giant cell arteritis, while it can affect the aorta and branches of the carotid arteries, is most known for involving the temporal artery (hence, the name, temporal arteritis) and can produce a headache and visual disturbances, from diplopia to blindness. The characteristic microscopic feature is granulomatous inflammation with damage to the elastic lamellae.

35. Correct: Takayasu's arteritis (A)

The vasculitides are systemic disorders for the most part, and patients will often have systemic complaints, including arthralgias, myalgias, fever and night sweats. Takayasu's arteritis can involve the aorta and subclavian arteries, with involvement of subclavian arteries leading to a thoracic aortic aneurysm.

36. Correct: Granulomatosis with polyangiitis (A)

Granulomatosis with polyangiitis, previously referred to as Wegener's granulomatosis, is known for involving the upper and lower respiratory tract (hence the history of sinusitis and the pulmonary infiltrates), and the kidney, presenting with nephritic syndrome, and microscopically may have necrotizing or crescentic glomerulonephritis.

37. Correct: Kawasaki's disease (E)

Children with Kawasaki's disease (also, mucocutaneous lymph node syndrome) present with fever (up to 104°F), cervical lymphadenopathy, rash, erythema of the oral mucosa, erythema and edema of the palms and soles, and desquamation of skin of palms, soles, and perineal region. One long-term complication is coronary artery aneurysms.

38. Correct: Thromboangiitis obliterans (B)

Patients present with ulcers of the fingers, feet, or toes, which are due to involvement of the radial and tibial arteries. The condition is essentially always associated with cigarette use. Patients can have severe pain, both with activity and at rest, due to the ulceration of the skin and likely involvement of the nerves.

8.11 Congenital Heart Disease—Answers and Explanations

Easy	Medium	Hard

39. Correct: Coarctation of the aorta (D)

Coarctation of the aorta would produce both hypertension (and resultant enlargement of the heart) and a murmur (**D**). Aortic stenosis due to a tricuspid aortic valve would present much later in life (**B**), and, although a bicuspid aortic valve can produce stenosis at a younger age, not usually by the age of 33 years (**A**). Neither a ventricular septal defect nor a thoracic aortic aneurysm is usually associated with such a marked elevation in blood pressure (**C, E**).

40. Correct: Measurement of blood pressure in both the upper and lower extremities (B)

See the explanation for question 39. Given that the blood pressure drops after the site of the coarctation, there should be a difference between the blood pressure in the upper and lower extremities (**B**). The other tests listed are not as useful in the diagnosis of coarctation of the aorta (**A, C-E**).

41. Correct: Tetralogy of Fallot (E)

The child has a cyanotic congenital heart defect. Of the listed conditions, only tricuspid atresia and tetralogy of Fallot cause cyanosis shortly after birth; of the two, tetralogy of Fallot is much more common (**C, E**). Initially, an ASD, VSD, and patent ductus arteriosus would not cause cyanosis, although if a right to left shunt develops later in life, they can, at that time, cause cyanosis (**A-B, D**).

42. Correct: Right ventricular hypertrophy (D)

See the explanation for question 41. In tetralogy of Fallot, the patient will have pulmonary stenosis leading to right ventricular hypertrophy, a ventricular septal defect, and an overriding aorta (**D**). Stenosis of the aorta would be coarctation, a noncyanotic lesion (**A**). (**B**) would be a patent ductus arteriosus, also a noncyanotic lesion. Neither anomalous origin of a coronary artery (**C**) or incomplete closure of the foramen ovale (E) would present at this age in this manner.

43. Correct: Eisenmenger's syndrome (A)

Although a ventricular septal defect is initially a noncyanotic congenital heart lesion, with time, and due to hypertrophy of the right ventricle with subsequent increased pressure, the shunt can reverse and become right to left, causing cyanosis. This transition is termed Eisenmenger's syndrome (**A**). The clinical scenario does not fit the other diagnosis (**B-E**).

44. Correct: The membranous portion of the interventricular septum (D)

An atrial septal defect does not usually produce a loud or even detectable murmur (**A, B**). A ductus arteriosus produces a continuous murmur as blood is always flowing through the connection between the aorta and pulmonary artery (**C**). The murmur is most likely, of the choices, produced by a ventricular septal defect, and, for ventricular septal defects, the most common location is within the membranous portion of the interventricular septum (**D, E**).

45. Correct: Ventricular septal defect (B)

The newborn has a cyanotic heart condition. The most common cause of a cyanotic congenital heart defect in this age group is tetralogy of Fallot, which includes as a component a ventricular septal defect (**B**). Tricuspid atresia is a very rare form of cyanotic congenital heart disease (**E**). An atrial septal defect, severe congenital aortic stenosis, and coarctation of the aorta would not cause cyanosis at this age (**A, C-D**).

46. Correct: Totally anomalous pulmonary venous return (C)

Of the conditions listed, only total anomalous pulmonary venous return would have flow between the left and right atrium through an atrial septal defect (**C**). None of the other conditions are usually associated with an atrial septal defect (**A-B, D-E**).

47. Correct: Tricuspid atresia (D)

Tricuspid atresia usually requires both an atrial septal defect and a ventricular septal defect, to allow blood to reach both circulations around blockage at the junction between the right atrium and right ventricle (**D**). However, if the tricuspid stenosis is lesser in nature, only one septal defect may be required. Total anomalous pulmonary venous return, transposition of the great arteries, and persistent truncus arteriosus require or may require one septal defect to allow blood to reach both circulations, but they do not routinely require both an ASD and a VSD (**B-C, E**). An atrial septal defect is not a normal component of tetralogy of Fallot (**A**).

8.12 Ischemic Heart Disease—Answers and Explanations

Easy	Medium	Hard

48. Correct: Thrombus overlying a ruptured atherosclerotic plaque resulting in occlusion of the vessel (D)

The clinical history of severe chest pain with elevated troponin is consistent with acute myocardial infarction. The pathophysiology of myocardial infarction is one of abrupt total occlusion of the vessel in the setting of thrombosis, almost always from a ruptured atherosclerotic plaque (**D**). A coronary artery dissection (**B**) or ruptured aneurysm of a coronary artery (**E**) could both cause an acute myocardial infarction but would be rare. Both (**A, C**) would be associated with stable angina, and, with (**C**), the patient would be expected to have well-developed collaterals.

49. Correct: Release of foamy macrophages into the lumen of the vessel leading to thrombus formation (A)

A vulnerable plaque is one with a very thin fibrous cap. These plaques are at most risk of rupture. Rupture will allow the contents of the atheromatous core to enter the lumen of the vessel, triggering thrombosis (**A**). For (**B-E**), see previous information.

50. Correct: A thin fibrous cap (D)

Lymphocytes release mediators that contribute to the breakdown of the fibrous cap and can lead to a thin fibrous cap, which has a high likelihood for rupture (**D**). Although (**A-C**) are complications that a plaque can develop, the T-lymphocytes contribute mostly to thinning of the cap. Granulomas would not be a common occurrence (**E**).

51. Correct: A coronary artery dissection (D)

The patient is presenting with symptoms typical for an acute myocardial infarct; however, she has no risk factors for atherosclerosis (**A, B**). A coronary artery aneurysm could rupture and cause an acute myocardial infarct, but these are the result of Kawasaki's disease, which would have affected her when she was young. Polyarteritis nodosa does not frequently involve the heart (**E**); however, coronary artery dissection is strongly associated with pregnancy (**D**).

52. Correct: C-reactive protein (D)

The patient has a clinical history consistent with stable angina. It would not be expected that he is having injury to the myocardium, and thus, especially given the time frame, (**A-B**) would not be elevated. An elevated d-dimer would not be an abnormal laboratory finding usually associated with this clinical scenario (**C**), and there is nothing that suggests a condition that would cause an elevated c-ANCA (**E**). As chronic inflammation is a component of atherosclerosis, the C-reactive protein can be elevated (**D**).

53. Correct: Thin fibrous cap with a large necrotic core (A)

As the man had an acute myocardial infarction, he most likely had some form of acute change in a coronary artery plaque that led to occlusion of the vessel. While an acute change can potentially occur in any plaque, those with a thin fibrous cap overlying a large necrotic core would be the most likely of the choices to rupture (**A**). Based on the clinical scenario, (**B-E**) are not the best explanation.

54. Correct: Coronary artery atherosclerosis (E)

The most common cause of ischemic heart disease is coronary artery atherosclerosis (**E**). (**A–C**) could all potentially cause ischemic heart disease; however, compared to atherosclerosis, they are very rare. Sarcoidosis (**D**) is not usually a cause of ischemic heart disease, as it does not usually affect the coronary arteries; however, fibrosis can be found in sarcoidosis associated with the granulomas.

55. Correct: A coronary artery dissection (C)

This woman has sustained a sudden death. With the exception of (**D**), all of the choices are strongly associated with sudden death. Given her lack of risk factors for atherosclerosis, and no history of hypertension, (**A, B**) are not likely. Although a young female would be a candidate for a hypertrophic cardiomyopathy, given that she has no family history of sudden death, hypertrophic cardiomyopathy is less likely (**E**). Coronary artery dissection is a cause of sudden death and is strongly associated with pregnancy (**C**). When people die suddenly of a coronary artery dissection, most often there is no family history of sudden deaths.

56. Correct: An occlusive thrombus superimposed on a 50% stenotic atherosclerotic plaque (C)

Given the description of the chest pain, and the history of hypertension and smoking, the patient is most likely having an acute myocardial infarction. An occlusive thrombus is more likely than a nonocclusive thrombus to cause an acute myocardial infarction, and cause sudden death (**A, B**). A 50% stenotic plaque would not be expected to have caused symptoms previously; however, if the plaque changes acutely, the degree of stenosis can become 100% in seconds. An 85% stenotic plaque would have been expected, especially given the lack of diabetes mellitus, to have caused symptoms before; thus, (**C**) is the correct choice and (**D**) is not. With the lack of family history of sudden death, other than due to atherosclerosis, (**E**) is unlikely.

57. Correct: An aortic dissection with hemorrhage into the retroperitoneal soft tissue with survival for three days in the hospital (D)

The heart has a subendocardial infarct involving the entire left ventricle. The coronary arterial distribution is very specific, with the anterior descending supplying the anterior wall, the circumflex supplying the lateral wall, and the right supplying the inferior wall. In about 10% of people, the circumflex coronary artery supplies the inferior wall. To infarct the entire left ventricle by the formation of a thrombus, the person would have to be left dominant, and the thrombus would have to be in the left main coronary artery, a situation that is not described (**A-C, E**); however, if there is generalized poor perfusion, the subendocardium, being the last portion of the myocardium to receive blood, could have ischemic injury. This situation could occur in shock, or generalized hypoperfusion, such as could occur with a dissection (D).

58. Correct: A lethal ventricular dysrhythmia (A)

Given his past medical history and symptoms, he is having an acute myocardial infarction. While all conditions listed are potential complications of an acute myocardial infarct, ruptures occur 1 day to 1 week after the infarct (**B, C**). Pericarditis accompanies a transmural myocardial infarct or can develop later (Dressler's syndrome); however, a constrictive pericarditis would require scarring and would not occur in this time frame. Ventricular aneurysms, the pathologic form, take much longer to develop, and, since they are fibrous, they do not easily rupture. The most common cause of death from an acute myocardial infarct in individuals outside the hospital is a lethal ventricular dysrhythmia (**A**).

59. Correct: Apparently normal cardiac myocytes (A)

After a myocardial infarct, coagulative necrosis may be visible as early as three hours, but more likely around six hours or more, and coagulative necrosis associated with a prominent neutrophilic infiltrate would be around 1 to 3 days (**B**), with macrophages appearing around day 3 (**C**), and cleaning up the dead cells for 3 to 7 days (**D**). Large patches of fibrosis would indicate the infarct occurred two months earlier (**E**). Most likely, at one hour, no changes would be seen (**A**).

60. Correct: A mural thrombus (C)

Of the choices, it is most likely that she developed a mural thrombus, which then embolized to the brain and caused the cerebral infarct (**C**). Although a ventricular aneurysm could be a source of a mural thrombus, it would not develop in the 10-day time frame (**B**). Rupture of the free wall would lead to a hemopericardium, not an embolus (**A**). Neither pericarditis nor a ventricular arrhythmia would lead to the infarct (**D, E**). If the patient had left atrial fibrillation, mural thrombi could form, but ventricular fibrillation often causes death. If ventricular fibrillation is sustained for a long enough period of time to cause a thrombus, it most likely will cause death.

61. Correct: Contractile dysfunction of one of the mitral valve papillary muscles (E)

The cause of a new murmur would be mitral insufficiency, and, while both contractile dysfunction and rupture of the papillary muscle could cause mitral insufficiency, given the time course of events, the correct answer is (**E**), as it is too soon for rupture to have occurred (**D**). The other conditions listed would not produce a murmur (**A-C**).

8.13 Cardiomyopathies— Answers and Explanations

Easy	Medium	Hard

62. Correct: Arrhythmogenic right ventricular dysplasia-cardiomyopathy (D)

The description of a dilated right ventricle with fat infiltration and fibrosis of a thinned wall is most consistent with the diagnosis of arrhythmogenic right ventricular dysplasia-cardiomyopathy (**D**). The other choices are incorrect (**A-C, E**).

63. Correct: A thickened interventricular septum (B)

Given the history of sudden cardiac death in the family, (**A-D**) are all possible. A bicuspid aortic valve is not usually considered hereditary, and, at the age of 24 years, it would be unlikely to present with severe calcification (**E**). Fibrosis in the left ventricular outflow tract corresponding to the anterior leaflet of the mitral valve is characteristic of hypertrophic cardiomyopathy. In hypertrophic cardiomyopathy the main gross feature is the thickened interventricular septum (**B**). (**A, C, D**) are not associated with left ventricular outflow tract fibrosis.

64. Correct: β-myosin heavy chain gene (B)

The most common mutation associated with hypertrophic cardiomyopathy is that of the β-myosin heavy chain gene (**B**). The other choices are not correct (**A, C-E**).

65. Correct: Recent switch from paroxetine to buproprion for his depression (A)

The microscopic appearance, eosinophils in a perivascular location, is characteristic of hypersensitivity myocarditis. Hypersensitivity myocarditis most commonly occurs because of a reaction to a medication or a change in the therapeutic regimen of an already prescribed medication (**A**). A coxsackievirus B infection would have lymphocytes (**B**), a mutation of the β myosin heavy chain gene would be associated with myocardial disarray (**C**), and recent heavy alcohol use does not produce a characteristic change in the myocardium (**E**). Although eosinophils are present, release of major basic protein is not the cause of the microscopic changes (**D**).

66. Correct: A past coxsackievirus B infection (A)

Given the fact that she does not have a history of sudden cardiac death in her family, a genetic mutation is less likely (**D, E**). The morphologic appearance of her heart is consistent with a dilated cardiomyopathy, and her symptoms correlate. A dilated cardiomyopathy can have a variety of underlying causes, but one is a past coxsackievirus B infection, which caused a lymphocytic myocarditis (**A**). Heavy alcohol use is a common cause of a dilated cardiomyopathy. Neither a past *S. pneumoniae* or group A streptococcal infection are typically associated with a dilated cardiomyopathy (**B, C**).

67. Correct: A mural thrombus in the left ventricle (B)

The gross and microscopic features of the heart are those of a dilated cardiomyopathy, a condition that is commonly associated with chronic alcoholics. Of the choices, mural thrombi are most frequently associated with dilated cardiomyopathy (**B**), as the enlarged heart, with poor contractility, can cause abnormal blood flow and resultant thrombi. The remainder of the conditions listed are not associated with a dilated cardiomyopathy (**A, C-E**), although a viral myocarditis (**E**) can ultimately lead to a dilated cardiomyopathy; however, the lymphocytic infiltrate would not still be present.

68. Correct: Myocyte disarray (E)

The clinical scenario (i.e., sudden death in a young adult) in combination with the thick interventricular septum identified at autopsy is consistent with the diagnosis of hypertrophic cardiomyopathy. Microscopic examination of the heart in this condition will reveal myocyte disarray (**E**). The other features listed are not typical of hypertrophic cardiomyopathy (**A-D**).

8.14 Miscellaneous Cardiovascular Disease— Answers and Explanations

Easy	Medium	Hard

69. Correct: Rupture with bleeding (C)

Varicose veins can rupture and bleed, and they have even been a cause of death in this fashion (**C**); however, they are not associated with the other complications (**A-B, D-E**).

70. Correct: A pulmonary thromboembolus (D)

Given the recent trauma and resultant relative immobility, this patient is a setup for a pulmonary thromboembolus. The episode of sharp chest pain and dyspnea was likely from a small thrombus that reached the periphery of the lung, whereas his death was caused by a saddle pulmonary thromboembolus (**D**). Although the other conditions (**A-C, E**) can cause sudden death, he has no risk factors for them.

71. Correct: Tumor in the pancreas (C)

Pancreatic tumors are a known risk factor for thrombosis, which can be a precursor to pulmonary thromboembolus (**C**). The other conditions listed, other than being a source of immobility, are not direct risk factors for pulmonary thromboembolus (**A-B, D-E**).

72. Correct: A patent foramen ovale (B)

Deep venous thrombi usually embolize to the lungs, since they arise in the venous circulation; however, with a patent foramen ovale the emboli can cross over to the systemic circulation and can cause a cerebral infarct, which is referred to as a paradoxical embolus (**B**). Although all of the other conditions listed could cause an acute cerebral infarct, none are the result of deep venous thrombi (**A, C-E**).

73. Correct: Embolic occlusion of the pulmonary artery (A)

The patient has clinical features consistent with a deep venous thrombus: swelling and erythema of the lower extremity and palpable cord in the lower extremity (i.e., the thrombus). A deep venous thrombus is a risk for a pulmonary thromboembolus, which can cause an embolic occlusion of a pulmonary artery (**A**). None of the other answers, without a patent foramen ovale, would result from a deep venous thrombus (**B-E**).

74.   Correct: History of recent long-distance travel by car (D)

In a young adult, the findings of sharp chest pain, dyspnea, and a cough with occasional blood are consistent with small pulmonary thromboemboli. As a saddle pulmonary thromboembolus could cause sudden death, it is very important to rule this diagnosis out, and thus, determine whether the patient has any risk factors for deep venous thrombi (**D**). The other choices are not correct (**A-C, E**).

75.   Correct: Accentuation of the pulmonic component of the second heart sound (C)

With the history of recent immobility, the history of dyspnea and sharp chest pain with a cough is most consistent with a pulmonary thromboembolus. Of the physical examination findings, only (**C**) is associated with a pulmonary thromboembolus. The respiratory rate would be increased (**E**). Pitting edema is associated with congestive heart failure; the edema associated with deep venous thrombi is not typically pitting (**A**). Neither a murmur nor retinal hemorrhages are usually associated with a pulmonary thromboembolus (**B, D**).

76.   Correct: D-dimer (C)

See the explanation in question 89. Of the listed tests, d-dimer is the most useful when diagnosing a pulmonary thromboembolus (**C**). Testing for Factor V Leiden would help determine whether the patient was at risk for a thrombus, but it would not help diagnosis the pulmonary thromboembolus, only the reason for the formation of the deep venous thrombus that preceded it (**B**). (**A, D-E**) are not useful or specific for the diagnosis of a pulmonary thromboembolus.

77.   Correct: A lung tumor (C)

The symptoms are consistent with superior vena cava syndrome, which results from compression of the superior vena cava by an apical pulmonary neoplasm. Given her smoking history, she is at risk for lung cancer, and her history of coughing up blood is consistent with a pulmonary tumor (**C**). The other conditions listed (**A-B, D-E**) are not typically associated with obstruction of the superior vena cava.

78.   Correct: Angiosarcoma (D)

Chronic lymphedema, as could occur following mastectomy and lymph node dissection, is a risk factor for development of angiosarcoma (**D**). The swelling of the right upper extremity is consistent with lymphedema. Lymphedema is not a risk factor for the other listed conditions (**A-C, E**).

79.   Correct: Acute lymphangiitis (C)

The clinical features are consistent with acute lymphangiitis (**C**), and none of the other choices (**A-B, D-E**).

80.   Correct: Glomus tumor (C)

A glomus tumor is known for causing pain and commonly is found underneath the fingernail (**C**). The other conditions listed are not usually painful and do not have a predilection for the subungual region (**A-B, D-E**).

81.   Correct: HHV-8 (D)

The gross and microscopic descriptions are consistent with Kaposi sarcoma, which is known to occur in HIV+ individuals, as well as those who are immunosuppressed for organ transplantation and other scenarios. The virus associated with Kaposi sarcoma is HHV-8 (**D**). HIV is not the direct cause of Kaposi sarcoma (**A**). HSV, HHV-6, and CMV are associated with a variety of conditions, but not Kaposi sarcoma (**B-C, E**).

82.   Correct: Rhabdomyoma (C)

Cardiac rhabdomyomas are associated with tuberous sclerosis (**C**), as are hypopigmented macules, Shagreen patch, cortical tubers, subependymal giant cell astrocytomas, lymphangiomyomatosis, and renal angiomyolipomas. Patients with tuberous sclerosis can get fibromas, but these are not typically cardiac in location, usually periungual (**B**). A myxoma would not produce a nodule in the myocardium (**A**), and metastatic melanoma and angiosarcoma (**D-E**) are not usually associated with tuberous sclerosis.

83.   Correct: Myxoma (B)

The description and location is classic for a cardiac myxoma, which is the most common primary tumor of the heart. Both papillary fibroelastoma and endocarditis could possibly occur at this location but would have a different texture, and their incidence would be rare (**A, E**). An angiosarcoma and lipoma would be most likely within the myocardium and have a different appearance (**C, D**).

84.   Correct: Healed endocarditis of the aortic valve, with a gaping defect in one leaflet (D)

There are two forms of hypertrophy of the heart: concentric and eccentric. Concentric hypertrophy is due to pressure overload, while eccentric hypertrophy is due to volume overload. The wall will be thin; however, the size of the chamber is increased. A perforation of an aortic valve leaflet would lead to insufficiency, which would cause volume overload and eccentric hypertrophy (**D**). An aldosterone-secreting adenoma of the adrenal gland and coarctation of the aorta would both cause hypertension and lead to concentric hypertrophy (**A, B**). Aortic stenosis due to a calcified bicuspid valve would also lead to concentric hypertrophy (**C**). Mitral stenosis should not lead to hypertrophy of the left ventricle, unless there is regurgitation as well (**E**).

85. Correct: Pulmonary fibrosis (D)

The patient has signs and symptoms of right-sided heart failure (i.e., hepatosplenomegaly and pitting edema), but not of left-sided heart failure, since there are no pleural effusions. In pure right-sided heart failure, the underlying cause is within the lungs; the pulmonary fibrosis could lead to right-sided heart failure (**D**). The other conditions listed would cause left-sided heart failure (**A-C, E**).

86. Correct: Pleural effusions (E)

The description is that of chronic passive congestion of the lungs, with the hemosiderin-laden macrophages being heart-failure cells. Of the choices, only pleural effusions are associated with left-sided heart failure (**E**). The other choices would be identified in right-sided heart failure (**A-D**).

87. Correct: Right ventricular hypertrophy (D)

With emphysema, there is a loss of vasculature in the heart, as the number of alveolar septa is decreased, which puts strain on the heart. This strain can lead to right ventricular hypertrophy (**D**), although most people with emphysema will not have right ventricular hypertrophy. None of the other choices is caused by a pulmonary process (**A-C, E**).

Chapter 9

Diseases of the Hematopoietic and Lymphoid Systems

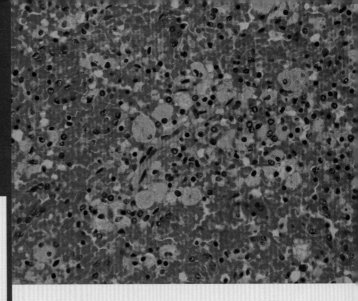

LEARNING OBJECTIVES

9.1 Anemia and Red Blood Cell Disorders

- List the causes of anemia.
- Describe the red blood cell morphology associated with various types of anemia.
- Discuss the clinical evaluation of a microcytic anemia to determine its underlying cause.
- Discuss the general mechanisms by which anemia occurs.
- Compare and contrast α- and β-thalassemia.
- List the laboratory abnormalities of β-thalassemia.
- Given a clinical scenario, distinguish between the types of microcytic anemia.
- Compare and contrast the forms of β-thalassemia.
- Describe the laboratory evaluation of microcytic anemia and iron deficiency anemia.
- Given laboratory testing, distinguish between the various types of microcytic anemia.
- Given a red blood cell morphology, identify diseases causing it and determine how to distinguish among them.
- Compare megaloblastic anemia due to folate or B12 deficiency.
- Given signs, symptoms, and laboratory evaluation, diagnosis and determine the underlying cause of anemia.
- Given signs, symptoms, and laboratory testing, diagnose hereditary spherocytosis.
- Describe the approach to diagnose iron deficiency in a patient over the age of 50 years old and the association with colon cancer.
- Describe the typical laboratory findings in anemia of chronic disease.
- Distinguish between folic acid deficiency and vitamin B12 deficiency and list the common causes of each.
- Given the clinical scenario, diagnose paroxysmal nocturnal hemoglobinuria and list its common complications.
- Diagnose hereditary spherocystosis.
- Diagnose glucose-6-phosphate dehydrogenase deficiency and recognize common precipitants.
- Diagnose acute chest syndrome in sickle cell disease.
- Diagnose thalassemia trait.

- Diagnose β-thalassemia major and describe the typical laboratory findings.
- Diagnose α-thalassemia minor and understand the typical laboratory findings.
- Diagnose warm antibody hemolytic anemia.
- Diagnose hereditary hemochromatosis.
- Describe the effects of the parvovirus infection on individuals with a predisposition to anemia.
- Describe the clinical presentation, epidemiology, and laboratory abnormalities associated with Fanconi anemia.
- Describe the clinical presentation, epidemiology, and laboratory testing for the diagnosis of ITP.
- Given the laboratory tests, distinguish between intravascular and extravascular hemolysis.
- List the causes of hemolytic anemia.
- Given the laboratory findings, diagnose hemolytic anemia.
- Distinguish between extravascular and intravascular hemolysis.
- List the features of thrombotic thrombocytopenic purpura.
- Given the laboratory findings, diagnose microcytic anemia, and list the forms of microcytic anemia and describe how to distinguish between them using laboratory testing.

9.2 Transfusion and Miscellaneous

- Given the signs and symptoms, diagnose acute pancreatitis, and list and describe the complications of acute pancreatitis.
- List the causes of schistocytes.
- Given the clinical scenario, diagnose transfusion-related acute lung injury (TRALI).

9.3 Lymphoid

- Given signs and symptoms, diagnose infectious mononucleosis.
- List pathologic changes associated with EBV virus infection.

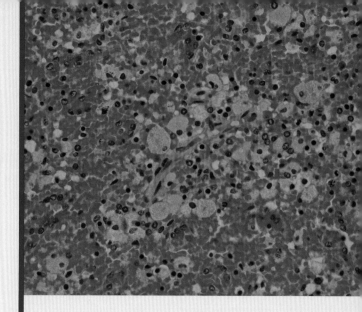

- ▶ List the viral causes of this disorder.
- ▶ List the common surface markers for myeloid and lymphoid cells.
- ▶ Describe the complications related to an infiltrative process of the bone marrow.
- ▶ List and describe laboratory tests useful in the diagnosis of leukemia.
- ▶ List the cellular markers associated with B- and T-cell neoplasms.
- ▶ List the genetic abnormalities associated with each form of acute and chronic myeloid and acute and chronic lymphoid neoplasms.
- ▶ Describe the physical examination, laboratory, and genetic findings of chronic lymphocytic leukemia.
- ▶ List causes and describe the complications of aplastic anemia.
- ▶ Given signs, symptoms, and laboratory testing, diagnose acute leukemia in children, and list the relative frequency of precursor B-cell lymphoblastic leukemia and precursor T-cell lymphoblastic leukemia.
- ▶ Given the clinical scenario and laboratory testing, diagnose myelofibrosis.
- ▶ Diagnose polycythemia vera and list the association with the JAK2 mutation.
- ▶ Given the clinical scenario, imaging, and laboratory evaluation, diagnose multiple myeloma.
- ▶ Describe the testing methods to diagnose multiple myeloma.
- ▶ Given the pathologic description and clinical scenario, diagnose a Burkitt lymphoma.
- ▶ Describe the epidemiology, etiology, and treatment of a Burkitt lymphoma.
- ▶ Given the clinical presentation and laboratory testing, diagnose CML, and list the cytogenetic abnormality associated with CML.

9.1 Anemia and Red Blood Cell Disorders–Questions

Easy	Medium	Hard

1. A 37-year-old white female presents to her family physician with complaints of fatigue and dizziness. The fatigue has been increasing in severity for several months. Physical examination reveals a temperature of 98.8°F, pulse of 106 bpm, respiratory rate of 18 breaths per minute, and blood pressure of 108/76 mm Hg. Physical examination is unremarkable other than slight pallor of the conjunctivae. Laboratory testing reveals a hemoglobin of 10.9 g/dL. Her stool is negative for occult blood. She has no family history of cancer, does not drink alcohol excessively, and eats a regular balanced diet. Of the following, what is the most likely cause of her symptoms?

A. Menstrual blood loss

B. Colonic adenocarcinoma

C. Warm autoimmune hemolytic anemia

D. Vitamin B12 deficiency

E. Sickle cell disease

Hematopoietic

2. A 53-year-old male presents to his family physician with complaints of fatigue and dizziness. The fatigue has been ongoing for several months and increasing in severity. Physical examination reveals a temperature of 98.6°F, a pulse of 109 bpm, and a respiratory rate of 20 breaths per minute. Laboratory testing reveals a hemoglobin of 9.8 g/dL and an MCV of 75 fL. Of the following, which is a blood smear most likely to reveal?

A. Teardrop cells

B. Rouleaux

C. Pencil cells

D. Leukemic blasts

E. Schistocytes

Hematopoietic

3. A 64-year-old male presents to his family physician with fatigue and dizziness, which started three months ago. Physical examination reveals a temperature of 98.6°F, a pulse of 113 bpm, and a respiratory rate of 22 breaths per minute. Laboratory testing reveals a hemoglobin of 9.5 g/dL and an MCV of 70 fL. Of the following, which test is most likely to help identify the source of the laboratory results?

A. A Coombs test

B. Osmotic fragility test

C. Testing for vitamin B12

D. Fecal occult blood test

E. Donath-Landsteiner antibody testing

Hematopoietic

4. A 63-year-old male presents to his family physician with complaints of fatigue. The fatigue has been developing for several months. He also reports being constipated over the past few weeks. He has a family history of colonic adenocarcinoma. Laboratory testing reveals a hemoglobin of 10.3 g/dL and an MCV of 71 fL. The patient is scheduled for a colonoscopy, which reveals a mass in the rectum. A biopsy reveals an invasive adenocarcinoma. Of the following, testing would most likely reveal?

A. Decreased ferritin, decreased serum iron, decreased TIBC

B. Increased ferritin, increased serum iron, increased TIBC

C. Decreased ferritin, increased serum iron, decreased TIBC

D. Increased ferritin, decreased serum iron, decreased TIBC

E. Decreased ferritin, decreased serum iron, increased TIBC

Hematopoietic

5. A 56-year-old female presents to her family physician with complaints of fatigue. Physical examination reveals a temperature of 98.6°F, a pulse of 109 bpm, and a respiratory rate of 20 breaths per minute. Laboratory testing indicates a hemoglobin of 9.9 g/dL. In the physician's differential diagnosis, he includes pure red cell aplasia and a warm autoimmune hemolytic anemia. Of the following tests, which is most useful for distinguishing between the two conditions?

A. MCV

B. RDW

C. Ferritin

D. Reticulocyte count

E. Total iron-binding capacity

Hematopoietic

6. A pathologist is examining the liver biopsy of a 22-year-old male with cirrhosis. A Prussian blue stain reveals extensive positivity. Laboratory testing does not reveal HbH or HbBarts. Of the following, what is the most likely diagnosis?

A. α-thalassemia

B. β-thalasssemia major

C. Severe iron deficiency anemia

D. Sideroblastic anemia

E. β-thalassemia minor

Liver, heme

7. A 36-year-old male, originally from Greece, emigrated to the United States with his family when he was a child. He presents to an acute care clinic after falling from a chair and hitting his head, producing a laceration of the scalp. On physical examination, his blood pressure is 112/68 mm Hg, his pulse is 109 bpm, and his temperature is 98.9°F. He has no past medical history. A complete blood count reveals a white blood cell count of 7,100 cells/μL, hemoglobin of 11 g/dL, and Hct of 34%. The MCV is 50 fL. Of the following, what is the most likely diagnosis?

A. Hereditary spherocytosis

B. β-thalassemia minor

C. Iron deficiency anemia

D. Anemia of chronic disease

E. Megaloblastic anemia

Heme

8. Given the previous clinical scenario, of the following, if laboratory testing is performed, which would be identified?

A. β4

B. β+/β+

C. b0/b

D. Mutation in spectrin

E. Valine for glutamic acid at 6th position in β-globulin chain

Heme

9. A 47-year-old female with a 26-year history of systemic lupus erythematosus is being seen by her family physician for a routine examination and refill of medications. She does relate that recently she has felt more fatigued and occasionally becomes short of breath when exercising at the gym. She is still menstruating. A physical examination reveals a temperature of 98.7°F, a pulse of 92 bpm, and a blood pressure of 108/65 mm Hg. Laboratory testing reveals a white blood cell count of 3,700 cells/μL, a hemoglobin of 10.2 g/dL, and Hct of 32%. The MCV is 71 fL. Her physician is concerned about the possibility of iron deficiency anemia or anemia of chronic disease. Which of the following tests would be the most help to confirm the diagnosis?

A. Serum iron

B. HbA2

C. Erythrocyte protoporphyrin

D. Ferritin

E. Blood smear

Heme

10. A 41-year-old female with a 17-year history of systemic lupus erythematosus is being seen by her family physician for a routine examination and refill of medication. She does relate that recently she has felt more fatigued and occasionally becomes short of breath when exercising at the gym. She is still menstruating. A physical examination reveals a temperature of 98.7°F, a pulse of 94 bpm, and a blood pressure of 103/67 mm Hg. Laboratory testing reveals a white blood cell count of 3,800/μL, a hemoglobin of 10.2 g/dL, and Hct of 32%. The MCV is 75 fL. Additional laboratory test reveals a TIBC of 630 μg/dL (normal is 255–450 μg/dL), a serum iron of 41 μg/dL (normal is 50–160 μg/dL), and a transferrin saturation of 15% (normal is 20–45%). Of the following, what is the most likely diagnosis?

A. Iron deficiency anemia

B. Warm autoimmune hemolytic anemia

C. Cold autoimmune hemolytic anemia

D. Anemia of chronic disease

E. Sideroblastic anemia

Heme

11. A medical technologist is examining a blood smear and notes many red blood cells that are decreased in size, are hyperchromatic, and lack a central pallor. The lab requisition form indicates a history of systemic lupus erythematosus. There is no family history of anemia. The medical technologist performs a direct Coombs test, which is positive. Of the following, what is the most likely diagnosis?

A. Warm autoimmune hemolytic anemia

B. Microangiopathic hemolytic anemia

C. Hereditary spherocytosis

D. G6PD deficiency

E. Iron deficiency anemia

Heme

12. A medical technologist is examining a blood smear and notes many spherocytes. She performs a monospecific direct Coombs test, which is negative. The laboratory requisition form indicates that the patient was seen in the clinic and was diagnosed with infectious mononucleosis. Of the following, what is the agent responsible for the change in the red blood cells?

A. IgG

B. IgM

C. IgE

D. IgD

E. IgA

Heme

13. A 47-year-old male is diagnosed with megaloblastic anemia by his family physician based on a complete blood count, peripheral blood smear, and MCV. Of the following, which feature would favor B12 deficiency as the cause of his anemia versus folate deficiency?

A. Hypersegmented neutrophils

B. Elevated concentration of homocysteine

C. Elevated concentration of methylmalonic acid

D. Pencil cells on peripheral smear

E. Teardrop cells on peripheral smear

Heme

14. A 48-year-old male presents to his family physician with complaints of fatigue. His vital signs are temperature of 98.7°F, pulse of 110 bpm, respiratory rate of 20 breaths per minute, and blood pressure of 131/85 mm Hg. Physical examination reveals pale conjunctivae and nail beds; however, the conjunctivae are slightly yellow discolored. A complete blood cell count reveals a hemoglobin of 8.5 g/dL. The MCV is 86 fL. Additional testing reveals an AST of 15 U/L, an ALT of 12 U/L, total bilirubin of 5.3 mg/dL, direct bilirubin of 0.2 mg/dL, and LDH of 210 U/L. Urinalysis identifies hemoglobin in the urine. Of the following, what is the most likely etiology for his low hemoglobin?

A. A remote cardiac valve replacement

B. A warm autoimmune hemolytic anemia

C. Aplastic anemia

D. Folate deficiency

E. Iron deficiency

Heme

15. A 36-year-old Caucasian female presents to the emergency room in acute distress, being pale, short of breath, and very easily fatigued. Her vital signs are temperature of 99.0°F, pulse of 130 bpm, respiratory rate of 28 breaths per minute, and blood pressure of 100/74 mm Hg. Physical examination reveals yellow discoloration of her conjunctivae and a palpable spleen. She has a history of a cholecystectomy at age 25, and knows that her father and paternal grandmother had a history of anemia; otherwise, she has no significant past medical history. Laboratory testing reveals a hemoglobin of 5.2 g/dL. Of the following, what is her most likely underlying diagnosis?

A. Hereditary spherocytosis

B. α-thalassemia trait

C. β-thalassemia minor

D. G6PD deficiency

E. Sickle cell anemia

Heme, spleen

16. Given the previous clinical scenario, of the following, which laboratory test will be most useful in diagnosing her underlying etiology?

A. Measurement of folate and B12 concentration

B. Hemoglobin electrophoresis

C. Direct Coombs test

D. Osmotic fragility testing

E. Ferritin concentration

Heme, spleen

17. A 56-year-old man with a history of well-controlled hypertension presents for an annual physical. He reports good health and no complaints. His vital signs and physical examination are normal. In addition to a fasting lipid profile and comprehensive metabolic panel, his physician orders a complete blood count, which showed 7.5×10^9 cells/L leukocytes, a hemoglobin of 9.1 g/dL, with a mean corpuscular volume of 76 fL and a platelet count of 425,000 cells/μL. Which of the following tests is indicated next?

A. Colonoscopy

B. Ferritin

C. Barium contrast enema

D. Vitamin B12 level

E. Flow cytometry

Hematologic

18. A 39-year-old female with poorly controlled rheumatoid arthritis presents to her family physician complaining of fatigue, worsening over the past 2 months. Her physical examination is unchanged from a year ago. A complete blood count is remarkable for a hemoglobin of 9.5 g/dL with a mean corpuscular volume of 78 fL. A serum ferritin level is 300 ng/mL. Which additional test would support the diagnosis of anemia of chronic disease in this patient rather than iron deficiency?

A. Increased total iron-binding capacity (TIBC)

B. Decreased transferrin saturation

C. Normal soluble transferrin receptor levels

D. Increased platelet count

E. Decreased leukocyte count

Hematologic

19. A 32-year-old Asian female is evaluated for anemia by her primary care physician. Her hemoglobin level is 8.7 g/dL with a mean corpuscular volume of 104 fL. Serum cobalamin levels are normal. Homocysteine levels are elevated, and her methylmalonic acid level is normal. Which of the following drugs is known to cause this condition?

A. Cephalosporins

B. Atorvastatin

C. Topiramate

D. Retinoic acid

E. Methotrexate

Hematologic

20. A 32-year-old man presents to his primary care physician complaining of blood in his urine, which he first noticed this morning. Other than fatigue, he is without complaint. Physical examination is normal except for scleral icterus. His urine is rose colored. A complete blood count shows a leukocyte count of 3.8 × 10⁹ cells/L, a serum hemoglobin of 8.2 g/dL, and platelet count is 92 × 10⁹ cells/L. Microscopic analysis of the urine reveals 1 red cell/hpf. Serum aminotransferases are normal, and the patient has a total bilirubin of 5.8 mg/dL with a direct bilirubin of 0.3 mg/dL. A direct antibody test is negative; however, flow cytometry demonstrates abnormally low expression of CD55 and CD59 on the patient's blood cells. Which of the following complications of this disease is this patient most likely to die from?

A. Sepsis

B. Hepatic vein thrombosis

C. Myocardial infarction

D. Acute leukemia

E. Intraabdominal hemorrhage

Hematologic

21. A 34-year-old woman is evaluated in the emergency for right upper quadrant pain. On examination she has right upper quadrant tenderness with a positive Murphy sign. There is a palpable mass in the left upper quadrant, and scleral icterus is present. Complete blood count reveals a leukocyte count of 14.5 × 10⁹ cells/L, a hemoglobin of 7.6 g/dL, and a platelet count of 75 × 10⁹ cells/L. The reticulocyte count is 13%. Serum AST is 410 U/L, and ALT is 350 U/L. Total bilirubin is 9.5 mg/dL with a direct bilirubin of 3.5 mg/dL. Which additional test result is likely to be seen in this patient?

A. A low mean cell hemoglobin concentration

B. A low mean corpuscular volume

C. A normal alkaline phosphatase

D. A normal right upper quadrant ultrasound

E. Howell-Jolly bodies within red blood cells on peripheral smear

Hematologic

22. A 33-year-old Caucasian male is seen in the emergency department for pain and redness of the right buttock. He is started on trimethoprim-sulfamethoxazole and doxycycline. He returns to his family physician four days later because of a yellowing of his eyes. His physical examination is unremarkable except for mild jaundice and scleral icterus. A complete blood count shows a leukocyte count of 10.2 × 10⁹ cells/L, a hemoglobin of 7.2 g/dL, and a platelet count of 260 × 10⁹ cells/L. Total bilirubin is 6.2 mg/dL and direct bilirubin is 0.3 mg/dL. Aminotransferases are normal. Serum haptoglobin is undetectable. A peripheral blood smear is likely to show which of the following?

A. Pencil cells

B. Spherocytes

C. Target cells

D. Sickle cells

E. Heinz bodies

Hematologic

23. A 26-year-old African American male presents to the emergency department with diffuse chest pain and shortness of breath, which started four hours prior to admission. His temperature is 102.3°F (39°C), pulse is 110/min, blood pressure 152/86 mm Hg and oxygen saturation is 85% on room air. On examination, he appears uncomfortable, heart sounds are normal, and crackles are heard in both lung fields. A complete blood count shows a leukocyte count of 16.5 × 10⁹ cells/L, a hemoglobin of 6.3 g/dL, and a platelet count of 525 × 10⁹ cells/L. A 12-lead electrocardiogram shows sinus tachycardia with a left axis deviation and no ST segment changes. A contrast CT of the chest shows bilateral infiltrates and no pulmonary embolism. Serum lactate dehydrogenase is 920 U/L, and total bilirubin is 9.2 mg/dL. A peripheral blood smear is likely to show which of the following?

A. Pencil cells

B. Spherocytes

C. Target cells

D. Sickle cells

E. Heinz bodies

Hematologic

24. A 26-year-old male African immigrant with no significant past medical history is referred to hematology for evaluation of anemia discovered incidentally on routine blood work. A complete blood count shows a leukocyte count of 3.6×10^9 cells/L and a hemoglobin of 10.1 g/dL. The mean cell hemoglobin concentration is 24 g/dL, and the mean corpuscular volume is 76 fL. His serum ferritin level is 460 ng/mL. A hemoglobin electrophoresis test shows elevated HbA2. A peripheral blood smear is likely to show which of the following?

A. Pencil cells

B. Spherocytes

C. Target cells

D. Sickle cells

E. Heinz bodies

Hematologic

25. A 4-year-old African American child is evaluated in a hematology clinic for anemia. The child has received multiple blood transfusions starting at the age of 10 months, but has not been transfused in the past 2 years due to social difficulties. On examination, the child has abnormally prominent cheekbones and forehead, a depressed nasal bridge, and dental malocclusion. Heart sounds are normal, but the point of maximal impulse is laterally displaced. His lungs are clear. The spleen is markedly enlarged. Which of the following laboratory results would be expected in this patient?

A. Low red cell distribution width

B. Low reticulocyte count

C. Increased serum ferritin

D. Increased mean corpuscular volume

E. Increased mean cell hemoglobin concentration

Hematologic

26. A 19-year-old male is evaluated in a hematology clinic for unexplained anemia discovered on routine blood work. The patient is of Asian descent, with no medical problems, and is asymptomatic. A peripheral smear shows a mild hypochromic, microcytic anemia with occasional target cells. A ferritin level is normal. His hemoglobin electrophoresis is normal and his HbA2 level is within the normal range. What is the most likely diagnosis?

A. Sickle cell anemia

B. Sickle cell trait

C. β-thalassemia minor

D. α-thalassemia minor

E. Glucose-6-phosphate dehydrogenase deficiency

Hematologic

27. A 65-year-old female presents to her primary care physician with pallor and fatigue. A complete blood count reveals a hemoglobin of 8.2 g/dL. The Total bilirubin is 6.4 mg/dL, and direct bilirubin is 0.2 mg/dL. Her lactate dehydrogenase is elevated, and a direct antibody test causes agglutination with anti-IgG. Her peripheral smear reveals spherocytes. What is the most likely diagnosis?

A. Hereditary spherocytosis

B. Glucose-6-phosphate dehydrogenase deficiency

C. Warm antibody hemolytic anemia

D. Cold antibody hemolytic anemia

E. Paroxysmal cold hemoglobinuria

Hematologic

28. A 56-year-old man presents complaining of fatigue and polyarthralgia. Laboratory testing for rheumatoid factor and anti-nuclear antibodies are normal. A complete blood count is performed, which shows a Hb of 19.2 mg/dL. His transferrin saturation is 65% and his serum ferritin is 1425 ng/mL. What additional testing is indicated?

A. Erythropoietin level

B. Chest radiograph

C. Genetic testing

D. Flow cytometry

E. CT abdomen with contrast

Hematologic

29. A 16-year-old female with sickle cell disease presents with a fever and severe fatigue that started two days ago. She takes hydroxyurea and has not had a sickle cell crisis in 2 years. A complete blood count reveals a leukocyte count of 3.3×10^9 cells/L, a hemoglobin of 4.2 g/dL, and a platelet count of 204×10^9 cells/L. The patient's reticulocyte count is 0.3%. A bone marrow biopsy is performed that shows giant pronormoblasts and a decrease in erythrocyte precursors. What is most likely to have caused this condition?

A. Hydroxyurea

B. Splenic sequestration

C. Parvovirus B19 infection

D. Myelodysplastic syndrome

E. Myelofibrosis

Heme

30. A 7-year-old boy is seen in a hematology clinic due to progressive pancytopenia associated with recurrent infections. The child was born with deformities of both thumbs. A complete blood count shows a leukocyte count of 2.1×10^9 cells/L, a hemoglobin of 6.3 g/dL and a platelet count of 47×10^9 cells/L. He has an older brother who suffered a similar illness and died at age 12 of acute myelogenous leukemia. What is the most likely diagnosis?

A. Thrombocytopenia-absent radii syndrome

B. Wiskott-Aldrich syndrome

C. Ataxia-telangectasia

D. Fanconi anemia

E. Diamond-Blackfand anemia

Heme

31. A 32-year-old female is evaluated by her primary care physician for bleeding gums. She first noticed the problem 3 weeks ago. She also reports two episodes of epistaxis during the same time. She denies any recent illnesses and takes no medication. A physical examination is normal except for the presence of multiple punctate red lesions on the skin, which do not blanch with pressure. There is no lymphadenopathy or splenomegaly. A complete blood count shows a leukocyte count of 7.2×10^9 cells/L, a serum hemoglobin of 11.5 g/dL, and a platelet count of 37×10^9 cells/L. Laboratory testing for HIV and a hepatitis panel are normal. A peripheral blood smear shows normal red cells and platelets with no schistocytes. What is the most likely diagnosis?

A. Hemolytic uremic syndrome

B. Thrombotic thrombocytopenic purpura

C. Hereditary hemorrhagic telangiectasia

D. Idiopathic thrombocytopenic purpura

E. Myelodysplastic syndrome

Heme

32. A 37 year-old male presents to his family physician with complaints of fatigue. A complete blood count is as follows: hemoglobin 11.7 g/dL, hematocrit of 34%, and MCV of 87 fL. Additional laboratory tests reveal a total bilirubin of 1.9 mg/dL, LDH of 563 U/L, and haptoglobin of 13 mg/dL. The urine is positive for both hemoglobin and hemosiderin. Of the following, what is the most likely diagnosis?

A. B12 deficiency

B. Hereditary spherocytosis

C. Warm autoimmune hemolytic anemia

D. Babesiosis

E. Iron deficiency anemia

Heme

33. A 39-year-old female is brought to the emergency room by her family. She has been complaining of fatigue, and most recently, prompting the visit to the emergency room, she became confused about what day it was and where she was at. Her vital signs include a temperature of 99.8°F. A complete blood count is as follows: hemoglobin 10.7 g/dL, hematocrit of 30%, platelet count of 91,000 cells/µL, and MCV of 87 fL. Additional laboratory tests reveal a total bilirubin of 1.8 mg/dL, LDH of 581 U/L, and haptoglobin of 12 mg/dL. The urine is positive for both hemoglobin and hemosiderin. Of the following, what would most likely be seen on the blood smear?

A. Elliptocytes

B. Spherocytes

C. Schistocytes

D. Target cells

E. Bite cells

Heme

34. A 38-year-old female presents to her family physician with complaints of fatigue. Laboratory testing reveals a total bilirubin of 0.4 mg/dL, an LDH of 267 U/L, haptoglobin of 101 mg/dL, hemoglobin of 10.8 g/dL, hematocit of 32%, and MCV of 76 fL. Total iron binding capacity is 545 mg/dL, and ferritin is 6 ng/mL. Of the following, what is the most likely cause of her presenting condition?

A. An autoimmune disorder

B. Undiagnosed thalassemia

C. Heavy menstrual bleeding

D. Sideroblastic anemia

E. Malaria

Heme

35. Given the previous clinical scenario, which of the following would a blood smear reveal?

A. Spherocytes

B. Organisms in the red blood cells

C. Schistocytes

D. Increased central pallor of red blood cells

E. Hypersegmented neutrophils

Heme

36. A 32-year-old female presents to her family physician with complaints of fatigue. Laboratory testing reveals a total bilirubin of 0.5 mg/dL, an LDH of 271 U/L, haptoglobin of 117 mg/dL, hemoglobin of 10.3 g/dL, hematocit of 30%, and MCV of 56 fL. Total iron-binding capacity is 293 µg/dL, and ferritin is 82 ng/mL. Of the following, what is the most likely diagnosis?

A. Iron deficiency anemia

B. Anemia of chronic disease

C. Thalassemia

D. Megaloblastic anemia

E. Warm autoimmune hemolytic anemia

Heme

37. Given the previous clinical scenario, of the following tests, which would be most useful in identifying the specific underlying cause of her presenting condition?

A. Anti-dsDNA

B. Serum folate concentration

C. Hemoglobin electrophoresis

D. Transferrin saturation

E. ANCA testing

Heme

9.2 Transfusion and Miscellaneous—Questions

| Easy | Medium | Hard |

38. A 43-year-old alcoholic presents to the emergency room with complaints of abdominal pain, which developed suddenly about one day ago and is in the epigastric region but also affects his back. Admission laboratory testing reveals a white blood cell count of 18,000 cells/µL, hemoglobin of 14 g/dL, hematocrit of 38%, ALT of 98 U/L, AST of 88 U/L, GGT of 121 U/L, alkaline phosphatase of 870 U/L, amylase of 332 U/L, and lipase of 650 U/L. Despite treatment, his condition worsens and he begins to ooze blood from needle puncture sites. Of the following, what is the most likely diagnosis?

A. Warm autoimmune hemolytic anemia

B. Cold autoimmune hemolytic anemia

C. Thrombotic thrombocytopenic purpura

D. Disseminated intravascular coagulation

E. Megaloblastic anemia

Pancreas

39. Given the previous clinical scenario, of the following, what cell type is most likely to be found on a blood smear?

A. Teardrop cells

B. Spherocytes

C. Macro-ovalocyte

D. Schistocyte

E. Ringed sideroblast

Pancreas, heme

40. A 38-year-old female receives 4 units of cross-matched blood after an intraoperative hemorrhage during a total abdominal hysterectomy. Two hours after the transfusion she becomes hypoxic with pulse oximetry of 86 to 89%. Her temperature is 99.9°F (37.7°C). A plain chest radiograph shows bilateral diffuse infiltrates with a normal cardiomediastinal sillouette. A direct antiglobulin (Coombs) test is performed and is negative. What is the most likely diagnosis?

A. Acute volume overload

B. Sepsis

C. Hemolytic transfusion reaction

D. Transfusion-related acute lung injury

E. Anaphylaxis

Hematologic

9.3 Lymphoid—Questions

| Easy | Medium | Hard |

41. A 19-year-old female college student presents to the campus medical clinic with complaints of fatigue that developed within the last few days. She also has a sore throat. She uses alcohol only occasionally. She does not use intravenous drugs or abuse prescription medication. Her past medical history is noncontributory. Her temperature is 99.9°F, pulse is 93 bpm, respiratory rate is 17 breaths per minute, and blood pressure is 100/75 mm Hg. A physical examination is noncontributory except for a palpable spleen and posterior cervical lymphadenopathy. Of the following, what is the most likely diagnosis?

A. Acute lymphocytic leukemia

B. Follicular lymphoma

C. Subacute bacterial endocarditis

D. Infectious mononucleosis

E. Systemic lupus erythematosus

Spleen, lymph nodes

42. A 20-year-old female college student develops a low-grade fever (99.7°F), fatigue, and a sore throat after a weekend visit from her boyfriend, who goes to school in another state. She presents to the clinic, where a physical examination reveals generalized lymphadenopathy and an enlarged spleen. Of the following, which is most likely to be identified on a blood smear?

A. Schistocytes

B. Blasts

C. Reed-Sternberg cells

D. Atypical lymphocytes

E. Rouleaux

Spleen, lymph nodes

43. Given the previous clinical scenario, of the following, which etiologic agent is the most likely source of her signs and symptoms?

A. HIV

B. HSV

C. EBV

D. *Streptococcus pneumoniae*

E. *Staphylococcus aureus*

Spleen, lymph nodes

44. A 20-year-old male college student presents to the campus clinic with complaints of fatigue, which started two days ago, and a sore throat. His vital signs are temperature of 99.7°F, pulse of 96 bpm, respiratory rate of 17 breaths per minute, and blood pressure of 110/78 mm Hg. A cursory physical examination reveals no murmurs or abnormal breathing sounds. The patient is prescribed amoxicillin. Shortly after beginning the antibiotic, he develops a morbilliform rash. Of the following, what physical finding was missed on physical examination?

A. A heart murmur

B. Rales in the upper lobes of the lungs

C. Cervical lymphadenopathy

D. Decreased bowel sounds

E. Splenomegaly

Hematology

45. A 21-year-old female college student develops fatigue and a low-grade fever after a visit by her boyfriend, who goes to a different college in another state. During a massage given to her by a friend, her friend notes small swellings on the back of her neck. The next day, she goes horseback riding with her friends and falls from a horse onto a large pile of hay. Several minutes after the fall, she becomes unresponsive, and ultimately dies. At autopsy, of the following, which is most likely to be identified by the forensic pathologist?

A. A ruptured coronary artery aneurysm

B. A lacerated kidney

C. A lacerated aorta

D. A ruptured spleen

E. A ruptured berry aneurysm

Spleen

46. A pathologist is examining a blood smear that has leukemic cells, and a bone marrow biopsy of the patient has a pronounced leukemic infiltrate. The morphology of the cells appears to be myeloid to the pathologist. If the cells are myeloid, which of the following markers is most likely to stain positive on the cells?

A. CD4

B. CD10

C. CD13

D. CD19

E. CD20

Heme

47. A 56-year-old male presents to his family physician with complaints of three weeks of fatigue with easy bleeding (he has noted multiple bruises on his upper and lower extremities that developed after minimal trauma), as well as five days of a productive cough and chills. His vital signs are temperature of 100.2°F, blood pressure of 131/87 mm Hg, and pulse of 112 bpm. A chest X-ray reveals an infiltrate in the lower lobe of the right lung. His hemoglobin is determined to be 9.7 g/dL. The doctor feels that all of his complaints are related to one underlying disease process. Of the following, which is most likely to reveal the underlying disease process?

A. A CT scan of the head

B. A bone marrow biopsy

C. A skin biopsy for fibroblast culture

D. Culture of the sputum

E. Routine urinalysis

Heme

48. Given the previous clinical scenario, of the following, which laboratory tests are most likely to assist in determining what this disease process is?

A. Urinalysis and culture

B. Culture of the sputum, with sensitivities of the organism

C. Complete blood count including blood smear

D. Liver panel

E. Anti-dsDNA, anti-SSA, and anti-SSB

Heme

49. Given the previous clinical scenario, after his hemoglobin is determined to be 9.7 g/dL, his white blood cell count is determined to be 83,000 cells/µL, with 80% blasts. A smear reveals white blood cells with a fine chromatin pattern that is homogeneous and evenly dispersed throughout the nucleus, and a very small rim of cytoplasm. The cells are CD19 positive, and genetic testing reveals a t(9;22). No Auer rods are identified. Of the following, what is the most likely diagnosis?

A. Acute lymphocytic leukemia

B. Chronic lymphocytic leukemia

C. Acute myeloid leukemia

D. Chronic myeloid leukemia

E. Myelodysplasia

Heme

50. A 50-year-old male presents to his family physician with complaints of fatigue, present for the past 2 months. During that time, he has also lost 20 lbs. without any change in his diet or exercise regimen. His vital signs are temperature of 99.5°F, pulse of 86 bpm, and blood pressure of 125/82 mm Hg. A physical examination reveals splenomegaly. Laboratory testing indicates a white blood cell count of 102,500 cells/µL, hemoglobin of 10.9 g/dL, and Hct of 33%. The blood smear has a prominence of meta-myelocytes and myelocytes. If genetic testing is performed, which of the following would most likely be identified?

A. t(8;14)

B. t(11;14)

C. t(14;18)

D. t(9;22)

E. t(15;17)

Heme

51. A 12-year-old boy is brought to the emergency room by his family. Over the past two weeks, he has developed marked fatigue, and his parents have noted pinpoint hemorrhages in his eyelids. On examination, the patient appears ill. His vital signs are temperature of 99.6°F, blood pressure of 100/65 mm Hg, and pulse rate of 102 bpm. The white blood cell count is 87,000 cells/µL, with 92% blasts, hemoglobin of 8.6 g/dL, and platelet count of 68,000 cells/µL. Of the following, which would genetic testing most likely reveal?

A. t(15;17)

B. t(9;22)

C. t(12;21)

D. t(11;14)

E. t(14;18)

Heme

52. A 53-year-old male presents to his family physician with complaints of fatigue, which has been slowly developing for about 3 months. In that time, he has also lost 24 lbs., without any change in his diet or exercise regimen. His vital signs are temperature of 99.7°F, pulse of 81 bpm, and blood pressure of 144/82 mm Hg. Laboratory testing indicates a white blood cell count of 145,000 cells/µL, hemoglobin of 10.6 g/dL, and Hct of 34%. The blood smear has a prominence of immature myeloid cells and occasional basophils. No blasts are identified. Of the following, what is a characteristic physical finding associated with this disease?

A. Splenomegaly

B. Systolic ejection murmur

C. Decreased breath sounds on the right side

D. Chvostek sign

E. Pitting edema of the lower extremities

Heme

53. A 31-year-old worker at a chemical factory is exposed to a large benzene spill. Following exposure, he is taken to the emergency room. Over the next several weeks, he develops fatigue and a generalized malaise. His friends take him to the emergency room, where he is noted to be acutely ill. His friends relate that he has been bleeding from his gums. A complete blood cell count reveals a hemoglobin of 7.9 g/dL and platelet count of 43,000 cells/µL. Of the following, what is the most likely diagnosis?

A. Acute lymphocytic leukemia

B. Anemia of chronic disease

C. Aplastic anemia

D. Warm autoimmune hemolytic anemia

E. Cold autoimmune hemolytic anemia

Heme

54. A 4-year-old female is brought to the emergency room by her parents. Over the past two months she has developed severe fatigue and shortness of breath, and has intermittent fevers, up to 99.9°F. She has had bleeding after brushing her teeth. Yesterday, she developed a bad headache and has been vomiting. Her vital signs are temperature of 99.8°F, pulse of 112 bpm, respiratory rate of 31 breaths per minute, and blood pressure of 105/78 mm Hg. A physical examination reveals cervical and inguinal lymphadenopathy as well as an enlarged spleen. A complete blood cell count reveals a hemoglobin of 9.7 g/dL, platelet count of 89,000 cells/μL, and white blood cell count of 93,000 cells/μL. Of the following, what is the most likely diagnosis?

A. Acute bacterial meningitis

B. Subarachnoid hemorrhage due to ruptured berry aneurysm

C. Precursor B cell lymphoblastic leukemia

D. Precursor T cell lymphoblastic leukemia

E. Infectious mononucleosis

Heme

55. A 65-year-old female presents complaining of severe fatigue, which began 4 months ago and has gradually worsened. On examination she has moderate hepatosplenomegaly with normal examination of the heart, lungs, and skin. A complete blood count shows a leukocyte count of 150×10^9 cells/L, hemoglobin level of 9.8 g/dL, and platelet count of 424×10^9 cells/L. A peripheral blood smear shows immature leukocyte forms as well as teardrop-shaped erythrocytes and nucleated red cells. Cytogenetic testing is negative for the BCR-ABL1 translocation. What is the most likely diagnosis?

A. Chronic myelogenous leukemia

B. Acute myelogenous leukemia

C. β-thalassemia major

D. Anemia of chronic disease

E. Myelofibrosis

Hematologic

56. A 76-year-old Caucasian man presents to his physician because of severe itching following warm baths and showering. These episodes are not associated with visible rash, and the patient reports trying multiple different soaps and shampoos with no change in the symptoms. On examination he appears to be his stated age, ruddy cyanosis of the face is noted, heart and lungs are normal to auscultation. His spleen is slightly enlarged. His serum leukocyte count is 14.3×10^9 cells/L, hemoglobin is 20.1 g/dL, and platelet count is 850×10^9 cells/L. Which of the following is likely to be demonstrated on additional testing?

A. Positive JAK2 mutation on reverse transcription PCR

B. 9,22 translocation on fluorescence in situ hybridization

C. Tartate-resistant acid phosphatase activity on peripheral blood film

D. Teardrop-shaped erythrocytes on peripheral blood smear

E. Myeloid precursors with Auer rods on peripheral blood smear

Hematologic

57. A 68-year-old male is evaluated in the emergency department after a fall. The patient reports striking his head, but that he did not lose consciousness. His neurologic examination is normal. Plain films of the skull reveal multiple lytic lesions. A complete blood count is normal except for a hemoglobin of 9.8 g/dL and mean corpuscular volume of 78 fL. A comprehensive metabolic panel shows an elevated creatinine with serum calcium of 12.0 mg/dL and total protein of 10.6 g/dL. What is the next step in the workup?

A. Technetium bone scan

B. Bone marrow biopsy

C. Urine and serum protein electrophoresis

D. MRI brain

E. Flow cytometry

Heme

58. A 7-year-old Nigerian child is treated at a regional medical center for a facial tumor. The mass is located within the mandible itself. Biopsy reveals sheets of medium-sized neoplastic cells that stain deep blue on Giemsa stain with numerous vacuoles in the cytoplasm, interspersed with macrophages. Which of the following is true regarding this patient's disease?

A. Most of the cases in HIV-positive patients are associated with Epstein-Barr virus infection.

B. This disease is caused by up-regulation of the *c-myc* oncogene.

C. Tumor lysis syndrome is uncommon in this disease.

D. The disease is usually unresponsive to chemotherapy.

E. Tumor cells are likely positive for TdT.

Heme

59. A 57-year-old man is brought to his physician by his wife because of weight loss. The man reports that his weight has declined from 222 lbs. (100 kg) to 195 lbs. (88 kg) over a two-month period without any change in his diet or activity level. He also reports severe fatigue and a discomfort in the upper abdomen. A complete blood count shows a leukocyte count of 83.2×10^9 cells/L, a hemoglobin of 7.1 g/dL, and a platelet count of 724×10^9 cells/L. On examination, pallor of the skin and mucous membranes is noted and the spleen is markedly enlarged. His peripheral blood smear reveals promyelocytes, myelocytes, and basophils. Of the following, what would most likely be found on cytogenetic analysis?

A. t (8;14)

B. t (8;21)

C. t (15;17)

D. t (12;21)

E. t (9;22)

Heme

60. A 62-year-old man is initially seen in the urgent care department because of a sore on the medial surface of the left ankle. On examination, the patient is afebrile. There is erythema and induration of the anterior portion of both lower extremities below the knee. The patient is diagnosed with cellulitis and observed in the hospital because of a serum leukocyte count of 20.3×10^9 cells/L. Despite receiving 48 hours of intravenous antibiotics his leukocyte count remains elevated. He is discharged and completes a ten-day course of oral clindamycin. He returns to the urgent care center for follow-up after completing the antibiotics. At that time the appearance of his lower extremities is unchanged, and his serum leukocyte count is 25×10^9 cells/L. A peripheral blood smear drawn at the time of his second visit is shown in the figure below. What is the most likely cause of his leukocytosis?

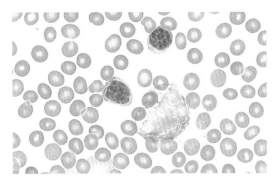

A. Sepsis with gram-negative bacteremia

B. Leukemoid reaction

C. Chronic lymphocytic leukemia

D. Myelodysplastic syndrome

E. Drug reaction

Heme

61. A 25-year-old man presents to his primary care doctor complaining of a lump on his neck, which he first noticed a week ago. He also reports intermittent low-grade fevers and a 5 lb. (2.2 kg) unintentional weight loss over the past month. On examination, there is a 3-cm, nontender lymph node anterior to the posterior border of the left sternocleidomastoid muscle on the left side. The remainder of his examination is unremarkable. A complete blood count shows a normal leukocyte count and a mild normocytic, normochromic anemia. An excisional biopsy is performed that shows fibrotic bands of collagen separating clusters of inflammatory cells and interspersed lacunar cells. What is the diagnosis?

A. Reactive lymphadenopathy

B. Chronic lymphocytic lymphoma

C. Hodgkin's lymphoma

D. Diffuse large B-cell lymphoma

E. Mantle cell lymphoma

Heme

9.4 Anemia and Red Blood Cell Disorders—Answers and Explanations

Easy	Medium	Hard

1. Correct: Menstrual blood loss (A)

The low hemoglobin is consistent with anemia, and anemia can cause fatigue and dizziness. Although all of the diseases listed could produce an anemia (**B-E**), given the clinical scenario, heavy menstrual bleeding would be the most likely underlying cause (**A**). At her young age and with her family history colonic adenocarcinoma is unlikely (**B**). Her normal diet and lack of other medical conditions exclude a B12 deficiency (**D**). And, given she is white, sickle cell disease is very unlikely (**E**). She has no risk factors for a warm autoimmune hemolytic anemia, including an autoimmune disorder or a white blood cell neoplasm (**C**).

2. Correct: Pencil cells (C)

The symptoms of fatigue and dizziness combined with the hemoglobin concentration of 9.8 mg/dL are consistent with anemia. The MCV of 75 fL indicates a microcytic anemia. A common cause of microcytic anemia is iron deficiency anemia, which is characterized by central pallor of the reticulocytes, also, elongated red blood cells called pencil cells can be found (**C**). Teardrop cells are associated with myelofibrosis (**A**), rouleaux with increased globulins or decreased albumin (**B**), and schistocytes with hemolytic processes, such as TTP (**E**). Leukemic blasts are found in leukemia (**D**).

3. Correct: Fecal occult blood test (D)

Based on the symptoms and laboratory testing, the patient has a microcytic anemia, which is characterized by the low MCV. One common cause of microcytic anemia is iron deficiency, which can occur secondary to occult blood loss from colonic adenocarcinoma, which could be suggested by a positive fecal occult blood test (**D**). A negative fecal occult blood test does not preclude the presence of an adenocarcinoma; however, of the tests listed, it would be the most useful. A Coombs test will help identify a warm autoimmune hemolytic anemia (**A**). An osmotic fragility test will help identify spherocytosis (**B**). A Donath-Landsteiner antibody is associated with paroxysmal cold hemoglobinuria (**E**). All are causes of anemia, but not characteristically a microcytic anemia. A B12 deficiency will lead to a macrocytic anemia (**C**).

4. Correct: Decreased ferritin, decreased serum iron, increased TIBC (E)

Based on the clinical scenario, the patient has an iron deficiency anemia due to colonic adenocarcinoma. Laboratory testing in patients with iron deficiency anemia will reveal a decreased ferritin (the storage form of iron), decreased serum iron, and increased iron-binding capacity (**E**). The other choices are incorrect (**A-D**).

5. Correct: Reticulocyte count (D)

Pure red cell aplasia is a disorder of the production of red blood cells, and warm autoimmune hemolytic anemia is a disorder characterized by the destruction of red blood cells. The reticulocyte count would be the most useful, as with destruction of red blood cells, the reticulocyte count would be expected to be increased, whereas it would be normal or decreased with a disorder of production (**D**). Both diseases would be normocytic, so MCV is not useful (**A**). Neither disorder is based on a deficiency of iron, so a ferritin concentration would not be useful (**C**). RDW can assist in iron deficiency anemia (**B**).

6. Correct: β-thalassemia major (B)

Individuals with β-thalassemia major require blood transfusions from the time of birth and can easily develop a secondary hemochromatosis, which could lead to cirrhosis of the liver (**B**). An individual with a significantly decreased production of α chains would have HbH (β tetramers) and HbBart (four γ chains) (**A**). None of the other diseases is a significant risk factor for cirrhosis (**C-E**).

7. Correct: β-thalassemia minor (B)

The patient has a microcytic anemia; however, the MCV is very low, out of proportion to the low hemoglobin. This is characteristic of a β-thalassemia, which is more common in a Mediterranean population (**B**). The other diseases would cause microcytic anemia as well, excluding megaloblastic anemia (**E**), but the history does not support any other choice (**A, C-D**).

8. Correct: b⁰/β (C)

The patient has a microcytic anemia; however, the MCV is very low, out of proportion to the low hemoglobin. This is characteristic of β-thalassemia, which is more common in a Mediterranean population. The fact he is presenting at the age of 36 years with an unrelated condition indicates the anemia is not severe (**C**). β^4 is associated with HbH disease (loss of three alpha genes) (**A**) and β^+/β^+ is thalassemia major (**B**), which is loss of both genes. Both would present much sooner, with thalassemia major presenting often at birth. A mutation in spectrin is associated with hereditary spherocytosis (**D**), and valine for glutamic acid with sickle cell anemia (**E**), neither of which cause a microcytic anemia.

9. Correct: Ferritin (D)

In iron deficiency anemia, ferritin is decreased, but in anemia of chronic disease, ferritin is increased (**D**). In both diseases serum iron is decreased (**A**) and erythrocyte protoporphyrin is increased (**C**). Although there are some findings on the blood smear that might help in a more severe case, the anemia is mild in this case (**E**). HbA2 helps to separate thalassemia trait from thalassemia minor (elevated in thalassemia minor) (**B**).

10. Correct: Iron deficiency anemia (A)

The patient has a microcytic anemia. Although WAIHA and CAIHA can cause anemia, it is usually normocytic (**B, C**). IDA, ACD, and sideroblastic anemia can cause a microcytic anemia. In iron deficiency anemia, the TIBC is increased and the transferrin saturation is decreased (**A**), whereas in sideroblastic anemia the transferrin saturation is increased (**E**), and in anemia of chronic disease, both these tests are normal (**D**).

11. Correct: Warm autoimmune hemolytic anemia (A)

Spherocytes are found in a variety of conditions, including hereditary spherocytosis and warm and cold autoimmune hemolytic anemias, but typically are not found in G6PD deficiency or iron deficiency anemia (**D, E**). Hereditary spherocytosis and microangiopathic hemolytic anemia will have a negative direct Coombs test (**B, C**), whereas warm autoimmune hemolytic anemia will have a positive direct Coombs test (**A**) because of IgG present on the surface of the red blood cells.

12. Correct: IgM (B)

Spherocytes are found in a variety of conditions, including hereditary spherocytosis and warm and cold autoimmune hemolytic anemias. Individuals with infectious mononucleosis can develop a cold autoimmune hemolytic anemia, which has a negative monospecific direct Coombs test. The underlying cause of the anemia is IgM antibody binding to red blood cells (**B**). The other choices (**A, C-E**) are incorrect.

13. Correct: Elevated concentration of methylmalonic acid (C)

Megaloblastic anemia due to either a folate or a B12 deficiency will have hypersegmented neutrophils and an elevated concentration of homocysteine (**A, B**); however, while the methylmalonic acid will be normal in folate deficiency, it will be elevated in B12 deficiency (**C**). Pencil cells are found in severe iron deficiency anemia (**D**), and teardrop cells are found when there is fibrosis of the bone marrow (**E**), and neither is characteristic of megaloblastic anemia. B12 is a necessary cofactor for the conversion of methylmalonyl-CoA to succinyl-CoA. Methylmalonyl-CoA builds up, and is converted to methylmalonic acid.

14. Correct: A remote cardiac valve replacement (A)

The patient has anemia, with hemoglobin of 8.5 g/dL. The anemia is normocytic, making iron deficiency (usually microcytic) and folate deficiency (associated with macrocytic anemia) less likely (**D, E**). The increased bilirubin and increased LDH indicate hemolysis, and the hemoglobin in the urine is consistent with intravascular hemolysis, which a defective or malfunctioning cardiac valve could cause (**A**). With extravascular hemolysis, such as would occur with a warm autoimmune hemolytic anemia (**B**), LDH and bilirubin can be increased, but hemoglobin would not be found in the urine. There is no history of a drug exposure or other risk factor to indicate aplastic anemia, and, it would not cause hemoglobin in the urine (**C**).

15. Correct: Hereditary spherocytosis (A)

Although sickle cell anemia is hereditary, it would be very rare in a Caucasian female, and patients with the disease can auto-infarct their spleen, so splenomegaly outside of childhood would be rare (**E**). G6PD deficiency is X-linked, so the likelihood of two females in three generations having the disease is highly unlikely (**D**). In hereditary spherocytosis, splenomegaly is common (**A**). The cholecystectomy was most likely for gallstones because of elevated bilirubin concentrations due to hemolysis of red blood cells. In most cases, hereditary spherocytosis is autosomal dominant. Given her presentation, α-thalassemia trait and β-thalassemia minor are unlikely (**B, C**).

16. Correct: Osmotic fragility testing (D)

Although sickle cell anemia is hereditary (as determined by hemoglobin electrophoresis), it would be very rare in a Caucasian female. Patients with the disease can auto-infarct their spleen, so splenomegaly outside of childhood would be rare. Therefore, hemoglobin electrophoresis is unlikely to be useful (**B**). Given the acute presentation and clinical history, a megaloblastic anemia is unlikely (**A**). Given the family history and acute presentation, iron deficiency anemia (ferritin concentration) is unlikely (**E**). As the anemia is not antibody related, a direct Coombs test is not useful (**C**). The requirement for a cholecystectomy was most likely for pigment stones from unconjugated hyperbilirubinemia. The history is consistent with hereditary spherocytosis, which can be detected with an osmotic fragility test (**D**).

17. Correct: Ferritin (B)

This man's red cell indices are consistent with iron deficiency. The diagnosis should be confirmed by checking a ferritin level (**B**). If indeed he is iron deficient, then evaluation for occult gastrointestinal blood would be the next step, by colonoscopy with or without esophagogastroduodenoscopy (**A**). The other choices are incorrect (**C-E**).

18. Correct: Normal soluble transferrin receptor levels (C)

Increased TIBC (**A**) is most consistent with iron deficiency anemia. Low transferrin saturation (**B**) can be seen in both iron deficiency and anemia of chronic disease, as can increased platelets (**D**). Soluble transferrin receptor (sTfR) levels can be useful in distinguishing between iron deficiency and anemia of chronic disease. sTfR level is usually low in iron-deficient states and normal in anemia of chronic disease (**C**). The use of a leukocyte count would not be useful (**E**).

19. Correct: Methotrexate (E)

Methotrexate causes folic acid deficiency by inhibiting dihydrofolate reductase (**E**). Other drugs known to cause folic acid deficiency include trimethoprim and phenytoin. The other drugs listed are not causes of folic acid deficiency (**A-D**).

20. Correct: Hepatic vein thrombosis (B)

This patient suffers from paroxysmal nocturnal hemoglobinuria. His urine is red-colored; however, he has only one red cell per hpf on urinalysis, suggesting hemoglobinuria rather than hematuria. Of the causes of death listed, the most likely is hepatic vein thrombosis (**B**). Other common sites of thrombosis include the inferior vena cava and cerebral veins. The other conditions listed (**A, C-E**) are not common causes of death for patients with paroxysmal nocturnal hemoglobinuria.

21. Correct: A low mean corpuscular volume (B)

This patient has laboratory and clinical evidence of acute choledocholithiasis (positive Murphy sign with abnormal aminotransferases and conjugated hyperbilirubinemia) as well as hypersplenism (left upper quadrant mass) and hemolytic anemia. The patient is likely to have evidence of gallstones and a dilated common bile duct on ultrasound as well as an elevated alkaline phosphatase. Furthermore, the concomitant unconjugated hyperbilirubinemia, anemia, the presence of gallstones, and splenomegaly are all highly suggestive of underlying hereditary spherocytosis. Due to red cell membrane loss in this condition, the mean cell hemoglobin concentration is increased (**A**) and the mean corpuscular volume is decreased (**B**). Howell-Jolly bodies, nuclear remnants seen within the red blood cells of asplenic individuals, would not be expected in this patient with an enlarged spleen (**E**). The alkaline phosphatase is likely to be elevated (**C**), and the right upper quadrant abdominal ultrasound would reveal the gallstones (**D**).

22. Correct: Heinz bodies (E)

The onset of unconjugated hyperbilirubinemia and anemia after exposure to sulfamethoxazole is highly suggestive of glucose-6-phosphate dehydrogenase (G6PD) deficiency. Pencil cells would be expected in iron deficiency anemia (**A**). Spherocytes and target cells are seen in hereditary spherocytosis and thalassemia respectively (**B, C**). Given the man's ethnicity, G6PD deficiency is more likely than sickle cell disease (**D, E**). Heinz bodies (**E**) are characteristic of G6PD deficiency.

23. Correct: Sickle cells (D)

The patient is suffering from acute chest syndrome from sickle cell anemia. The blood smear would likely show active sickling (**D**). Target cells are classically seen in thalassemia (**C**), and would be unlikely unless the patient has sickle HbC (HbSC) or sickle-β-thalassemia (Hb Sβ⁺ or Hb Sb⁰). These disease entities, while not rare, are less common than homozygous sickle C disease (HbSS), and in the case of Hb SC and Hb Sβ⁺, less likely to produce clinically severe disease. Pencil cells, spherocytes, and Heinz bodies (**A, B, E**) would not be expected.

24. Correct: Target cells (C)

This patient has β-thalassemia minor. Unlike β-thalassemia major, patients with β-thalassemia minor usually only have a mild hypochromic, microcytic anemia that resembles iron deficiency. A peripheral blood smear would be expected to show some target cells (**C**). The other options are associated with other diseases (**A-B, D-E**).

25. Correct: Increased serum ferritin (C)

The patient has classic facies of thalassemia major. The disease is characterized by a microcytic (hence low MCV), hypochromic (hence low MCHC) anemia with anisocytosis (hence elevated RDW) (**A, D-E**). Ongoing red cell destruction results in an increased reticulocyte count, although the reticulocyte count is lower than would be expected given the severity of anemia due to ineffective erythropoiesis (**B**). The ineffective erythropoiesis suppresses hepcidin, leading to excessive iron absorption. The combination of excessive absorption and repeated iron loading due to transfusions produces iron overload in these patients. The ferritin in this case would be expected to be increased (**C**).

26. Correct: α-thalassemia minor (D)

The most likely diagnosis is α-thalassemia minor (**D**). Patients with α-thalassemia minor are often asymptomatic and have a mild hypochromic, microcytic anemia. Target cells may be observed, but unlike the β-thalassemias, HbA2 is normal (**C**). Because α-thalassemia is caused by an absence or decrease in production of the α-globin chain, an abnormal hemoglobin electrophoresis is not observed (**A, B**). The clinical scenario is not consistent with G6PD deficiency (**E**).

27. Correct: Warm antibody hemolytic anemia (C)

This patient's laboratory studies are consistent with a hemolytic anemia. The positive direct antibody test indicates an autoantibody as the cause. The most common autoimmune hemolytic anemia is warm antibody hemolytic anemia, caused by IgG autoantibodies against red cell antigens (**C**). Red cell hemolysis in warm antibody disease occurs primarily in the spleen. In the spleen, phagocytes phagocytize portions of the opsonized membranes of the red cells, causing spherocytosis. The laboratory test results are not consistent with (**A-B, D-E**).

28. Correct: Genetic testing (C)

The patient's complaints of fatigue and arthralgias as well as his polycythemia and abnormally elevated transferrin saturation and ferritin levels are all highly suggestive of hemochromatosis. The diagnosis can be confirmed in most cases by genetic testing for *HFE* gene mutations, although liver biopsy stained for iron is still considered the gold standard in diagnosing hemochromatosis (**C**). The other tests (**A-B, D-E**) would not be of use in formulating the diagnosis of hereditary hemochromatosis.

29. Correct: Parvovirus B19 infection (C)

The complete blood count and the bone marrow biopsy findings are consistent with aplastic crisis. Parvovirus B19 infections are the most common cause of aplastic crises (**C**). The other conditions listed are, based on the clinical scenario, not likely, although each could potentially cause various forms of cytopenias (**A-B, D-E**).

30. Correct: Fanconi anemia (D)

This patient's presentation is most consistent with Fanconi anemia, an X-linked inherited aplastic anemia, more common in persons of Ashkenazi Jewish descent (**D**). Similar to other heritable aplastic anemia such as Schwachman-Diamond, Diamond-Blackfand, and thrombocytopenia-absent radii (TAR) syndromes, Fanconi anemia is associated with radial defects. TAR and Diamond-Blackfand anemia tend to present with transfusion-dependent anemia in the neonatal period (**A, E**), whereas Fanconi anemia tends to present after age 6. Neither Wiskott-Aldrich nor ataxia-telangectasia is consistent with this patient's clinical presentation (**B, C**).

31. Correct: Idiopathic thrombocytopenic purpura (D)

This patient has idiopathic thrombocytopenic purpura (**D**). The absence of features of hemolytic anemia make hemolytic uremic syndrome and thrombotic thrombocytopenic purpura unlikely (**A, B**). Myelodysplastic syndromes are uncommon in patients this young (**E**), and the clinical scenario is inconsistent with hereditary hemorrhagic telangiectasia (**C**).

32. Correct: Babesiosis (D)

The patient has anemia, as indicated by the low hemoglobin, which is normocytic, as indicated by the MCV. The elevated total bilirubin, elevated LDH, and decreased haptoglobin indicate hemolysis, and the presence of hemoglobin and hemosiderin in the urine indicates intravascular hemolysis. Hereditary spherocytosis and warm autoimmune hemolytic anemia cause extravascular hemolysis (**B, C**). Iron deficiency anemia would be a microcytic anemia (**E**). B12 deficiency would produce a megaloblastic anemia (**A**). Babesiosis causes intravascular hemolysis (**D**).

33. Correct: Schistocytes (C)

The patient has a hemolytic anemia, indicated by the low hemoglobin, elevated total bilirubin, elevated LDH, and decreased haptoglobin. The presence of hemoglobin and hemosiderin in the urine indicates the hemolysis is intravascular. The findings of anemia, thrombocytopenia, fever, and metal status changes are four of the five features of TTP, with the fifth being renal failure. In TTP, the characteristic finding on blood smear is schistocytes (**C**). The other cell types listed (**A-B, D-E**) are not characteristic of TTP.

34. Correct: Heavy menstrual bleeding (C)

The patient has a microcytic anemia, with low hemoglobin and low MCV. The increased TIBC and decreased ferritin are consistent with an iron deficiency anemia. The most common cause of iron deficiency anemia listed would be heavy menstrual bleeding (**C**). Other causes of a microcytic anemia that are listed are sideroblastic anemia, undiagnosed thalassemia, and anemia of chronic disease in an autoimmune disorder; however, none have a decreased ferritin (**A-B, D**). Malaria would cause an intravascular hemolysis, and there is no evidence of a hemolysis (**E**).

35. Correct: Increased central pallor of red blood cells (D)

The laboratory findings are consistent with a microcytic anemia. The lack of elevations of total bilirubin and LDH and lack of decreased concentration of haptoglobin indicate that the anemia is not due to hemolysis. Spherocytes, organisms in the red blood cells (e.g., malaria, babesia), and schistocytes would be present in various types of hemolytic anemias (**A-C**). Hypersegmented neutrophils are found in megaloblastic anemia, which has an increased MCV (**E**). The patient has iron deficiency anemia, based on the decreased ferritin and increased TIBC, and the characteristic feature of red blood cells in a smear is increased central pallor (**D**), and also, the marked anisocytosis and the appearance of pencil cells, which are elongated red blood cells.

119

36.   Correct: Thalassemia (C)

The patient has a microcytic anemia, as evidenced by the decreased hemoglobin and MCV of less than 80 fL. The total bilirubin, LDH, and haptoglobin are normal, indicating there is no laboratory evidence of hemolysis. The TIBC and ferritin are normal, ruling out iron deficiency anemia and anemia of chronic disease (**A-B**), which normally have alterations in these two lab tests. In thalassemia, often there is a marked decrease in the MCV that is out of proportion to the decrease in hemoglobin. Megaloblastic anemia would have an increased MCV (**D**), and warm autoimmune hemolytic anemia would have laboratory evidence of hemolysis (**E**).

37.   Correct: Hemoglobin electrophoresis

The patient has a microcytic anemia. The normal ferritin and TIBC rule out an iron deficiency anemia and anemia of chronic disease. The patient may have either an α-thalassemia trait or a β-thalassemia minor. A hemoglobin electrophoresis would identify increased hemoglobin A2 in patients with β-thalassemia and thus would serve to distinguish these two entities (**C**). Anti-dsDNA would help in an evaluation of lupus and serum folate in megaloblastic anemia, neither of which are in the differential diagnosis (**A, B**). Transferrin saturation would not contribute anything beyond the normal TIBC and ferritin studies (**D**). An ANCA testing would have essentially no purpose in this case (**E**).

9.5 Transfusion and Miscellaneous—Answers and Explanations

Easy	Medium	Hard

38.   Correct: Disseminated intravascular coagulation (D)

The patient has the signs and symptoms of acute pancreatitis. One complication of acute pancreatitis is disseminated intravascular coagulation, which could cause blood to ooze at needle puncture sites, because there is widespread use of clotting factors, which leaves none available for local clotting needs (**D**). Acute pancreatitis is not directly a cause of warm autoimmune hemolytic anemia (**A**), cold autoimmune hemolytic anemia (**B**), thrombotic thrombocytopenic purpura (**C**), or megaloblastic anemia (**E**).

39.   Correct: Schistocyte (B)

The patient has the signs and symptoms of acute pancreatitis. One complication of acute pancreatitis is disseminated intravascular coagulation, which would cause a patient to ooze blood from puncture sites. The characteristic cell type found on the blood smear is a schistocyte (**B**). Teardrop cells are found in bone marrow fibrosis (**A**), macro-ovalocytes in megaloblastic anemia (**C**), spherocytes in autoimmune hemolytic anemia and hereditary spherocytosis (**D**), and ringed sideroblasts in sideroblastic anemia (**E**).

40.   Correct: Transfusion-related acute lung injury (D)

The onset of hypoxia within two hours of transfusion with bilateral infiltrates on plain chest radiograph is highly suggestive of transfusion-related acute lung injury (TRALI) (**D**). This clinical scenario is rarely caused by volume overload (**A**) or acute heart failure, though frequently misdiagnosed as such. The use of cross-matched blood and the negative Coomb's test make a hemolytic transfusion reaction unlikely (**C**). The exact cause of TRALI is unknown; however, evidence points toward activation of neutrophils in the transfusion recipient by donor blood. TRALI is the leading cause of transfusion-related mortality in the United States. The scenario is not consistent with sepsis (**B**) or anaphylaxis (**E**).

9.6 Lymphoid—Answers and Explanations

Easy	Medium	Hard

41.   Correct: Infectious mononucleosis (D)

The patient has signs and symptoms consistent with infectious mononucleosis (**D**). Although a neoplastic process could cause fatigue, a low-grade fever, and splenomegaly, it would be much less likely than infectious mononucleosis given the clinical scenario, and it would not usually be the cause of a sore throat (**A, B**). Subacute endocarditis usually isn't associated with splenomegaly (**C**), and the findings are not supportive of SLE (**E**).

42.   Correct: Atypical lymphocytes (D)

This patient has signs and symptoms consistent with infectious mononucleosis. On blood smear, patients with infectious mononucleosis will have atypical lymphocytes, which are lymphocytes with abundant cytoplasm and a large nucleus (**D**). Schistocytes would be consistent with intravascular fragmentation of red blood cells, such as due to an artificial aortic valve, or intravascular clotting, such as in disseminated intravascular coagulation (**A**). Blasts would be typical for leukemia (**B**), and Reed-Sternberg cells for Hodgkin's lymphoma, although Reed-Sternberg cells would be seen in tissue sections and not on a blood smear (**C**). The atypical lymphocytes in a lymph node can mimic a Reed-Sternberg cell. Rouleaux indicate increased globulins, such as in multiple myeloma (**E**).

43. Correct: EBV (C)

The patient's signs and symptoms are most consistent with infectious mononucleosis, which is caused by EBV (**C**). CMV can also produce infectious mononucleosis, and distinguishing between the two viruses as to the underlying cause would require serologic methods. Primary HIV can present with an infectious mononucleosis–like clinical scenario, but would be much less common (**A**). HSV, *Streptococcus pneumoniae*, and *Staphylococcus aureus* would not usually cause splenomegaly (**D, E**).

44. Correct: Cervical lymphadenopathy (C)

The patient presents with signs and symptoms of infectious mononucleosis, which, because of the sore throat, can mimic streptococcal pharyngitis. Patients with infectious mononucleosis will have lymphadenopathy, which is most often prominent in the posterior cervical region (**C**). Not all individuals with infectious mononucleosis will have splenomegaly (**E**). Infectious mononucleosis would not normally cause a heart murmur (**A**), rales (**B**), or decreased bowel sounds (**D**).

45. Correct: A ruptured spleen (D)

The patient has signs and symptoms consistent with infectious mononucleosis, with the swellings noted by her friend being posterior cervical lymphadenopathy. Many people with infectious mononucleosis develop splenomegaly, and the spleen is more fragile and can rupture after minor trauma (**D**). Although the other conditions listed could cause death, none are consistent with the clinical scenario (**A-C, E**).

46. Correct: CD13 (C)

CD13 is a marker for myeloid cells (**C**). The remainder of the cells would indicate a lymphoid cell of B-cell origin (CD10, CD19, and CD20) or T-cell origin (CD4) (**A-B, D-E**).

47. Correct: Bone marrow biopsy (B)

The patient has signs and symptoms indicating problems with red blood cells (anemia), platelets (easy bruisability), and white blood cells (infection); this constellation of conditions would indicate an abnormality of the bone marrow, possibly a leukemia or another infiltrative process. Of the choices, a bone marrow biopsy would be best at determining the underlying pathology (**B**). If the underlying cause of the patient's symptoms is leukemia, the other choices (**A, C-E**) would not be useful in making the diagnosis.

48. Correct: Complete blood count including blood smear (C)

The patient has signs and symptoms indicating problems with red blood cells (anemia), platelets (easy bruisability), and white blood cells (infection); this constellation of conditions would indicate an abnormality of the bone marrow, possibly a leukemia or another infiltrative process. Of the choices, a complete blood count including blood smear would be the most likely test to have positive results related to the underlying disease process, in the form of an elevated white blood cell count and identification of leukemic cells in the blood (**C**). The other tests listed (**A–B, D–E**), if the diagnosis is leukemia, would not be as useful as a complete blood count and blood smear.

49. Correct: Acute lymphocytic leukemia (A)

The patient has signs and symptoms indicating problems with red blood cells (anemia), platelets (easy bruisability), and white blood cells (infection); this constellation of conditions would indicate an abnormality of the bone marrow, possibly a leukemia or another infiltrative process. The white blood cell count, and blast count is consistent with a leukemia (**E**); given the sudden onset, an acute leukemia is most likely (**B, D**). Although a t(9;22) is commonly associated with CML, it also occurs in adult ALL. The CD19 positivity is consistent with a B-cell neoplasm (**A, C**).

50. Correct: t(9;22) (D)

The patient has signs and symptoms consistent with chronic myelogenous leukemia, which could present with fatigue, weight loss, fever, and splenomegaly. The blood smear is consistent with a leukemia, and the description is that of a chronic myeloid leukemia, with more mature leukemia cells (i.e., not blasts). Of the translocations, the t(9;22) is found in CML (**D**). t(8;14) is found in Burkitt's lymphoma (**A**), t(11;14) in mantle cell lymphoma (**B**), t(14;18) in follicular lymphoma (**C**), and t(15;17) in acute myeloid leukemia (**E**).

51. Correct: t(12;21) (C)

The patient has acute lymphocytic leukemia. The symptoms and signs are consistent with an infiltrative process in the bone marrow, and the differential indicates an acute leukemia. In children, the majority (around 75%) of the acute leukemias are acute lymphocytic leukemia, so, although other forms of leukemia are possible, the most common would be ALL. t(12;21), which translocates the *TEL1* and *AML1* genes, is characteristic of acute lymphocytic leukemia (**C**). t(9;22) can be found in ALL, but most commonly in adult ALL (**B**). Of the translocations, t(11;14) is found in mantle cell lymphoma (**D**), t(14;18) in follicular lymphoma (**E**), and t(15;17) in acute myeloid leukemia (**A**).

52. Correct: Splenomegaly (A)

The signs and symptoms are consistent with a leukemia. The blood smear is consistent with chronic myelogenous leukemia. Patients with chronic myelogenous leukemia frequently have splenomegaly (**A**), which commonly causes decreased breathing sounds at the left lung base due to elevation of the left hemidiaphragm (**C**). Chvostek sign is associated with hypocalcemia (**D**). Pitting edema is associated with congestive heart failure (**E**). CML does not normally, on its own, produce a systolic ejection murmur (**B**).

53. Correct: Aplastic anemia (C)

The patient has symptoms related to both anemia and thrombocytopenia; thus, anemia of chronic disease and warm and cold autoimmune hemolytic anemia are unlikely, as they would be expected to produce only anemia (**B, D-E**). An acute lymphocytic leukemia would explain his signs and symptoms, but this disease is less likely in an adult (**A**). Benzene can cause damage to the bone marrow, leading to aplastic anemia, which can then present with complications due to a pancytopenia. Given the time course of events, aplastic anemia due to the benzene exposure is the most likely diagnosis (**C**).

54. Correct: Precursor B-cell lymphoblastic leukemia (C)

Given the clinical scenario, with evidence of anemia, bleeding disorder, and fever, and the white blood cell count, the most likely diagnosis among the choices is a leukemia. Of the two choices, precursor B-cell lymphoma is more common than precursor T-cell lymphoma (**C, D**). Both acute bacterial meningitis and a subarachnoid hemorrhage due to a ruptured berry aneurysm (which do occur in children) could present suddenly with headache and vomiting (due to increased intracranial pressure) but would not explain the entire clinical scenario (**A, B**). Infectious mononucleosis would be unlikely in this young age and would not easily explain the bleeding or the markedly elevated white blood cell count (E).

55. Correct: Myelofibrosis (E)

The finding of hepatosplenomegaly with teardrop-shaped erythrocytes (dacryocytes) and nucleated red cells in a patient this age is most consistent with the diagnosis of myelofibrosis (**E**). The clinical presentation is inconsistent with thalassemia and anemia of chronic disease (**C, D**), and chronic myelogenous leukemia is less likely given the absence of the Philadelphia chromosome (**A**). Given the more chronic presentation, over the course of 4 months, acute myelogenous leukemia is unlikely (**B**).

56. Correct: Positive JAK2 mutation on reverse transcription PCR (A)

The patient's elevated hemoglobin, history of pruritus with bathing, and ruddy appearance all suggest polycythemia. 95% of all patients with polycythemia

vera are positive for the JAK2 mutation (**A**). The other tests listed are more consistent with CML (**B**), hair cell leukemia (**C**), myelofibrosis (**D**), and acute promyelocytic leukemia (**E**).

57. Correct: Urine and serum protein electrophoresis (C)

In a patient with multiple lytic lesions of the cranium and elevated serum creatinine, calcium, and protein, the most likely diagnosis is multiple myeloma. The next indicated study in this patient's workup is a urine and serum electrophoresis with immunofixation to evaluate for the presence of a monoclonal protein (**C**). A bone marrow biopsy would not be performed before a protein electrophoresis (**B**). There is little role for a nuclear bone scan in the evaluation of myeloma (**A**). The lack of osteoblastic lesions in myeloma makes these scans negative and adds little information. In the absence of a monoclonal protein however, a bone scan might be useful. Neither an MRI of the brain nor flow cytometry would be performed as the next diagnostic step in his evaluation (**D, E**).

58. Correct: This disease is caused by up-regulation of the *c-myc* oncogene (B)

Translocation between the *c-myc* gene and immunoglobulin genes is the defining feature of a Burkitt lymphoma (**B**). In 80% of cases the translocation, t(8;14), is between *c-myc* and the immunoglobulin heavy chain gene. The remainder of the cases involve translocation of *c-myc* with immunoglobulin light chain genes. Epstein-Barr virus is involved in almost all cases of African (endemic) Burkitt lymphoma, but fewer than 30% of sporadic or immunodeficiency-related cases (**A**). This malignancy has one of the highest turnover rates known, making it extremely fast growing but also very chemosensitive (**D**). Because of this fact, the risk of tumor lysis syndrome is very high (**C**). The neoplastic cells in Burkitt lymphoma do not express terminal deoxynucleotidyl transferase (TdT), distinguishing it from acute lymphoblastic leukemia (**E**).

59. Correct: t (9;22) (E)

The clinical history and peripheral smear are characteristic of chronic myelogenous leukemia. This disease is caused by the presence of the BCR-ABL fusion gene, which causes production of a constitutively active tyrosine kinase. In the vast majority of these cases this fusion gene is the result of a translocation between chromosomes 9 and 22 (Philadelphia chromosome) (**E**). The other choices are incorrect (**A-D**).

60. Correct: Chronic lymphocytic leukemia (C)

The photo shown is of smudge cells, cellular remnants of fragile neoplastic lymphocytes characteristically seen on the peripheral blood smears of patients with chronic lymphocytic leukemia (CLL). In this case the patient's lower extremity skin changes, which are bilateral and associated with an ulcer, are due to venous stasis rather than cellulitis, and the leukocytosis is caused by previously undiagnosed and clinically inapparent CLL (**C**). The image is inconsistent with the other conditions listed (**A-B, D-E**).

61. Correct: Hodgkin's lymphoma (C)

The microscopic description is that of a nodular sclerosing variant Hodgkin's lymphoma (HL). Classic Reed-Sternberg cells are not seen in this, the most common HL variant. Instead, lacunar cells, neoplastic cells with multilobed or folded nuclei surrounded by an artifactual clear area are seen (**C**). In contrast to the other diseases listed (**A-B, D-E**), Hodgkin's lymphoma is common in younger patients.

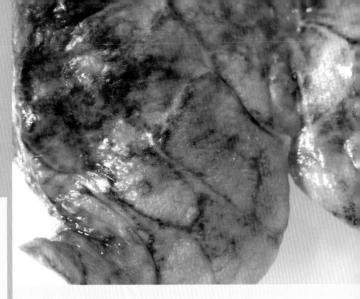

Chapter 10

Diseases of the Respiratory System

LEARNING OBJECTIVES

10.1 Obstructive Lung Disease

- ▸ Diagnosis chronic obstructive pulmonary disease
- ▸ Diagnose chronic bronchitis
- ▸ Diagnose asthma and describe the associated pulmonary function testing, etiology, and complications
- ▸ Diagnose asthma; describe the histologic findings of asthma
- ▸ Diagnose chronic obstructive pulmonary disease and list the associated physical findings and describe the associated histologic features
- ▸ Diagnose asthma and describe the pulmonary function testing and immunologic mechanism of asthma

10.2 Restrictive Lung Disease

- ▸ Diagnosis and list the underlying causes of a pneumothorax
- ▸ Distinguish between obstructive and restrictive lung disease
- ▸ Diagnose asbestos-related lung disease
- ▸ List the pathologic findings associated with asbestos-related lung disease
- ▸ Diagnose interstitial lung disease and list the etiologies
- ▸ Diagnose interstitial lung disease; describe the etiologies, physical examination findings, and histology
- ▸ Describe the histologic features of hypersensitivity pneumonitis and list the common etiologies
- ▸ Diagnose restrictive lung disease, list the various forms of restrictive lung disease, and describe the histologic findings of chronic hypersensitivity pneumonitis

10.3 Pulmonary Infections

- ▸ Diagnose acute bronchopneumonia
- ▸ Diagnose lobar pneumonia and list the common bacterial cause of lobar pneumonia
- ▸ Describe the association between splenectomy and infections with certain types of bacteria
- ▸ Diagnose acute bronchopneumonia and describe complications that arise from acute bronchopneumonia
- ▸ Diagnose lobar pneumonia and list the common etiologic agent for this condition
- ▸ Diagnose interstitial pneumonia and list the etiologic agents that produce an interstitial pneumonia

10.4 Pulmonary Neoplasms

- ▸ Describe the causes of hypercalcemia and describe the histologic appearance of pulmonary neoplasms
- ▸ Diagnose hypercalcemia and list the complications of hypercalcemia
- ▸ Describe how the location of laryngeal tumors affects their prognosis
- ▸ Given the gross appearance of a pleural neoplasm, diagnose mesothelioma
- ▸ Diagnose superior vena cava syndrome
- ▸ Diagnose a pathologic fracture
- ▸ Diagnose Cushing's syndrome and list the paraneoplastic syndromes associated with the various lung tumors
- ▸ Compare the treatment of small cell versus non-small cell carcinoma
- ▸ Diagnose bronchial obstruction due to a neoplasm
- ▸ Diagnose a pulmonary neoplasm and describe the complications of a pulmonary neoplasm

10.5 Disease of Pleura

- ▸ List the types of atelectasis and provide an example of a condition causing each type
- ▸ List the types of atelectasis, and describe the pathologic changes associated with each one
- ▸ Diagnose a pneumothorax
- ▸ Diagnose a tension pneumothorax

10.6 Miscellaneous Pulmonary Disease

- ▸ Diagnose a pulmonary thromboembolus, and list the associated pathologic findings
- ▸ Diagnose pulmonary thromboembolus; describe the clinical diagnosis of a pulmonary thromboembolus
- ▸ Diagnose a pleural effusion
- ▸ Diagnose tension pneumothorax
- ▸ Diagnose pulmonary thromboembolus
- ▸ Describe the gross and microscopic findings of a pulmonary thromboembolus
- ▸ Diagnose a pulmonary thromboembolus and list the risk factors for the condition
- ▸ Describe the use of the D-dimer test in the evaluation of a possible pulmonary thromboembolus
- ▸ Diagnose foreign body aspiration

10.1 Obstructive Lung Disease—Questions

Easy	Medium	Hard

1. A 66-year-old male is being followed by his family physician for shortness of breath, which began several years ago and has progressively worsened. The shortness of breath occurs with exertion and ends quickly after the cessation of exertion. Nitroglycerin does not affect the course of the shortness of breath. The shortness of breath is occasionally accompanied by a cough, but he has never had any other associated symptoms. Of the following, what is the most likely diagnosis?

A. Chronic obstructive pulmonary disease

B. Chronic interstitial pneumonia

C. Severe coronary artery atherosclerosis

D. Pulmonary thromboemboli

E. Granulomatosis with polyangiitis

Lungs

2. Given the previous clinical scenario, which of the following is the most likely underlying cause of his disease process?

A. Asbestos

B. α-1-antitrypsin deficiency

C. Cigarette smoke

D. c-ANCA

E. *Mycobacterium tuberculosis*

Lung

3. A 56-year-old male with a 65-pack-per-year smoking history presents to his family physician for a checkup. He has not seen a doctor in 15 years. His vital signs are temperature of 98.7°F, respiratory rate of 16 breaths per minute, heart rate of 85 bpm, and blood pressure of 159/85 mm Hg. During the history, he relates that he has been coughing up thick yellow-green material for about the last three years, on and off, but more frequently for at least half of the year. Physical examination reveals some ronchi, but no crackles. His fingernail beds are slightly blue, and a pulse oximeter reveals an oxygen saturation of 88%. He does not report having difficulty breathing. Of the following, what is the most likely diagnosis?

A. Emphysema

B. Chronic bronchitis

C. Lobar pneumonia

D. Granulomatosis with polyangiitis

E. Chronic eosinophilic pneumonia

Lung

4. Given the previous clinical scenario, a histologic section of his lung would most likely reveal which of the following?

A. Noncaseating granulomas and transmural neutrophilic vasculitis

B. Hypertrophy of smooth muscle in the airways

C. Alveolar macrophage infiltrate throughout all alveolar airspaces

D. Hypertrophy of mucous glands in the airways

E. Patchy fibrosis of the alveolar septa

Lung

5. A 24-year-old male is brought to the emergency room by his roommate for evaluation of an acute episode of shortness of breath and wheezing. His roommate reports that he has had attacks such as this in the past. When he was coughing, he did not cough anything up. Of the following, which is correct regarding this condition?

A. Pulmonary function tests will reveal a normal FEV1/FVC ratio.

B. It is due to heavy cigarette use.

C. Prior to this episode, the patient likely had an upper respiratory tract infection.

D. The causative agent is IgA.

E. It has an increased risk for the development of adenocarcinoma.

Lung

6. A 36-year-old male is brought to the emergency room by his roommate. While driving around, he began to cough and developed shortness of breath and wheezing. His roommate reports that he has had multiple attacks like this in the past. When he was coughing, he did not cough anything up. Of the following, which would histologic examination of the lungs likely reveal?

A. Asteroid bodies

B. Lepidic growth

C. Charcot-Leyden crystals

D. Oxalic acid crystals

E. Ferruginous bodies

Lung

7. A 61-year-old male with a 60-pack-per-year smoking history presents to an acute care clinic, not having seen a physician in 20 years. He says that he is having increased difficulty with breathing. Over the past several years, he has frequently had a cough that lingered, and in which he would cough up phlegm. Which of the following findings, which is related to his presenting condition, is most likely to be identified?

A. A systolic murmur

B. A diastolic murmur

C. Xanthelasmas

D. Enlarged anteroposterior dimension of the chest

E. Coarse rales throughout the lungs

Lung

8. Given the previous clinical scenario, of the following, which would histologic examination of the lungs most likely reveal?

A. Keratin pearls

B. Lepidic growth

C. Eosinophilic infiltrates in wall of airways

D. Loss of alveolar septa in the upper lobes

E. Granulomas

Lung

9. A 13-year-old male is brought to the emergency room by his parents. While helping them clean out the attic, he quickly developed difficulty breathing and was wheezing. Physical examination revealed wheezing and pulsus paradoxus. He has had two similar episodes before, but of much less severity, and lasting for only a short time. Of the following, which is true regarding this condition?

A. Pulmonary function testing would reveal a normal FEV1/FVC ratio.

B. The underlying mechanism is a type II hypersensitivity reaction.

C. Gross changes can include hyperinflation of the lungs and mucous plugging.

D. The disease is associated with Hirschsprung disease.

E. It is unlikely to involve a cough.

Lung

10. Given the previous clinical scenario, in ten years, if the patient died during a car accident and an autopsy was performed, of the following which would histologic examination of the lung most likely reveal?

A. Granulomatous inflammation

B. Loss of pulmonary parenchyma in the apices

C. Hypertrophy of airway smooth muscle

D. Multifocal collections of lymphocytes

E. Polarizable foreign material

Lung

10.2 Restrictive Lung Disease—Questions

Easy	Medium	Hard

11. A 68-year-old male with a 75-pack-per-year smoking history, who has been experiencing dyspnea on exertion for the past two years, not associated with chest pain, becomes acutely short of breath while eating dinner with friends. He is transported to the emergency room, where auscultation reveals diminished breath sounds on the right side. A chest X-ray reveals marked radiolucency of the right pleural cavity. Of the following, what is the most likely etiology for his acute shortness of breath?

A. Erosion of neoplasm through pleural surface

B. Erosion of bronchial wall by tuberculous granuloma

C. Aspiration of foreign body

D. Rupture of bulla

E. Trauma of the chest wall

Lung

12. A 63-year-old retired male went to his family physician with complaints of increasing difficulty with breathing. He says the symptoms started a few years ago but have progressed to the point where he has difficulty breathing with even mild physical exertion. As part of his examination, his physician performs pulmonary function tests. His FEV1 is 72% of predicted and his FVC is 75% of predicted with a normal FEV_1/FVC ratio. Of the following, what is his most likely diagnosis?

A. Centriacinar emphysema

B. Panacinar emphysema

C. Asthma

D. Bronchiectasis

E. Interstitial lung disease

Lung

13. A 71-year-old retired plumber dies after several years of a disease characterized by difficulty breathing for multiple years and accelerated by the presence of an aggressive neoplasm, which was diagnosed 8 months prior to his death. At autopsy, which was requested by his family, the pathologist identifies thick white pleural plaques and a neoplasm that essentially encases the right lung. Microscopic examination of the lungs reveals fibrosis and thickening of the alveolar septa. Of the following, what is the most likely diagnosis?

A. Coal worker's pneumoconiosis

B. Chronic silicosis

C. Asbestos-related lung disease

D. Sarcoidosis

E. Cryptogenic organizing pneumonia

Lung

14. Given the previous clinical scenario, of the following, what would microscopic examination of the lungs also reveal?

A. Rod-shaped accumulations of hemosiderin

B. Extensive finely stippled black pigment

C. Charcot-Leyden crystals

D. Giant cells associated with fibrosis

E. Asteroid bodies

Lung

15. A 46-year-old male presents to a primary care physician complaining of a persistent nonproductive cough that has worsened steadily over the past two years as well as progressive exertional dyspnea. He is worried because a friend of his recently died from a heart attack. His vital signs are temperature of 98.9°F, pulse of 89 bpm, and blood pressure of 131/79 mm Hg. Physical examination reveals bibasilar end-inspiratory crackles. There is no lower extremity edema. Auscultation of the chest does not reveal an S3, and jugular venous pressure is measured at 2 cm H_2O. Of the following, which is the most likely etiology for his disease?

A. Undiagnosed hypertension

B. Hypercholesterolemia

C. Exposure to silica

D. Factor V Leiden mutation

E. Gastroesophageal reflux

Lung

16. Given the previous clinical scenario, of the following, what is true about his condition?

A. Pulmonary function testing would reveal a normal vital capacity.

B. The condition is almost always due to tobacco use.

C. Hilar lymph nodes would have caseating granulomas.

D. Histologic examination of the lung would reveal smooth muscle hypertrophy of airway walls.

E. Digital clubbing may be present.

Lung

17. A 56-year-old male presents to a primary care physician. He says that over the past two and a half years he has had increasing shortness of breath that is accompanied by a dry cough at times. He works as a computer programmer. He does have a significant past medical history, with cardiac problems in the past as well as chronic pain. His vital signs are temperature of 98.6°F, pulse of 93 bpm, and blood pressure of 129/82 mm Hg. Physical examination reveals bibasilar end-inspiratory crackles. A lung biopsy is performed, which reveals both areas of normal lung and areas of diseased lung. Within the diseased lung, there is honeycomb change and fibroblastic foci. Of the following, what is the diagnosis?

A. UIP

B. DIP

C. NSIP

D. LIP

E. COP

Lung

18. Given the previous clinical scenario, of the following, which medication has this patient received that is the source of his presenting condition?

A. Amiodarone

B. Lisinopril

C. Penicillin

D. Morphine

E. Omeprazole

Lung

19. A pathologist is reviewing a lung biopsy from a 51-year-old male who presented with dyspnea. On the biopsy, she sees granulomas throughout the alveolar septa, some associated with fibrosis. Stains for acid-fast bacilli are negative. Of the following, what is the most likely occupation of the patient?

A. Farmer

B. Coal miner

C. Railroad engineer

D. Concrete pourer

E. Chimney sweep

Lung

20. A 35 year-old male with chronic nonproductive cough, and shortness of breath, who has uveitis, and, on histologic examination of the lungs, foci of inflammation associated with asteroid bodies.

A. Acute interstitial pneumonia

B. Usual interstitial pneumonitis (UIP)

C. Sarcoidosis

D. Chronic silicosis

E. Chronic hypersensitivity pneumonitis

Lung

21. A 70-year-old retired railroad worker with chronic shortness of breath with exertion and a nonproductive cough, who has a history of pleural plaques.

A. Respiratory bronchiolitis-interstitial lung disease

B. Desquamative interstitial pneumonitis

C. Sarcoidosis

D. Goodpasture's syndrome

E. Asbestosis

Lung

22. A 43-year-old female develops a chronic cough and dyspnea on exertion over the course of a few years. A lung biopsy reveals areas of honeycomb change, areas with fibroblastic foci, and areas of normal lung parenchyma.

A. Usual interstitial pneumonitis (UIP)

B. Sarcoidosis

C. Acute interstitial pneumonia

D. Nonspecific interstitial pneumonitis (NSIP)

E. Goodpasture's syndrome

Lung

23. A 58-year-old male with an 80-pack-per-year smoking history has developed over several years a nonproductive cough and worsening dyspnea on exertion. A biopsy of the lung reveals essentially all alveolar airspaces to contain finely pigmented macrophages.

A. Respiratory bronchiolitis-interstitial lung disease

B. Chronic silicosis

C. Chronic hypersensitivity pneumonitis

D. Desquamative interstitial pneumonitis

E. Usual interstitial pneumonitis (UIP)

Lung

24. A 47-year-old pigeon breeder presents with a slowly-developing dyspnea on exertion. A lung biopsy reveals granulomas in the alveolar septa.

A. Sarcoidosis

B. Nonspecific interstitial pneumonitis (NSIP)

C. Chronic hypersensitivity pneumonitis

D. Acute interstitial pneumonia

E. Asbestosis

Lung

25. A 53-year-old male with a history of worsening difficulty breathing that has developed over 1 year finally presents these changes to his family physician. He has a past medical history of systemic hypertension, treated with an ACE inhibitor, and type 2 diabetes mellitus, which developed 3 years ago, and is treated by dietary restrictions. He works as an accountant and raises pigeons in his spare time. He has never smoked. His vital signs are temperature of 98.7°F, pulse of 101 bpm, respiratory rate of 20 breaths per minute, and blood pressure of 110/68 mm Hg. Physical examination reveals diffuse crackles. There is no pitting edema or jugular venous distention. Pulmonary function testing reveals a decreased FVC, and an FEV1/FVC ratio that is essentially normal. Of the following, what would biopsy of the lung be most likely to reveal?

A. Alveolar septal fibrosis and hemosiderin-laden macrophages

B. Essentially all alveolar airspaces filled with pigment-laden macrophages

C. Small granulomas scattered throughout the biopsy in the alveolar septa

D. Infiltrating small neoplastic cells

E. Alveolar airspaces filled with neutrophils

Lung

10.3 Pulmonary Infections—Questions

Easy	Medium	Hard

26. A 63-year-old female presents to her family physician complaining of shortness of breath, which has developed over the last two days. In addition, she complains of chills and a cough productive of thick green-yellow mucous. Her vital signs are temperature 100.2°F, pulse 89 bpm, respiratory rate 23 breaths per minute, and blood pressure 100/79 mm Hg. Auscultation of the chest reveals rales in the lower right side, and an X-ray reveals an infiltrate in the lower lobe of the right lung. Of the following, what is her most likely diagnosis?

A. Chronic bronchitis

B. Acute bronchopneumonia

C. Pulmonary thromboembolus

D. Granulomatosis with polyangiitis

E. Adenocarcinoma in situ

Lung

27. A 21-year-old female is brought to the emergency room by her parents. Over the past two days, she has developed a fever of 101°F according to her parents, chills, a productive cough, and occasional sharp chest pain. An X-ray reveals consolidation of the upper lobe of the right lung. Of the following, which organism would a culture of the lung most likely grow?

A. Viridans streptococci
B. *Hemophilus influenzae*
C. *Streptococcus pneumoniae*
D. *Klebsiella pneumoniae*
E. *Mycoplasma pneumoniae*

Lung

28. A 28-year-old male presents to the emergency room with complaints of chills and a productive cough that have been ongoing for 3 days. His vital signs are temperature of 101°F, pulse of 111 bpm, respiratory rate of 23 breaths per minute, and blood pressure of 121/80 mm Hg. An X-ray reveals an infiltrate in the right lower lobe of the lung. A culture of his sputum grows *Streptococcus pneumoniae*. Of the following, which was a significant risk factor in his development of this specific organism?

A. Occupational use of a respirator
B. Past history of chest trauma
C. Remote splenectomy
D. Intravenous drug abuse
E. Recent travel to South America

Lung

29. A 61-year-old female with a history of metastatic ductal carcinoma of the breast is brought to the emergency room by her family. Over the past week, she has developed difficulty breathing and has coughed up green-yellow mucoid sputum. She has no history of hypertension, diabetes mellitus, or hypercholesterolemia and has never smoked. Her vital signs are temperature of 101°F, pulse of 107 bpm, and blood pressure of 105/67 mm Hg. Physical examination reveals crackles and decreased breathing sounds on the right side of her chest. Of the following, what is the most likely diagnosis?

A. Congestive heart failure
B. Chronic bronchitis
C. Acute bronchopneumonia
D. Pulmonary metastases
E. Desquamative interstitial pneumonitis

Lung

30. Given the previous clinical scenario, of the following, what is a complication of her disease process?

A. Cerebral infarction due to septic emboli
B. Myocardial rupture
C. Hyperplasia of bronchial mucous glands
D. Empyema
E. Pulmonary emphysema

Lung

31. A 15-year-old girl is brought to the emergency room by her parents. Over the past two days, she has developed some difficulty breathing and cough productive of yellow-green sputum. Her temperature at home prior to arrival was 101.2°F. An X-ray in the emergency room reveals consolidation of the entire lower lobe of the left lung. Of the following, what is the most likely diagnosis?

A. Acute bronchopneumonia
B. Lobar pneumonia
C. Interstitial pneumonia
D. Usual interstitial pneumonia
E. Sarcoidosis

Lung

32. Given the previous clinical scenario, of the following, what is the most likely etiologic agent?

A. *Staphylococcus aureus*
B. *Pseudomonas aeruginosa*
C. *Streptococcus pneumoniae*
D. *Mycoplasma pneumoniae*
E. *Influenza A*

Lung

33. A pathologist is examining the microscopic slide of a section of lung taken at autopsy. In the interstitium, she identifies patchy collections of lymphocytes. The infiltrates are present in both the right upper and left lower lobes of the lung. Of the following, what is the most likely etiologic agent?

A. *Streptococcus pneumoniae*
B. *Staphylococcus aureus*
C. *Mycobacterium tuberculosis*
D. *Mycoplasma pneumoniae*
E. *Strongyloides stercoralis*

Lung

10.4 Pulmonary Neoplasms—Questions

Easy	Medium	Hard

34. A 63-year-old female with an 80-pack-per-year smoking history has been complaining to her husband of feeling weak and being constipated. She also has abdominal pain. He brings her to the emergency room because she has started to act very odd including acting paranoid. While in the emergency room, she has a seizure. Laboratory testing reveals a total calcium of 13.0 mg/dL. On chest X-ray, she has a probable mass in the left upper lobe of the lung near the hilum. Of the following, what would a biopsy of the mass most likely reveal?

A. Neoplastic glands
B. Small neoplastic cells with a high nuclear to cytoplasm ratio
C. Keratin pearls
D. Noncaseating granulomas
E. Cartilage

Lung

35. Given the previous clinical scenario, of the following, what is she at most risk for developing?

A. A parathyroid gland adenoma
B. Kidney stones
C. Sarcoidosis of the lungs
D. Glioblastoma multiforme
E. Paget's disease

Lung

36. A 63-year-old male with an 80-pack-per-year smoking history is diagnosed with a laryngeal tumor. His physician informs him that he has an excellent prognosis. Of the following choices, what was the most likely tumor type and what was its location?

A. Squamous cell carcinoma/supraglottic
B. Squamous cell carcinoma/glottic
C. Squamous cell carcinoma/subglottic
D. Adenocarcinoma/supraglottic
E. Adenocarcinoma/glottic
F. Adenocarcinoma/subglottic

Larynx

37. A 67-year-old male presents to his family physician because of complaints of increasing difficulty breathing over the last several months. A chest X-ray reveals a mass in the right side of the chest, apparently surrounding the lung. An exploratory thoracotomy confirms the radiologic impression of a neoplasm encasing the right lung. Of the following, which is the most correct statement regarding this neoplasm?

A. It has an excellent prognosis
B. It produces PTH
C. It produces ADH
D. Examination of the underlying lung will likely reveal ferruginous bodies
E. Asteroid bodies will be found throughout the tumor

Lung

38. A 66-year-old male with a clinical history of systemic hypertension, emphysema, and an 80-pack per year smoking history is brought to the emergency room by his family. The emergency room physician examining him notes marked congestion of his head, neck, and upper extremities. Of the following, what is the most likely diagnosis?

A. Horner's syndrome
B. Aortic dissection
C. Allergic reaction to medication
D. Superior vena cava syndrome
E. Bullous pemphigoid

Lung

39. A 64-year-old male is brought to the emergency room by his family after he falls and develops pain in his right thigh. His past medical history is significant for hypertension and emphysema, and he has a 60-pack-per-year smoking history. Over the past 6 months, he has developed a persistent nonproductive cough and occasionally coughs up blood. An X-ray of the right thigh reveals a fracture of the diaphysis of the femur associated with a mass. The mass does not communicate with the medullary cavity. Of the following, what is the most likely diagnosis?

A. Ewing sarcoma
B. Chondrosarcoma
C. Osteochondroma
D. Metastatic lung carcinoma
E. Osteoporosis

Lung

40. A 67-year-old male over the course of about 6 months gains about 30 lbs., develops hypertension, sustains a fracture of his hip and is diagnosed with osteoporosis, and develops glucose intolerance. A chest X-ray reveals a pulmonary mass. Of the following, what is the most likely diagnosis?

A. Squamous cell carcinoma

B. Adenocarcinoma

C. Large cell carcinoma

D. Small cell carcinoma

E. Adenocarcinoma in situ

Lung

41. A 68-year-old male who presented to the clinic with a cough, occasionally with blood, and was ultimately diagnosed with a lung cancer is undergoing a resection. The surgeon asks for a frozen section on the resected mass and a thin rim of pulmonary tissue. A diagnosis of small cell carcinoma is made. Of the following choice, what will the surgeon most likely do?

A. Expand the margins of his original resection by 1.0 cm

B. Resect the entire lobe in which the mass is located

C. Resect the entire lung in which the mass is located

D. Remove any involved lymph nodes

E. Stop the surgery

Lung

42. A 71-year-old male presents to his family physician because of difficulty breathing, which has been ongoing for several weeks but greatly worsened in the last two days. He has a 50-pack-per-year smoking history; however, other than mild hypertension he has no significant past medical history. Physical examination reveals decreased breathing sounds on the right side, decreased resonance, and decreased fremitus. An X-ray reveals deviation of the trachea to the right side of the body. Of the following, what is the most likely diagnosis?

A. Right-side tension pneumothorax

B. Lobar pneumonia

C. Bronchogenic carcinoma in right bronchus

D. Congestive heart failure with right pleural effusion

E. Aortic dissection with hemothorax

Lung

43. A 57-year-old female with a history of systemic lupus erythematosus and systemic hypertension presents to her family physician because of a lingering nonproductive cough after an upper respiratory tract infection. She occasionally coughs up a tiny amount of blood. Physical examination reveals a palpable nodule above her right clavicle. A chest X-ray reveals a mass in the periphery of the left lung. Of the following, what is a complication of her presenting disease?

A. Cardiac dysrhythmia due to interventricular septal involvement

B. Cirrhosis of the liver

C. Kidney stones

D. Hoarseness

E. Hashimoto thyroiditis

Lung

10.5 Disease of Pleura— Questions

Easy	Medium	Hard

44. A 27-year-old male is stabbed in the chest, with the blade transecting his right internal mammary artery. Shortly thereafter, he develops shortness of breath and collapses. Emergency medical services responds and transports him to the emergency room, where a chest tube is placed, which results in 1 L of blood being removed from his right pleural cavity. Of the following, which condition is occurring in his right lung?

A. Compressive atelectasis

B. Obstructive atelectasis

C. Contraction atelectasis

D. Centrilobular emphysema

E. Bullous emphysema

Pleural space

45. At the time of autopsy, an X-ray of the chest reveals a mediastinal shift toward the right lung. When the pathologist examines the right lung at autopsy, he notices that the surface is wrinkled and the underlying parenchyma appears more solid. Microscopic examination of the lung reveals collapse of the alveoli. Of the following, which is the most likely cause of these changes in the lung?

A. Blood in the right pleural cavity

B. A foreign body in the right bronchus

C. Asbestosis

D. A ruptured bulla of the right lung

E. *Mycoplasma* infection

Lung

46. A 68-year-old male with a 75-pack-per-year smoking history, who has been experiencing dyspnea on exertion for the past two years, not associated with chest pain, becomes acutely short of breath while eating dinner with friends. He is transported to the emergency room, where auscultation reveals diminished breathing sounds on the right side. A chest X-ray reveals marked radiolucency of the right pleural cavity. Of the following, what is the most likely diagnosis?

A. Hemothorax

B. Pneumothorax

C. Chylothorax

D. Empyema

E. Congestive heart failure

Pleura

47. A 41-year-old male is brought to the emergency room because of a sudden onset of chest pain and worsening difficulty of breathing. His vital signs are temperature of 99.0°F, pulse of 105, respiratory rate of 30 breaths per minute, and blood pressure of 92/60 mm Hg. Physical examination reveals decreased breathing sounds on the right side of the chest and hyper-resonance to percussion. Of the following, what is the most likely diagnosis?

A. Pulmonary thromboembolus

B. Acute myocardial infarct

C. Tension pneumothorax

D. Ruptured pulmonary neoplasm

E. Acute asthma

Lung

10.6 Miscellaneous Pulmonary Disease—Questions

| Easy | Medium | Hard |

48. A 28-year-old female presents to the emergency room. She has had a sudden onset of chest pain and difficulty breathing, and she is concerned because her father died unexpectedly at the age of 34 years. She describes the chest pain as relatively sharp. Her vital signs are temperature of 98.9°F, pulse of 103 bpm, respiratory rate of 26 breaths per minute, and blood pressure of 124/85 mm Hg. Her past medical history is noncontributory, except that she was in a skiing accident two weeks before, where she severely sprained her ankle and she is still not getting around well. She does not smoke or have high cholesterol. Of the following, what is the most likely diagnosis?

A. Acute myocardial infarction

B. Pulmonary thromboembolus

C. Hypertrophic cardiomyopathy

D. Status asthmaticus

E. Fat embolus

Lung

49. Given the previous clinical scenario, if she died suddenly, which of the following would be identified at autopsy?

A. A thrombus in one of the epicardial coronary arteries

B. A thick interventricular septum in the heart

C. Microscopic fat in the pulmonary vasculature

D. A thromboembolus in the pulmonary veins

E. A thromboembolus in the pulmonary artery

Lung

50. Given the previous clinical scenario, of the following, which test is most likely to be positive?

A. Troponin I

B. Genetic testing for mutation of the β-myosin heavy chain gene

C. D-dimer

D. Culture of sputum

E. Urinary metanephrines

Lung

51. A 68-year-old female presents to the emergency room with her family who brought her in because she has had a cold for multiple days but, to them, appears to be worsening, and, she has been coughing up green-yellow material. She is otherwise healthy, with only a past medical history of hypothyroidism treated with hormone replacement and mild osteoporosis. Vital signs are temperature of 100.8°F, pulse of 106 bpm, and respiratory rate of 24 breaths per minute. Auscultation reveals decreased breathing sounds on the right side and decreased resonance to percussion on the right side. Of the following, what is the cause for the diminished breath sounds in the right hemithorax?

A. Congestive heart failure

B. Pleural effusion

C. Chronic obstructive pulmonary disease

D. Pulmonary thromboembolus

E. *Mycobacterium tuberculosis*

Lung

52. A 36-year-old male is brought to the emergency room by friends because he suddenly developed shortness of breath and is complaining of sharp chest pain that is worse when he breathes deeply. His vital signs are temperature of 98.7°F, pulse of 135 bpm, respiratory rate of 33 breaths per minute, and blood pressure of 81/58 mm Hg. Physical examination reveals percussion resonance, which is increased on the left side of his chest, and distended jugular veins. Of the following, what is the next most appropriate step?

A. X-ray his chest

B. Performs a helical CT scan

C. Insert an open-bore needle or catheter in his left chest

D. Give the patient oxygen

E. Give the patient an aspirin

Lung

53. A 54-year-old male develops sharp chest pain and shortness of breath suddenly while in the hospital recovering from a surgical repair of a fractured ankle. He has no other past medical history. On physical examination by an attending physician, his vital signs are pulse of 115 bpm, respiratory rate of 30 breaths per minute, and blood pressure of 100/70 mm Hg. A pulse oximeter reveals an oxygen saturation of 85%. An ECG shows sinus tachycardia and some right ventricular strain. While being examined, he goes into cardiac arrest and cannot be resuscitated. Of the following, what is the most likely diagnosis?

A. Cerebral infarct

B. Acute myocardial infarct

C. Pulmonary thromboembolus

D. Aortic dissection

E. Foreign body aspiration

Lung

54. Given the previous clinical scenario, of the following, what would most likely be identified at autopsy, either grossly or microscopic?

A. Thrombus in a coronary artery

B. Lines of Zahn

C. Empyema

D. Foreign body in the airway

E. Red infarct in the lung

Lung

55. A 37-year-old obese female is ambulating for the first time in three days since undergoing an exploratory laparotomy for abdominal pain, which did not disclose an identifiable abnormality, when she suddenly develops sharp chest pain and difficulty breathing. A nurse responds to her and, taking her vital signs, notes a pulse rate of 134 bpm and a respiratory rate of 31 breaths per minute. She has no significant past medical history. Of the following, what is the most likely diagnosis?

A. Acute myocardial infarct

B. Tension pneumothorax due to spontaneous rupture of pleural bleb

C. Pulmonary thromboembolus

D. Peritonitis due to a perforated peptic ulcer

E. Fat emboli syndrome

Lung

56. Given the previous clinical scenario, of the following conditions, which one is most likely for her to also have?

A. Undiagnosed B-cell lymphoma

B. Factor V Leiden mutation

C. Pulmonary emphysema

D. Pancreatic carcinoma

E. Cirrhosis of the liver

Lung

57. A 36-year-old female has sudden onset of difficulty breathing and sharp chest pain. For the past two weeks, she has had decreased mobility from injuries sustained in a motor vehicle accident. One of her siblings died three years ago, and an autopsy found thrombi in the lung. Of the following, which laboratory tests can essentially exclude the possibility of a pulmonary thromboembolus in this patient?

A. Normal PT

B. Normal PTT

C. Normal D-dimer

D. Normal fibrinogen

E. Normal troponin I

Lung

58. Four days after a transcontinental plane flight, a 43-year-old male suddenly develops chest pain and difficulty breathing while walking with his wife. He collapses. Medical services are summoned, but unable to revive him. An autopsy is performed. He has no past medical history other than gastroesophageal reflux effectively treated with omeprazole. Of the following, what is the pathologist most likely to identify?

A. Extension of a hepatocellular carcinoma into the inferior vena cava

B. Pale discoloration of the anterior wall of the left ventricle

C. Alveolar airspaces filled with neutrophils

D. A foreign body in the airway

E. Thrombus at the pulmonary artery bifurcation

Lung

59. A 2-year-old child is playing on the floor near her parents who are watching television, when she suddenly starts coughing and having difficulty breathing. Prior to this episode, she did not have any symptoms. Her parents rush her to the emergency room. On physical examination, the doctor identifies stridor. She has no past medical history. Her mother and father have been married since the summer of high school and have had no other sexual partners. Of the following, what is the most likely diagnosis?

A. Pulmonary artery embolus

B. Occult head trauma

C. Foreign body in the airway

D. Laryngeal polyp

E. Lobar pneumonia

Lung

10.7 Obstructive Lung Disease—Answers and Explanations

Easy	Medium	Hard

1. Correct: Chronic obstructive pulmonary disease (A)

The most common causes of shortness of breath in the elderly are chronic obstructive pulmonary disease, congestive heart failure, and asthma (**A**). Chronic interstitial pneumonia, pulmonary thromboemboli, and granulomatosis with polyangiitis could all cause shortness of breath but are much less common than COPD (**B, D, E**). And, with no history of accompanying chest pain despite several years of symptoms, severe coronary artery atherosclerosis is not likely (**C**).

2. Correct: Cigarette smoke (C)

The most common causes of shortness of breath in the elderly are chronic obstructive pulmonary disease, congestive heart failure, and asthma. Chronic obstructive pulmonary disease is most commonly due to tobacco use (**C**). Asbestosis, emphysema due to α-1-antitrypsin deficiency, granulomatosis with polyangiitis (associated with c-ANCA), and *Mycobacterium tuberculosis* are associated with shortness of breath but are not as common (**A-B, D-E**).

3. Correct: Chronic bronchitis (B)

Of the diseases listed, emphysema and chronic bronchitis are the most common (**A, B**). With chronic bronchitis, patients have a productive cough for several months in two consecutive years (**B**). Physical examination can reveal ronchi and signs of hypoxemia, with dyspnea occurring later in the course of the disease, whereas in emphysema, dyspnea occurs earlier ("pink puffers"). Without a fever, lobar pneumonia is not likely, and the time course is too long (**C**). (**D, E**) are possible, but rarer.

4. Correct: Hypertrophy of mucous glands in the airways (D)

This patient has signs and symptoms consistent with chronic bronchitis. With chronic bronchitis, patients have a productive cough for several months in two consecutive years. Physical examination can reveal ronchi and signs of hypoxemia, with dyspnea occurring later in the course of the disease; whereas, in emphysema, dyspnea occurs earlier ("pink puffers"). The histologic finding of chronic bronchitis is hypertrophy of the mucous glands in the airways (**D**). The other histologic features are not typical of chronic bronchitis (**A-C, E**).

5. Correct: Prior to this episode, the patient likely had an upper respiratory tract infection. (C)

The patient has the signs and symptoms of asthma: nonproductive cough, shortness of breath, and wheezing, with a past history of the same. The FEV1/FVC ratio is decreased (**A**). The causative agent is IgE (**D**), and there is no increased risk of adenocarcinoma (**E**). Heavy cigarette use, while it could exacerbate asthma, is not the underlying cause of asthma (**B**); however, patients can have a history of a recent upper respiratory tract infection as an inciting cause of a symptomatic episode (**C**).

6. Correct: Charcot-Leyden crystals (C)

The patient has the signs and symptoms of asthma: nonproductive cough, shortness of breath, and wheezing, with a past history of the same. Charcot-Leyden crystals are a feature of asthma (**C**), asteroid bodies are found in giant cells and associated with sarcoidosis (**A**), lepidic growth is the growth pattern for adenocarcinoma in situ (**B**), oxalic acid crystals are

135

found in the kidney in ethylene glycol overdose and are associated with *Aspergillus* infections (**D**), and ferruginous bodies are associated with asbestosis (**E**).

7.   Correct: Enlarged anteroposterior dimension of the chest (D)

The clinical history is consistent with chronic obstructive pulmonary disease. Of the listed findings, an enlarged anteroposterior dimension of the chest (i.e., barrel chest) is most consistent with the diagnosis (**D**). COPD does not cause a murmur (**A, B**); xanthelasmas are associated with high cholesterol (**C**), and coarse rales are not a feature of COPD (**E**).

8.   Correct: loss of alveolar septa in the upper lobes (D)

The clinical history is consistent with chronic obstructive pulmonary disease. The histologic features of chronic obstructive pulmonary disease are hyperplasia of mucous glands (the chronic bronchitis component) and the loss of alveolar septa (the emphysema component) (**D**). Keratin pearls are found in squamous cell carcinoma, and lepidic growth in adenocarcinoma in situ (**A, B**). Asthma has eosinophilic infiltrates in the wall of the airways (**C**), and granulomas are found in sarcoidosis, tuberculosis, hypersensitivity pneumonitis, and others (**E**).

9.   Correct: Gross changes can include hyperinflation of the lungs and mucous plugging (C)

The clinical scenario is consistent with asthma, with a child developing dyspnea and wheezing after exposure to dust and other potential allergens that an attic might contain. During an asthmatic attack, patients can have pulsus paradoxus. Pulmonary function testing would reveal a decreased FEV1/FVC ratio (**A**), as asthma is an obstructive lung disease. Asthma in this situation would most likely be due to a type I hypersensitivity reaction (**B**). Asthma is not usually associated with Hirschsprung disease (**D**), and a nonproductive cough is characteristic of the disorder (**E**). Gross changes including hyperinflation of the lung (due to obstruction) and mucous plugging are characteristic pathologic features (**C**).

10.   Correct: Hypertrophy of airway smooth muscle (C)

Given the clinical scenario, dyspnea and wheezing developing after exposure to allergens, the most likely diagnosis, especially given past episodes of similar symptoms, is asthma. The histologic features of asthma are smooth muscle hypertrophy, collagen deposition under the basement membrane, an eosinophilic infiltrate, and presence of Charcot-Leyden crystals (collections of major basic protein), and Curschmann spirals (sloughed epithelial cells cast in the shape of airways) (**C**). The other histologic changes listed are not characteristic features of asthma (**A-B, D-E**).

10.8 Restrictive Lung Disease—Answers and Explanations

Easy	Medium	Hard

11.   Correct: Rupture of bulla (D)

Based on the patient's age, history of tobacco use, and symptoms prior to the acute event, his most likely underlying diagnosis is chronic obstructive pulmonary disease. In patients with emphysema, which is one component of chronic obstructive pulmonary disease, subpleural bullae can form. If one ruptures, the patient can develop a pneumothorax (**D**). Although the other listed conditions could have the potential for causing a pneumothorax, these are much less likely with tuberculosis or aspiration of foreign body. None listed are as common as COPD (**A-C, E**).

12.   Correct: Interstitial lung disease (E)

This individual has a reduced FEV1 and FVC, but a normal or elevated FEV1/FVC ratio. This testing is consistent with a restrictive lung disease (**E**). The other choices are obstructive lung diseases and would have a decreased FEV1/FVC ratio (**A-D**).

13.   Correct: Asbestos-related lung disease (C)

The pleural plaques, neoplasm encasing the lung (a mesothelioma), and fibrosis of the alveolar septa are most consistent with asbestos exposure (**C**). Pleural mesotheliomas are highly characteristic of asbestos exposure; pleural plaques can be seen with asbestos exposure (as well as other conditions), and the lung changes are consistent with interstitial lung disease. While CWP, silicosis and sarcoidosis can cause interstitial lung disease, they are not associated with pleural plaques or mesothelioma (**A-B, D**). Cryptogenic organizing pneumonia would be more of an acute to subacute process (**E**).

14.   Correct: Rod-shaped accumulation of hemosiderin (A)

Asbestos bodies are fibers of asbestos (note that the fibers themselves are not visible with standard H&E stain) engulfed by macrophages and coated with iron (**A**). The other pathologic findings described at the autopsy are consistent with asbestos exposure. Extensive finely stippled black pigment could be seen in coal workers or heavy smokers (**B**), Charcot-Leyden crystals in asthma (**C**), giant cells associated with fibrosis in sarcoidosis (**D**), and asteroid bodies are found within giant cells and are frequently associated with sarcoidosis (**E**).

15. Correct: Exposure to silica (C)

The gradual onset of a cough and dyspnea, in a patient with no signs or symptoms to suggest congestive heart failure, and with bibasilar crackles is consistent with interstitial lung disease. Silica exposure is one cause of interstitial lung disease (**C**). The other things listed are not risk factors by themselves for interstitial lung disease (**A-B, D-E**).

16. Correct: Clubbing of the fingers may be present. (E)

The gradual onset of a cough and dyspnea, in a patient with no signs and symptoms to suggest congestive heart failure, and with bibasilar crackles, is consistent with interstitial lung disease. Digital clubbing can occur in some forms of the disease (**E**). The vital capacity would be decreased (**A**). Only a few forms of interstitial lung disease are associated with tobacco use (**B**). In sarcoidosis, the hilar lymph nodes would have noncaseating granulomas (**C**). The smooth muscle of the airways is not hypertrophied (**D**).

17. Correct: UIP (A)

UIP is characterized by patchy changes, unlike NSIP, which is diffuse (**A, C**). The changes include both acute (fibroblastic foci) and chronic (honeycomb change) findings, which is consistent with the temporally heterogenous nature of the disease. DIP has prominent alveolar macrophages (**B**), LIP a lymphocytic infiltrate (**D**), and COP is an acutely presenting condition with fibroblastic plugs in the airways (**E**).

18. Correct: Amiodarone (A)

The slow onset of a cough and dyspnea, in a patient with nothing else to suggest congestive heart failure, and with bibasilar crackles is consistent with interstitial lung disease. Of the drugs listed, amiodarone is most commonly associated with interstitial lung disease (**A**). The other choices are not correct (**B-E**)

19. Correct: Farmer (A)

The microscopic findings are consistent with a chronic hypersensitivity pneumonitis, of which farmer's lung, due to exposure to thermophilic *Actinomyces* is one common form (**A**). The other choices are less likely (**B-E**).

20. Correct: Sarcoidosis (C)

Sarcoidosis can cause interstitial fibrosis leading to a restrictive lung disease, which can present with chronic cough and shortness of breath. People with sarcoidosis can have extrapulmonary manifestations including uveitis and erythema nodosum. Histologic examination will reveal granulomas, and the giant cells can contain asteroid bodies. Also found in sarcoidosis are Schaumann bodies, which are concentrically calcified microscopic bodies.

21. Correct: Asbestosis (E)

Asbestos exposure can lead to several pathologic findings, including pleural mesothelioma, pleural plaques, and asbestosis. Asbestosis is an interstitial lung disease, characterized by fibrosis of the pulmonary parenchyma, and is associated with ferruginous bodies. Some forms of asbestos exposure can lead to marked fibrosis of the pleural cavities. In addition to mesothelioma, asbestos exposure is a risk factor for bronchogenic carcinoma.

22. Correct: Usual interstitial pneumonitis (UIP) (A)

Usual interstitial pneumonitis is one form of restrictive lung disease, which can present with a slowly-developing chronic cough and dyspnea on exertion. The characteristic histologic features are temporally heterogeneous changes—both honeycomb change and fibroblastic foci, and areas of unaffected lung interspersed between areas of affected lung (i.e., patchy distribution). NSIP is temporally homogenous, and the pulmonary parenchyma is diffusely affected.

23. Correct: Desquamative interstitial pneumonitis (DIP) (D)

Desquamative interstitial pneumonitis is one form of restrictive lung disease and can present with a slowly developing chronic cough and dyspnea on exertion. It is strongly associated with tobacco use, and the histologic feature is alveolar airspaces filled with pigment-laden macrophages (the pigment being carbonaceous material from the tobacco use). Respiratory bronchiolitis with interstitial lung disease occurs under a similar clinical scenario (i.e., a tobacco user presenting with dyspnea on exertion and chronic cough), but has patchy involvement of the pulmonary parenchyma and not diffuse involvement.

24. Correct: Chronic hypersensitivity pneumonitis (C)

Although sarcoidosis can present with dyspnea on exertion, and patients can have granulomas on lung biopsy, the fact that the patient is a pigeon breeder presenting with those symptoms and having that histologic appearance is consistent with chronic hypersensitivity pneumonitis.

25. Correct: Small granulomas scattered throughout the biopsy in the alveolar septa (C)

With an insidious onset of difficulty breathing, and pulmonary function testing revealing an essentially normal FEV1/FVC ratio, the most likely diagnosis is a restrictive lung disease. Given the history of working with pigeons, one possible cause is chronic hypersensitivity pneumonitis, which would have small granulomas identified on biopsy (**C**). Alveolar septal fibrosis with hemosiderin-laden macrophages would be consistent with congestive heart failure, for which he has essentially no risk factors (**A**), given his hypertension is apparently well treated. Desquamative interstitial pneumonitis is characterized by alveolar airspaces filled with pigment-laden macrophages and essentially always occurs in smokers (**B**). Neither a tumor nor bronchopneumonia is supported by the clinical scenario (**D-E**).

10.9 Pulmonary Infections— Answers and Explanations

Easy	Medium	Hard

26.   Correct: Acute bronchopneumonia (B)

With a productive cough, shortness of breath, chills, a fever, and a chest infiltrate, the most likely diagnosis is acute bronchopneumonia (**B**). The other diseases could cause shortness of breath and some of the other findings (e.g., chronic bronchitis could cause productive cough; pulmonary thromboembolus could cause an infiltrate with a red infarct; granulomatosis with polyangiitis could cause an infiltrate and fever; adenocarcinoma in situ could cause an infiltrate and fever), but not the combination seen in this patient and not with the commonness of acute bronchopneumonia (**A, C-E**).

27.   Correct: *Streptococcus pneumoniae* (C)

This patient has signs, symptoms, and radiologic evaluation consistent with the diagnosis of lobar pneumonia. The most common organism causing a lobar pneumonia is *Streptococcus pneumoniae* (**C**). The other choices are incorrect (**A-B, D-E**).

28.   Correct: Remote splenectomy (C)

Individuals who have had a splenectomy have an increased risk for the development of infections by encapsulated bacteria, such as *Streptococcus pneumoniae* and *Neisseria meningitidis* (**C**). None of the other factors listed, at the age of 28 years, provide a known significant risk factor for *S. pneumoniae* pneumonia (**A-B, D-E**).

29.   Correct: Acute bronchopneumonia (C)

Given her presentation of dypsnea, associated with fever and productive cough, the most likely diagnosis is acute bronchopneumonia (**C**). She has no risk factors for congestive heart failure, and the associated crackles should be bilateral (**A**). Chronic bronchitis produces a productive cough, but the diagnosis requires symptoms to occur over time, and this is an acute event (**B**). Although pulmonary metastases may be an underlying cause of the bronchopneumonia, they would not, by themselves, produce the symptoms identified (**D**). Desquamative interstitial

pneumonitis would present with a more insidious course, and, given the patient has never smoked, is highly unlikely (**E**).

30.   Correct: Empyema (D)

Given the clinical scenario, the most likely diagnosis is an acute bronchopneumonia. One complication of acute bronchopneumonia is an empyema, if the inflammation extends into the pleural cavity (**D**). Septic emboli are not usually associated with bronchopneumonia, although sepsis can definitely occur (**A**). Hyperplasia of bronchial mucous glands is a feature of chronic bronchitis (**C**). Myocardial rupture is not a complication of acute bronchopneumonia. Pulmonary emphysema is not a complication of bronchopneumonia (**E**).

31.   Correct: Lobar pneumonia (B)

The clinical scenario and radiographic findings are consistent with lobar pneumonia, which most commonly affects one entire lobe (**B**). Acute bronchopneumonia essentially always arises in individuals who have another underlying medical condition, such as cancer or Alzheimer's disease (**A**). Both interstitial and bronchopneumonia have patchy infiltrates on X-ray and do not involve one entire lobe (**A, C**). Usual interstitial pneumonia presents in older adults, is associated with a more insidious onset, and does not usually have a high fever (C). Sarcoidosis and UIP would be rare in a child, would present with a more insidious onset, and are unlikely to have a high fever (**D, E**).

32.   Correct: *Streptococcus pneumoniae* (C)

The clinical scenario is characteristic for lobar pneumonia. The most common etiologic agent of lobar pneumonia is *Streptococcus pneumoniae*, although other organisms can also cause the condition (**C**). Influenza A is commonly associated with a bacterial superinfection, commonly *Staphylococcus aureus* (**A, E**). *Mycoplasma pneumoniae* would not present in this manner (**D**), and *Pseudomonas aeruginosa* would be a rare community-acquired cause of lobar pneumonia (**B**).

33.   Correct: *Mycoplasma pneumoniae* (D)

The pathologic description is that of an interstitial pneumonia, which is most commonly associated with viruses and *Mycoplasma* (**D**). *Mycobacterium tuberculosis* would produce caseating granulomas (**C**), and *Streptococcus* and *Staphylococcus* would be characterized by alveolar airspaces filled with neutrophils (**A, B**). When *Strongyloides* migrates through the lung, there can be an eosinophilic infiltrate (Löffler's syndrome) (**E**).

10.10 Pulmonary Neoplasms—Answers and Explanations

Easy	Medium	Hard

34. Correct: Keratin pearls (C)

The patient has symptoms consistent with hypercalcemia: weakness, constipation, abdominal pain, and psychiatric symptoms. Seizures can also occur. Squamous cell carcinoma, which has keratin pearls, can produce a parathyroid-hormone-like protein that will result in hypercalcemia (**C**). Adenocarcinoma (**A**) and small cell carcinoma (**B**) are not usually associated with PTH production. The mass is not a pulmonary hamartoma (**E**) or sarcoidosis (**D**).

35. Correct: Kidney stones (B)

The patient has symptoms consistent with hypercalcemia, weakness, constipation, abdominal pain, and psychiatric symptoms. Seizures can also occur. The laboratory testing confirms this diagnosis. Individuals with hypercalcemia are at risk for fractures and kidney stones (**B**). Nothing in the clinical history supports a diagnosis putting her at risk for the other conditions that are listed (**A, C-E**).

36. Correct: Squamous cell carcinoma/glottis (B)

The most common tumor of the larynx in a heavy tobacco user would be a squamous cell carcinoma (**A-F**). Tumors that develop on the glottis are more likely to be identified earlier in their course than supra- or subglottic tumors (and, hence, have a better prognosis) because even a small tumor on the vocal cords can cause a voice change and cause the patient to seek medical attention (**B**). Subglottic tumors have to grow to sufficient size to obstruct the airway to cause symptoms (**C, F**), and supraglottic tumors are more likely to metastasize early because of the lymphatic circulation, and also would produce obstruction later (**A, D**).

37. Correct: Examination of the underlying lung may reveal ferruginous bodies. (D)

The gross description of the tumor is consistent with a mesothelioma. The histologic diagnosis of a mesothelioma can be difficult for an inexperienced pathologist, but the gross appearance is characteristic. Pleural mesotheliomas are essentially always due to asbestos exposure. One histologic finding of asbestos-related lung disease is ferruginous bodies (**D**). Mesotheliomas have a poor prognosis (**A**). Squamous cell carcinomas of the lung are most known for producing a PTH-like protein (**B**), and small cell carcinomas of the lung are most known for producing ADH, ACTH, and other substances (**C**). Asteroid bodies are found in giant cells and are a feature often associated with sarcoidosis (**E**).

38. Correct: Superior vena cava syndrome (D)

Superior vena cava syndrome is caused by a lung tumor that compresses the superior vena cava, resulting in obstruction of return blood flow to the heart from the head and upper extremities, leading to congestion (**D**). Horner's syndrome can also be associated with lung tumors but involves compression or damage to the cervical sympathetic nerves, producing ptosis and miosis (**A**). An aortic dissection, allergic reaction to medication, and bullous pemphigoid would not produce such changes (**B, C, E**).

39. Correct: Metastatic lung carcinoma (D)

In adults, the most common tumors of the bones are metastases (**D**). The location is typical for Ewing sarcoma, but these tumors occur in children (**A**). The location is not typical for chondrosarcoma (**B**). As osteochondromas likely represent a development abnormality, it is highly unlikely that a tumor present for his entire life would now produce a pathologic fracture, and osteochondromas communicate with the medullary cavity (**C**). Metastases to bone often result in pathologic fractures (**D**). Osteoporosis can cause a pathologic fracture; however, there would not be a mass in the diaphysis associated with osteoporosis (**E**).

40. Correct: Small cell carcinoma (D)

The patient has features of Cushing's syndrome. Cushing's syndrome can occur due to ectopic production of ACTH. Of lung tumors, small cell carcinoma is the most recognized for producing ACTH (**D**). It can also produce ADH, while squamous cell carcinoma is most recognized for producing a PTH-like hormone. The other tumors listed do not commonly produce ACTH (**A-C, E**).

41. Correct: Stop the surgery (E)

At the time of diagnosis, small cell carcinoma is assumed to have metastasized, thus the surgeon will not usually resect an entire lobe or an entire lung, and instead the patient will receive chemotherapy (**A-D**). Non–small cell carcinomas (squamous cell, adenocarcinoma, and large cell) are not assumed to have metastasized, and therefore the surgeon will often attempt complete resection of the tumor. Although a specific ultimate diagnosis is important (e.g., squamous cell versus adenocarcinoma), at the time of surgery, the most important distinction is small cell versus non-small cell, as it directs the course of the surgery.

42. Correct: Bronchogenic carcinoma in the right bronchus (C)

A bronchogenic carcinoma in the right bronchus will block air flow into the right lung, which will lead to absorptive atelectasis. Atelectasis will lead to decreased breathing sounds and decreased resonance. The trachea will shift toward the side of the lesion, as the left lung is still filling with air whereas the right lung is not (**C**). A right-sided tension pneumothorax would have decreased breathing sounds because of the air between the chest wall and lung, but also increased resonance for the same reason, and deviation of the trachea toward the left side, because of the pressure in the right pleural cavity (**A**). An aortic dissection can hemorrhage into the pleural cavity, but the left pleural cavity would be affected (**E**). Given the long time course, a lobar pneumonia is unlikely (**B**), and congestive heart failure usually causes bilateral pleural effusions, and, given his minimal past medical history, this diagnosis is much less likely (**D**).

43. Correct: Hoarseness (D)

The clinical scenario is consistent with a pulmonary neoplasm, with the palpable nodule above the right clavicle being a Virchow node, which is concerning for a pulmonary neoplasm. Given the peripheral location of the tumor and no mention of smoking history, a diagnosis of adenocarcinoma is most likely. One complication of pulmonary neoplasms is hoarseness due to involvement of the recurrent laryngeal nerve (**D**). A cardiac dysrhythmia due to septal involvement could occur in sarcoidosis; however, the clinical scenario is more consistent with a pulmonary neoplasm (**A**). Cirrhosis of the liver, kidney stones, and Hashimoto thyroiditis are not consequences of a pulmonary neoplasm (**B-C, E**)

10.11 Disease of Pleura—Answers and Explanations

Easy	Medium	Hard

44. Correct: Compressive atelectasis (A)

The blood in the right pleural cavity will compress the right lung, not allowing air to enter the alveoli, and result in collapse of the alveolar airspaces, or compressive atelectasis (**A**). Obstructive atelectasis occurs due to blockage of the airway (e.g., a swallowed foreign body) (**B**), and contraction atelectasis occurs due to scarring impairing the ability of the airways to expand (**C**). Centrilobular and bullous emphysema are chronic processes (**D, E**).

45. Correct: A foreign body in the right bronchus (B)

The right lung is atelectatic. When the mediastinal shift is toward the lung that is atelectatic, the type of atelectasis is most likely obstructive in nature, such as would be caused by a foreign body in the right bronchus (**B**). Blood or air in the right pleural cavity would cause a mediastinal shift toward the left lung

(**A, D**). Although asbestosis can be associated with atelectasis, a mediastinal shift would most likely not be apparent, as the disease affects both lungs equally, similar to a *Mycoplasma* infection (**C, E**).

46. Correct: Pneumothorax (B)

While either air or fluid in the pleural cavity could lead to diminished breath sounds, air is radiolucent (**B**), while the remainder of the causes listed would be more radiodense (**A, C-E**).

47. Correct: Tension pneumothorax (C)

The decreased breathing sounds and hyperresonance to percussion are due to air filling the right pleural cavity. With a tension pneumothorax, with every breath the patient increases the amount of air in the pleural cavity and none can escape (**C**). This condition can lead to hypotension and cyanosis, and emergent treatment via needle or catheter insertion into the affected pleural cavity is needed. The other conditions could present with chest pain and increasing dyspnea, but they would not have the same physical examination, except if bleeding into the pleural cavity occurred with a ruptured neoplasm, and then decreased breathing sounds could be present; however, this would be a rare complication of a pulmonary neoplasm, and, given his age, a neoplasm would be unlikely (**A-B, D-E**).

10.12 Miscellaneous Pulmonary Disease—Answers and Explanations

Easy	Medium	Hard

48. Correct: Pulmonary thromboembolus (B)

This patient has signs and symptoms, combined with the clinical history, consistent with a thromboembolus (**B**). The fact her father died at an early age indicates the probable presence of a hereditary thrombophilia, such as factor V Leiden. Although coronary artery atherosclerosis leading to an acute myocardial infarct and hypertrophic cardiomyopathy are inherited, the signs and symptoms are not most consistent with these two conditions, as the chest pain is pleuritic in nature (**A, C**). A fat embolus can occur days to weeks after a long bone fracture, but not a sprain, and this would not explain the hereditary component (**E**). Other than shortness of breath, the clinical scenario does not suggest asthma (**D**)

49. Correct: A thromboembolus in the pulmonary artery (D)

This patient has signs and symptoms, combined with the clinical history, consistent with a thromboembolus (**D**). The fact her father died at an early age indicates the probable presence of a hereditary thrombophilia, such as factor V Leiden. The pathologic finding is a thromboembolus in the pulmonary artery, not vein (**E**). The cause of her symptoms is not coronary artery disease, hypertrophic cardiomyopathy, or a fat embolus (**A, B, C**).

50. Correct: D-dimer (C)

This patient has signs and symptoms, combined with the clinical history, consistent with a thromboembolus. The fact her father died at an early age indicates the probable presence of a hereditary thrombophilia, such as factor V Leiden. Although a troponin I test might be performed to rule out an acute myocardial infarct, the history is not as consistent with this diagnosis (**A**). Genetic testing for mutation of the β-myosin heavy chain gene would be performed in hypertrophic cardiomyopathy (**B**), culture of sputum if concerned for pneumonia (**D**), and urinary metanephrines, commonly for the diagnosis of pheochromocytoma (**E**). A D-dimer is highly sensitive, but not specific. Thus, while a negative D-dimer may help rule out a pulmonary thromboembolus, a positive D-dimer test can result from a variety of conditions (**C**).

51. Correct: Pleural effusion (B)

The findings on physical examination are consistent with a pleural effusion. Given that it is unilateral and that she has no risk factors for congestive heart failure, congestive heart failure is unlikely (**A**). The clinical scenario would be consistent with a pleural effusion, possibly an empyema, related to a bronchopneumonia (**B**). The clinical scenario is not as consistent with the other choices (**C-E**).

52. Correct: Insert a needle in his left chest (C)

The patient has the signs and symptoms of a tension pneumothorax, including sudden onset of shortness of breath, sharp chest pain, tachypnea, tachycardia, hypotension, and distended jugular veins. Needle thoracostomy, which can be accomplished by insertion of an open-bore needle or a catheter in the chest to release the air, is indicated given the unstable presentation (**C**). The other choices are incorrect, as the condition requires immediate treatment (**A-B, D-E**).

53. Correct: Pulmonary thromboembolus (C)

The signs and symptoms of a pulmonary thromboembolus (sharp chest pain, shortness of breath, hypoxia), in association with the background for the condition (i.e., immobile patient), are consistent with the diagnosis (**C**). The patient has no risk factor for atherosclerosis, other than age and sex; thus, the likelihood of a cerebral or a myocardial infarct are smaller, and with no history of hypertension, limited risk for aortic dissection (**A-B, D**). Because there are no neuromuscular difficulties, foreign body aspiration is unlikely (**E**).

54. Correct: Lines of Zahn (B)

The signs and symptoms of a pulmonary thromboembolus (sharp chest pain, shortness of breath, hypoxia), in association with the background for the condition (i.e., an immobile patient), are consistent with the diagnosis. The patient has no risk factor for atherosclerosis, other than age and sex; thus a thrombus in a coronary artery is less likely (**A**). Not being febrile or otherwise ill, an empyema is very unlikely (**C**). Because he is not neuromuscularly impaired, aspiration of a foreign body is highly unlikely (**D**). Lines of Zahn are found in thrombi, and in the lung, would be a thromboembolus (**B**). Although red infarcts are associated with pulmonary thromboemboli, it would not occur in such a setting, as it would take time to develop after the initial symptoms (**E**).

55. Correct: Pulmonary thromboembolus (C)

Given that the patient is obese and has been nonmobile due to recovering from a surgery, she is at risk for the development of deep venous thrombi, which can embolize to the lung, and characteristically present with sharp chest pain and tachypnea and tachycardia (**C**). Given she has no risk factors, an acute myocardial infarction is unlikely, also sharp chest pain would be unusual (**A**). A tension pneumothorax can cause sudden sharp chest pain, tachypnea, and tachycardia; however, in comparison to a pulmonary thromboembolus in the given clinical scenario, it is not very likely (**B**). Fat emboli syndrome can develop after trauma of a long bone, or can be associated with pancreatitis, but would not occur in the described situation (**E**). Given the time course, it is unlikely that she perforated a peptic ulcer and presents later with peritonitis (**D**).

56. Correct: Factor V Leiden mutation (B)

The clinical scenario, i.e., sudden onset of sharp chest pain and dyspnea, in an obese nonmobile individual, is consistent with a pulmonary thromboembolus resulting from deep venous thrombi. Individuals with factor V Leiden mutations, a relatively common mutation, are at increased risk for deep venous thrombi and subsequent pulmonary thromboemboli due to an increased propensity for clotting (**B**). Pancreatic carcinoma is associated with an increased risk for thrombi; however, it is not a very likely diagnosis in a young female (**D**). Cirrhosis of the liver, which can result in decreased production of clotting factors, would not be a significant risk factor for deep venous thrombi (**E**). Given her age and the clinical scenario, pulmonary emphysema and an undiagnosed B-cell lymphoma lack support (**A, C**).

57.   Correct: Normal D-dimer (C)

Although D-dimer is not specific for pulmonary thromboembolus, it is quite sensitive; therefore, while an elevated D-dimer may have many different causes, essentially all patients with a pulmonary thromboembolus will have an elevated D-dimer, so a normal D-dimer essentially excludes a pulmonary thromboembolus (**C**). A pulmonary thromboembolus is not typically a cause of an increased, or decreased, PT, PTT, or fibrinogen; therefore, normal concentrations of these proteins do not exclude a pulmonary thromboembolus (**A-B, D**). While a pulmonary thromboembolus can cause an elevated troponin I, a normal troponin I does not exclude the diagnosis of a pulmonary thromboembolus (**E**).

58.   Correct: Thrombus at the pulmonary artery bifurcation (E)

Given the clinical scenario of a long period of relative immobility followed by sharp chest pain and dyspnea, the most likely diagnosis of those listed is pulmonary thromboembolus (**E**). Because he has no neuromuscular disease or intoxication, and as he had no stridor, a foreign body is not very likely (**D**). He has no risk factors for an acute myocardial infarct, and, given the time frame, no gross change in the myocardium would be apparent, as those take around 12 to 24 hours to develop, and sharp chest pain is not characteristic of a myocardial infarct (**B**). His story is inconsistent with pneumonia (**C**). Without listed risk factors for cirrhosis, hepatocellular carcinoma with extension into the inferior vena cava is very unlikely (A).

59.   Correct: Foreign body in the airway (C)

Given the age of the patient and her mobility, a pulmonary thromboembolus is not very likely, nor is head trauma (**A, B**). Given no exposure to human papilloma virus, a laryngeal polyp is very unlikely (**D**). With no previous symptoms, a lobar pneumonia is not likely (**E**). In a mobile infant on the floor, ingestion of a foreign body with subsequent inhalation is a concern and would present as described (**C**).

Chapter 11

Diseases of the Kidney and Urinary Tract

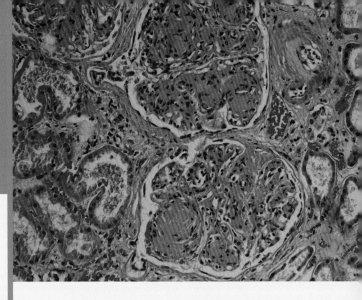

LEARNING OBJECTIVES

11.1 Glomerular Disease

- ▶ Describe the histopathologic abnormalities found in the various glomerular diseases causing nephrotic and nephritic syndrome
- ▶ Diagnose nephrotic syndrome
- ▶ List the causes of nephrotic syndrome by age category
- ▶ Describe how to diagnose the causes of nephrotic syndrome
- ▶ List the signs, symptoms, and laboratory abnormalities associated with nephritic syndrome
- ▶ Describe the laboratory findings in nephrotic and nephritic syndrome
- ▶ Describe the pathophysiologic mechanism of the glomerular diseases
- ▶ List the type of urine cast associated with nephrotic syndrome
- ▶ Diagnose Henoch-Schonlein purpura
- ▶ Diagnose minimal change disease
- ▶ Describe the pathology associated with minimal change disease
- ▶ Diagnose focal segmental glomerulosclerosis
- ▶ List the causes and clinical features of nephrotic syndrome
- ▶ List the causes of primary nephrotic syndrome
- ▶ List the etiologic agent associated with the collapsing variant of FSGS
- ▶ Diagnose membranous glomerulonephropathy
- ▶ List the causes of a secondary membranous glomerulonephropathy

11.2 Tubular and Interstitial Disease

- ▶ Describe the clinical presentation of an individual with pre-renal failure due to dehydration
- ▶ List the laboratory testing results found in pre-renal acute renal failure
- ▶ Describe the clinical presentation of acute renal failure

- ▶ List the laboratory test results commonly associated with acute renal failure
- ▶ List the causes of post-renal acute renal failure
- ▶ Describe the laboratory tests associated with pre-renal azotemia
- ▶ List the causes of pre-renal azotemia
- ▶ Describe the physical examination findings of use in distinguishing the causes of acute renal failure
- ▶ Distinguish between pre-renal and intrinsic renal failure
- ▶ List the causes of intrinsic renal failure and describe their histologic findings
- ▶ List the general causes of acute tubular necrosis
- ▶ List the types of casts associated with various renal diseases
- ▶ Describe the pathway of ethylene glycol in the body
- ▶ List the metabolic abnormalities occurring with acute renal failure

11.3 Renal Tumors, Cysts, and Calculi

- ▶ List the testing best utilized to distinguish post-renal azotemia from pre-renal and renal azotemia
- ▶ Diagnose renal cell carcinoma
- ▶ List the radiographic appearance of the various types of kidney stones
- ▶ List the underlying causes of kidney stones
- ▶ List the risk factors for the development of nephrolithiasis
- ▶ Diagnose *Schistosoma haematobium* infection of the bladder

11.1 Glomerular Disease— Questions

| Easy | Medium | Hard |

1. A 42-year-old male presents to an acute care clinic. He reports that he has developed swelling of his eyelids over the past several weeks, which has progressed to the point that he has difficulty seeing. He also describes that during this time period he has felt nauseated and occasionally vomited. His past medical history includes intravenous use of heroin, which he stopped about 2 years ago. His vital signs are temperature of 98.6°F, blood pressure of 125/81 mm Hg, and pulse of 83 bpm. A physical examination reveals track marks on the arm and edema of the eyelids. Laboratory testing reveals total cholesterol of 230 mg/dL and albumin of 1.8 g/dL. He is scheduled for a renal biopsy. Of the following, which would a biopsy of the kidney, without the use of electron microscopy, most likely reveal?

A. Glomerular crescents

B. A tram-track appearance on silver stain

C. A lumpy-bumpy pattern on silver stain

D. Nothing

E. Segmental sclerosis of some glomeruli

Kidney

2. Given the previous clinical scenario, which of the following would immunofluorescence staining of the kidney most likely reveal?

A. IgG positivity with a granular pattern

B. IgG and IgM positivity with a granular pattern

C. IgG positivity with a linear pattern

D. IgM positivity with a linear pattern

E. Entrapped IgM

Kidney

3. A 4-year-old child is brought to her pediatrician by her parents. Over the past several days, they have noticed swelling of her eyelids, and she has vomited twice in the past two days. She has no significant past medical history. Her vital signs are a temperature of 98.6°F, blood pressure of 97/62 mm Hg, and pulse of 76 bpm. Laboratory testing reveals an albumin of 2.2 gm/dL and total cholesterol of 243 mg/dL. A urine dipstick is positive for protein and negative for red blood cells and white blood cells. She is admitted to the hospital. Of the following, which would further testing most likely reveal?

A. Urine osmolality of 500 mOsm/kg

B. Urine output of 300 mL in one day

C. 4.0 g/day of protein in the urine

D. Red blood cell casts

E. Leukocyte esterase positivity in the urine

Kidney

4. Given the previous clinical scenario, of the following, which would further testing most likely reveal?

A. Minimal change disease

B. Focal segmental glomerulosclerosis

C. Membranous glomerulonephropathy

D. Rapidly progressive glomerulonephritis

E. Membranoproliferative glomerulonephritis

Kidney

5. A 37-year-old female presents to an acute care clinic. Over the past several days, she has noticed swelling of her eyelids and she has experienced nausea and vomiting several times in the past two days. She has no significant past medical history. Her vital signs are a temperature of 98.6°F, blood pressure of 97/62 mm Hg, and pulse of 91 bpm. Laboratory testing reveals an albumin of 2.2 gm/dL and total cholesterol of 243 mg/dL. A urinalysis is positive for protein, negative for red blood cells, and white blood cells. She is admitted to the hospital. Overnight testing reveals 4.1 g/24 hrs of protein in the urine. Of the following, what is the best method to diagnosis her condition?

A. Urine culture

B. Renal ultrasound

C. Renal artery angiogram

D. Renal biopsy

E. Cystography

Kidney

6. Given the previous clinical scenario, a renal biopsy is performed. Immunofluorescence staining reveals granular IgG positivity, and electron microscopy reveals subepithelial immune complexes. Of the following, what is the diagnosis?

A. Minimal change disease

B. Focal segmental glomerulosclerosis

C. Membranous glomerulonephropathy

D. Postinfectious glomerulonephritis

E. Type I membranoproliferative glomerulonephritis

Kidney

7. A medical technologist is examining a urine specimen from a child, age 8 years. The technologist identifies 1 white blood cell/high-power field, 20 red blood cells/high-power field, no bacteria, and occasional red blood cell casts. Of the following, what is the most likely diagnosis?

A. Minimal change disease

B. Membranous glomerulonephropathy

C. Post-infectious glomerulonephritis

D. Recent bladder trauma

E. Wilms tumor

Kidney

8. Given the previous clinical scenario, of the following, which would be the most likely mechanism of the disease process?

A. Effacement of podocyte foot processes

B. Formation of C5b-9 membrane attack complex

C. Subendothelial immune complex deposits only

D. Autoimmune-type reaction to group A streptococcus infection

E. Infiltration of neoplastic cells

Kidney

9. A 46-year-old male with a history of diabetes mellitus diagnosed when he was 12 years old presents to his family physician because he has noticed swelling of his eyelids and swelling of his lower extremities. His vital signs are a temperature of 98.7°F, pulse of 81 bpm, and blood pressure of 114/71 mm Hg. Physical examination reveals periorbital edema and edema of the lower extremities. Laboratory testing reveals a BUN of 43 mg/dL, creatinine of 3.7 mg/dL, albumin of 1.8 g/dL, and total cholesterol of 256 mg/dL. Of the following, what might microscopic examination of the urine reveal?

A. Red blood cell casts

B. White blood cell casts

C. Pigmented granular casts

D. Fatty casts

E. Cellular casts

Kidney

10. A 7-year-old male is brought by his parents to his pediatrician. He just got over a streptococcal pharyngitis and now is complaining of abdominal pain and pain in his joints. His parents also relate that he has been having some blood in his bowel movements. In addition, he has developed a rash consisting of raised red bumps on his lower extremities and buttocks. Of the following, what is the most likely diagnosis?

A. Dermatitis herpetiformis

B. Acute rheumatic fever

C. Henoch-Schonlein purpura

D. Lyme disease

E. Rocky Mountain spotted fever

Kidney

11. A 6-year-old male is brought to his pediatrician by his parents. They say that over the past week he has been sick, complaining of nausea and occasionally vomiting. They thought it was a stomach flu, but they noticed that his eyes appear swollen. Other than periorbital edema and edema of other locations of the body, his physical examination is essentially normal. A urinalysis reveals a pH of 6.0, 4+ protein, and no nitrites, leukocyte esterase, or hemoglobin. Of the following, what is the most likely mechanism of his disease process?

A. Subepithelial immune complexes

B. A thin basement membrane

C. Sclerosis of glomeruli

D. Infection of the kidney

E. Effacement of podocyte foot processes

Kidney

12. A pathologist is examining a kidney biopsy and notes that some of the glomeruli have sclerosis of a portion of the glomerulus. Of the following, what feature was most likely identified in the patient prior to the biopsy?

A. Blood pressure of 171/93 mm Hg

B. Proteinuria of 2.5 g/day

C. Tinnitus

D. Red blood cell casts

E. Increased serum concentration of lipoprotein(a)

Kidney

13. A 44-year-old male presents to his family physician. He says that over the past several weeks, he has been feeling nauseated and thought it was a stomach flu, as friends had similar symptoms. However, his symptoms lingered longer, and now he has noticed his eyelids are swelling. His vital signs are a temperature of 98.7°F, pulse of 87 bpm, and blood pressure of 121/80 mm Hg. A urinalysis reveals a pH of 6.8 and 4+ protein and is negative for hemoglobin, glucose, and urobilinogen. A few hyaline casts are present. The patient's only past medical history is a hernia repair at age 28 and rib fractures sustained in a skiing accident. Of the following, what is the most likely diagnosis?

A. Postinfectious glomerulonephritis

B. Rapidly progressive glomerulonephritis

C. Focal segmental glomerulosclerosis

D. Cryptogenic cirrhosis of the liver

E. Acute pancreatitis

Kidney

14. Given the previous clinical scenario, of the following, what condition is he most likely to have?

A. Recent infection with *Streptococcus pneumoniae*

B. Chronic CMV infection

C. HIV infection

D. Granulomatosis with polyangiitis

E. Polyarteritis nodosa

Kidney

15. A 35-year-old male presents to his family physician because of complaints of weight gain and decreased vision, which have been developing over the past few months. His vital signs are a temperature of 98.6°F, pulse of 86 bpm, and blood pressure of 119/68 mm Hg. On physical examination, his physician noted periorbital edema as well as edema at other locations of the body. A urinalysis reveals 4+ proteinuria and no glucose or hemoglobin. The medical technologist notes that the urine appears frothy. Shortly thereafter, the patient undergoes a renal biopsy, which reveals subepithelial immune complexes. Of the following, what is the most likely diagnosis?

A. Minimal change disease

B. Focal segmental glomerulosclerosis

C. Membranous glomerulonephropathy

D. Postinfectious glomerulonephritis

E. Rapidly progressive glomerulonephritis

Kidney

16. Given the previous clinical scenario, of the following, serologic testing for what agent is most likely to be positive?

A. Hepatitis B

B. *Borrelia burgdoferi*

C. HIV

D. *Clostridium difficile*

E. Epstein-Barr virus

Kidney

11.2 Tubular and Interstitial Disease—Questions

Easy	Medium	Hard

17. A 25-year-old male presents to the emergency room, brought in by his friends, who are concerned for his well-being. They say that over the past few days he has been easily fatigued and has grown lethargic in the last day, which prompted their visit. His vital signs are a temperature of 98.7°F, pulse of 128 bpm, and blood pressure of 81/52 mm Hg. A physical examination reveals decreased capillary refill. Further questioning of the friends indicates that they have been working in the heat for the past 5 days. Of the following, what will laboratory testing most likely reveal?

A. BUN:creatinine ratio of > 20

B. Urine osmolality of < 500 mOsm/kg

C. Urine specific gravity of < 1.020

D. Urine Na+ > 20 mEq/L

E. Cellular casts

Kidney

18. A 68-year-old male is brought to an acute care clinic by his wife. Over the past few days, he has developed fatigue, and in the last day, he has become lethargic. She says that over the past few days, he has been going to the bathroom less. His vital signs are temperature 98.7°F, pulse of 87 bpm, and blood pressure of 131/85 mm Hg. Laboratory testing reveals a blood urea nitrogen of 29 mg/dL and creatinine of 2.0 mg/dL. Six months ago, he also had a BUN and creatinine performed and they were 12 mg/dL and 0.8 mg/dL respectively. The subsequent placement of a Foley catheter reveals 845 mL of urine in the bladder. Of the following, what is the most likely cause of his presenting state?

A. Sepsis

B. Dehydration

C. Recent ingestion of antifreeze

D. Focal segmental glomerulonephritis

E. Benign prostatic hyperplasia

Prostate

19. A 35-year-old female is having her yearly physical examination. She reports no major changes since last year, although in the last few months sometimes she feels a little more fatigued, but attributes the change to her job, which has become more stressful. Physical examination reveals a bruit during auscultation of the left side of her back. Her vital signs are a temperature of 98.5°F, pulse of 91 bpm, and blood pressure of 158/97 mm Hg. Routine laboratory testing reveals a hemoglobin of 13 g/dL, Hct of 40%, MCV of 91 fL, BUN of 42 mg/dL, and creatinine of 1.8 mg/dL. Of the following, what is the most likely diagnosis?

A. An abdominal aortic aneurysm

B. Renal artery stenosis

C. Staghorn calculus of the left kidney

D. Endometriosis

E. Iliac artery atherosclerosis

Kidney

20. A 62-year-old male presents to an acute care clinic with complaints of fatigue, which has developed over the past few weeks. His vital signs are a temperature of 98.8°F, blood pressure of 129/87 mm Hg, and pulse of 93 bpm. Laboratory testing reveals a hemoglobin of 15.1 g/dL, Hct of 46%, MCV of 92 fL, BUN of 37 mg/dL, and creatinine of 2.3 mg/dL. The patient is asked to urinate, after which a catheter is placed, which reveals a post-void residual of 450 mL. Of the following, which physical examination finding is most likely to reveal the underlying cause of his elevated serum creatinine?

A. A holosystolic murmur

B. Bilateral coarse rales

C. Decreased bowel sounds

D. A nodular prostate on rectal exam

E. Pitting edema of the lower extremities

Prostate

21. A 36-year-old male is brought to an acute care clinic by friends, who report that over the past several days he has been complaining of nausea and fatigue and, over the past day, has become lethargic and has difficulty remembering the time of the day or place he is at. No one is aware of any significant past medical history. His vital signs are a temperature of 98.7°F, blood pressure of 101/64 mm Hg, and pulse of 102 bpm. Laboratory testing reveals a hemoglobin of 14.8 g/dL, hematocrit of 42%, MCV of 87 fL, BUN of 108 mg/dL, and creatinine of 8.4 mg/dL. Of the following, what other test abnormality is most likely to be found?

A. Fractional excretion of Na+ of < 1%

B. Normal urine sediment

C. Specific gravity of > 1.020

D. Urine Na+ of < 20 mEq/L

E. Urine osmolality of < 400 mOsm/kg

Kidney

22. A 29-year-old male is brought to an acute care clinic by his girlfriend, who reports that over the past several days he has been complaining of nausea and fatigue, and over the past day, has become lethargic and has difficulty remembering the time of the day or place he is at. His past medical history is significant for a motor vehicle accident when he was 16 years old. His vital signs are a temperature of 98.6°F, blood pressure of 99/62 mm Hg, and pulse of 107 bpm. A physical examination reveals a holosystolic murmur. Laboratory testing reveals a hemoglobin of 14.6 g/dL, hematocrit of 41%, MCV of 86 fL, BUN of 112 mg/dL, and creatinine of 8.7 mg/dL. Additional testing reveals a fractionated excretion of sodium of 6% and a urine osmolality of 272 mOsm/kg. Of the following, which is the most likely cause of the patient's presenting condition?

A. A kidney stone

B. Congestive heart failure

C. Acute tubular necrosis

D. Renal cell carcinoma

E. Renal artery stenosis

Kidney

23. Given the previous clinical scenario, of the following, which histologic change would explain his presenting condition?

A. Neutrophilic infiltrate in the wall of the bladder

B. Infiltrating neoplastic glands in the kidneys

C. Hyperplastic glands in the prostate

D. Coagulative necrosis of renal tubular epithelial cells

E. Granulomas in the wall of the ureter

Kidney

24. A 24-year-old female is involved in a motor vehicle accident, during which she fractures both femurs. She is taken to the hospital by way of an ambulance. On presentation, her blood pressure is 60 mm Hg palpable, and her pulse is 130 bpm. She is treated with fluid resuscitation and receives multiple units of O- blood. She is taken to surgery and subsequently admitted to the hospital. One day later, she is noted to have a urine output of only 200 mL/day. Of the following, which laboratory test results are most consistent with her disease process?

A. BUN of 16 mg/dL and creatinine of 0.8 mg/dL

B. BUN of 40 mg/dL and creatinine of 1.9 mg/dL

C. BUN of 52 mg/dL and creatinine of 5.3 mg/dL

D. Positive c-ANCA

E. Positive p-ANCA

Kidney

147

25. Given the previous clinical scenario, of the following, which type of cast would most likely be identified in the urine sediment?

A. Pigmented granular casts

B. Broad waxy casts

C. Fatty casts

D. Red blood cell casts

E. White blood cell casts

Kidney

26. A 25-year-old male is found in his bedroom by his parents after he stayed in his room for an entire day without coming out. On his nightstand are a suicide note and a glass with remnants of fluorescent yellow-green fluid. In the emergency room, laboratory testing reveals a blood urea nitrogen of 67 mg/dL and a creatinine of 5.8 mg/dL. Of the following, which enzyme is responsible for causing his present condition?

A. Myeloperoxidase

B. Alcohol dehydrogenase

C. Superoxide dismutase

D. Aspartate transaminase

E. Acetylcholinesterase

Kidney

27. A 46-year-old female presents to an acute care clinic. Over the past several days, she has developed severe fatigue associated with nausea. Her vital signs are a temperature of 98.7°F, blood pressure of 106/72 mm Hg, and pulse of 87 bpm. Laboratory testing reveals a hemoglobin of 12.9 g/dL, BUN of 31 mg/dL, and creatinine of 3.2 mg/dL. Of the following, which laboratory abnormality is most likely present?

A. Hypernatremia

B. Hyperkalemia

C. Hypercalcemia

D. Hypophosphatemia

E. Metabolic alkalosis

Kidney

11.3 Renal Tumors, Cysts, and Calculi—Questions

Easy	Medium	Hard

28. A 37-year-old male is brought to the emergency room by his friends, because over the past few days he has developed fatigue, and in the last day, become lethargic. His only past medical history is kidney stones, having passed one several years ago. His vital signs are a temperature of 98.8°F, blood pressure of 110/73 mm Hg, and pulse of 94 bpm. Laboratory testing reveals a hemoglobin of 14.6 g/dL, BUN of 33 mg/dL, and creatinine of 1.9 mg/dL. Of the following, which is the best choice to begin his evaluation?

A. Renal biopsy

B. Culture of the throat

C. Renal ultrasound

D. Culture of the stool

E. Culture of the urine

Kidney

29. A 62-year-old male smoker presents to his family physician because he has noticed blood in his urine. A review of his systems also reveals back pain. His vital signs are a temperature of 98.6°F, pulse of 84 bpm, and blood pressure of 124/82 mm Hg. Laboratory testing reveals BUN of 13 mg/dL and creatinine of 0.7 mg/dL. Urinalysis reveals 3+ red blood cells, but no red blood cell casts. He is admitted to the hospital for two days. His urine output is 1 L/day. Additional laboratory testing reveals an albumin of 4.0 g/dL. Of the following, what is the most likely diagnosis?

A. Focal segmental glomerulosclerosis

B. Rapidly progressive glomerulonephritis

C. Renal cell carcinoma

D. Ischemic acute tubular necrosis

E. Post-renal azotemia

Kidney

30. A 35-year-old male presents to the emergency room with complaints of severe flank pain that radiates into his groin and is associated with some nausea and vomiting. He has also noticed blood in his urine. He has no significant past medical history. His vital signs are a temperature of 99.7°F, blood pressure of 139/85 mm Hg, and pulse of 104 bpm. Physical examination reveals costovertebral angle tenderness. Of the following, what is the most likely diagnosis?

A. Ruptured abdominal aortic aneurysm

B. Aortic dissection

C. Acute prostatitis

D. Nephrolithiasis

E. Psoas muscle abscess

Kidney

31. A 37-year-old female presents to an acute care clinic with complaints of severe flank pain that radiates into her groin. She also reports nausea, and, while waiting for her appointment, she vomits. Other than mild hypothyroidism treated with hormone replacement, she has no significant past medical history. Her vital signs are a temperature of 99.9°F, blood pressure of 142/91 mm Hg, and pulse of 109 bpm. Physical examination reveals costovertebral angle tenderness. An X-ray of the abdomen does not reveal an abnormality. Of the following, which would be consistent with these findings?

A. Calcium oxalate kidney stone

B. Calcium phosphate kidney stone

C. Uric acid kidney stone

D. Struvite kidney stone

E. Cystine kidney stone

Kidney

32. Given the previous clinical scenario, an intravenous pyelogram reveals an obstruction in the left ureter. Of the following, which would be most likely to cause this patient's condition?

A. Sarcoidosis

B. Diffuse large B-cell lymphoma

C. *Proteus vulgaris* infection

D. Parathyroid gland hyperplasia

E. Bone metastases

Kidney

33. A 51-year-old male presents to the emergency room complaining of sudden onset of colicky severe pain in his lower back. Associated with the pain he has blood in his urine. His past medical history includes hypertension treated with a β-blocker and gout. He has never smoked cigarettes. His vital signs are a temperature of 98.8°F, pulse of 112 bpm, and blood pressure of 132/85 mm Hg. Of the following, what is the most likely diagnosis?

A. Renal cell carcinoma

B. Acute myocardial infarction

C. Aortic dissection

D. Nephrolithiaisis

E. Transitional cell carcinoma of the bladder

Kidney

34. Given the previous clinical scenario, of the following, which is most correct regarding his presenting condition?

A. It is a significant risk factor for renal cell carcinoma.

B. Some forms are associated with *Proteus mirabilis* infection.

C. The condition most likely arose from foreign travel.

D. An ultrasound would be unlikely to identify the pathologic lesion.

E. He has no risk for acute renal failure.

Kidney

35. A 37-year-old male presents to his family physician with complaints of blood in his urine. A urinalysis reveals 4+ blood, with microscopic clots identified. The patient returned home 4 months ago after a missionary trip to Africa. He does not smoke nor drink alcohol. He has no family history of hereditary disorders. Of the following, what is the most likely diagnosis?

A. Transitional cell carcinoma of the bladder

B. Renal cell carcinoma

C. *Schistosoma haematobium* infection of the bladder

D. Membranous glomerulonephropathy

E. Post-infectious glomerulonephritis

Kidney

11.4 Glomerular Disease—Answers and Explanations

Easy	Medium	Hard

1. Correct: Segmental sclerosis of some glomeruli (E)

The patient has features of nephrotic syndrome (edema, hyperlipidemia, and hypoalbuminemia). Minimal change disease, which would have no abnormalities on H&E staining or silver stain (**D**), is most common in children, whereas focal segmental glomerulosclerosis is the most common cause of primary nephrotic syndrome in adults (**E**). Membranoproliferative glomerulonephritis (tram-track), post-infectious glomerulonephritis (lumpy-bumpy pattern), and rapidly progressive glomerulonephritis (crescents) cause nephritic syndrome (**A-C**). Heroin use is associated with focal segmental glomerulosclerosis.

2. Correct: Entrapped IgM (E)

The patient has features of nephrotic syndrome (edema, hyperlipidemia, and hypoalbuminemia). Minimal change disease, which would have no abnormalities on H&E staining or silver stain, is most common in children, whereas focal segmental glomerulosclerosis (FSGS) is the most common cause of primary nephrotic syndrome in adults. FSGS has entrapped IgM and C3 noted by immunofluorescence staining (**E**). IgG positivity with a granular pattern is seen in membranous glomerulonephropathy (**A**), IgG and IgM positivity in postinfectious glomerulonephritis (**B**), and IgG positivity with a linear pattern in type I rapidly progressive glomerulonephritis (**C**). IgM positivity with a linear pattern is not normally described in diseases of the kidney (**D**).

149

3. Correct: 4.0 g/day of protein in the urine (C)

With the edema of the eyelids, hyperlipidemia, and hypoalbuminemia, the most likely diagnosis is nephrotic syndrome. The fourth component of nephrotic syndrome is proteinuria of > 3.5 g/day (**C**). The likeliest diagnosis in a pediatric patient with nephrotic syndrome is minimal change disease. A urine output of 300 mL/24 hours would only be expected in acute renal failure, which would be less common in pediatric nephrotic syndrome and of which there is no evidence to suggest this in the clinical scenario (**B**). A urine osmolality of 500 mOsm/kg would only be expected in the setting of hypovolemia, which again, is not suggested in the clinical scenario (**A**). Red blood cell casts are consistent with nephritic rather than nephrotic syndrome (**D**), and leukocyte esterase is found in urinary tract infections (**E**).

4. Correct: Minimal change disease (A)

Based on the signs and symptoms, and laboratory testing of proteinuria, hypoalbuminemia, and hyperlipidemia, the diagnosis is nephrotic syndrome. The most common cause of nephrotic syndrome in children is minimal change disease (**A**). Focal segmental glomerulosclerosis and membranous glomerulonephropathy also cause nephrotic syndrome, but would be rarer in children (**B, C**). Rapidly progressive glomerulonephritis and membranoproliferative glomerulonephritis cause nephritic syndrome (**D, E**).

5. Correct: Renal biopsy (D)

Based on the signs and symptoms (edema), and laboratory testing identifying proteinuria, hypoalbuminemia, and hyperlipidemia, the diagnosis is nephrotic syndrome. Determination of the form of glomerular disease causing the nephrotic syndrome requires a renal biopsy (**D**). The other testing methods (**A-C, E**) would not be useful in making the final diagnosis.

6. Correct: Membranous glomerulonephropathy (C)

Based on the signs and symptoms (edema), and laboratory testing identifying proteinuria, hypoalbuminemia, and hyperlipidemia, the diagnosis is nephrotic syndrome. Minimal change disease, focal segmental glomerulosclerosis, and membranous glomerulonephropathy are causes of nephrotic syndrome. Minimal change disease has no immune complex deposits (**A**). FSGS can have positive immunofluorescence due to entrapped IgM and C3 but has no immune complex deposits (**B**). Membranous glomerulonephropathy has granular IgG positivity and subepithelial immune complex deposits (**C**). Post-infectious glomerulonephritis can have granular IgG positivity and subepithelial immune complexes, but also intramembranous and subendothelial immune complex deposits, and causes nephritic syndrome (**D**). Type I membranoproliferative glomerulonephritis causes nephritic syndrome and has subendothelial immune complex deposits (**E**).

7. Correct: Postinfectious glomerulonephritis (C)

Red blood cell casts indicate glomerular bleeding. Although a Wilms tumor or recent bladder trauma could cause blood to be in the urine, they would not normally cause red blood cell casts to be formed (**D, E**). The finding of blood in the urine and red blood cell casts is not consistent with nephrotic syndrome, which is what minimal change disease or membranous glomerulonephropathy would produce (**A, B**). Post-infectious glomerulonephritis would cause nephritic syndrome, which is associated with red blood cell casts (**C**).

8. Correct: Autoimmune-type reaction to group A streptococcus infection (D)

Red blood cell casts indicate glomerular bleeding and are found in nephritic syndrome. Effacement of podocyte foot processes occurs in minimal change disease, which causes nephrotic syndrome (**A**). Formation of the C5b-9 membrane attack complex is the mechanism of the disease process in membranous glomerulonephropathy, which causes nephrotic syndrome (**B**). Red blood cell casts are characteristic of nephritic syndrome and not nephrotic syndrome. Given the age, the most likely cause is post-infectious glomerulonephritis due to a group A streptococcal pharyngitis, which has subepithelial, intramembranous, and subendothelial immune complexes (**C, D**). An infiltrating tumor would not likely cause red blood cell casts (**E**).

9. Correct: Fatty casts (D)

The patient has the features of nephrotic syndrome (generalized edema, hypoalbuminemia, and hyperlipidemia, and a 24-hour urine sample would reveal > 3.5 grams of protein). Red blood cell casts are associated with nephritic syndrome, white blood cell casts with pyelonephritis (**A, B**), and pigmented granular casts with acute tubular necrosis (**C**). Fatty casts are associated with nephrotic syndrome (**D**). Either red blood cells or white blood cells could be cellular casts (**E**).

10. Correct: Henoch-Schonlein purpura (C)

The combination of abdominal pain, arthralgias, and gastrointestinal bleeding occurring following a streptococcal pharyngitis and associated with palpable purpura on the buttocks and lower extremities is consistent with Henoch-Schonlein purpura (**C**). Although acute rheumatic fever can present similarly, it is not commonly associated with GI bleeding and has a different skin rash (erythema marginatum) (**B**). Lyme disease could also present similarly, but the rash is erythema chronicum migrans (**D**). Dermatitis herpetiformis is associated with celiac disease and presents on the extensor surfaces of the body (**A**). Given the time frame after the pharyngitis, and lack of exposure, Rocky Mountain spotted fever is not likely (**E**).

11. Correct: Effacement of podocyte foot processes (E)

The patient has features of nephrotic syndrome, presenting with nausea and vomiting, and having periorbital edema, and proteinuria. The most common cause of nephrotic syndrome in children is minimal change disease, which is characterized by effacement of foot processes (**E**). Subepithelial immune complexes are found in post-infectious glomerulonephritis, which causes nephritic syndrome (**A**). Thin basement membrane disease can cause nephrotic syndrome, but is not a common cause of nephrotic syndrome in children (**B**). Focal segmental glomerulosclerosis is a cause of nephrotic syndrome, but not as common as minimal change disease in children (**C**). Focal segmental glomerulosclerosis is the second most common cause of nephrotic syndrome in children. The history, including the lack of leukocyte esterase in the urine, is not consistent with pyelonephritis (**D**).

12. Correct: Increased serum concentration of lipoprotein(a) (E)

The pathologic description is that of focal segmental glomerulosclerosis, which is a cause of nephrotic syndrome. Hypertension and red blood cell casts are associated with nephritic syndrome (**A, D**). Proteinuria is found in both nephrotic and nephritic syndrome; however, with nephrotic syndrome, the amount of proteinuria is > 3.5 g/day (**B**). Tinnitus is not commonly associated with either syndrome (**C**). Nephrotic syndrome causes hyperlipidemia, and the concentration of lipoprotein(a) can be elevated (**E**).

13. Correct: Focal segmental glomerulosclerosis (C)

The patient has signs, symptoms, and laboratory findings consistent with nephrotic syndrome, with nausea, vomiting, periorbital edema, and proteinuria. The main primary cause of nephrotic syndrome in adults is focal segmental glomerulosclerosis (**C**). Post-infectious glomerulonephritis and rapidly progressive glomerulonephritis cause nephritic syndrome, which would be associated with hypertension and blood in the urine, including red blood cell casts (**A, B**). Given the lack of abdominal pain and risk factors, in combination with the proteinuria, acute pancreatitis is unlikely (**E**). Although cirrhosis could cause nonspecific symptoms, the patient has no risk factors, and, although cirrhosis could cause hypoalbuminemia and edema, it should not be the sole presenting symptom (**D**).

14. Correct: HIV infection (C)

The patient has the signs and symptoms of nephrotic syndrome: periorbital edema and proteinuria not associated with hypertension or hematuria. The most common primary cause of nephrotic syndrome in adults is focal segmental glomerulosclerosis (FSGS). The collapsing variant of FSGS is associated with rapidly progressive renal insufficiency. This form of FSGS can be seen in patients with HIV (**C**). Post-streptococcal glomerulonephritis and granulomatosis with polyangiitis would present with a nephritic syndrome (**A, D**). Chronic CMV infection and polyarteritis nodosa, while each could affect the kidney, do not usually present with either a nephrotic or a nephritic syndrome (**B, E**).

15. Correct: Membranous glomerulonephropathy (C)

The patient has the signs and symptoms of nephrotic syndrome: periorbital edema and proteinuria not associated with hypertension or hematuria. Post-infectious glomerulonephritis and rapidly progressive glomerulonephritis cause nephritic syndrome (**D, E**). Minimal change disease and focal segmental glomerulosclerosis are not associated with immune complex deposition (**A, B**). In membranous glomerulonephropathy, subepithelial deposits are most characteristic, but deposits in other locations can be seen as well. The complexes will produce a granular pattern on immunofluorescence and stain with IgG (**C**).

16. Correct: Hepatitis B (A)

Membranous glomerulonephropathy can be secondarily associated with a variety of conditions, including drug use (NSAIDs), autoimmune disorders (SLE), and various types of cancer and infections; however, the infection most commonly associated with membranous glomerulonephropathy is hepatitis B (**A**). Given the results of the biopsy, focal segmental glomerulosclerosis is not the diagnosis, and the chance of a collapsing variant of FSGS associated with HIV infection is less (**C**). The other organisms listed are not commonly associated with membranous glomerulonephropathy (**B, D-E**).

11.5 Tubular and Interstitial Disease—Answers and Explanations

Easy	Medium	Hard

17. Correct: BUN:creatinine ratio of > 20 (A)

Given the clinical history combined with the symptoms (fatigue, lethargy, hypotension, and tachycardia), the patient is most likely dehydrated. Dehydration can cause pre-renal failure, and a patient will have a BUN:creatinine ratio of > 20 (**A**), urine osmolality of > 500mOsm/kg, urine specific gravity of > 1.020, Urine Na+ of < 20 mEq/L, and a bland urinary sediment (**B-E**).

18. Correct: Benign prostatic hyperplasia (E).

This patient has the signs and symptoms of acute renal failure, and laboratory testing confirms azotemia, with an elevated BUN and creatinine. The ratio is < 20:1, so sepsis and dehydration would be less likely (**A, B**). Although both recent ingestion of antifreeze and focal segmental glomerulonephritis have the potential to cause acute renal failure (**C, D**), as the patient had a large amount of urine in his bladder, benign prostatic hyperplasia is the most likely cause of his presenting state (**E**).

19. Correct: Renal artery stenosis (B)

The patient has azotemia, and, based on the BUN:creatinine ratio of > 20:1, would favor a pre-renal azotemia. A bruit can be heard from atherosclerosis, or stenosis of a blood vessel. Atherosclerosis of the iliac artery would not be heard during auscultation of the back, and would not cause pre-renal azotemia (**E**); however, renal artery stenosis would, and is more common in younger females (**B**). The other choices would not cause a bruit, and would not normally present with pre-renal azotemia (**A, C, D**).

20. Correct: A nodular prostate on rectal exam (D)

The presenting symptom, fatigue, is general; however, people in acute renal failure can have fatigue among other symptoms, and they can be asymptomatic. The BUN:creatinine ratio would not favor a pre-renal azotemia, such as would occur with congestive heart failure (**E**). The post-void residual favors a post-renal azotemia, and of these, obstruction due to an enlarged prostate would be one cause (**D**). None of the other choices (**A-C**) directly link to the underlying cause of the elevated creatinine.

21. Correct: Urine osmolality of < 400 mOsm/kg (E)

Based on the clinical scenario, the patient has acute renal failure, which can present with nausea, fatigue, lethargy, and mental status changes. The BUN:Cr ratio is < 20:1, which is supportive of a diagnosis of intrinsic acute renal failure. Of the tests, only a urine osmolality of < 400 mOsm/kg is also supportive of an intrinsic acute renal failure (**E**), the remainder support a pre-renal acute renal failure (**A-D**).

22. Correct: Acute tubular necrosis (C)

The patient has the signs, symptoms, and laboratory testing consistent with acute renal failure. The BUN:Cr ratio is < 20:1, which supports an intrinsic renal failure and is confirmed by the fractionated excretion of sodium and urine osmolality. Of the choices, acute tubular necrosis causes intrinsic renal failure (**C**), and the others do not (**A-B, D-E**).

23. Correct: Coagulative necrosis of renal tubular epithelial cells (D)

The patient has the signs, symptoms, and laboratory testing consistent with acute renal failure. The BUN:Cr ratio is < 20:1, which supports an intrinsic renal failure and is confirmed by the fractionated excretion of sodium and urine osmolality. One cause of intrinsic renal failure is acute tubular necrosis, which would have coagulative necrosis of renal tubular epithelial cells as a histologic finding (**D**). Infections of the bladder and ureter and benign prostatic hyperplasia could cause a post-renal azotemia (**A, C-D**), and a renal cell carcinoma is not commonly a cause of intrinsic renal failure (**B**).

24. Correct: BUN of 52 mg/dL and creatinine of 5.3 mg/dL (C)

Given the clinical scenario, extensive blood loss, and resultant acute renal failure, with elevated BUN and creatinine and oliguria, the most likely cause of the condition is acute tubular necrosis of ischemic origin (**C**). Acute tubular necrosis is an intrinsic form of acute renal failure and is characterized by a BUN:Cr ratio of < 20:1 (**A-C**). ANCA testing would be unnecessary (**D-E**).

25. Correct: Pigmented granular casts (A)

Given the clinical scenario, extensive blood loss, and resultant acute renal failure, with elevated BUN and creatinine and oliguria, the most likely cause of the condition is acute tubular necrosis of ischemic origin. Acute tubular necrosis is an intrinsic form of acute renal failure and is characterized by a BUN:Cr ratio of < 20:1. The urine can contain pigmented granular ("muddy-brown") casts (**A**). Broad waxy casts are found in chronic renal failure (**B**), fatty casts in nephrotic syndrome (**C**), red blood cell casts in renal bleeding, most commonly of glomerular origin (**D**), and white blood cell casts in infections, such as pyelonephritis or interstitial nephritis (**E**).

26. Correct: Alcohol dehydrogenase (B)

Given the scenario and descriptions, this patient most likely ingested antifreeze, leading to acute tubular necrosis and acute renal failure. Ethylene glycol, found in antifreeze, does not itself damage the body; however, through the action of alcohol dehydrogenase (**B**), the compound is broken down into oxalic acid, which accumulates in the kidney and causes renal failure. The other answers are incorrect (**A, C-E**).

27. Correct: Hyperkalemia (B)

Given the signs, symptoms, and laboratory testing, the most likely diagnosis is acute renal failure. During acute renal failure, patients can develop hyponatremia (due to the inability to excrete water) (**A**), hyperkalemia (**B**), hypocalcemia (due to high phosphate concentrations in the blood) (**C**), hyperphosphatemia (**D**), and metabolic acidosis (due to the inability to excrete waste products) (**E**).

11.6 Renal Tumors, Cysts, and Calculi—Answers and Explanations

Easy	Medium	Hard

28. Correct: Renal ultrasound (C)

Given the symptoms of fatigue and lethargy and the elevated BUN and creatinine, he is in acute renal failure. Given his past history of kidney stones, obstruction causing post-renal azotemia and renal failure is a distinct possibility, and such obstruction could be ruled out by ultrasound (**C**). Cultures of the throat, stool, and urine would not be the next best step (**B, C-D**). A renal biopsy is not appropriate (**A**).

29. Correct: Renal cell carcinoma (C)

Renal cell carcinomas can cause hematuria, back pain, and, on physical examination, a palpable mass can sometimes be appreciated (**C**). Given the normal BUN and creatinine, normal urine output, and lack of hypertension, the patient does not have nephritic syndrome, ruling out rapidly progressive glomerulonephritis (**B**). Given the normal BUN and creatinine and normal urine output, acute renal failure is not present, ruling out ischemic acute tubular necrosis (**D**). With urine output normal and without renal azotemia, post-renal azotemia is not possible (**E**). Focal segmental glomerulosclerosis would have hypoalbuminemia and would not usually have red blood cells in the urine (**A**).

30. Correct: Nephrolithiasis (D)

An abdominal aortic aneurysm that has ruptured can cause abdominal pain, but not normally hematuria (**A**). While an aortic dissection and psoas muscle abscess could cause flank pain, they would not normally be associated with hematuria (**B, E**). Acute prostatitis could cause pelvic or abdominal pain, but not commonly flank pain, and would not likely produce gross hematuria (**C**). Nephrolithiasis will produce a flank pain that radiates into the groin and is associated with nausea and vomiting, and patients can have hematuria (**D**).

31. Correct: Uric acid kidney stone (C)

All kidney stones, except for uric acid stones, are radiopaque and should show up on an abdominal X-ray (**A-B, D-E**). However, uric acid stones are radiolucent and may be missed on X-ray (**C**). The findings of severe flank pain radiating into the groin and associated with nausea and vomiting, hematuria, and costovertebral angle tenderness are consistent with nephrolithiasis.

32. Correct: Diffuse large B cell lymphoma (B)

Uric acid stones occur in association with gout and tumors with a rapid cellular turnover, such as leukemia and lymphoma (**B**). Sarcoidosis and parathyroid gland hyperplasia could produce a hypercalcemia, and would be associated with calcium oxalate or calcium phosphate stones, which are radiopaque (A, D). Bone metastases could also cause hypercalcemia (E). *Proteus vulgaris* infections are associated with struvite stones (C).

33. Correct: Nephrolithiasis (D)

The clinical scenario is consistent with nephrolithiasis (**D**). With the history of gout, the patient may have a uric acid stone. Renal cell carcinoma and transitional cell carcinoma of the bladder can both cause hematuria but are not likely to present acutely with severe flank pain (**A, E**). An acute myocardial infarction should always be considered in a middle-age to older male with hypertension, but it would not cause hematuria (**B**). An aortic dissection can cause sudden onset of severe sharp back pain, but hematuria would be very unusual (**C**).

34. Correct: Some forms are associated with *Proteus mirabilis* infection. (B)

Given the signs and symptoms, the most likely diagnosis is nephrolithiasis. Although the patient's history of gout indicates that the type of stone he may have is a uric acid stone, staghorn calculi, or struvite stones, which are associated with *Proteus mirabilis* infection (**B**). Nephrolithiasis is not a significant risk factor for renal cell carcinoma (**A**). Foreign travel can result in infections with certain parasites, such as schistosomiasis, which can infect the bladder and cause hematuria; however, foreign travel is not necessary for the formation of kidney stones (**C**). Ultrasound can be used to diagnose kidney stones (**D**), and if the stone causes obstruction of the urinary tract, the patient is at risk for postrenal renal failure (**E**).

35. Correct: *Schistosoma haematobium* infection of the bladder (C)

Given the recent travel history to Africa and work as a missionary, followed by hematuria, a *Schistosoma* infection is the most likely of the choices, as this parasite is found in Africa, it infects the bladder, and can present with hematuria (**C**). Transitional cell carcinoma of the bladder and renal cell carcinoma can cause hematuria with blood clots; however, he has no risk factors for either, and given his young age, they are unlikely (**A, B**). Membranous glomerulonephropathy does not cause hematuria (**D**), and post-infectious glomerulonephritis does cause hematuria, but the characteristic feature is red blood cell casts, and microscopic clots would not be formed (**E**).

Chapter 12

Diseases of the Mouth and Gastrointestinal Tract

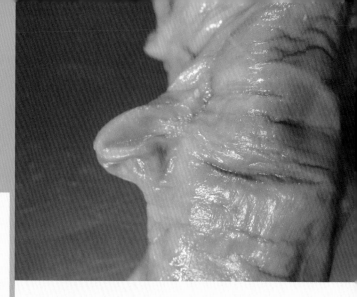

LEARNING OBJECTIVES

12.1 Diseases of the Esophagus
- Describe the types and locations of esophageal carcinoma, and list the risk factors for esophageal neoplasms
- List the risk factors for esophageal carcinoma
- Given the signs, symptoms, and laboratory testing, diagnose Plummer-Vinson's syndrome, and list the conditions associated with it.
- Describe esophageal varices and their complications, and list the risk factor for esophageal varices.
- List the causes of cirrhosis and their relative frequency of occurrence.
- Given the signs and symptoms, diagnose esophageal carcinoma.

12.2 Diseases of the Stomach
- Given the signs and symptoms, diagnose pyloric stenosis.
- Describe the pathological change in congenital pyloric stenosis.
- Given the signs and symptoms, diagnosis celiac disease.
- List the gastrointestinal tumors associated with Heliobacter pylori infection.
- List the causes of upper gastrointestinal hemorrhage, and given a clinical scenario, determine the most likely etiology.
- Describe the appearance of gastric carcinoma, gross and microscopic.
- Given the signs and symptoms, diagnose peritonitis, and list its causes.
- Given the clinical history, diagnose a peptic ulcer.
- Given the signs and symptoms, diagnose peritonitis, listing causes.
- Given the clinical history, diagnose peptic ulcer.
- Describe the mechanism of formation of a peptic ulcer.
- Given the signs and symptoms, diagnose gastric adenocarcinoma, and list the risk factors associated with it.
- Describe the histologic appearance of chronic gastritis.
- Given the signs, symptoms, and biopsy results, diagnose chronic gastritis.

- Compare and contrast chronic gastritis due to Heliobachter pylori and due to autoimmune gastritis.
- Given the signs, symptoms, and biopsy results, diagnose chronic gastritis.
- List the complications of autoimmune gastritis.
- List the underlying causes of gastrointestinal bleeding.
- Compare and contrast the listed sources of gastrointestinal bleeding and the types of symptoms they would produce.

12.3 Diseases of the Small Intestine
- Describe the histologic features of the small and large intestine.
- List the location where various vitamins and minerals are absorbed in the intestine, and list the pathologic conditions associated with vitamin and mineral deficiencies.
- List the causes of pancreatitis.
- List the complications of pancreatitis.
- Given the signs and symptoms, diagnose a vitamin deficiency.
- Given the signs and symptoms, diagnose Whipple's disease, and list the causative agent.
- Given the signs and symptoms, diagnose carcinoid syndrome.
- Given the signs and symptoms, diagnose carcinoid tumor, and list the common features associated with this neoplasm.
- Given the signs and symptoms, diagnose acute appendicitis.
- Describe the histologic findings of acute appendicitis.
- Given the gross description, diagnose pseudomyxoma peritonei, and list its causes.
- Given the signs and symptoms, diagnose a bowel obstruction.
- List the common causes of a bowel obstruction and the gross and microscopic features of each.

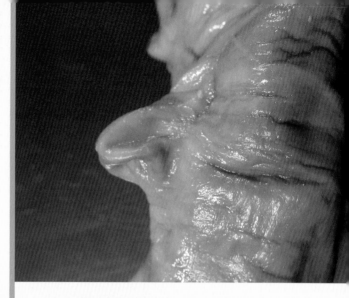

- ▶ Given the gross description, diagnose Meckel's diverticulum, and list the histological features associated with this lesion.
- ▶ Given the signs and symptoms, diagnose lactose deficiency.
- ▶ Given the stool electrolyte and osmolality testing, distinguish between osmotic and nonosmotic diarrhea.
- ▶ Given the signs and symptoms, diagnose Zollinger-Ellison's syndrome, and describe its features.
- ▶ Given the clinical scenario, diagnose Zollinger-Ellison's syndrome.
- ▶ Describe the location of the tumor type responsible for Zollinger-Ellison's syndrome.
- ▶ List the type of MEN syndrome associated with Zollinger-Ellison syndrome, and list other tumor types found.
- ▶ Given the clinical scenario, diagnose celiac disease, describing its epidemiologic, genetic, serologic, and histologic features.
- ▶ Given the clinical scenario, diagnose lactose intolerance, describing its histologic features.
- ▶ Describe the epidemiologic, gross and microscopic features of a Meckel's diverticulum.
- ▶ Given the clinical scenario, diagnose intestinal obstruction, and list the causes of intestinal obstruction.
- ▶ List the conditions commonly associated with prematurity.
- ▶ List the conditions premature infants are most prone to develop.

12.4 Diseases of the Large Intestine

- ▶ Given the signs and symptoms, diagnose Hirschsprung's disease.
- ▶ List the blood supply for the various regions of the gastrointestinal tract.
- ▶ Given a pathologic description, identify intestinal ischemia and determine its cause.
- ▶ Describe the normal histologic features of the small and large intestines, and distinguish normal histologic findings in the gastrointestinal tract from pathologic findings.
- ▶ Given the signs and symptoms, diagnose gastroesophageal reflux, and list the potential complications if left untreated.
- ▶ Given the signs and symptoms, diagnose inflammatory bowel disease and list the appropriate methods to confirm the diagnosis.
- ▶ Given the signs, symptoms, and radiologic studies, diagnose Crohn's disease, and list its histologic features and extraintestinal manifestations.

- ▶ Given the signs, symptoms, and laboratory testing, diagnose colonic adenocarcinoma, and list the histologic features of the disease.
- ▶ Given the pathologic description and clinical scenario, diagnose colonic adenocarcinoma.
- ▶ Describe the precursor lesions of colonic adenocarcinoma.
- ▶ Given the pathologic description, diagnose familial adenomatous polyposis, and list the gene mutation associated with the disease.
- ▶ Describe the common locations for tubular adenomas.
- ▶ Describe the histologic features of the tubular adenoma.
- ▶ Given the signs and symptoms, diagnose diverticulitis, describing its gross and microscopic appearance.
- ▶ Given the clinical scenario, diagnose Clostridium difficile colitis, and describe its pathologic features.
- ▶ List the extraintestinal manifestations of ulcerative colitis and the serologic findings associated with it and primary sclerosing cholangitis.
- ▶ Describe the gross and microscopic pathologic features of ulcerative colitis, comparing and contrasting its appearance with familial adenomatous polyposis.
- ▶ Compare and contrast the gross and microscopic features of Crohn's disease and ulcerative colitis.
- ▶ List complications of ulcerative colitis, describing pyoderma gangrenosum.
- ▶ Describe the microscopic features of Crohn's disease, including the distribution of lesions in it.
- ▶ Given the clinical scenario, diagnose diverticular disease, and describe its complications.
- ▶ Given the clinical scenario, diagnose a right-sided colonic adenocarcinoma.

12.1 Diseases of the Esophagus—Questions

Easy	Medium	Hard

1. A 54-year-old male presents to an acute care clinic. He has not seen a doctor in 10 years. He reports that over the last 6 months, he has had increasing difficulty swallowing food and has lost 30 lbs. He has a 50-pack-per-year smoking history. When asked, he says that he has never really had a problem with heartburn. An upper endoscopy is scheduled and performed. A mass is identified in the middle third of the esophagus. Of the following, what is a biopsy likely to reveal?

A. Neoplastic glandular cells

B. Neoplastic squamous cells

C. Neoplastic smooth muscle cells

D. Neoplastic skeletal muscle cells

E. Neoplastic cartilage

Esophagus

2. Given the previous clinical scenario, which of the following is a risk factor for this disease process?

A. Cirrhosis of the liver

B. Chronic pancreatitis

C. *Helicobacter pylori* infection

D. Diverticulum

E. Ascending cholangitis

Esophagus

3. A 34-year-old female presents to her primary care physician for her yearly checkup and reports that over the past several months, she has developed some difficulty with swallowing, which she attributed to nerves related to her job as a grocery clerk. She has also had increased fatigue, which she also attributes to her job. She also reports heavy menstrual periods. Her vital signs are temperature of 98.7°F, pulse of 110 bpm, and blood pressure of 98/65 mm Hg. Physical examination reveals pallor of the oral mucosa, increased pigmentation of the oral mucosa, and a few ulcers of the oral mucosa. Laboratory testing indicates a hemoglobin of 7.1 g/dL. Of the following, what is the most likely diagnosis?

A. Plummer-Vinson syndrome

B. Addison's disease

C. Zollinger-Ellison syndrome

D. Whipple's disease

E. Peutz-Jeghers syndrome

Mouth, esophagus

4. Given the previous clinical scenario, which of the following is the most likely cause of her dysphagia?

A. Achalasia

B. Esophageal diverticulum

C. Esophageal web

D. Gastroesophageal junction neoplasm

E. Anxiety

Mouth, esophagus

5. A 51-year-old male was brought to the emergency room by ambulance after an episode of hematemesis. His vital signs are temperature of 97.8°F, pulse of 126 bpm, and blood pressure of 92/60 mm Hg. Laboratory testing reveals a hemoglobin of 8.2 g/dL. During his treatment, an emergent EGD is performed, revealing dilated veins in the distal esophagus, one of which ruptured. Of the following, what is the most likely underlying etiology of his presenting disease process?

A. Hepatitis A infection

B. Antimitochondrial antibodies (with titer of > 1:40)

C. Excessive alcohol consumption

D. Hepatocellular carcinoma

E. Herpes simplex virus infection

Liver

6. A 62-year-old male presents to an acute care clinic. He says that over the past 6 months, he has had difficulty swallowing, which has progressively gotten worse. In this time, he has lost 25 lbs. His past medical history is significant for hypertension and diabetes mellitus type 2. He has consumed up to 12 cans of beer per day for the last 25 years and has a 50-pack-per-year smoking history. Prior to the last 6 months, he had occasional heartburn for the last 20 years, but otherwise, no gastrointestinal complaints. Of the following, what is the most likely diagnosis?

A. Gastroesophageal reflux disease

B. Boerhaave's syndrome

C. Esophageal adenocarcinoma

D. Achalasia

E. CREST syndrome

Esophagus

12.2 Diseases of the Stomach—Questions

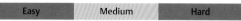

7. A 15-day-old male is brought to the emergency room by his parents. They are concerned because he started projectile vomiting. While he is in the emergency room, he vomits, and the emergency room physician notes that the fluid is not bile stained. Palpation of the abdomen reveals a mass in the left upper quadrant of the abdomen. Of the following, what is the most likely diagnosis?

A. Gastrointestinal stromal tumor

B. Congenital pyloric stenosis

C. Congenital pancreatic cyst

D. Choledochal cyst

E. Duodenal atresia

Stomach

8. Given the previous clinical scenario, of the following, what would a biopsy of the mass reveal?

A. Adipose tissue

B. Skeletal muscle

C. Smooth muscle

D. Lymphoma cells

E. Invasive adenocarcinoma

Stomach

9. A 7-month-old female is brought to her pediatrician by her parents. They report that over the past two weeks, she has been irritable, has lost 2 lbs., and has had diarrhea. The mother reports that she was breastfeeding their baby until about 3 weeks ago, when they introduced formula to her diet. Of the following, what is the most likely underlying mechanism for the patient's symptoms?

A. Aganglionosis of the colon

B. Hypertrophied muscle in the pylorus of the stomach

C. Absence of smooth muscle in the wall of the duodenum

D. Antigliadin antibodies

E. Congenital hypertrophy of Brunner's glands

Small intestine

10. A 35-year-old male is seen by a gastroenterologist for complaints of recurrent bouts of abdominal pain, felt to represent some form of gastritis. The gastroenterologist performs an EGD and identifies no abnormalities, other than possibly some patchy erythema of the gastric mucosa. Biopsies are taken and read by the pathologist as "chronic gastritis" with a description of chronic inflammation in the submucosa and a Warthin-Starry stain that identifies *Helicobacter pylori*. Of the following, which is the man most at risk for if his condition is not treated?

A. Celiac disease

B. Gastrointestinal stromal tumor

C. Marginal zone B-cell lymphoma

D. Mantle cell lymphoma

E. Chronic pancreatitis

Stomach

11. A 37-year-old male is brought to the emergency room by his wife because he started to vomit bright red blood at home. Over the past year, he has frequently complained of abdominal pain while eating a meal, and, as such, has lost about 40 lbs. He has no past medical history and is on no medications. He consumes about 1 beer per day and has a 10-pack-per-year history of smoking. Of the following, what is the most likely source of his bleeding?

A. Esophageal varices

B. Eroded gastric adenocarcinoma

C. Gastric peptic ulcer

D. Dieulafoy's lesion

E. Mallory-Weiss laceration

Stomach

12. Given the previous clinical scenario, which of the following is the most likely significant underlying etiology for his condition?

A. Alcohol use

B. Tobacco use

C. Infection with *Helicobacter pylori*

D. Use of NSAIDs

E. Recent lye ingestion

Stomach

13. A 47-year-old male has had abdominal pain for about 4 months. His primary care physician has prescribed omeprazole, which has not apparently worked. He presents to his primary care physician again, this time complaining of a nodule at his umbilicus. He has no other significant past medical history. Biopsy of the nodule reveals neoplastic cells with a signet ring appearance. He undergoes an exploratory laparotomy. Of the following, which is the surgeon likely to find?

A. A large ulcerated mass in the body of the stomach

B. Diffuse thickening of the wall of the stomach

C. A red and yellow mass in the cortex of a kidney

D. A mass in one of the adrenal glands

E. An ulcerated mass in the large intestine

Stomach

14. A 41-year-old male is brought to the emergency room by his wife. He had been complaining of a dull ache in his stomach region yesterday, but the pain suddenly worsened and now he has sharp severe pain throughout his abdomen, which is worsened when he moves. He has had abdominal pain in the past, but never this bad, and it had always been alleviated with antacids. He has not vomited. He has no past medical history and has not had any surgeries. Physical examination reveals rigidity of the abdominal wall. Of the following, what is the most likely diagnosis?

A. Intestinal obstruction

B. Perforated peptic ulcer

C. An aortic dissection

D. Acute cholecystitis

E. Acute pancreatitis

Stomach

15. Given the previous clinical scenario, which of the following is the most likely mechanism of the disease process?

A. Increased blood pressure

B. Infiltration by neoplastic cells

C. Unbalanced gastric acid effects on mucosa

D. Obstruction of venous blood flow

E. Overproduction of gastrin

Stomach

16. A 57-year-old male presents to his family physician. He describes that over the past 6 months, he has had occasional abdominal pain that he describes as dull. He has lost 20 lbs. in the preceding six months because he has had decreased appetite and early satiety. With increasing frequency, he has had episodes of nausea and vomiting. Other than systemic hypertension controlled with an ACE inhibitor, he has no significant past medical history. He has an 80-pack-per-year smoking history. His vital signs are temperature of 99.2°F, pulse of 91 bpm, and blood pressure of 131/82 mm Hg. A physical examination reveals vague left upper quadrant tenderness. Palpation of the left supraclavicular region reveals a nontender, nonmobile mass. A fecal occult blood test is positive. Of the following, what is the most likely diagnosis?

A. Peptic ulcer

B. Gastric adenocarcinoma

C. Chronic pancreatitis

D. Acute cholecystitis

E. Cirrhosis of the liver

Stomach

17. Given the previous clinical scenario, biopsy of the stomach performed one year prior to the onset of symptoms would most likely have shown which of the following?

A. Lymphocytic infiltration and intestinal metaplasia

B. Granulomatous inflammation

C. Chronic ulcer

D. Eosinophilic infiltrate with squamous metaplasia

E. Neutrophilic infiltration and intestinal metaplasia

Stomach

18. A 36-year-old male presents to his family physician with complaints of indigestion and a burning abdominal pain. An EGD is scheduled. A biopsy reveals lymphocytic infiltration of the gastric mucosa associated with mucosal atrophy. The number of parietal cells is not significantly reduced. Of the following, what is one mechanism of the disease process?

A. Autoantibodies against intrinsic factor

B. *MYC* translocation

C. Achlorhydria

D. Urease production

E. Production of C3a and C5a

Stomach

19. A 41-year-old female with a history of Hashimoto's thyroiditis requiring thyroid replacement therapy presents to her physician with complaints of gnawing epigastric pain that occurs intermittently. It is not associated with exertion, and she has no shortness of breath with the pain. A biopsy of the stomach reveals a mucosal lymphocytic infiltrate and a decreased number of parietal cells. Of the following, what does her presenting condition put her at increased risk for?

A. Megaloblastic anemia

B. Gastrointestinal stromal tumor

C. Meningitis

D. Cirrhosis of the liver

E. Chronic pyelonephritis

Stomach

20. A 37-year-old male presents to his family physician with complaints of fatigue and abnormal bowel movements. He describes his feces as often being dark red-black and tenacious. A fecal occult blood test is positive. Of the following, what is the most likely source of the change in his feces?

A. A gastric peptic ulcer

B. A proximal jejunal peptic ulcer

C. A colonic adenocarcinoma

D. Angiodysplasia

E. Diverticulosis

Stomach

12.3 Diseases of the Small Intestine—Questions

Easy	Medium	Hard

21. A pathology resident is examining a histologic section underneath the microscope of a segment of small intestine removed during surgery on a 19-year-old male who was involved in a car accident, and sustained an injury of the intestine. The resident sees glands within the submucosa. Given that a large segment of the portion of the intestine represented by the slide was removed, of the following, which disease is the man at risk for?

A. Megaloblastic anemia

B. Invasive adenocarcinoma

C. Iron deficiency anemia

D. Celiac disease

E. Crohn's disease

Small intestine

22. A 41-year-old chronic alcoholic presents to an acute care clinic. He says that over the past several months, he has had very greasy bowel movements, and he reports they stick to the toilet bowl. He has had multiple admissions in the past for severe abdominal pain, but he cannot remember the diagnoses. Additional history reveals that he feels that he bleeds much more easily than normal after a minor cut than he did years before. Of the following, what other conditions might he develop if his condition remains untreated?

A. Peripheral neuropathy

B. Glossitis

C. Dementia combined with dermatitis

D. Congestive heart failure

E. Decreased visual acuity

Intestine, pancreas

23. A 67-year-old male who lives in Montana and does not travel outside the state is brought to the emergency room by his family because he has become disoriented in the past few days, not knowing who he was or where he was at. They say that over the past several months, he has had some difficulty in remembering events from the day, including what he had for meals, which was a behavior that they just ascribed to old age. Also, for about the past year, he has complained to them of intermittent diarrhea and joint pain. Prior to the past year, he has been relatively healthy, only diagnosed with hypertension, which has been controlled with medication. Of the following, which is the most likely cause of his symptoms?

A. *Streptococcus pneumoniae*

B. Enterohemorrhagic *Escherichia coli*

C. *Borrelia burgdorferi*

D. *Tropheryma whipplei*

E. *Listeria monocytogenes*

Small intestine, brain, joints

24. A 51-year-old male presents to his family physician. Over the last 6 months he has had multiple episodes of nonbloody diarrhea. He has also felt flushed often and often wheezes when he exerts himself. His past medical history is significant only for hypertension, first diagnosed 5 years ago, which has been controlled with an ACE inhibitor. He has no history of smoking. His vital signs are temperature of 98.7°F, pulse of 89 bpm, and blood pressure of 121/81 mm Hg. Of the following, what is the most likely diagnosis?

A. Acute myocardial infarct

B. Asthma

C. Carcinoid syndrome

D. Inflammatory bowel disease

E. Pemphigus vulgaris

Liver, appendix

25. Given the previous clinical scenario, which of the following features is most characteristic of the disease process?

A. The neoplasm responsible most commonly arises in the liver.

B. The symptoms are due to release of somatostatin.

C. The neoplasm responsible is aggressive.

D. The patient could develop a peptic ulcer of the jejunum.

E. Endocardial fibrosis affecting the aortic valve is common.

Appendix, liver

26. A 24-year-old female presents to the emergency room with abdominal pain. She states that over the past three days she has had steady, cramping abdominal pain around her umbilicus, and the pain has now moved down to the right side of her abdomen, just above her hip. Associated with the pain, she has felt nausea and occasionally vomited. Her past medical history is significant only for a fractured left radius, which occurred while skiing. Her mother died from metastatic colonic adenocarcinoma at the age of 67 years. Her vital signs are temperature of 101.5°F, pulse of 102 bpm, and blood pressure of 119/76 mm Hg. Physical examination reveals rebound tenderness. Of the following, what is the most likely diagnosis?

A. Perforated cecum due to colonic adenocarcinoma

B. Volvulus

C. Intussusception

D. Acute appendicitis

E. Diverticulitis

Appendix

27. Given the previous clinical scenario, of the following, what is the most likely anatomic site for her symptoms, and what would be the histologic finding?

A. Appendix; neutrophilic infiltration of the wall

B. Appendix: granulomatous inflammation of the wall

C. Appendix; lymphocytic infiltration of the wall

D. Right kidney: neutrophilic infiltration of the cortex and medulla

E. Right kidney; granulomatous inflammation of the cortex and medulla

F. Right kidney: lymphocytic infiltration of the wall

Appendix

28. A 66-year-old male presents to his family physician, complaining of bloating, which has developed over the course of several weeks. After evaluation, an exploratory laparotomy is performed. When the peritoneum is entered, the surgeon finds a large amount of gelatinous material. Of the following, what is the most likely anatomic site for the condition causing this change?

A. Lung

B. Liver

C. Stomach

D. Appendix

E. Large intestine

F. Prostate

Appendix

29. A 54-year-old female presents to the emergency room, stating that over the past three days her abdomen has become distended and painful, and that she has been unable to pass gas or defecate. Over the past two days, she has vomited several times. Her past medical history is only significant for acute appendicitis, requiring an appendectomy, and a gastric bypass for weight reduction. Her vital signs are a temperature of 99.3°F, pulse of 105 bpm, and blood pressure of 132/83 mm Hg. A physical examination reveals hyperactive and high-pitched bowel sounds. An X-ray reveals air fluid levels in the gastrointestinal tract. Of the following, what is the pathologic feature of the most likely etiology underlying her presenting condition?

A. Neutrophilic infiltrate

B. Collagen deposition

C. Granulomatous inflammation

D. Infiltration of neoplastic glands

E. Cholesterol

Intestine

30. A pathologist is conducting an autopsy on a 35-year-old female who died in a motor vehicle accident as the result of blunt force injuries. When removing the small and large intestine, the pathologist identifies an outpouching of the wall of the small intestine near the ileocecal valve. Of the following, what is true regarding this lesion?

A. It is a false diverticulum.

B. They commonly become infected and present like acute appendicitis.

C. Gastric or pancreatic tissue may be present.

D. It is a remnant of the urachus.

E. Almost all will eventually develop an adenocarcinoma.

Small intestine

31. A 28-year-old white male presents to his family physician. Over the past 6 months, he has had multiple episodes of watery diarrhea. The diarrhea has been associated with bloating, excessive flatulence, and some abdominal cramps. The symptoms occur frequently in the late morning, after he eats breakfast. Most frequently for breakfast he has cereal and a piece of fruit. His physician orders a 24-hour stool collection specimen for electrolytes and osmolality. The test results from the collection are that his sodium is 8.1 mmol/24 hr, his potassium is 19.3 mmol/24 hr, and his measured osmolality is 123.3 mmol/24. Of the following, what is the most likely cause of the patient's symptoms?

A. Celiac disease

B. VIPoma

C. Disaccharidase deficiency

D. Inflammatory bowel disease

E. Rotavirus

Gastrointestinal

32. A 36-year-old male is brought to the emergency room by his wife because of acute onset of lower GI bleeding. He also has bright red blood in his stool. Both an EGD and colonoscopy fail to identify a source of bleeding; however, the EGD does identify a healed ulcer in the duodenum. Exploratory surgery identifies a peptic ulcer in the proximal portion of the jejunum. Of the following, what is the most likely mechanism for his lesion?

A. Lodged foreign body

B. Neoplastic infiltration of the wall of the small intestine

C. *Helicobacter pylori* infection

D. Increased gastrin production

E. *Entamoeba histolytica* infection

Small intestine

33. Given the previous clinical scenario, of the following, where is the location of the underlying lesion responsible for his presenting condition?

A. Liver

B. Kidney

C. Brain

D. Pancreas

E. Prostate

Jejunum

34. Given the previous clinical scenario, of the following, although not the lesion directly responsible for the patient's condition, what tumor type, associated with the patient's presenting condition, may be identified?

A. Medullary thyroid carcinoma

B. Pancreatic adenocarcinoma

C. Cholangiocarcinoma

D. Parathyroid adenoma

E. Tubulovillous adenoma

Jejunum

35. A 35-year-old male presents to his family physician. Over the past 6 months, he has had recurrent bouts of diarrhea and has lost 40 lbs. He describes the stool as appearing greasy and difficulty to flush. He also notes that he has developed an itchy rash on his elbows and back. He has no significant past medical history, never having used cigarettes and only drinking about 1 to 2 beers per month. He has not traveled outside the United States. Physical examination reveals a vesicular rash on the elbows and his lower back. Of the following, which statement is true regarding his disease process?

A. It is more common in African Americans.

B. It is associated with HLA-B27.

C. Serology would reveal antimitochondrial antibodies.

D. The disease is due to a reaction to corn in his diet.

E. Biopsy of the duodenum would confirm the diagnosis.

Small intestine

36. A 39-year-old Asian female presents to her family physician complaining of recent development of increased abdominal bloating, passing gas, and slight abdominal pain. She describes that the symptoms commonly occur after she ingests milk products. Her family physician refers her to a gastroenterologist, who schedules an EGD. The gastroenterologist, takes biopsies of her duodenum. Of the following, what will the biopsy reveal?

A. Flattened villi and lymphocytic infiltrate

B. Granulomatous inflammation

C. Pseudopolyps

D. Infiltrating neoplastic cells

E. Normal mucosa

Duodenum

37. A 19-year-old female presents to the emergency room. Over the past two days, she has developed severe abdominal pain associated with bloating of her abdomen. She has been vomiting multiple times, and has been unable to pass gas or feces. Physical examination reveals hyperactive and high-pitched bowel sounds. Her past medical history is significant only for a fractured left tibia sustained in a car accident 4 years ago. She is taken to surgery, and a lesion is removed from the terminal ileum. On microscopic examination, the pathologist identifies gastric mucosa in the lesion. Of the following, which statement is true regarding her lesion?

A. It is due to abdominal trauma sustained in the car accident.

B. Ileocecal regurgitation produced the gastric metaplasia.

C. It is a remnant of the omphalomesenteric duct.

D. It is a significant risk factor for carcinoma.

E. It most commonly presents in an older population.

Small intestine

38. A several-days-old infant develops abdominal distension and failure to pass fecal material. A diagnosis of necrotizing enterocolitis is made by the attending pediatrician. Of the following, what was the most direct risk factor for this condition?

A. Maternal syphilis

B. Maternal parvovirus infection

C. Prematurity

D. Congenital hepatic neuroblastoma

E. Large for gestational age

Large intestine

39. A male is born prematurely at 25 weeks estimated gestational age. In the days following delivery, he develops necrotizing enterocolitis and hyaline membrane disease. Of the following, which other condition is he at most risk for developing?

A. Extrahepatic biliary atresia

B. Congenital hypothyroidism

C. Intraventricular hemorrhage

D. Hydronephrosis

E. Pancreatic dysplasia

Brain

12.4 Diseases of the Large Intestine—Questions

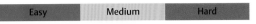

| Easy | Medium | Hard |

40. A newborn male who failed to pass meconium at birth was brought to the emergency room by his parents because he had not passed stool since they left the hospital. Of the following, what is the most likely diagnosis?

A. Diverticulitis

B. Hirschsprung's disease

C. Intussusception

D. Meckel's diverticulum

E. Galactosemia

Large intestine

41. Given the previous clinical scenario, of the following, what is the underlying cause of the disease process?

A. Abnormal migration of neural crest cells

B. Abnormal migration of alveolar crest cells

C. Abnormal migration of ectodermal cells

D. Abnormal migration of mesodermal cells

E. Abnormal migration of endodermal cells

Large intestine

42. A pathology resident is performing an autopsy on a 67-year-old male who died in the hospital and notes that the serosal surface of the large intestine at the splenic flexure is red-brown discolored. Microscopic examination of this segment of his bowel would later reveal extravasated red blood cells in the mucosa. Of the following, what is the most likely cause of these abnormalities?

A. An occlusive thrombus of the celiac trunk

B. An occlusive thrombus of the superior mesenteric artery

C. An occlusive thrombus of the inferior mesenteric artery

D. A ruptured thoracic aortic aneurysm, with three days of survival

E. A ruptured thoracic aortic aneurysm, with no survival

Large intestine

43. A pathology resident is examining a section of the distal ileum under the microscope. The segment of small bowel was obtained at the autopsy of a 56-year-old male who died suddenly at home and who had a history of hypertension and diabetes mellitus. In the submucosa, she identifies numerous large clusters of lymphocytes. Of the following, what was the individual's most likely cause of death?

A. Follicular lymphoma

B. Acute lymphocytic leukemia

C. Hodgkin's lymphoma

D. Atherosclerotic coronary artery disease

E. Glioblastoma multiforme

Small intestine

44. A 67-year-old female presents to the emergency room with a two-day history of abdominal pain, which started suddenly and has gotten worse over the past two days. During her evaluation in the emergency room, she becomes unresponsive, and, despite aggressive resuscitation, is unable to be revived. At autopsy, her small and large intestine, from the proximal jejunum to the midportion of the transverse colon, is observed to be dark red and discolored. In addition, she has 1,200 mL of cloudy yellow fluid in her peritoneal cavity and fibrinous adhesions between loops of intestine. Of the following, what is the most likely diagnosis?

A. Giant cell arteritis involving the superior mesenteric artery

B. Giant cell arteritis involving the inferior mesenteric artery

C. Thrombosis of an atherosclerotic plaque in the superior mesenteric artery

D. Thrombosis of an atherosclerotic plaque in the inferior mesenteric artery

E. Spontaneous dissection of the superior mesenteric artery

F. Spontaneous dissection of the inferior mesenteric artery

Small intestine, large intestine

45. A 63-year-old female presents to the emergency room with a two-day history of abdominal pain, which started suddenly and has gotten worse over the past two days. She was brought in by her sister, as she was too sick to drive, and because her sister was concerned for her health, not thinking she had a stomach flu. Despite treatment, she dies. At autopsy, her small and large intestine, from the proximal jejunum to the midportion of the transverse colon, is observed to be dark red and discolored. In addition, she has 1,400 mL of cloudy yellow fluid in her peritoneal cavity and fibrinous adhesions between loops of intestine. Of the following, what is the most likely diagnosis?

A. Giant cell arteritis involving the superior mesenteric artery

B. Spontaneous dissection of the superior mesenteric artery

C. Dysplasia of the superior mesenteric artery

D. Thrombosis of an atherosclerotic plaque of the superior mesenteric artery

E. Angiosarcoma of the renal artery compressing the superior mesenteric artery

Small intestine, large intestine

46. A 50-year-old male presents to a walk-in clinic. For several years, he has had what he describes as heartburn, which he says is often worse when he lies down. His wife has told him that at night he quite frequently coughs, although he is a very sound sleeper and doesn't notice. A physical examination reveals a pulse of 76 bpm and blood pressure of 110/70 mm Hg. The man has no other medical conditions and reports that his family is quite healthy, with most living into their 90s. Which of the following causes of death would be directly related to his disease process if it remains untreated?

A. Acute myocardial infarction

B. A thoracic aortic dissection

C. Boerhaave's syndrome

D. Metastatic adenocarcinoma

E. GI bleed due to ruptured esophageal varices

Esophagus

47. A 42-year-old male has, over the past year, presented to his family physician with complaints of intermittent diarrhea and abdominal pain and received a variety of diagnoses, from acute gastritis to presumed diverticulosis. During this time, he has lost 20 lbs. and developed arthritis involving multiple joints. He is referred to a gastroenterologist who performs a barium enema and identifies narrowed regions of the large intestine intermingled with normal regions. Of the following, what is the diagnosis?

A. Colonic adenocarcinoma

B. Diverticulitis

C. Diverticulosis

D. Ulcerative colitis

E. Crohn's disease

Large intestine

48. A 40-year-old male has, over the past year, presented to his family physician with complaints of intermittent diarrhea and abdominal pain and received a variety of diagnoses, from acute gastritis to presumed diverticulosis. During this time, he has lost 20 lbs. and developed arthritis involving multiple joints. He now presents to the emergency room with complaints of cramping lower abdominal pain with bloody stools. His vital signs are temperature of 98.7°F, pulse of 92 bpm, and blood pressure of 113/80 mm Hg. His serum leukocyte count is normal. Of the following, what diagnostic study would be most likely to confirm his diagnosis?

A. Exploratory laparotomy with removal of appendix

B. Stool culture

C. Barium enema

D. EGD

E. Peritoneal tap

Large intestine

49. A 43-year-old male has, over the past year, presented to his family physician with complaints of intermittent diarrhea, which is occasionally bloody, and abdominal pain, and received a variety of diagnoses, from acute gastritis to presumed diverticulosis. During this time, he has lost 15 lbs. He is referred to a gastroenterologist who performs a barium enema and identifies narrowed regions of the large intestine intermingled with normal regions. Of the following, what would a biopsy of the large intestine likely show?

A. Crypt abscesses and ulcers

B. Amoeba with engulfed red blood cells

C. Noncaseating granulomas

D. Invasive neoplastic glands

E. Coagulative necrosis and an eosinophilic infiltrate

Large intestine

50. Given the previous clinical scenario, of the following, which condition is this patient most likely to develop?

A. Primary sclerosing cholangitis

B. Primary biliary cirrhosis

C. Glaucoma

D. Uveitis

E. Autoimmune hepatitis

Large intestine

51. A 61-year-old male presents to his family physician because of complaints of fatigue. Occasionally, he has also noticed blood in his stool. His significant past medical history is hypertension, diagnosed 10 years ago, and effectively treated with an ACE inhibitor. His vital signs are a temperature of 98.8°F, pulse of 99 bpm, and blood pressure of 119/71 mm Hg. A physical examination reveals an obese male, who readily admits his diet is high in fat and carbohydrates, in no apparent distress. A fecal occult blood test is positive. Laboratory testing reveals a hemoglobin of 12.5 g/dL, hematocrit of 37%, and MCV of 76 fL. Of the following, what is the most likely diagnosis?

A. Adenocarcinoma of the distal ileum

B. Colonic adenocarcinoma

C. B12 deficiency

D. Inflammatory bowel disease

E. *Giardia lamblia*

Colon

52. Given the previous clinical scenario, of the following choices, which would be true regarding his most likely underlying etiology?

A. Pseudopolyps are a common feature.

B. Organisms with engulfed red blood cells could be identified histologically.

C. Depth of invasion in the muscularis propria is an important prognostic feature.

D. Signet ring cells are a common histologic feature.

E. Patients will often have increased pigmentation of the lips and oral mucosa.

Colon

53. A 62-year-old male presents to the emergency room with abdominal distention and severe constipation, not having been able to defecate for 8 days. After disimpaction, a barium enema reveals an apple-core-like lesion in the rectum. He undergoes a colectomy two weeks later, and a 4.0-cm ulcerated mass is identified in the rectum. He has no family history of gastrointestinal lesions. Of the following, what was the most likely precursor lesion?

A. Hyperplastic polyp

B. Peutz-Jeghers polyp

C. Tubular adenoma

D. Villous adenoma

E. Leiomyoma

Colon

54. A pathology resident is examining a colectomy specimen. The colonic mucosa has a 3.0-cm invasive neoplasm, and in the surrounding mucosa are an estimated 300 polyps. Of the following, the mutation of which gene produced these findings?

A. *APC*

B. *MYC*

C. Cyclin D1

D. *BAX*

E. *BAD*

Colon

55. A pathology resident is looking at biopsy specimens underneath the microscope in preparation for the next morning's signout with her attending physician. She identifies one biopsy as being of a tubular adenoma. Of the following, which organ was she most likely examining, and what histologic feature was present to account for the diagnosis?

A. Small intestine; metaplasia

B. Small intestine; dysplasia

C. Small intestine; neoplasia

D. Large intestine; metaplasia

E. Large intestine; dysplasia

F. Large intestine; neoplasia

Colon

56. A 41-year-old female is brought to the emergency room by her husband. Over the past several days, she has had cramping pain on the lower left side of her abdomen, and has been nauseated and vomited several times in the past two days. Also, she has been constipated and has not passed stool in two days. Her past medical history is significant for systemic lupus erythematosus, diagnosed 15 years ago. Her family history is significant for a mother who died at the age of 68 years from breast cancer and a father who died at the age of 60 years from a myocardial infarct. Her vital signs are a temperature of 99.9°F, pulse of 108 bpm, and blood pressure of 121/82 mm Hg. An X-ray after a barium enema reveals an apple-core type lesion. A colectomy reveals a segment of colon with a thickened wall, but no mucosal lesion. Of the following, which is correct regarding her presenting illness?

A. The symptoms are caused purely by diverticulosis.

B. The symptoms are caused purely by diverticulitis.

C. The surgeon failed to resect her colonic adenocarcinoma.

D. The surgeon failed to resect her intestinal obstruction.

E. Her children are highly likely to develop a similar condition.

Large intestine

57. A 41-year-old woman presents to the emergency room. She has had two days of abdominal pain and diarrhea, and, starting today, she has seen blood in the diarrhea, which prompted her visit to the emergency room. Associated with the diarrhea she has felt malaise and fatigue. Her past medical history includes systemic lupus erythematosus. Also, she was diagnosed with a urinary tract infection two weeks ago and placed on ciprofloxacin by her primary care doctor. Her vital signs are a temperature of 99.7°F, pulse of 108 bpm, and blood pressure of 116/72 mm Hg. Of the following, what is the most likely cause of her diarrhea?

A. *Salmonella*

B. *Entamoeba histolytica*

C. Crohn's disease

D. *Clostridium difficile*

E. Inflammatory bowel disease

Colon

58. Given the previous clinical scenario, which of the following would examination of the colon most likely reveal?

A. Flask-shaped ulcers

B. Pseudopolyps

C. Marked dilation

D. Pseudomembranes

E. Diverticula

Colon

59. A 32-year-old male has had multiple presentations to his family physician and an acute care clinic with complaint of intermittent diarrhea, which occasionally contains blood. He has also lost 20 lbs. over the past several months. Associated with these symptoms, he frequently has abdominal pain. A barium enema identifies three strictures in the large intestine. Of the following, what is the most likely diagnosis?

A. Pseudomembranous colitis

B. Familial adenomatous polyposis

C. Crohn's disease

D. Ulcerative colitis

E. Diverticulitis

Large intestine

60. A 33-year-male is seeing his family physician because his skin has become yellow. At the same time, he has felt febrile and occasionally had chills and abdominal pain. His medical history is significant for ulcerative colitis. He does not smoke or use intravenous illicit drugs; he does drink 1 to 2 beers per day. Of the following, what serologic test is most likely to be positive?

A. c-ANCA

B. p-ANCA

C. Antiendomysial antibodies

D. Antimitochondrial antibodies

E. Anti-smooth muscle antibodies

Colon

61. A pathologist is examining a segment of colon resected from a patient. The mucosa has multiple polypoid projections. Microscopic examination of the polypoid projections reveals relatively normal mucosa, with some mucosal and submucosal inflammation at the edges. Of the following, what is the diagnosis?

A. Familial adenomatous polyposis

B. Ulcerative colitis

C. Pseudomembranous colitis

D. Celiac disease

E. Polyarteritis nodosa

Colon

62. A 28-year-old female presented to her family physician because of ongoing complaints of intermittent watery diarrhea and some abdominal pain. Quite frequently, there is blood in the diarrhea and, occasionally, mucus. A gastroenterologist performs a colonoscopy and, in the distal portion of the rectum, identifies roughened and reddened mucosa, with a biopsy showing mucosal crypts filled with neutrophils. A diagnosis was made. One year later, she presented to her family physician because of the development of an ulcer on her right lower extremity. She thought she had banged her leg against something, which caused redness; however, it did not heal, and progressed. What are her underlying and most current diagnoses?

A. Crohn's disease/erythema nodosum

B. Crohn's disease/pyoderma gangrenosum

C. Crohn's disease/bullous pemphigoid

D. Ulcerative colitis/erythema nodosum

E. Ulcerative colitis/pyoderma gangrenosum

F. Ulcerative colitis/bullous pemphigoid

Colon

63. A 28-year-old male presented to his family physician with complaints of intermittent diarrhea. An EGD and a colonoscopy were scheduled and performed and biopsies were taken. The biopsies revealed transmural lymphocyte aggregates and occasional noncaseating granulomas. Of the following, where was the biopsy most likely taken from?

A. Esophagus

B. Stomach

C. Duodenum

D. Ascending colon

E. Rectum

Colon

64. A 61-year-old female presented to her family physician with complaints of bright red blood in her stool about 3 years ago, and was told that it was benign and not to worry. A colonoscopy performed 6 months ago revealed no mucosal masses. She presents now with complaints of pain in the left lower quadrant, which is associated with nausea and occasional vomiting. Her past medical history is significant only for Hashimoto's thyroiditis and mild osteoarthritis. She has had no surgeries. Her vital signs are a temperature of 100.1°F, pulse of 107 bpm, and blood pressure of 129/83 mm Hg. Of the following, what is the most likely diagnosis?

A. Acute appendicitis

B. Diverticulitis

C. Colonic adenocarcinoma

D. Ulcerative colitis

E. Intestinal ischemia

Colon

65. Given the previous clinical scenario, of the following, what is she most at risk for?

A. Cirrhosis of the liver

B. Metastatic disease to the liver

C. Pneumaturia

D. Primary sclerosing cholangitis

E. Acute myocardial infarction

Colon

66. A 66-year-old male presents to his family physician with complaints of fatigue. After determining that the fatigue is not psychogenic in origin, his physician conducts a physical examination and notes some slight pain with pressure in the right lower quadrant of the abdomen and a positive fecal occult blood test. Laboratory testing reveals a hemoglobin of 10.4 mg/dL. A barium enema does not reveal any abnormalities but illustrates only the transverse and descending segments of the large intestine. The patient has no history of changes in bowel habits. Of the following, what is the most likely diagnosis?

A. Acute appendicitis

B. Diverticulosis

C. Volvulus

D. Colonic adenocarcinoma

E. Celiac disease

Colon

12.5 Diseases of the Esophagus—Answers and Explanations

| Easy | Medium | Hard |

1. Correct: Neoplastic squamous cells (B)

The history and endoscopy are consistent with an esophageal neoplasm. Given the location and the history of alcohol use and cigarette smoking, but the absence of heartburn, the most likely tumor type is squamous cell carcinoma (**B**). Adenocarcinomas most often arise from Barrett's esophagus, due to reflux (**A**). The other choices are possible, but not very likely (**C-E**).

2. Correct: Diverticulum (D)

The history and endoscopy are consistent with an esophageal neoplasm. Given the location and the history of alcohol use and cigarette smoking, but the absence of heartburn, the most likely tumor type is squamous cell carcinoma. Adenocarcinomas most often arise from Barrett's esophagus, due to reflux. Risk factors for esophageal squamous cell carcinoma include, other than smoking and alcohol use, achalasia, diverticuli, esophageal webs, and a hereditary component (**D**). Cirrhosis of the liver, chronic pancreatitis, *H. pylori* infection, and ascending cholangitis are not by themselves risk factors for esophageal carcinoma (**A-C, E**).

3. Correct: Plummer-Vinson syndrome (A)

The classic triad of Plummer-Vinson syndrome is iron deficiency anemia, which is the most likely cause of anemia in a patient with heavy menstrual periods;

glossitis, which is manifested by the oral mucosal changes; and dysphagia, which is due to esophageal webs (**A**). While Addison's disease and Peutz-Jeghers syndrome are associated with mucocutaneous hyperpigmentation, they are not a normal cause of dysphagia or iron deficiency anemia (**B, E**). Zollinger-Ellison syndrome and Whipple's disease are not common causes of any of the listed symptoms (**C, D**).

4. Correct: Esophageal web (C)

The classic triad of Plummer-Vinson syndrome is iron deficiency anemia, which is the most likely cause of anemia in a patient with heavy menstrual periods; glossitis, which is manifested by the oral mucosal changes; and dysphagia, which is due to esophageal webs (**C**). While the other conditions listed could produce dysphagia, they are not associated with oral mucosal changes or iron deficiency anemia (**A-B, E**), with the exception of a neoplasm, which, with blood loss, could produce iron deficiency anemia. However, oral mucosal changes are not associated with a neoplasm, and with the lack of reflux in the history, and the lack of risk factors for esophageal carcinoma, it is unlikely (D).

5. Correct: Excessive alcohol consumption (C)

The patient has an upper GI bleed due to esophageal varices. Esophageal varices most commonly develop as a complication of cirrhosis of the liver. Chronic alcoholism is a common cause of cirrhosis of the liver (although most chronic alcoholics do not develop cirrhosis of the liver) (**C**). Hepatitis A does not have a chronic stage and would not lead to cirrhosis (**A**). Antimitochondrial antibodies of a high titer most commonly indicate primary biliary cirrhosis, which is a cause of cirrhosis and potentially varices, but not as common of a cause as chronic alcoholism (**B**). Hepatocellular carcinoma is a complication of cirrhosis but would not itself contribute to the development of varices (**D**). An HSV can infect the esophagus but would not commonly cause massive bleeding and is not associated with the development of varices (**E**).

6. Correct: Esophageal adenocarcinoma (C)

Given the clinical scenario, of the choices, esophageal carcinoma is the most likely answer of the choices, as patients can have progressive difficulty swallowing and weight loss, and alcohol consumption and tobacco use are significant risk factors (**C**). GERD would be very unlikely to cause progressive dysphagia unless a stricture developed (**A**). Boerhaave's syndrome is a rupture of the esophagus and would present as an emergency, not over the course of 6 months (**B**). Both achalasia and sclerosis associated with CREST syndrome could present with chronic dysphagia; however, given his risk factors, including the long-term heart burn, likely leading to Barrett's esophagus, and ultimately to esophageal adenocarcinoma, achalasia and CREST syndrome are much less likely (**D, E**).

12.6 Diseases of the Stomach—Answers and Explanations

Easy	Medium	Hard

7. Correct: Congenital pyloric stenosis (B)

The signs and symptoms are typical for congenital pyloric stenosis, which is also more common in males than females (**B**). It is found in children with Turner's syndrome and trisomy 18. A gastrointestinal stromal tumor would be very unlikely in a child and would not be associated with projectile vomiting (**A**). Duodenal atresia causes vomiting, but the vomiting is bilious and occurs during the first 24 hours after birth (**E**). The other conditions can occur in children and could potentially produce a palpable mass, but are not associated with projectile vomiting (**C, D**).

8. Correct: Smooth muscle (C)

The signs and symptoms are typical for congenital pyloric stenosis. Congenital pyloric stenosis is due to hypertrophied smooth muscle (**C**). The other answers are incorrect (**A-B, D-E**).

9. Correct: Antigliadin antibodies (D)

This infant has the classic features of celiac disease, occurring due to exposure to gluten after its introduction to her diet. The underlying mechanism for celiac disease is antigliadin antibodies (**D**). Aganglionosis of the colon would be found in Hirschsprung's disease (**A**), and hypertrophied muscle in the pylorus would be found in pyloric stenosis (**B**). The remainder of the choices are not characteristic of any specific disease (**C, E**). Although not listed as a possible choice, the most common cause of the patient's presenting condition would be a milk allergy.

10. Correct: Marginal zone B-cell lymphoma (C)

Chronic gastritis due to *Helicobacter pylori* is associated with peptic ulcers, gastric polyps, gastric adenocarcinoma, and extranodal marginal zone B-cell lymphoma (in the GI tract, referred to as lymphoma of mucosa-associated lymphoid tissue, or MALToma) (**C**). *H. pylori* infections are not associated with the remainder of the conditions listed (**A-B, D-E**).

11. Correct: Gastric peptic ulcer (C)

Although all of the conditions can cause upper GI bleeding, with no past medical history, esophageal varices, normally associated with cirrhosis, are unlikely (**A**); an eroded tumor is not likely to cause bright red blood hemorrhage of a significant amount; and given his young age, a gastric adenocarcinoma is less likely (**B**). Dieulafoy's lesion is rare (**D**), and without a history of prolonged vomiting prior to the GI bleed, a Mallory-Weiss laceration is unlikely (**E**).

12. Correct: Infection with *H. pylori* (C)

Although sources of upper gastrointestinal hemorrhage are numerous, one of the most common sources is a peptic ulcer. Given the clinical scenario, and symptoms consistent with an ulcer, and with no competing causes, it is the most likely cause. For gastric ulcers, *Helicobacter pylori* is the underlying etiology in about 70%, and for duodenal ulcers it is essentially always the underlying cause (**C**). NSAID use is a common cause of gastric peptic ulcers, but not nearly as common as *H. pylori* infection (**D**). Although alcohol use and tobacco use can contribute to the risk for development of an ulcer, they are not as important as an *H. pylori* infection (**A, B**). Recent lye ingestion could cause GI hemorrhage; however, it would be rare (**E**).

13. Correct: Diffuse thickening of the wall of the stomach (B)

Signet ring cell morphology is characteristic of a form of aggressive gastric adenocarcinoma. Patients can develop a subcutaneous nodule around the umbilicus (a Sister Mary Joseph nodule), and the stomach can appear diffusely thickened, termed linitis plastica (**B**). The findings are most consistent with an aggressive gastric adenocarcinoma, confirmed by the signet ring cells. These findings do not match those of an intestinal-type gastric adenocarcinoma (**A**), a renal cell carcinoma (**C**), an adrenal tumor (**D**), or a colonic adenocarcinoma (**E**). Gastric adenocarcinomas with intestinal morphology, as opposed to signet ring cell morphology, usually present with bulky tumor growth.

14. Correct: Perforated peptic ulcer (B)

Given the characterization of the pain (severe sharp pain throughout his abdomen, worse with movement), peritonitis is the most likely cause, and while all of the choices could potentially cause peritonitis, the history of previous abdominal pain relieved with antacids is consistent with a peptic ulcer (**B**), and acute cholangitis and acute pancreatitis, by themselves, would not normally cause abdominal pain affecting the entire abdomen (**D-E**). Given the lack of vomiting, and history of no surgeries, an intestinal obstruction is not likely (**A**). With no history of hypertension, an aortic dissection is unlikely (**C**).

15. Correct: Unbalanced gastric acid effects on mucosa (C)

The patient is presenting with peritonitis, which can cause diffuse sharp abdominal pain that is worsened by movement. The physical finding of rigidity is consistent with peritonitis. Given the lack of significant past medical history, but a history of abdominal pain in the past relieved by antacids, the most likely cause of the peritonitis is a ruptured peptic ulcer. The underlying mechanism is unbalanced effect of gastric acid on the gastric mucosa (**C**). In the stom-

169

ach, most peptic ulcers are due to *Helicobacter pylori* infection, but NSAIDs are another common cause; whereas essentially all duodenal peptic ulcers are due to *H. pylori* infection. The development of peptic ulcers occurs when the normal defenses against gastric acid (mucus secretion, bicarbonate secretion, and prostaglandin production) are inadequate to counteract the effect of gastric acid. While the other choices do represent the potential mechanism of a disease process that could result in peritonitis or cause abdominal pain, each is much less likely than a peptic ulcer given the clinical scenario (**A-B, D-E**).

16.   Correct: Gastric adenocarcinoma (B)

The weight loss, early satiety, nausea and vomiting, evidence of a gastrointestinal hemorrhage, and the presence of a palpable lymph node, consistent with a metastasis, is most consistent with a gastric adenocarcinoma (**B**). The location of the abdominal pain is not as consistent with acute cholecystitis, and, given the lack of significant risk factors, chronic pancreatitis and cirrhosis of the liver are less likely (**C-E**). Although a peptic ulcer could produce a similar clinical scenario, lymphadenopathy would not be an associated finding (**A**).

17.   Correct: Lymphocytic infiltration and intestinal metaplasia (A)

The weight loss, early satiety, nausea and vomiting, and evidence of a gastrointestinal hemorrhage, and the presence of a palpable lymph node, consistent with a metastasis, is most consistent with a gastric adenocarcinoma. Risk factors for gastric adenocarcinoma include diets with nitrites and smoked food, cigarette use, and chronic gastritis with intestinal metaplasia. Chronic gastritis is characterized by lymphocytic infiltrates and intestinal metaplasia (a premalignant condition) can develop (**A**). Peptic ulcers rarely develop into a malignant neoplasm (**C**). Granulomatous inflammation can occur in some disease processes but would be rare compared to chronic gastritis and intestinal metaplasia (**B**). In chronic gastritis, the infiltrate is neither eosinophilic nor neutrophilic (**D-E**).

18.   Correct: Urease production (D)

The clinical history and biopsy findings are consistent with chronic gastritis. Chronic gastritis is most often due to *H. pylori* infection. Mechanisms of *H. pylori*–induced damage of the gastric mucosa include urease production (D), production of IL-8 (which recruits neutrophils), enhancement of gastric acid secretion and decreased bicarbonate production, and production of VacA (a passive urea transporter). Autoantibodies to parietal cells lead to autoimmune gastritis, which has a similar histologic appearance, except the number of parietal cells is decreased (**A**). Autoimmune gastritis can result in hypochlorhydria or achlorhydria (**C**). *MYC* translocation and produc-

tion of C3a and C5a play roles in neoplasia and acute inflammation and are not significant factors in the mechanism by which *H. pylori* produces chronic gastritis (**B, E**).

19.   Correct: Megaloblastic anemia (A)

The patient has symptoms of dyspepsia, and, associated with the biopsy, it is consistent with chronic gastritis. The decreased number of parietal cells is consistent with autoimmune gastritis, and the past history of Hashimoto's thyroiditis is also supportive of this diagnosis, as patients with one autoimmune condition often will develop others. Autoimmune gastritis is due to antibodies against parietal cells. A decreased number of parietal cells will result in decreased production of intrinsic factor and decreased absorption of vitamin B12, leading to megaloblastic anemia (**A**). Autoimmune gastritis is not a significant risk factor for gastrointestinal stromal tumors, meningitis, cirrhosis of the liver, or chronic pyelonephritis (**B-E**).

20.   Correct: A gastric peptic ulcer (A)

The patient is having rectal bleeding, which is confirmed by the positive fecal occult blood test, which is testing for heme in the stool. Given the appearance of the blood in the stool, the source of the hemorrhage is upper GI, which rules out a colonic adenocarcinoma, angiodysplasia, and diverticulosis (**C-E**). Angiodysplasia, a condition with dilated blood vessels in the distal small intestine and colon, would present with bright red blood per rectum. And, although heavy bleeding from a colonic adenocarcinoma and diverticulosis would be less likely, the blood should be bright red. Both a gastric peptic ulcer and a proximal jejunal peptic ulcer could present with digested blood; however, the gastric peptic ulcer is far more common in occurrence (**A, B**).

12.7 Diseases of the Small Intestine—Answers and Explanations

Easy	Medium	Hard

21.   Correct: Iron deficiency anemia (C)

The resident is seeing Brunner's glands, which are found in the duodenum. The duodenum is the site at which iron is absorbed. Poor absorption of iron could lead to iron deficiency anemia (**C**). A lack of folate (absorbed in jejunum) or B12 (absorbed in ileum) could lead to megaloblastic anemia (**A**). While celiac disease and Crohn's disease could lead to malabsorption, they are not caused by a lack of vitamins or minerals (**D, E**).

22. Correct: Decreased vision (E)

In a chronic alcoholic with recurrent bouts of abdominal pain, recurrent pancreatitis is a likely diagnosis. Chronic pancreatitis can lead to malabsorption, specifically of fat and fat-soluble vitamins. Vitamin K deficiency would lead to bleeding defects. A peripheral neuropathy may be due to B12 deficiency (**A**), glossitis due to B6 deficiency (**B**), dementia and dermatitis due to niacin deficiency (**C**), and congestive heart failure due to B1 deficiency (thiamine deficiency) (**D**), which are all water-soluble vitamins. Vitamin A, which is fat soluble, if deficient, can lead to blindness (**E**).

23. Correct: *Tropheryma whipplei* (D)

Whipple's disease, caused by *Tropheryma whipplei,* can present with diarrhea, arthritis, and CNS diseases, manifested in a variety of ways including delirium, cognitive impairment, hypersomnia, and abnormal movements (e.g., myoclonus, choreiform movements). Patients often have nonspecific symptoms such as arthritis, fever, or diarrhea for months to years before the diagnosis is made (**D**). *Borrelia burgdorferi,* which is associated with CNS symptoms and arthritis, is only rarely associated with diarrhea and is not found in Montana (**C**). The other entities would not present with the constellation of symptoms (**A-B, E**).

24. Correct: Carcinoid syndrome (C)

Flushing, diarrhea, and wheezing are consistent with carcinoid syndrome (**C**). Given the time frame, it is not an acute myocardial infarct, and none of the symptoms are frequently associated with an acute myocardial infarct (**A**). Although asthma can cause wheezing, it is not commonly associated with diarrhea (**B**). Inflammatory bowel disease could cause diarrhea, but is not commonly associated with wheezing (**D**). The patient has no features of pemphigus vulgaris (**E**).

25. Correct: The patient could develop a peptic ulcer of the jejunum. (D)

The signs and symptoms are consistent with a carcinoid tumor. Carcinoid tumors most frequently arise in the appendix (**A**); however, they can metastasize to the liver, which allows hormones secreted to bypass the liver and enter the circulation system, subsequently causing systemic effects. Diarrhea, flushing, and wheezing result from serotonin entering the systemic circulation (**B**). The tumors are relatively benign (**C**) but can metastasize. They can potentially secrete gastrin, which can lead to Zollinger-Ellison syndrome, where a patient can have multiple ulcers, including in unusual locations such as the jejunum (**D**). Patients with carcinoid syndrome can develop right-sided valvular lesions, not of the aortic (**E**).

26. Correct: Acute appendicitis (D)

The signs and symptoms are classic for acute appendicitis, with pain starting around the umbilicus and moving to the right lower quadrant of the abdomen (**D**). Although all of the other choices could cause a peritonitis, each would be much less likely compared to acute appendicitis (**A-C, E**).

27. Correct: Appendix; neutrophilic infiltration of the wall (A)

The patient has symptoms classic for acute appendicitis, with abdominal pain starting around the umbilicus, and progressing to the right lower quadrant of the abdomen, and associated with nausea, some vomiting, and fever. Although acute pyelonephritis could present in this age group and could present with a fever, the pain is usually flank pain (**D-F**). The histologic appearance would be neutrophilic infiltration of the wall, the finding of an acute inflammatory process (**A**). Although there are disease processes that involve the appendix and can cause a granulomatous or lymphocytic infiltrate, the clinical scenario is characteristic for acute appendicitis, which would have a neutrophilic infiltrate (**B-C**).

28. Correct: Appendix (D)

The description is that of pseudomyxoma peritonei. The gross features are associated with both benign and malignant neoplasms, and the classification and naming of the lesion is controversial; however, in a vast majority of cases, the neoplasm responsible for the changes in the peritoneal cavity is found in the appendix (**D**). Although a variety of neoplasms could give rise to the finding of pseudomyxoma peritonei, neoplasms in the appendix are by far the most common source, which indicates that the other answers (**A-C, E-F**) are not the best choice.

29. Correct: Collagen deposition (B)

The signs and symptoms are consistent with a bowel obstruction. The most common cause of a bowel obstruction is a fibrous adhesion or hernia occurring after surgery. The fibrous adhesion would be composed of collagen (**B**). The other features listed could also be associated with a bowel obstruction, causes of which can include a neoplasm (**D**), gallstones (**E**), and others (**A, C**); however, the most common cause is adhesions.

30. Correct: Gastric or pancreatic tissue may be present. (C)

The lesion is a Meckel's diverticulum, which is a remnant of the omphalomesenteric duct (or, vitelline duct) (**D**), and can contain ectopic gastric or pancreatic tissue (**C**). It is a true diverticulum, having all four layers of the bowel in their wall (**A**). The risk of infection or developing cancer is not significantly increased (**B, E**).

171

31. Correct: Disaccharidase deficiency (C)

The finding of a gap between the calculated stool osmolality [2(Na+K)] and measured serum osmolality is consistent with an osmotic diarrhea, and is a way to distinguish an osmotic diarrhea from a nonosmotic diarrhea. The only condition listed that causes an osmotic diarrhea is disaccharidase deficiency, which is most commonly lactase deficiency (**C**). The symptoms are consistent with lactase deficiency. As the other choices would produce a nonosmotic diarrhea, they are incorrect (**A-B, D-E**).

32. Correct: Increased gastrin production (D)

The patient has two ulcers, and one is in an unusual location, being in the jejunum instead of the stomach or duodenum. Patients with Zollinger-Ellison syndrome, which is due to a gastrin-secreting tumor, often have multiple ulcers, and they can have ulcers in unusual locations, such as the jejunum (**D**). *Helicobacter pylori* infections are associated with gastric and duodenal ulcers (**C**). *Entamoeba histolytica* infections cause a flask-shaped ulcer but occur in the large intestine (**E**). A lodged foreign body and a tumor would produce an ulcer at one location, and given his young age, a neoplasm is less likely, and small intestinal neoplasms are rare (**A, B**).

33. Correct: Pancreas (D)

The patient has two ulcers, and one is in an unusual location, being in the jejunum instead of the stomach or duodenum. Patients with Zollinger-Ellison syndrome, a condition caused by a gastrin-secreting tumor, often have multiple ulcers, and they can have ulcers in unusual locations, such as the jejunum. The tumor is usually located in the region of the 2nd or 3rd part of the duodenum, the junction of the head and neck of the pancreas, and the cystic duct (**D**). The other locations are incorrect (**A-C, E**).

34. Correct: Parathyroid adenoma (D)

Although the gastrinoma causing Zollinger-Ellison can occur sporadically, in many cases it occurs as a component of multiple endocrine neoplasia type I (MEN I). Of the listed tumors, parathyroid adenomas are found in MEN I (**D**), and also pituitary adenomas and pancreatic endocrine tumors. The other tumors are not usually associated with MEN type I (**A-C, E**).

35. Correct: Biopsy of the duodenum would confirm the diagnosis. (E)

The patient has malabsorption, with historical evidence of steatorrhea, indicating malabsorption of fat. Given his history, celiac disease is the most likely diagnosis. The rash on the elbows represents dermatitis herpetiformis, which is associated with celiac disease. A biopsy of the duodenum can confirm the diagnosis, and the changes seen are flattened villi, a lymphocytic infiltrate, and crypt hyperplasia (**E**). The disease is more common in whites (**A**), is associated with HLA-DQ2 and -DQ8 (**B**), antigliadin, antitissue transglutaminase, and antiendomysial antibodies are found (**C**), and it is a reaction to gluten, which is in wheat, rye, or barley, and not corn (**D**).

36. Correct: Normal mucosa (E)

Given the clinical scenario, the most likely diagnosis is lactose intolerance (a disaccharidase deficiency), which commonly occurs in Asian patients. The biopsy is negative in this disease (**E**). Flattened villi and lymphocytic infiltrate are found in celiac disease (**A**), granulomatous inflammation could be found in Crohn's disease (**B**), and pseudopolyps are associated with ulcerative colitis (**C**), which would not occur in the duodenum. The history does not suggest a neoplastic process, and given her young age, no reported family history, and a biopsy of the duodenum, and the rarity of tumors at this location, infiltrating neoplastic cells are highly unlikely (**D**).

37. Correct: It is a remnant of the omphalomesenteric duct. (C)

The patient has a Meckel's diverticulum, which is a relatively common congenital lesion and can present with intestinal obstruction. The clinical scenario and physical examination are consistent with an intestinal obstruction. Meckel's diverticulum can contain both gastric and pancreatic tissue, but not due to a metaplastic process as described (**B**). It is not a significant risk factor for carcinoma (**D**), and more frequently presents in a younger population (**E**). Meckel's diverticulum does not result from trauma (**A**).

38. Correct: Prematurity (C)

Premature infants are at risk for several conditions, including necrotizing enterocolitis (**C**). The other conditions listed are not direct risk factors commonly associated with necrotizing enterocolitis, although each could potentially be associated with prematurity, none are a risk factor for necrotizing enterocolitis (**A-B, D-E**).

39. Correct: Intraventricular hemorrhage (C)

Three conditions commonly associated with premature infants are necrotizing enterocolitis, hyaline membrane disease, and intraventricular hemorrhage (**C**). Hyaline membrane disease is due to a deficiency of surfactant. Intraventricular hemorrhage occurs because the subependymal regions of the cerebral ventricles are highly vascular but have delicate vasculature, which, with prematurity, is prone to rupture. The other conditions listed are not commonly associated with prematurity (**A-B, D-E**).

12.8 Diseases of the Large Intestine—Answers and Explanations

Easy	Medium	Hard

40. Correct: Hirschsprung's disease (B)

The signs and symptoms are consistent with Hirschsprung's disease (**B**). The condition is more common in males than in females and is due to aganglionosis of the large intestine. Diverticulitis occurs in adults (**A**). Intussusception occurs in older children and is associated with vomiting and currant jelly stools (**C**). Galactosemia leads to cirrhosis (**E**) and would not produce constipation at birth. Although a Meckel's diverticulum is a congenital malformation and could present immediately after birth, it would be highly unlikely (**D**).

41. Correct: Abnormal migration of neural crest cells (A)

The signs and symptoms are consistent with Hirschsprung's disease. Hirschsprung's disease is due to abnormal migration of neural crest cells, resulting in aganglionosis of either the entire large intestine, or the rectum and sigmoid colon (**A**). The other answers are incorrect (**B-E**).

42. Correct: A ruptured thoracic aortic aneurysm, with three days of survival (D)

The pathologic changes, gross and microscopic, are consistent with an ischemic infarct. The splenic flexure is a watershed area, receiving blood from both the superior and inferior mesenteric arteries (**A-C**). Therefore, with low blood flow and hypotension, as would occur with a ruptured aneurysm, the area is underperfused. If the event causing the hypotension causes immediate death, no pathologic changes would have developed (**E**); however, with a period of survival, the ischemic injury would be manifested grossly and microscopically (**D**).

43. Correct: Atherosclerotic coronary artery disease (D)

The microscopic findings are Peyer's patches, which are a normal histologic feature of the terminal ileum. Of the causes of death listed, and given the history of hypertension and diabetes mellitus, atherosclerotic coronary artery disease is by far the most common (**D**). The histologic findings are not indicative of a lymphoma or leukemia (**A-C**). In contrast to atherosclerotic cardiovascular disease as a cause of death, a glioblastoma multiforme would be rare (**E**).

44. Correct: Thrombosis of an atherosclerotic plaque in the superior mesenteric artery (C)

The clinical presentation and gross description of the pathologic changes fits that of ischemia of the large intestine. The distribution is within that of the superior mesenteric artery. Of the three conditions, all could cause ischemia; however, thrombosis of an atherosclerotic plaque would be the most common cause (**A-F**).

45. Correct: Thrombosis of an atherosclerotic plaque of the superior mesenteric artery (D)

The clinical scenario and pathologic description fits that of ischemia of the large intestine. The distribution is within that of the superior mesenteric artery. Of the conditions listed, all can involve the vasculature and result in ischemia; however, giant cell arteritis of the superior mesenteric artery would be very rare, as would a spontaneous dissection or dysplasia (**A-C**). The most common cause of ischemic colitis would be atherosclerosis (**D**). An angiosarcoma could compress the superior mesenteric artery and lead to ischemia, but it would be a very rare cause (**E**).

46. Correct: Metastatic adenocarcinoma (D)

The patient has the symptoms of gastroesophageal reflux. With reflux, his lower esophagus can undergo glandular metaplasia, which has an increased risk for the development of adenocarcinoma (**D**). Given his history and the presentation, this is unlikely to be cardiac angina (**A**). With no other past medical history, the likelihood of a thoracic aortic aneurysm is low (**B**); Boerhaave's syndrome would be due to violent vomiting, which is not associated with reflux (**C**), and he has no risk factors for cirrhosis (**E**).

47. Correct: Crohn's disease (E)

The barium enema shows sites of narrow and skip lesions, which are characteristic of Crohn's disease, as there is multifocal involvement of the GI tract in this disease process (**E**). Although colonic adenocarcinoma and diverticulitis could present with a narrowing, it should be in only one location (**A, B**). Diverticulosis by itself would not present with a narrowing of the large intestine—only if it became inflamed and diverticulitis resulted would that occur (**C**). Ulcerative colitis does not produce skip lesions (**D**). Ulcerative colitis involves the entire mucosa starting distally in the large intestine and proceeding proximal. Pseudopolyps can occur, but not skip lesions.

48. Correct: Barium enema (C)

In the absence of fever or leukocytosis, the main differential diagnosis is Crohn's disease or ulcerative colitis. A barium enema can help distinguish between Crohn's disease and ulcerative colitis (**C**). Crohn's disease would be expected to produce skip lesions and cobblestoning, whereas ulcerative colitis typically involves contiguous sections of colon and lacks the mural thickening seen in Crohn's disease. Given the past history of abdominal complaints, the likelihood that his current symptoms represent an acute appendicitis or infectious process are not likely, and therefore, an exploratory laparotomy or stool culture are not necessary (**A, B**). A peritoneal tap could reveal ascites, peritonitis, or hemorrhage, which, given the clinical scenario, are not useful since he has no history of trauma or risk factors for cirrhosis, and, given the duration of the symptoms, peritonitis is unlikely (**E**). The symptoms are consistent with a lower gastrointestinal tract process; therefore, an EGD would be very low yield (**D**).

49. Correct: Noncaseating granulomas (C)

Given the clinical signs, symptoms and radiologic findings, Crohn's disease is the diagnosis. Histologically Crohn's disease has noncaseating granulomas, lymphoid aggregates, and transmural inflammation (**C**). Crypt abscesses and ulcers are more characteristic of ulcerative colitis (**A**). An amoeba with engulfed red blood cells is consistent with *Entamoeba histolytica* (**B**). Coagulative necrosis with an eosinophilic infiltrate is not characteristic of a large intestinal disease presenting in this fashion (**E**). Given his young age coupled with the results of the barium enema, a colonic adenocarcinoma is not likely (**D**).

50. Correct: Uveitis (D)

Given the clinical scenario and testing, Crohn's disease is the diagnosis. Individuals with Crohn's disease can develop other manifestations outside of the intestine, including migratory polyarthritis, erythema nodosum, ankylosing spondylytis, and uveitis (**D**). Primary sclerosing cholangitis and pyoderma gangrenosum are more characteristic of ulcerative colitis (**A**), whereas primary biliary cirrhosis, glaucoma, and autoimmune hepatitis are not commonly associated with inflammatory bowel disease (**B, C, E**).

51. Correct: Colonic adenocarcinoma (B)

The patient most likely has fatigue due to iron deficiency anemia, with the laboratory testing indicating a microcytic anemia. With the positive fecal occult blood test, and given the age, of the choices, a colonic adenocarcinoma is the most likely (**B**). Adenocarcinoma of the small intestine is rare compared to colonic adenocarcinoma (**A**). Inflammatory bowel disease would have most likely present at a younger age (**D**), and *Giardia lamblia* most frequently produces a watery diarrhea (**E**). A vitamin B12 deficiency would be associated with a macrocytic and not a microcytic anemia (**C**).

52. Correct: Depth of invasion in the muscularis propria is an important prognostic features. (C)

Given the signs and symptoms, a significantly possible diagnosis is colonic adenocarcinoma. With colonic adenocarcinoma, depth of invasion into the muscularis propria is an important prognostic feature (**C**). Pseudopolyps are associated with ulcerative colitis (**A**), *Entamoeba histolytica* can engulf red

blood cells (**B**), signet ring cells are associated with high-grade gastric adenocarcinoma (**D**), and individuals with Peutz-Jeghers polyps can have pigmentation of the lips and oral mucosa (**E**).

53. Correct: Villous adenoma (D)

Based on the description, the patient has an invasive colonic adenocarcinoma. While adenomas are benign, large adenomas have a higher chance of harboring an invasive tumor, and villous adenomas are more likely to harbor an invasive adenocarcinoma than tubular adenomas (**C, D**). Hyperplastic polyps are not commonly associated with a risk for adenocarcinoma (**A**). Peutz-Jeghers syndrome is rare and is autosomal dominant (**B**). Leiomyomas are benign smooth muscle tumors and very rarely develop a malignant component (**E**).

54. Correct: *APC* (A)

The patient has familial adenomatous polyposis, which is due to a mutation of the *APC* gene (**A**). APC promotes the degradation of β-catenin. Normally, β-catenin activates the *MYC* and cyclin D1 genes. The other choices, while associated with various types of neoplasms, are not the main cause of familial adenomatous polyposis.

55. Correct: Large intestine; dysplasia (E)

Tubular adenomas can occur in various parts of the gastrointestinal tract, but are most common in the large intestine and would be rare in the small intestine (**A-C**). The histologic feature of tubular adenomas are glands with enlarged, hyperchromatic nuclei interspersed between submucosal-type tissue, which represents a dysplastic process (**D-F**).

56. Correct: The symptoms are caused purely by diverticulitis. (B)

Inflammation of a diverticulum can result in diverticulitis (**A**), which can present with the symptoms that the patient had and can mimic an invasive adenocarcinoma by producing an apple-core lesion on barium enema (**B**). With diverticulitis, the wall of the colon would be expected to be thickened by the inflammation, but there would be no mucosal lesion (**C, D**). Diverticular disease is caused by herniation of mucosa and submucosa through a defect in the muscular layer. An individual can have diverticular disease and never develop diverticulitis; her children would not necessarily be likely to develop the same condition (**E**).

57. Correct: *Clostridium difficile* (D)

All of the possible answers are associated with diarrhea, and all but IBD can cause bloody diarrhea (**E**); however, given the history that she was just prescribed antibiotics, the most likely etiology is *Clostridium difficile*, which can result from both out-patient and inpatient use of antibiotics, can occur about 1 week after starting the antibiotic, and is associated most strongly with fluoroquinolones, cephalosporins, and clindamycin (**D**). Given the clinical scenario, (**A-C**) are much less likely.

58. Correct: Pseudomembranes (D)

The clinical scenario fits that of *Clostridium difficile* colitis, which occurs most commonly after antibiotic usage. The pathologic finding is pseudomembranes (**D**). Pseudomembranes can occur in other conditions, including some bacterial infections, such as *Staphylococcus* infections, and with ischemic injury. Flask-shaped ulcers are typical for *Entamoeba histolytica* (**A**), and pseudopolyps are found in ulcerative colitis (**B**), which would not likely have an acute presentation and would not be associated with recent antibiotic use. A markedly dilated colon (toxic megacolon) can occur in a variety of conditions, including ulcerative colitis, but is not associated with antibiotic use (**C**). Diverticula can cause some bleeding but are less commonly associated with diarrhea and would not have the temporal association with antibiotic use (**E**).

59. Correct: Crohn's disease (C)

Pseudomembranous colitis would have a more acute presentation and is not normally associated with strictures (**A**). Familial adenomatous polyposis is not normally associated with strictures, unless a neoplasm developed (**B**). Diverticulitis can produce a stricture and can mimic a rectal adenocarcinoma, but it would not be multifocal except in rare cases (**E**). Ulcerative colitis affects the mucosa and submucosa and does not normally produce strictures (**D**). Crohn's disease can present in this age group commonly; it is associated with diarrhea and abdominal pain, and, because the inflammation is transmural, can produce strictures (**C**).

60. Correct: p-ANCA (B)

Given the patient's medical history, the onset of jaundice can indicate primary sclerosing cholangitis, which is quite frequently associated with ulcerative colitis. p-ANCA is associated with both primary sclerosing cholangitis and ulcerative colitis (**B**). Anti-endomysial antibodies are associated with celiac disease (**C**), antimitochondrial antibodies with primary biliary cirrhosis (**D**), and anti–smooth muscle antibodies with autoimmune hepatitis (**E**). c-ANCA is associated with granulomatosis with polyangiitis (**A**).

61. Correct: Ulcerative colitis (B)

The polyps occurring in ulcerative colitis are actually pseudopolyps formed by residual mucosa, with loss of mucosa from the inflammatory infiltrate intervening (**B**). If the diagnosis were familial adenomatous polyposis, the mucosa of the polyps would be dysplastic (**A**). None of the other conditions would present a similar gross and microscopic appearance (**C-E**).

62. Correct: Ulcerative colitis/pyoderma gangrenosum (E)

The clinical presentation is consistent with inflammatory bowel disease, with ulcerative colitis more frequently having bright red blood via the rectum. Crypt abscesses (mucosal crypts filled with neutrophils) are typical of ulcerative colitis and not Crohn's disease (**A-C**). One complication of ulcerative colitis is pyoderma gangrenosum, which can appear as cellulitis and progress to ulceration with a violaceous rim (**E**). Bullous pemphigoid is not usually associated with ulcerative colitis (**F**), and the appearance of erythema nodosum is different (**D**).

63. Correct: Ascending colon (D)

The biopsy results are consistent with Crohn's disease, which causes transmural inflammation, noncaseating submucosal granulomas, and mural thickening (which would not be identified with only a biopsy). The history is consistent with Crohn's disease. Although Crohn's disease can potentially involve the entire GI tract (**A-C**), it most commonly involves the terminal ileum, colon, or both (**D**). Crohn's disease spares the rectum (**E**).

64. Correct: Diverticulitis (B)

Given the fact that she had bright red blood via her rectum three years ago and is now presenting acutely, she most likely has diverticular disease, which caused the bleeding and is now causing diverticulitis (**B**). Given her past workups, the development of a colonic adenocarcinoma from normal mucosa to an obstructing lesion in 6 months is highly unlikely (**C**). She has no risk factors for intestinal obstruction or ischemic bowel disease (**E**). Given her age of presentation, ulcerative colitis is unlikely (**D**), and the long clinical history is not consistent with acute appendicitis (**A**).

65. Correct: Pneumaturia (C)

Patients with diverticulitis are at risk for fistulas, and a fistula between the colon and the bladder can result in air in the bladder (**C**). Diverticular disease and diverticulitis are not risk factors for cirrhosis of the liver, a neoplasm with resultant metastases, primary sclerosing cholangitis, or acute myocardial infarction (**A-B, D-E**).

66. Correct: Colonic adenocarcinoma (D)

Given the lack of changes in bowel habit and nonacute presentation of the patient, volvulus is not likely, nor is acute appendicitis (**A, C**). Also, an acute appendicitis would not adequately explain the decreased hemoglobin. With no change in bowel habits, celiac disease is not a reasonable diagnosis, although celiac disease could cause a slight decrease in hemoglobin (**E**). Diverticulosis should be identified by barium enema (**B**). The most likely diagnosis from the choices is a colonic adenocarcinoma, with the carcinoma involving the right side of the colon (**D**).

Chapter 13

Diseases of the Liver, Gallbladder, and Biliary Tract

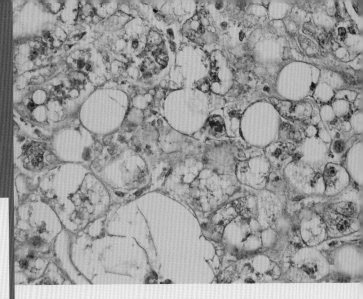

LEARNING OBJECTIVES

13.1 Cirrhosis and Its Complications
▶ Given the signs and symptoms, diagnose cirrhosis, and list its complications, etiologies, and identify the histologic changes associated with alcoholic liver disease.

▶ Diagnose spontaneous bacterial peritonitis.

▶ Describe the mechanism of formation of ascites in patients with cirrhosis.

▶ Given the clinical scenario, diagnose hepatocellular carcinoma.

▶ Given the clinical scenario, diagnose hepatocellular carcinoma, describing its gross and microscopic appearance, risk factors for development, and common complications.

▶ Given the clinical scenario, diagnose esophageal varices.

▶ Given the clinical scenario, diagnose bleeding due to esophageal varices, describing the mechanism by which they form.

13.2 Viral, Alcohol, and Metabolic Liver Disease
▶ Given the clinical scenario, diagnose Gilbert's syndrome.

▶ Given the signs and symptoms, diagnose Dubin-Johnson's syndrome.

▶ Describe the relationship between hepatitis B virus and hepatitis D virus

▶ Describe the difference in serologic testing for patients infected with hepatitis B virus and for those who are vaccinated against it.

▶ Given the clinical scenario, diagnose α-1-antitrypsin deficiency, describing its pathologic features, both gross and microscopic.

▶ List the diseases commonly presenting with an elevated AST and ALT.

▶ List the causes of nonalcoholic steatohepatitis, describing its microscopic pathologic features.

▶ List the diseases of the liver that can produce elevated AST and ALT, discussing the various laboratory tests used to distinguish between these entities.

▶ List the common autoantibodies associated with autoimmune hepatitis.

▶ Describe the use of the AST/ALT ratio when formulating a diagnosis of alcohol-related liver disease.

▶ Given the laboratory test results, diagnose hemochromatosis, and listening its complications and the gene mutation most commonly associated with hereditary hemochromatosis.

▶ Describe the pathologic changes of hemochromatosis, including the type of stain used in its diagnosis.

▶ Given the clinical scenario, diagnose acute viral hepatitis, listing the risk factors associated with the different types.

▶ Given the clinical scenario, including the laboratory testing, diagnose Wilson's disease, describing the pathologic changes associated with it, including its genetic inheritance and underlying gene.

13.3 Diseases of the Biliary Tract
▶ Given signs and symptoms, diagnose primary biliary cirrhosis, listing the antibody associated with the disease process.

▶ Given the signs, symptoms, and clinical history, diagnose primary sclerosing cholangitis, list the antibody associated with it.

▶ Given the signs and symptoms, diagnose chronic cholecystitis, listing the risk factors for chronic cholecystitis.

▶ Describe the gross and microscopic pathologic features of chronic cholecystitis.

▶ List the etiologies of jaundice.

▶ Describe how to use laboratory testing to narrow the differential diagnosis for jaundice.

▶ Given laboratory testing, differentiate between a conjugated and unconjugated hyperbilirubinemia.

▶ List the causes of conjugated and unconjugated hyperbilirubinemia, and describe their pathologic findings.

▶ Given the clinical scenario and laboratory testing, diagnose choledocholithiasis.

▶ Given the clinical scenario, diagnose an extrahepatic cholestasis, describing the association between primary sclerosing cholangitis and ulcerative colitis.

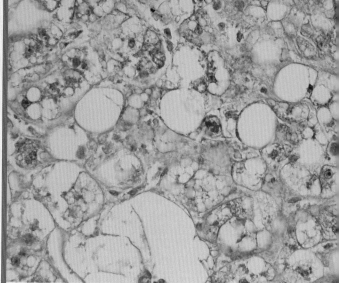

▶ Given the clinical scenario, diagnose primary sclerosing cholangitis, describing its histologic appearance.

▶ Given the signs and symptoms, diagnose acute calculous cholecystitis.

▶ Describe Murphy's sign.

▶ Describe the two types of gallstones with regard to appearance, composition, and underlying risk factors for formation.

13.4 Miscellaneous Liver Diseases

▶ Describe centrilobular necrosis of the hepatocytes, listing the etiologies for this histologic finding.

▶ List the etiologies for massive hepatic necrosis.

▶ Describe the reference range for laboratory tests.

▶ Given the signs, symptoms, and laboratory testing, diagnose autoimmune hepatitis, describing the demographics, histology, and risk for cirrhosis for this condition and listing the antibody associated with the disease.

▶ Given the signs, symptoms, and laboratory testing, diagnose acetaminophen toxicity.

▶ Given the signs, symptoms, and laboratory testing, diagnose acetaminophen overdose, describing the pathologic changes induced.

▶ Determine the etiology of elevated concentrations of AST and ALT.

▶ Given the clinical scenario and laboratory testing, distinguish between the causes of unconjugated hyperbilirubinemia .

▶ Given the signs, symptoms, and laboratory testing, diagnose a hemolytic anemia.

▶ Compare and contrast warm and cold autoimmune hemolytic anemia.

▶ Given the clinical scenario, diagnose a warm autoimmune hemolytic anemia, describing its underlying causes and mechanism.

▶ Given a description, diagnose a cholangiocarcinoma, describing its risk factors and clinical course of cholangiocarcinoma.

▶ Given the clinical scenario, diagnose Budd-Chiari's syndrome.

▶ List the possible causes of an elevated alkaline phosphatase.

▶ Describe the use of GGT concentrations to determine the underlying etiology of alkaline phosphatase elevations.

13.1 Cirrhosis and its Complications—Questions

Easy	Medium	Hard

1. A 43-year-old chronic alcoholic who has a past history of intravenous drug abuse is brought to the emergency room by his friends because of bright red hematemesis. He has no significant past medical history. He does not smoke, but drinks 8 to 12 cans of beer daily and has for the past 20 years. His vital signs are a temperature of 98.5°F, pulse of 140 bpm, and blood pressure of 91/60 mm Hg. Physical examination reveals abdominal distension with a fluid wave. Of the following, which is the most likely source of his GI bleed?

A. An esophageal carcinoma

B. Esophageal varices

C. Mallory-Weiss tear

D. Peptic ulcer

E. Fistula between common bile duct and small intestine

Liver

2. Given the previous clinical scenario, of the following, which is another complication this patient may develop due to the underlying disease process?

A. Primary biliary cirrhosis

B. Sclerosing cholangitis

C. Pancreatic adenocarcinoma

D. Hepatocellular carcinoma

E. Adenocarcinoma of the gallbladder

Liver

3. A 44-year-old male who lives by himself is brought to the emergency room by EMTs who were summoned to the apartment after a welfare check by police, which was initiated by the landlord. Upon arrival, he is noted to be unkempt. Vital signs are temperature of 99.1°F, blood pressure of 100/70 mm Hg, and pulse of 82 bpm. Physical examination reveals a golden yellow discoloration of the skin and conjunctivae, the abdomen is distended and a fluid wave is present, and small spider-like red discolorations are present on the skin. Of the following, what is the most likely cause of his underlying condition?

A. Chronic alcohol use

B. Obstruction of bile ducts

C. Congestive heart failure

D. Inflammation of the pancreas

E. Excessive aspirin consumption

Liver

4. Given the previous clinical scenario, of the following, what is most likely to be identified on microscopic examination of the liver?

A. Asteroid bodies

B. Howell-Jolly bodies

C. Mallory's hyaline

D. Targetoid lesions of the bile ducts

E. Bile lakes

Liver

5. A 46-year-old chronic alcoholic with a known history of cirrhosis is brought to the emergency room by his friends, who state that he has been really "out-of-it" for two days. His vital signs are a temperature of 101.1°F, blood pressure of 82/60 mm Hg, and pulse of 134 bpm. A physical examination reveals yellow discoloration of the conjunctivae and rebound tenderness with palpation of the abdomen, combined with guarding. Despite the abbreviated abdominal exam, a fluid wave is identified. Laboratory testing reveals a white blood cell count of 27,000 cells/μL, a hemoglobin of 9.9 g/dL, and a platelet count of 160,000 cells/μL. A peritoneal tap reveals a cloudy fluid in the abdominal cavity. He has no other significant past medical history. Of the following, what is the most likely diagnosis?

A. Perforated peptic ulcer

B. Acute pancreatitis

C. Acute appendicitis

D. Spontaneous bacterial peritonitis

E. Autoimmune hepatitis

Liver

6. A 42-year-old male with cirrhosis of the liver due to chronic alcoholism presents to his family physician because of increasing weight gain and a sensation of abdominal fullness. Physical examination reveals an abdominal fluid wave. Of the following, which laboratory testing would best correlate with the mechanism for the physical examination findings?

A. AST

B. ALT

C. GGT

D. Albumin

E. Immunoglobulin

Liver

7. A 44-year-old male with a history of significant alcohol consumption (about 10-12 beers per day for the last 20 years) and hepatitis C positivity presents to an acute care clinic with a history of abdominal pain and increased fullness, which has developed over several weeks to months. He has lost 30 lbs. in the last 5 months. Physical examination reveals some abdominal pain with palpation, and a negative stool occult blood test. Laboratory testing reveals an AST of 130 U/L, an ALT of 117 U/L, and α-fetoprotein of 723 ng/mL. An ultrasound reveals a single mass in the right lobe of the liver. Of the following, what is the most likely diagnosis?

A. Cavernous hemangioma

B. Focal nodular hyperplasia

C. Hepatocellular carcinoma

D. Metastatic colonic adenocarcinoma

E. Hepatoblastoma

Liver

8. Given the previous clinical scenario, of the following, what is characteristic for the mass?

A. It has a central scar.

B. Exposure to vinyl chloride is a commonly associated risk factor.

C. Use of corticosteroids is a significant risk factor.

D. Portal vein invasion with resultant thrombosis is a complication.

E. Patients are likely to develop a warm autoimmune hemolytic anemia.

Liver

9. A 43-year-old male with a history of chronic alcoholism and hepatitis C infection is brought to the emergency room by his friends because he has twice vomited large amounts of blood. Other than the two episodes of bleeding, he had not otherwise been vomiting. Of the following, what is the most likely mechanism of his bleeding?

A. Acute alcohol toxicity

B. Tear of the esophagus

C. Rupture of a dilated vein

D. Hemorrhage from a neoplasm

E. Trauma from a foreign object

Liver

10. Given the previous clinical scenario, of the following, what is the most likely mechanism for the development of the lesion causing his bleeding?

A. Increased hydrostatic pressure

B. Decreased interstitial oncotic pressure

C. Portal hypertension

D. Increased concentrations of ammonia

E. Hyperbilirubinemia

Liver

13.2 Viral, Alcohol, and Metabolic Liver Disease—Questions

Easy	Medium	Hard

11. A 37-year-old male presents to an acute care clinic with complaints of abdominal pain, which began a few days ago. His vital signs are a temperature of 98.7°F, pulse of 101 bpm, respiratory rate of 19 breaths per minute, and blood pressure of 129/82 mm Hg. A physical examination reveals an enlarged and tender liver. Laboratory testing reveals an AST of 271 U/L, ALT of 46 U/L, GGT of 190 U/L, and alkaline phosphatase of 210 U/L. Of the following, what is the most likely diagnosis?

A. Viral hepatitis

B. Alcoholic hepatitis

C. Acetaminophen toxicity

D. Acute cholecystitis

E. Ascending cholangitis

Liver

12. A 19-year-old male presents to his family physician. He reports that whenever he becomes very stressed, sometimes the whites of his eyes will turn somewhat yellow. His vital signs are temperature of 98.8°F, pulse of 72 bpm, respiratory rate of 17 breaths per minute, and blood pressure of 108/72 mm Hg. Physical examination reveals no abnormalities. Laboratory testing reveals an AST of 23 U/L, ALT of 19 U/L, alkaline phosphatase of 57 U/L, GGT of 27 U/L, and total bilirubin of 2.8 mg/dL. The direct bilirubin is 0.3 mg/dL. Urinalysis reveals no bilirubin. Of the following, what is the most likely diagnosis?

A. Gilbert's syndrome

B. Crigler-Najjar syndrome

C. Dubin-Johnson syndrome

D. Rotor's syndrome

E. Acute viral hepatitis

Liver

Liver

13. A 20-year-old male presents to his family physician. He reports that whenever he becomes very stressed, sometimes the whites of his eyes will turn somewhat yellow. His vital signs are a temperature of 98.7°F, pulse of 76 bpm, respiratory rate of 18 breaths per minute, and blood pressure of 110/71 mm Hg. A physical examination reveals no abnormalities. Laboratory testing reveals an AST of 23 U/L, ALT of 19 U/L, alkaline phosphatase of 57 U/L, GGT of 27 U/L, and total bilirubin of 2.8 mg/dL. The direct bilirubin is 2.6 mg/dL. Urinalysis reveals bilirubin. Of the following, what is the most likely diagnosis?

A. Gilbert's syndrome

B. Crigler-Najjar syndrome

C. Dubin-Johnson syndrome

D. Galactosemia

E. Acute viral hepatitis

Liver

14. A 43-year-old male presents to an acute care clinic because of yellowing of his eyes, fatigue, and malaise. After his evaluation, his physician suspects an infection with hepatitis D virus. Of the following, what other test must be positive, or be elevated, to justify serologic testing for hepatitis D virus?

A. Anti-HCV

B. HBsAg

C. Anti-Hbs

D. Serum ferritin

E. Anti–smooth muscle antibody

Liver

15. A 34-year-old female presents to her family physician complaining of new exertional dyspnea. She is a nonsmoker and has a past history of consistent mild elevations of AST and ALT. Past serologic tests for hepatitis, EBV, and CMV have been negative. She is only a social drinker, consuming about 1 drink per week. At her current admission, her physician performs pulmonary function tests, which reveal a slightly increased FVC but a decreased FEV1. Of the following, what would histologic examination of the liver most likely reveal?

A. PAS-positive globules in the hepatocytes

B. Portal lymphocytic infiltrate associated with bile duct damage

C. Cholestasis

D. Mallory's hyaline

E. Scattered enlarged cells with intranuclear inclusions

Liver, lung

16. A 37-year-old male is being evaluated by his family physician. Initial laboratory results indicated an AST of 78 U/L and an ALT of 64 U/L. The laboratory results were repeated in one month, and the AST and ALT were still elevated. A creatine kinase was 45 U/L. Additional testing was as follows: anti-HCV, HBsAg, serum iron, TIBC, ferritin, ceruloplasmin, and SPEP, which were all normal. An ultrasound of the liver revealed increased echogenicity. The patient is not on any medication, and he reportedly drinks about 1 to 2 beers per week socially with friends. A biopsy of the liver reveals macrovesicular steatosis with occasional fat vacuoles rimmed with neutrophils. Of the following, what would physical examination also reveal?

A. Elevated blood pressure

B. Abdominal fluid wave

C. Hyperactive bowel sounds

D. Body mass index of 36 kg/m^2

E. Decreased deep tendon reflexes

Liver

17. A 39-year-old female is being evaluated by her family physician. Initial laboratory results indicated an AST of 84 U/L and an ALT of 68 U/L. The laboratory results were repeated in one month, and the AST and ALT were still elevated. A creatine kinase was 105 U/L. A urine pregnancy test was negative. Additional testing was as follows: anti-HCV, HBsAg, serum iron, TIBC, ferritin, and ceruloplasmin, which were all normal. A serum protein electrophoresis revealed an increased amount of protein in the γ region. An ultrasound of her liver revealed no abnormality. The patient is not on any medication, and she consumes about 1 alcoholic beverage per month. Of the following, what additional laboratory testing is most likely to identify the disease?

A. Anti–smooth muscle antibodies

B. Anti–tissue transglutaminase antibodies

C. Serum glucose

D. Serologic testing for CMV infection

E. X-ray of the skull

Liver

18. A 35-year-old male is being evaluated by his family physician. Physical examination reveals him to be 176 lbs. and have a blood pressure of 113/71 mm Hg. Initial laboratory results indicated an AST of 105 U/L and an ALT of 51 U/L. The laboratory results were repeated one month later, and the AST and ALT were still elevated. A creatine kinase was 85 U/L. Additional testing was as follows: anti-HCV, HBsAg, serum iron, TIBC, ferritin, ceruloplasmin, and serum protein electrophoresis, which were all normal. The patient is not on any medication. Of the following, what is most likely to reveal the underlying cause of his elevated AST and ALT?

A. CT scan of the head

B. Antimitochondrial antibody testing

C. Family history

D. Social history

E. Ultrasound of the liver

Liver

19. A 42-year-old male is being evaluated by his family physician. Initial laboratory results indicated an AST of 78 U/L and an ALT of 64 U/L. The laboratory results were repeated one month later, and the AST and ALT were still elevated. A creatine kinase was normal. Additional test performed and results were as follows: anti-HCV, HBsAg, ceruloplasmin, and SPEP, which were all normal. Results of a third round of tests were serum iron of 201 µg/dL, ferritin of 289 ng/mL, and transferrin saturation of 53%. The patient is not on any medication, and he reportedly drinks about 1 to 2 beers per week socially with friends. Of the following, what test would most likely confirm his diagnosis?

A. Mutation analysis of *HFE* gene

B. Testing for *AAT* gene mutation

C. Testing for Factor V Leiden

D. Anti-neutrophil cytoplasmic antibody testing

E. Anti-DNAse II antibody testing

Liver

20. Given the previous clinical scenario, which of the following is a complication of the disease process?

A. Kidney stones

B. Gallstones

C. Intracerebral hemorrhage

D. Diabetes mellitus

E. Emphysema

Liver, pancreas

21. Given the previous clinical scenario, if the patient undergoes a liver biopsy, which of the following stains is most likely to be positive?

A. Wright-Giemsa

B. Congo red

C. Gram

D. Prussian blue

E. Oil-red-O

Liver

22. A 24-year-old male presents to an acute care clinic, complaining of the relative sudden onset of yellowing of his skin associated with nausea, vomiting, fatigue, and muscle aches. He has no significant medical history. He works at a daycare facility and, for meals at home, frequently consumes raw oysters. A physical examination reveals jaundice, but no track marks or other signs of intravenous drug abuse. Laboratory testing reveals an AST of 1313 U/L, ALT of 1289 U/L, total bilirubin of 2.9 mg/dL, and direct bilirubin of 2.1 mg/dL. Of the following, what is his most likely diagnosis?

A. Hepatitis A infection

B. Hepatitis B infection

C. Hepatitis C infection

D. Hepatitis D infection

E. Influenza A infection

Liver

23. A 23-year-old male is being evaluated by his family physician. He has no past medical history and appears to be well-nourished. Initial laboratory results indicated an AST of 72 U/L and an ALT of 73 U/L. The laboratory results were repeated in one month, and the AST and ALT were still elevated. A creatine kinase was 44 U/L. Additional tests and the results are as follows: anti-HCV, HBsAg, and SPEP, which were all normal. An ultrasound of the liver reveals no abnormality. The serum ceruloplasmin is 17 mg/dL, and serum copper is 57 µg/dL. The patient is not on any medication, and he reportedly drinks about 1 to 2 beers per week socially with friends. Of the following, what is the most likely diagnosis?

A. Autoimmune hepatitis

B. α-1-antitrypsin deficiency

C. Rhabdomyolysis

D. Wilson's disease

E. Huntington's chorea

Liver

24. Given the previous clinical scenario, which of the following is most characteristic of his disease process?

A. It is autosomal dominant.

B. Copper accumulation in the lens can occur.

C. The mutated gene is *ATP7B*.

D. CNS involvement is rare.

E. It is associated with c-ANCA.

Liver

13.3 Diseases of the Biliary Tract—Questions

Easy	Medium	Hard

25. A 41-year-old female has been followed by a physician for several years. Originally, she presented to her primary care physician with episodes of itching. Today she is being seen for fatigue. On physical examination, her physician notes that her conjunctivae are yellow. Other than mild hypothyroidism requiring hormone replacement, she has no other significant past medical history. She has no family history of liver disease. Of the following, what is her most likely diagnosis?

A. α-1-antitrypsin deficiency

B. Galactosemia

C. Primary sclerosing cholangitis

D. Primary biliary cirrhosis

E. Chronic cholecystitis

Liver

26. Given the previous clinical scenario, which of the following is the most likely mechanism causing her disease process?

A. Alcohol toxicity

B. c-ANCA

C. Antimitochondrial antibody

D. Anti-JAK antibody

E. Anti-smooth muscle antibody

Liver

27. A 53-year-old male presents to his family physician with complaints of fever, chills, and abdominal pain. He reports that he has had past episodes of a similar nature, but has not chosen to seek treatment. He has a past medical history of ulcerative colitis and had a colectomy 5 years ago for Stage I colonic adenocarcinoma, which has been in remission. An ERCP reveals strictures in the extrahepatic bile ducts. Of the following, what is the most likely diagnosis?

A. Choledocholithiasis

B. Metastatic colonic adenocarcinoma

C. Pancreatic adenocarcinoma

D. Primary sclerosing cholangitis

E. Budd-Chiari syndrome

Liver

28. Given the previous clinical scenario, of the following, what antibody is often associated with this disease?

A. c-ANCA

B. p-ANCA

C. Antimitochondrial antibody

D. Anti–smooth muscle antibody

E. Anti-gliadin antibody

Liver

29. A 42-year-old female presents to her family physician complaining of abdominal pain. She states that she has had the pain on and off for about 1 year. The pain usually comes on after a meal, increases in intensity for a few minutes and then subsides after about an hour or two. Occasionally, she feels nauseated. She has been married for 20 years, and has five children. Her vital signs are a temperature of 98.7°F, blood pressure of 132/82 mm Hg, and pulse of 82 bpm. A physical examination reveals her to be obese (weight of 230 lbs). Her conjunctivae are not discolored. Her chest is clear to auscultation, and the heart has a regular rate and rhythm. Abdominal examination reveals vague right upper quadrant abdominal pain. Of the following, what is the most likely diagnosis?

A. Viral hepatitis

B. Chronic cholecystitis

C. Acute appendicitis

D. Metastatic ovarian surface epithelial carcinoma

E. Ascending acute cholangitis

Gallbladder

30. Given the previous clinical scenario, of the following, what is a possible complication of her presenting disease process?

A. Small bowel obstruction

B. Hepatocellular carcinoma

C. Peptic ulcer of the duodenum

D. Focal nodular hyperplasia

E. Acute appendicitis

Gallbladder

31. Given the previous clinical scenario, pathologic examination of the affected organ would reveal which of the following?

A. Epithelium down-pouching into the muscularis

B. Extensive neutrophilic infiltrate in the wall

C. Invasive neoplastic glandular epithelium

D. Extensive eosinophilic infiltrate in the wall

E. Squamous metaplasia of the epithelium

Gallbladder

32. A 66-year-old male presents to his family physician with complaints of itching, pale-colored stool, and fatigue. He has been recently diagnosed with a follicular lymphoma. Physical examination reveals yellow discoloration of the conjunctivae. Laboratory testing reveals a hemoglobin of 10 g/dL. Of the following, which test would be elevated?

A. AST

B. ALT

C. Alkaline phosphatase

D. Total bilirubin

E. Direct bilirubin

Liver

33. A 43-year-old male presents to an acute care clinic because of yellowing of his eyes. Laboratory testing reveals a total bilirubin of 3.5 mg/dL, and the direct bilirubin is 0.2 mg/dL. A urine dipstick reveals no bilirubin. Of the following, what would a biopsy of the liver most likely reveal?

A. Portal tract lymphocytic invasion

B. Fibrous bridging between portal tracts

C. Necrosis of hepatocytes

D. Increased iron

E. Normal parenchyma

Liver

34. A 40-year old female presents to an acute care clinic with complaints of pain on the upper right side of her abdomen and slight yellowing of her eyes. Review of her systems indicates that she has had similar episodes of similar pain in the past, but none accompanied by yellowing of the eyes. Laboratory testing reveals an AST of 40 U/L, an ALT of 28 U/L, and an alkaline phosphatase of 512 U/L. An abdominal ultrasound reveals dilated extrahepatic bile ducts. Of the following, what is the most likely diagnosis?

A. Cirrhosis of the liver

B. Autoimmune hepatitis

C. Choledocholithiasis

D. Duodenal ulcer

E. Ovarian neoplasm

Gallbladder, liver

35. A 35-year-old male with a history of ulcerative colitis presents to an acute care clinic. In the last three weeks he has twice had a fever, up to 100°F, accompanied by chills, abdominal pain, and some yellow discoloration of his eyes. He is still in the third episode. A physical examination reveals scleral icterus. Laboratory testing reveals an AST of 24 U/L, ALT of 19 U/L, total bilirubin of 2.3 mg/dL, direct bilirubin of 1.8 mg/dL, and alkaline phosphatase of 329 mg/dL. An ultrasound reveals dilated bile ducts. He has no history of gallstones or alcohol use, other than social consumption of a few beers each month. Of the following, what is the most likely diagnosis?

A. Gilbert's syndrome

B. α-1-antritrypsin deficiency

C. Viral hepatitis

D. Warm autoimmune hemolytic anemia

E. Primary sclerosing cholangitis

Liver

36. Given the previous clinical scenario, of the following, what would a liver biopsy reveal?

A. Centrilobular lymphocyte infiltration

B. Granulomatous inflammation of the portal tracts

C. Fibrosis around the bile ducts in the portal tracts

D. Fibrous scarring of hepatic parenchyma forming nodules

E. Eosinophilic infiltrate of the portal tracts

Liver

37. A 41-year-old obese female presents to an acute care clinic with complaints of pain on the right side of her abdomen that started suddenly a few hours ago and has been increasing in severity. She also reports that she is nauseated and has vomited three times. She does not smoke, uses alcohol only occasionally, and does not use IV drugs. She has been married for 20 years and has five children. Her only past medical history is a fractured right radius during childhood. She has had no surgeries. Her vital signs are a temperature of 99.3°F, pulse of 109 bpm, and blood pressure of 131/81 mm Hg. Physical examination reveals slight scleral icterus. Of the following, what is the most likely diagnosis?

A. Acute hepatitis

B. Acute appendicitis

C. Intestinal obstruction

D. Acute calculous cholecystitis

E. Acquired pyloric stenosis

Gallbladder

38. Given the previous clinical scenario, on physical examination, the doctor palpates her right upper quadrant, which causes her to stop breathing. What is the term for this physical finding?

A. Courvoisier's sign

B. Murphy's sign

C. Chvostek's sign

D. Guarding

E. Homans' sign

Gallbladder

39. A 37-year-old female presents to her physician with complaints of abdominal pain. She is subsequently diagnosed with chronic cholecystitis, and her gallbladder is removed surgically. The pathologist examining the gallbladder identifies multiple small black stones in her gallbladder. Of the following, what underlying condition/factor did she most likely have?

A. Acute hepatitis

B. Multiple live born children

C. Hemolytic anemia

D. Acute pancreatitis

E. Hodgkin's lymphoma

Gallbladder

13.4 Miscellaneous Liver Disease—Questions

Easy	Medium	Hard

40. A pathologist is examining a section of a liver from an autopsy and notes that the centrilobular hepatocytes are eosinophilic and that nuclei are not visible, especially when compared to the more basophilic hepatocytes in the area around the portal tracts. Of the following, which is the most likely etiology for this change?

A. Alcohol binge

B. Recent hepatitis C infection

C. Delayed hospital death from aortic dissection

D. Immediate hospital death from pulmonary thromboembolus

E. Iron overload from repeat transfusions

Liver

41. A 19-year-old female is found unresponsive by her parents in her bedroom. 9-1-1 is called. On arrival to the hospital, she is comatose. Her parents report that she was doing fine yesterday morning, but that she wanted to stay in her room and study all day for an upcoming test, to forget about her boyfriend breaking up with her. The family reports that she has no underlying medical conditions that they know of. Despite medical care, she dies two days later and an autopsy is performed. Of the following, what will most likely be identified at autopsy?

A. Massive hepatic necrosis

B. Coronary artery dissection

C. Ruptured hepatic hemangioma

D. Acute pancreatitis

E. Ruptured berry aneurysm

Liver

42. A female laboratory worker at a state crime lab has her yearly testing for hepatitis B and C and also has a complete blood cell count, a liver panel, and a kidney panel (with 20 total tests performed). Her AST is slightly elevated at 45 U/L. She has no medical background and goes to the medical examiner to consult in private. Of the following, what should the ME say?

A. I suspect hepatitis, I recommend a viral panel.

B. I suspect alcohol-related injury, I suggest no binge drinking on the weekend.

C. I suspect chronic cholecystitis, I recommend an ultrasound.

D. I suspect a hereditary abnormality; I would have your children tested as well.

E. The reference range only covers 95% of individuals, do not worry.

Liver

43. A 37-year-old white female presents to an acute care clinic. Over the past week, she has developed abdominal pain and noticed that the whites of her eyes and skin are yellow. She also has fatigue and malaise. Her past medical history includes Hashimoto's thyroiditis, for which she takes hormone replacement. Her vital signs are a temperature of 98.6°F, pulse of 74 bpm, and blood pressure of 101/67 mm Hg. Physical examination reveals mild hepatomegaly and scleral icterus. Laboratory testing reveals ALT of 430 U/L, AST of 389 U/L, total bilirubin of 6.7 mg/dL, and direct bilirubin of 2.3 mg/dL. The physician also orders serum IgG, which is 2,130 mg/dL. She reports no alcohol use or intravenous drug use. Of the following, what is the most likely diagnosis?

A. Alcoholic hepatitis

B. Acute sclerosing cholangitis

C. Autoimmune hepatitis

D. Acute cholecystitis

E. Hepatic lymphoma

Liver

44. Given the previous clinical scenario, of the following, what is true regarding the presenting condition?

A. It is more common in males than females.

B. The most common cause is alcohol use.

C. It is likely to progress to cirrhosis.

D. The prominent histologic feature is granulomas.

E. It is most common in Northern Europeans.

Liver

45. Given the previous clinical scenario, of the following, what laboratory test is likely to be positive?

A. Anticentromere antibodies

B. Anti–cyclic citrullinated peptide antibodies

C. Anti-Jo-1 antibodies

D. Anti-liver, kidney microsome 1 antibodies

E. Anti–topoisomerase I antibodies

Liver

Liver

46. A 28-year-old female is found unresponsive in her bedroom by her parents, with whom she lives. An ambulance is called, and she is taken to the emergency room. In the emergency room, she is not responsive to questions and only slightly responsive to a sternal rub. Laboratory testing reveals an AST of 3,180 U/L and an ALT of 2,956 U/L. Her parents report that she has no significant past medical history, other than depression treated with paroxetine. She had an uneventful day, the day previously. Of the following tests, which is most likely to identify the cause of her current state?

A. A CT scan of the head

B. Bronchoscopy with culture

C. Serum toxicology testing

D. Pelvic exam with culture for group B streptococcus

E. CT angiogram of the coronary arteries

Liver

47. Given the previous clinical scenario, of the following, what would a histologic examination of the liver most likely reveal?

A. Marked neutrophilic infiltrate and Mallory's hyaline

B. Marked sinusoidal congestion

C. Extensive centrilobular necrosis

D. Infiltrating tumor cells

E. Fungal hyphae

Liver

48. A 62-year-old male is seen in the emergency room. His laboratory testing reveals an AST of 120 U/L, an ALT of 27 U/L, and a creatine kinase of 305 U/L. Which of the following conditions would be most expected to cause this pattern of laboratory abnormalities?

A. Hepatitis A

B. Hepatitis C

C. Acute myocardial infarct

D. Colonic adenocarcinoma

E. Encephalitis

Heart

49. A 73-year-old female who is on warfarin for a mechanical heart valve, implanted to treat degenerative calcified aortic stenosis, falls and sustains a large hematoma of her left buttocks and thigh, extending from just above her left hip to just above her left knee. Of the following, what laboratory test would be most likely to be elevated in the following few weeks?

A. Hemoglobin

B. Direct bilirubin

C. Total bilirubin

D. Albumin

E. ALT

Liver

50. A 52-year-old male has complaints of fatigue and yellowing of his eyes. His past medical history includes hypertension, treated with an ACE inhibitor, and gout. A physical examination reveals pallor of the conjunctivae. Laboratory testing reveals AST of 24 U/L, ALT of 17 U/L, total bilirubin of 3.2 mg/dL, and direct bilirubin of 0.2 mg/dL. A urine dipstick is negative for glucose, ketones, hemoglobin, and bilirubin. A complete blood count reveals a hemoglobin of 9.1 g/dL. A Coombs test is positive. Of the following, what is the most likely diagnosis?

A. ABO incompatible blood transfusion

B. Warm autoimmune hemolytic anemia

C. Cold autoimmune hemolytic anemia

D. Hereditary spherocytosis

E. Polycythemia

Red blood cells

51. Given the previous clinical scenario, of the following, which statement is correct regarding his disease process?

A. I and i antigens on red blood cells are the target for antibodies.

B. P antigen on red blood cells is the target for antibodies.

C. It frequently occurs after a *Mycoplasma pneumoniae* infection.

D. It occurs in patients with a B-cell lymphoma.

E. The urine can have hemosiderin.

Red blood cells

52. A 52-year-old male presents to his family physician with complaints of vague abdominal pain and a sensation of fullness. A CT scan of the abdomen reveals a mass in the right upper quadrant. The patient is scheduled for resection, and a pathologist examining the tumor identifies it as being derived from bile ducts. Of the following, which is a characteristic of this tumor?

A. It rarely occurs in association with cirrhosis.

B. It has an excellent prognosis.

C. It frequently produces an elevation of α-fetoprotein.

D. One complication of ulcerative colitis is a significant risk factor for the tumor.

E. One complication of peptic ulcers is a significant risk factor for the tumor.

Liver

187

53. A 23-year-old pregnant female presents to the emergency room complaining of pain in the upper portion of the right side of her abdomen. Physical examination reveals a fluid wave and hepatomegaly, with her liver palpable 6 cm below the costal margin. Laboratory testing reveals an AST of 213 U/L, ALT of 178 U/L, and alkaline phosphatase of 52 mg/dL. A complete blood count reveals a hemoglobin of 13.4 mg/dL and a platelet count of 224×10^3 cells/µL. Of the following, what is the most likely diagnosis?

A. Placenta accreta

B. HELLP syndrome

C. Budd-Chiari syndrome

D. Acetaminophen toxicity

E. Hepatocellular carcinoma

Liver

54. A patient was twice identified to have an elevated alkaline phosphatase, both times around 290 mg/dL. A GGT was 110 U/L. An ultrasound of the abdomen revealed no masses. Of the following, what is the most likely diagnosis?

A. Paget's disease

B. Celiac disease

C. Metastatic colonic adenocarcinoma

D. Placenta accreta

E. Wernicke's encephalopathy

Liver

13.5 Cirrhosis and its Complications—Answers and Explanations

Easy	Medium	Hard

1. Correct: Esophageal varices (B)

With the history of alcoholism and IV drug use, the patient has two main risk factors for cirrhosis, and the fluid wave is a physical examination consistent with ascites, which also supports a diagnosis of cirrhosis. One complication of cirrhosis is esophageal varices, which can rupture and cause a GI bleed (**B**). Esophageal carcinomas can cause bleeding and do occur in alcoholics, but they would be a less common cause of massive bleeding and not as common in alcoholics as cirrhosis, and he has no other risk factors for esophageal carcinoma (**A**). With no history of vomiting, a Mallory-Weiss is unlikely (**C**). Neither a peptic ulcer nor a fistula between the common bile duct and small intestine would cause ascites (**D, E**).

2. Correct: Hepatocellular carcinoma (D)

Cirrhosis of the liver is a risk factor for hepatocellular carcinoma. In adults, hepatocellular carcinoma rarely occurs without the background of cirrhosis (**D**). Cirrhosis itself does not increase the risk for any of the other tumors or conditions. (**A-C, E**).

3. Correct: Chronic alcohol use (A)

The patient has signs and symptoms consistent with cirrhosis: spider angiomas, jaundice, and a fluid wave indicating ascites. The most common cause of cirrhosis is chronic alcoholism. Although a relatively small number of chronic alcoholics develop cirrhosis, chronic alcoholism is a very common condition (**A**). Both obstruction of bile ducts and congestive heart failure are causes of cirrhosis, but less commonly a cause than alcohol use (**B, C**). Inflammation of the pancreas and excessive alcohol consumption are not associated with cirrhosis (**D, E**)

4. Correct: Mallory's hyaline (C)

The patient has signs and symptoms consistent with cirrhosis: spider angiomas, jaundice, and a fluid wave indicating ascites. The most common cause of cirrhosis is chronic alcoholism. Of the choices, the microscopic finding most commonly associated with alcoholic liver disease is Mallory's hyaline (**C**). Asteroid bodies are found in giant cells and associated with sarcoidosis (**A**). Bile lakes are found in people with bile duct obstruction (**E**). Howell-Jolly bodies are not found in the liver, and targetoid lesions of the bile ducts are not associated with alcohol use (**D, E**).

5. Correct: Spontaneous bacterial peritonitis (D)

Patients with cirrhosis can develop an infection of the ascitic fluid, which is referred to as spontaneous bacterial peritonitis (**D**). The other conditions are not by themselves normally associated with a significant amount of infected intra-abdominal fluid (**A-C, E**).

6. Correct: Albumin (D)

The history and physical examination are consistent with the diagnosis of ascites. Ascites develops due to increased hydrostatic pressure in the abdominal vasculature caused by portal hypertension, which develops due to the cirrhosis, and also due to decreased plasma oncotic pressure, due to decreased production of albumin by the liver. Although the other tests may have abnormal concentrations detected on laboratory testing of a patient with cirrhosis, they are not the direct cause of the increased fluid volume in the peritoneal cavity (**A-C, E**).

7. Correct: Hepatocellular carcinoma (C)

Given the history, the patient most likely has cirrhosis of the liver, and has developed a hepatocellular carcinoma. α-fetoprotein is often elevated in patients with hepatocellular carcinoma, but it is not specific, also being seen in acute and chronic liver disease; however, the ultrasound confirms a mass (**C**). Liver metastases can cause an elevated α-fetoprotein; however, given there is a solitary mass and the stool occult blood test is negative, metastatic colonic adenocarcinoma is not likely (**D**). Cavernous hemangiomas and focal nodular hyperplasia would occur as a single mass in the liver but are not commonly associated with an increased α-fetoprotein (**A, B**). Hepatoblastomas occur in children (**E**).

8. Correct: Portal vein invasion with resultant thrombosis is a complication. (D)

Given the clinical scenario (risk factors of chronic alcoholism and hepatitis C infection, elevated AST and ALT and α-fetoprotein, and mass), this patient most likely has cirrhosis of the liver and has developed hepatocellular carcinoma (in adults, hepatocellular carcinoma essentially always occurs in the background of cirrhosis). A central scar is characteristic of focal nodular hyperplasia (**A**), exposure to vinyl chloride is a known risk factor for angiosarcoma (**B**), hepatic adenomas are associated with use of oral contraceptives, and use of corticosteroids is not a commonly recognized risk factor for hepatocellular carcinoma (**C**). Patients are not necessarily likely to develop a warm autoimmune hemolytic anemia, as these anemias are most likely to develop in people with an abnormal immune response (e.g., SLE, lymphoma) (**E**). Hepatocellular carcinomas are well known for invasion of the portal vein (**D**).

9. Correct: Rupture of a dilated vein (C)

Given the clinical history of chronic alcoholism and hepatitis C infection, the patient most likely has cirrhosis of the liver, which has caused the development of esophageal varices. Rupture of esophageal varices is a common cause of death in individuals with cirrhosis. The rupture site is not easily tamponaded, and patients with cirrhosis of the liver may have decreased concentrations of clotting factors, causing them to bleed even more easily (**C**). Although alcoholics can tear the esophagus (and hemorrhage), which is a Mallory-Weiss tear, the hemorrhage is preceded by prolonged vomiting (**B**). Any of the other choices, with the exception of acute alcohol toxicity, could also potentially cause an individual to vomit blood, but none would be as common in an alcoholic as ruptured esophageal varices (e.g., trauma or hemorrhage from neoplasm), nor necessarily as likely to bleed as much (**A, D-E**).

10. Correct: Portal hypertension (C)

Based on the clinical scenario, the patient most likely has cirrhosis of the liver, due to alcohol use and hepatitis C infection, and has developed esophageal varices, which are bleeding. Esophageal varices develop due to portal hypertension. The increased pressure in the portal system shunts blood back to the heart through other routes, including veins in the esophagus (producing varices), the body wall (producing caput medusae), and the anal region (producing hemorrhoids) (**C**). The other mechanisms listed do not contribute to the development of esophageal varices (**A-B, D-E**). Increased hydrostatic pressure does contribute to the development of ascites.

13.6 Viral, Alcohol, and Metabolic Liver Disease—Answers and Explanations

Easy	Medium	Hard

11. Correct: Alcoholic hepatitis (B)

The individual has laboratory evidence of liver damage, with elevated AST, ALT, GGT, and alkaline phosphatase. The AST:ALT ratio is around 6:1, which is most characteristic of an alcoholic hepatitis (**B**). Other forms of liver disorder have a lower ratio (**A, C-E**).

12. Correct: Gilbert's syndrome (A)

Gilbert's syndrome causes an unconjugated bilirubinemia, which could be manifested by the elevated total bilirubin but normal direct bilirubin concentrations (**A**). Dubin-Johnson and Rotor's syndrome cause a conjugated bilirubinemia, and there may be bilirubin in the urine (**C-D**). Crigler-Najjar would not be asymptomatic, and the total bilirubin should be more elevated (**B**). Given the lack of elevation of AST and ALT, acute viral hepatitis is not likely (**E**).

13. Correct: Dubin-Johnson syndrome (C)

Dubin-Johnson and Rotor's syndrome cause an asymptomatic conjugated hyperbilirubinemia, which is exhibited by the elevated total bilirubin and elevated direct bilirubin (**C**). Dubin-Johnson syndrome is autosomal recessive. The condition results from impaired excretion of conjugated bilirubin. The liver is black due to a melanin-like substance in the cells. This diagnosis requires biopsy. Rotor's syndrome presents in a similar fashion to Dubin-Johnson, with similar lab testing, but without a pigmented liver. The clinical scenario is not consistent with the other choices (**A-B, D-E**).

14. Correct: HBsAg (B)

To develop an infection with hepatitis D virus, a patient must be coinfected with hepatitis B. Anti-HBs is not a confirmation of infection with the hepatitis B virus, as those people who have been vaccinated have anti-HBs (**C**). Anti-HCV and anti–smooth muscle antibody can indicate other reasons for liver disease but are not risk factors for infection with the hepatitis D virus (**A, E**). Testing for serum ferritin is not related to the evaluation of hepatitis D (**D**).

189

15. Correct: PAS-positive globules in the hepatocytes (A)

The patient has testing indicative of an obstructive lung disease, combined with evidence of liver damage. The combination of emphysema and cirrhosis occurs in patients with α-1-antitrypsin deficiency. The portal lymphocytic infiltrate associated with bile duct damage would be seen in primary biliary cirrhosis, which does not normally affect the lungs (**B**). Mallory's hyaline is seen in alcoholic liver disease, which does not normally affect the lungs (**D**). Scattered enlarged cells with intranuclear inclusions is consistent with CMV infection, which she tested negative for (**E**). Patients with α-1-antitrypsin deficiency will have PAS-positive, diastase-resistant globules in the hepatocytes, evidence of accumulation of the abnormal protein (**A**). Cholestasis occurs in a variety of conditions but is not characteristic for α-1-antitrypsin deficiency (**C**).

16. Correct: Body mass index of 36 kg/m² (D)

The persistently elevated AST and ALT must be explained. The battery of tests essentially rules out hepatitis B and C, hemochromatosis, Wilson's disease, autoimmune hepatitis, and α-1-antitrypsin deficiency. The history does not indicate medication use or alcohol consumption as a cause. The biopsy is consistent with nonalcoholic steatohepatitis, which can be seen most commonly in diabetes mellitus and obesity (**D**). None of the other signs would be expected on physical examination (**A-C, E**).

17. Correct: Anti–smooth muscle antibodies (A)

Given the presentation, a young woman with elevated AST and ALT, with no risk for medication or alcohol being the cause, autoimmune hepatitis is one consideration. Patients with autoimmune hepatitis will often have a hypergammaglobulinemia, which can cause an SPEP (serum protein electrophoresis) to have an increased amount of protein in the γ region. Patients with autoimmune hepatitis can have positive serologic testing for ANAs, anti-liver/kidney microsomal antibodies, and anti–smooth muscle antibodies (**A**). Anti-tissue transglutaminase antibodies are characteristic of celiac disease, which can present with an elevated AST and ALT, but would not have an abnormal SPEP (**B**). Autoimmune hepatitis would not cause an elevated serum glucose (**C**), and serologic testing for CMV and an X-ray of the skull would be negative (**D, E**).

18. Correct: Social history (D)

An elevated AST and ALT can be caused by a variety of conditions. When the AST/ALT ratio is 2:1, although not specific for, the finding is characteristic for alcohol-related liver disease. The creatine kinase indicates that the AST and ALT elevation was not muscular in origin. The laboratory tests rule out hepatitis B and C, hemochromatosis, Wilson's disease, and α-1-antitrypsin deficiency and, given the scenario, autoimmune hepatitis. In patients with an elevated AST and ALT, social history to include the amount of alcohol used is important (**D**). The most likely cause of an elevated AST and ALT when other causes have been ruled out would be alcohol use; although (**B-C, E**) could identify possible conditions of the liver, alcohol use would be most likely. A CT scan of the head would not be useful in determining this patient's underlying medical condition (**A**).

19. Correct: Mutation analysis of the *HFE* gene (A)

Hemochromatosis is a cause of elevated AST and ALT. With additional laboratory testing, elevated serum iron, elevated ferritin, and increased transferrin saturation would be identified, and the diagnosis of hemochromatosis confirmed via genetic analysis (**A**). Although α-1-antitrypsin is a cause of increased AST and ALT, the disease would not cause an increased serum iron, ferritin, or transferrin saturation (**B**). Also, the serum protein electrophoresis would have an increased amount of protein. The clinical scenario does not fit with a clotting disorder (**C**), a vasculitis that is positive for c-ANCA, most likely granulomatosis with polyangiitis or p-ANCA, possibly microscopic polyarteritis (**D**), or a defect associated with an antibody against DNAse II (**E**).

20. Correct: Diabetes mellitus (D)

Given the laboratory testing, specifically the elevated AST and ALT and elevated ferritin, serum iron, and transferrin saturation, and the other tests and clinical history being noncontributory, the most likely diagnosis is hemochromatosis. Hemochromatosis is a risk factor for cirrhosis of the liver, cardiomyopathy (variably described as causing either a dilated cardiomyopathy, a restrictive cardiomyopathy, or both), and diabetes mellitus (**D**). These changes are due to iron accumulation in the liver, heart, and pancreas. The other conditions listed are not routinely associated with hemochromatosis (**A-C, E**).

21. Correct: Prussian blue (D)

Given the laboratory testing, the most likely diagnosis is hemochromatosis. Patients with hemochromatosis develop complications due to organ damage from accumulated iron. The organs damaged include the heart, liver, and pancreas. A Prussian blue would stain the iron (**D**). A Wright-Giemsa stain is used for blood and bone marrow smears (**A**), a Congo red will stain amyloid (**B**), a Gram stain is for bacteria (**C**), and an oil-red-O stain is for fat (**E**).

22. Correct: Hepatitis A infection (A)

The clinical scenario (nausea, vomiting, fatigue, myalgia, jaundice, and elevated concentrations of AST, ALT, and conjugated bilirubin) is consistent with acute viral hepatitis. The only risk factors listed—history of eating raw oysters and working at a daycare facility—are most consistent with a hepatitis A infection (**A**). Although hepatitis B and C are possible, the clinical scenario best indicates hepatitis A (**B, C**). Hepatitis D only occurs in a coinfection with hepatitis B (**D**). The degree of liver damage as evidenced by the laboratory testing would not be usual for an influenza A infection (**E**).

23. Correct: Wilson's disease (D)

The clinical scenario, given the elevated liver enzymes and decreased serum ceruloplasmin and serum copper, is consistent with Wilson's disease (**D**). Decreased serum ceruloplasmin can also occur in fulminant hepatitis, malnutrition, and malabsorption, and malnutrition and other conditions can lead to decreased serum copper; however, of the listed conditions, the diagnosis of Wilson's disease is the most appropriate (**A-C, E**).

24. Correct: The mutated gene is *ATP7B*. (C)

The clinical scenario, given the elevated liver enzymes and decreased serum ceruloplasmin and serum copper, is consistent with Wilson's disease. Wilson's disease is autosomal recessive (**A**), with the *ATP7B* gene having the mutation (**C**). Copper accumulation in the cornea does occur (producing Keyser-Fleischer rings) (**B**), and CNS involvement is common with patients developing psychiatric symptoms (**D**), and extrapyramidal signs due to involvement of the basal ganglia. The disease is not associated with c-ANCA (**E**).

13.7 Diseases of the Biliary Tract—Answers and Explanations

| Easy | Medium | Hard |

25. Correct: Primary biliary cirrhosis (D)

Primary biliary cirrhosis is most common in middle-aged females, and patients will often present with pruritus due to cholestasis, which can evolve to cirrhosis of the liver (**D**). Jaundice is a sign of liver failure, and thus, among the choices, α-1-antitrypsin and galactosemia could cause fatigue, but they are not commonly associated with pruritus; also, galactosemia would affect younger ages (**A, B**). Although biliary cirrhosis can be secondary to gallstones in the bile duct (choledocholithiasis), stones present in the gallbladder itself (cholelithiasis) would not (**E**). Primary sclerosing cholangitis is associated with ulcerative colitis (**C**).

26. Correct: Antimitochondrial antibody (C)

Primary biliary cirrhosis is most common in middle-aged females, and patients will often present with pruritus (due to cholestasis), which can evolve to cirrhosis of the liver, which is associated with jaundice. Given the clinical scenario, primary biliary cirrhosis is a likely diagnosis, and this condition is associated with antimitochondrial antibodies (**C**). Although JAK is a signaling protein, there is no disease commonly associated with an antibody against it (**D**). Anti–smooth muscle antibodies are associated with autoimmune hepatitis (**E**). Pruritus would not be common in alcohol-induced liver damage (**A**), and c-ANCA associated with granulomatosis with polyangiitis is not associated with liver damage (**B**).

27. Correct: Primary sclerosing cholangitis (D)

The signs, symptoms, and history, combined with the results of the ERCP, are most consistent with primary sclerosing cholangitis (**D**). Choledocholithiasis would not normally produce multiple strictures of the bile ducts but could cause a focal obstruction of the bile ducts (**A**). Budd-Chiari syndrome is thrombosis of the hepatic veins (**E**). A metastatic colonic adenocarcinoma and potentially pancreatic adenocarcinoma could produce a stricture of an extrahepatic bile duct depending on its position but would not likely produce multiple strictures. Also, given the extended history of past episodes of the presenting symptoms, an aggressive neoplasm is unlikely (**B, C**).

28. Correct: p-ANCA (B)

The signs, symptoms, and history, combined with the results of the ERCP, are most consistent with primary sclerosing cholangitis. p-ANCA is associated with primary sclerosing cholangitis (**B**). c-ANCA is associated with granulomatosis with polyangiitis (**A**). Antimitochondrial antibody is associated with primary biliary cirrhosis (**C**). Anti–smooth muscle antibody is associated with autoimmune hepatitis, which is more common in females than males and is often associated with another autoimmune disorder (**D**). Anti-gliadin antibody is found in celiac disease (**E**).

29. Correct: Chronic cholecystitis (B)

This patient has signs and symptoms and risk factors consistent with chronic cholecystitis (right upper quadrant pain, female, obesity, multiple children, age) (**B**). She has no risk factors for viral hepatitis (**A**), and given the chronic nature of the problem, acute appendicitis and ascending acute cholangitis are not consistent (**C, E**). While metastatic ovarian surface epithelial carcinoma could present with abdominal pain, it would not likely be consistently after meals, and this condition would be uncommon compared to chronic cholecystitis (**D**).

30. Correct: Small bowel obstruction (A)

This patient has signs and symptoms and risk factors consistent with chronic cholecystitis (right upper quadrant pain, female, obesity, multiple children, age). One complication of chronic cholecystitis is a choledochoduodenal fistula, formed between the bile duct and the duodenum. If a gallstone enters the small intestine, it is possible for it to produce an obstruction (**A**). Chronic cholecystitis is not a risk factor for the other conditions (**B-E**).

191

31. Correct: Epithelium down-pouching into the muscularis (A)

This patient has signs, symptoms, and risk factors consistent with chronic cholecystitis (right upper quadrant pain, female, obesity, multiple children, age). Histologically, chronic cholecystitis is characterized by down-pouching of the epithelium into the muscularis, referred to as Rokitansky-Aschoff sinuses (**A**). The clinical features are not consistent with an acute inflammatory process such as acute cholecystitis (**B, D**). Squamous metaplasia is not a common finding in chronic cholecystitis or in the gallbladder in general (**E**), and, while an adenocarcinoma of the gallbladder could present similar to chronic cholecystitis, its incidence is much less common (**C**).

32. Correct: Total bilirubin (D)

The patient has anemia, most likely a warm autoimmune hemolytic anemia secondary to the follicular lymphoma. In patients with a hemolytic anemia, the amount of unconjugated bilirubin is elevated; therefore total bilirubin is elevated (**D**). The amount of conjugated hemoglobin is not increased, so direct bilirubin is not elevated (**E**). As there is no evidence of liver or gallbladder disease, AST, ALT, and alkaline phosphatase are not elevated (**A-C**).

33. Correct: Normal parenchyma (E)

The laboratory testing is consistent with an unconjugated hyperbilirubinemia, which can be due to hemolysis or abnormalities of liver conjugating enzymes among a few other causes; however, the liver biopsy would always be essentially negative (**E**). All of the other descriptions—hepatitis (**A**), cirrhosis (**B**), ischemic injury (**C**), and hemochromatosis (**D**)— would have a conjugated hyperbilirubinemia. With unconjugated hyperbilirubinemia, the urine dipstick is negative for bilirubin, whereas in a conjugated hyperbilirubinemia it can be positive.

34. Correct: Choledocholithiasis (C)

A duodenal ulcer would normally cause pain on the left side of the upper abdomen and is not usually associated with an increased alkaline phosphatase (**D**). Both autoimmune hepatitis and cirrhosis would be expected to have higher elevations of AST and ALT in comparison to alkaline phosphatase, when this patient has the opposite (**A, B**). Choledocholithiasis could present with jaundice due to obstruction and result in an elevated alkaline phosphatase, which is out of proportion to the increases in AST and ALT (**C**). The past episodes of abdominal pain are most likely due to cholelithiasis and chronic cholecystitis. An ovarian neoplasm would not, with rare exception, cause dilated extrahepatic bile ducts (**E**).

35. Correct: Primary sclerosing cholangitis (E)

The laboratory results are consistent with an extrahepatic cholestasis. The finding of an elevated conjugated bilirubin is inconsistent with Gilbert's syndrome and warm autoimmune hemolytic anemia, which would cause an increased unconjugated bilirubin (**A, D**). The finding of normal AST and ALT in association with an increased alkaline phosphatase is consistent with a cholestatic process and not a hepatocellular process, ruling out α-1-antitrypsin deficiency and viral hepatitis (**B, C**). Primary sclerosing cholangitis is commonly associated with ulcerative colitis (**E**).

36. Correct: Fibrosis around the bile ducts in the portal tracts (C)

In a patient with ulcerative colitis, the presenting symptoms and laboratory findings are consistent with primary sclerosing cholangitis. The histologic feature of primary sclerosing cholangitis is fibrosis around bile ducts in the portal tract (**C**). There can also be strictures of the extrahepatic bile ducts, producing a beaded appearance when an ERCP is performed. Some granulomatous inflammation of the portal tracts can be seen in primary biliary cirrhosis and is associated with a lymphocytic infiltrate (**B**). Fibrous scarring of the hepatic parenchyma forming nodules is cirrhosis of the liver (**D**). The other two features do not describe a specific disease entity (**A, E**).

37. Correct: Acute calculous cholecystitis (D)

This patient has four risk factors for gallstones: female sex, greater than age 40 years, five children (i.e., fertile), and obesity. Right upper quadrant pain that is sudden in onset and increases in severity is the choice characteristic for acute calculous cholecystitis (**D**). The patient has no risk factors for hepatitis, and a sudden onset of severe pain would be less likely (**A**). She has had no surgeries, and thus her risk for intestinal obstruction, most commonly due to adhesions, is less (**C**). The pain of acute appendicitis is not normally in the right upper quadrant (**B**). Acquired pyloric stenosis is not a commonly described entity. Also, pyloric stenosis is usually congenital and presents in infants, but not with severe pain (**E**).

38. Correct: Murphy's sign (B)

When palpation of the right upper quadrant causes respiratory arrest, it is most commonly associated with acute calculous cholecystitis and is referred to as Murphy's sign (**B**). Courvoisier's sign is a palpable gallbladder, commonly associated with obstruction due to pancreatic carcinoma, but can occur due to other conditions (**A**). Chvostek's sign is related to calcium concentrations (**C**), and Homans' sign is related to deep venous thrombi (**E**). Guarding would occur in patients with peritonitis (**D**).

39. Correct: Hemolytic anemia (C)

The patient has pigment stones. The other form of gallstone is cholesterol stones, which have the risk factors of female sex, fertility, age > 40 years, and obesity (**B**). Pigment stones are composed of bilirubin and calcium salts and occur with a background of hemolysis (**C**). Acute hepatitis is not commonly indicated as a risk factor for cholelithiasis, and acute pancreatitis, while caused by cholelithiasis, is not commonly listed as a cause (**A, D**). Hodgkin's lymphoma, by itself, is not a risk factor for gallstones (**E**).

13.8 Miscellaneous Liver Disease—Answers and Explanations

Easy	Medium	Hard

40. Correct: Delayed hospital death from aortic dissection (C)

The description is that of coagulative necrosis. In the liver, blood flows from the portal tract to the central veins, and thus these hepatocytes are the last to receive oxygenated blood and are at most risk for ischemic injury. In a low-flow state, such as would occur with an aortic dissection, these hepatocytes become ischemic and, given enough time for histologic changes to develop, will manifest coagulative necrosis (**C**). None of the other conditions listed would produce this change (**A-B, D-E**).

41. Correct: Massive hepatic necrosis (A)

Given the scenario, a suicide is a very likely possibility. When Tylenol (acetaminophen) is used to commit suicide, the pathologic finding is massive hepatic necrosis, with loss of around 80% or more of the hepatocytes (**A**). Although the other conditions listed could cause sudden death, the patient is not pregnant (a risk factor for coronary artery dissection) (**B**), is not an alcoholic, and does not have gallstones (risk factors for acute pancreatitis) (**C**). Both a ruptured hepatic hemangioma and ruptured berry aneurysm are possible causes of a sudden unexplained death, but a ruptured hemangioma would be very rare, and, given the lack of associated symptoms such as a headache, a ruptured aneurysm is not likely, and they are not the best fit to the clinical scenario (**C, E**)

42. Correct: The reference range only covers 95% of individuals, do not worry. (E)

The reference range for a laboratory test lists the range of values between which a given lab test is expected to fall for any particular patient; however, the reference range only covers 95% of individuals, and 5% are expected to fall outside that range. In a battery of 20 tests, it would be expected that a patient may be outside the reference range on one test (**E**). The other choices, while each could be the statement made by the consulted physician, are each not based upon an understanding of the statistical values associated with laboratory testing (**A-D**).

43. Correct: Autoimmune hepatitis (C)

Autoimmune hepatitis is a disease that occurs most commonly in females and Northern Europeans. The disease is associated with immune dysfunction (i.e., the elevated IgG concentration), and patients often have another autoimmune disorder (**C**). An elevated serum IgG would not be expected in alcoholic hepatitis (**A**). Acute sclerosing cholangitis occurs in patients with ulcerative colitis most frequently, but is not in the patient's past medical history (**B**). An elevated serum IgG would not be expected in acute cholecystitis, and the patient would be more likely to be febrile (**D**). A hepatic lymphoma would be very rare (**E**).

44. Correct: It is most common in Northern Europeans. (E)

Autoimmune hepatitis is a disease that occurs most commonly in females and Northern Europeans (**A, E**). The disease is associated with immune dysfunction (i.e., the elevated IgG concentration), and patients often have another autoimmune disorder. Because of the liver damage, ALT, AST, total bilirubin, and direct bilirubin may all be elevated. It is not likely to progress to cirrhosis, and the histologic features are lymphocytes in the portal tract (**C, D**). The condition is not associated with alcohol use (**B**).

45. Correct: Anti-liver, kidney microsome 1 antibodies (D)

Autoimmune hepatitis is a disease that occurs most commonly in females, and Northern Europeans. The disease is associated with immune dysfunction (i.e., the elevated IgG concentration), and patients often have another autoimmune disorder. Because of the liver damage, ALT, AST, total bilirubin, and direct bilirubin may all be elevated. It is not likely to progress to cirrhosis and the histologic features are lymphocytes in the portal tract. Anti-liver, kidney microsome 1 antibodies are associated with autoimmune hepatitis, as are antinuclear antibodies and anti–smooth muscle antibodies (**D**). Anticentromere antibodies are associated with systemic sclerosis (**A**), anti–cyclic citrullinated peptide antibodies are associated with rheumatoid arthritis (**B**), anti-Jo-1 antibodies are associated with polymyositis/dermatomyositis (**C**), and anti-topoisomerase I antibodies are associated with systemic sclerosis (**E**).

46. Correct: Serum toxicology testing (C)

The markedly elevated AST and ALT are most consistent with a drug or other toxic exposure, or ischemia-induced hepatic injury. Given her history of depression, absence of other medical history, and lack of other symptoms, it is highly likely that she overdosed with acetaminophen, of which a serum toxicology analysis would aid in the diagnosis (**C**). The other testing methods would not be of use (**A-B, D-E**) in directly diagnosing the cause of her unresponsiveness.

47. Correct: Extensive centrilobular necrosis (C)

The markedly elevated AST and ALT are most consistent with a drug or other toxic exposure or ischemia-induced hepatic injury. Given her history of depression, absence of other medical history, and lack of other symptoms, it is highly likely that she overdosed with acetaminophen. The liver would have extensive centrilobular necrosis (**C**). A neutrophilic infiltrate and Mallory's hyaline would be seen in alcoholic hepatitis, which is unlikely to raise the AST and ALT so markedly, and given this fact in combination with the history, it is unlikely (**A**). An incidental tumor would not raise the AST and ALT so high (**D**), and a fungal infection of a young female with no significant past medical history would be exceptionally rare (**E**). Marked sinusoidal congestion would not produce the markedly elevated AST and ALT (**B**).

48. Correct: Acute myocardial infarct (C)

An acute myocardial infarct will result in an elevation of AST and of creatine kinase (**C**). When AST is elevated and ALT is normal, the disease process causing the change is often not the liver, as AST can be found in a wide number of organs (including the heart, skeletal muscle, kidneys, and brain), and diseases of the liver will not normally produce an increase in creatine kinase (**A, B**). Neither colonic adenocarcinoma (unless it has metastases to the liver) or encephalitis would be expected to have an elevation of AST; however, encephalitis could cause an elevation of creatine kinase (**D, E**).

49. Correct: Total bilirubin (C)

With a fall resulting in a large hematoma, a large amount of blood is going to have to be broken down, similar to hemolysis. The amount of hemoglobin and resultant breakdown products produced can overwhelm the liver's ability to conjugate, and thus, the amount of unconjugated bilirubin, reflected by an increase in total bilirubin without an increase in direct bilirubin, would rise (**B, C**). If anything, the hemoglobin would be decreased (**A**), and the albumin and ALT, since the liver is otherwise healthy, should not be elevated (**D, E**).

50. Correct: Warm autoimmune hemolytic anemia (B)

The patient has evidence of hemolysis, with an elevated total bilirubin but normal direct bilirubin, indicating an increased amount of unconjugated bilirubin. The lack of hemoglobin in the urine indicates the hemolysis is not occurring intravascularly, as an ABO-incompatible blood transfusion would cause (**A**). A Coombs positive test indicates there are IgG antibodies bound to the red blood cells, which occurs in a warm autoimmune hemolytic anemia (**B**). In a cold autoimmune hemolytic anemia, the antibody bound to red blood cells is IgM and the Coombs test is negative (**C**). With polycythemia, the hemoglobin would be expected to be elevated (**E**), and hereditary spherocytosis would not be associated with a positive Coombs test (**D**).

51. Correct: It occurs in patients with a B-cell lymphoma. (D)

The patient has evidence of hemolysis causing an unconjugated hyperbilirubinemia, with no evidence of the liver as a source. The lack of hemoglobin in the urine is consistent with his hemolysis being extravascular. In intravascular hemolysis, the urine can have hemoglobin and hemosiderin (**E**). Extravascular hemolysis, with a positive Coombs test and with no history of a blood transfusion, is consistent with a warm autoimmune hemolytic anemia, which can be seen in patients with SLE and B-cell lymphomas among other causes (**D**). I and i antigens are the target in a cold autoimmune hemolytic anemia, which can follow a *Mycoplasma pneumoniae* infection (**A, C**), and the P antigen is the target in a paroxysmal cold hemoglobinuria (**B**). IgM antibodies are not detected in the standard Coomb test.

52. Correct: One complication of ulcerative colitis is a significant risk factor for the tumor. (D)

The tumor derived from bile ducts is a cholangiocarcinoma, which commonly occurs in cirrhotic livers, often in combination with hepatocellular carcinoma (**A**). The tumor has a poor prognosis (**B**). Hepatocellular carcinomas are most frequently associated with an elevation of α-fetoproteins; in fact, patients with cirrhosis of the liver, a risk factor for the development of hepatocellular carcinoma, can be followed with serial α-fetoproteins to monitor for the possible development of the tumor (although ultrasound imaging is preferred) (**C**). Primary sclerosis cholangitis, which occurs in a large proportion of patients with ulcerative colitis, is a significant risk factor for cholangiocarcinoma, along with *Opisthorchis sinensis* infection (**D**). Peptic ulcers are not a risk factor for the development of cholangiocarcinoma (**E**).

53. Correct: Budd-Chiari syndrome (C)

Budd-Chiari syndrome is due to thrombosis of the hepatic veins or inferior vena cava. Risk factors include pregnancy, use of oral contraceptives, Factor V Leiden, and other coagulation disorders. Patients can develop ascites due to the acute increased pressure in the portal system (C). HELLP (hemolysis, elevated liver enzymes, and low platelets) syndrome occurs in pregnant females, but the laboratory testing is not consistent with this disorder, as the patient is not thrombocytopenic (B). Acetaminophen toxicity would be expected to have much higher elevations of AST and ALT (D), and there are no risk factors listed for an intentional overdose. Hepatocellular carcinoma and placenta accreta are not consistent with the clinical diagnosis (A, E).

54. Correct: Metastatic colonic adenocarcinoma (C)

An elevated alkaline phosphatase can represent disease of the hepatobiliary system, bone, placenta, or intestine; however, an elevated GGT would confirm that the underlying etiology is one of the hepatobiliary system. Tumor metastases to the liver can cause an elevated alkaline phosphatase and GGT. Metastatic colonic adenocarcinoma frequently involves the liver (C). An elevated alkaline phosphatase can occur in Paget's disease; however, the GGT would not be elevated (A). Wernicke's encephalopathy occurs in alcoholics, and as such, indirectly the GGT could be elevated, but the alkaline phosphatase would not be (E). Celiac disease and placenta accreta are not commonly associated with an elevated alkaline phosphatase (B, D).

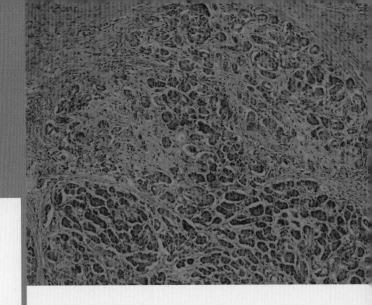

Chapter 14

Diseases of the Pancreas

LEARNING OBJECTIVES

14.1 Diseases of the Pancreas

▶ List the symptoms of pancreatic carcinoma, correlating the location of a pancreatic tumor with possible symptoms.

▶ Given the signs, symptoms, and laboratory testing, diagnose acute pancreatitis.

▶ List the signs, symptoms, and laboratory findings associated with pancreatic carcinoma.

▶ Given the signs, symptoms, and laboratory findings, diagnose pancreatic carcinoma, describing its complications.

14.1 Diseases of the Pancreas–Questions

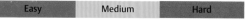

1. A 56-year-old male is diagnosed with pancreatic adenocarcinoma. He undergoes a Whipple procedure and has a 20-year postoperative survival, with no recurrence of the tumor. Of the following, what was the most likely site of the tumor?

A. Head of the pancreas

B. Proximal body of the pancreas

C. Distal body of the pancreas

D. Tail of the pancreas

E. Ectopic pancreatic tissue in the spleen

Pancreas

2. A 43-year-old alcoholic presents to the emergency room with complaints of abdominal pain, which developed suddenly about one day ago and is in the epigastric region but also affects his back. Admission laboratory testing reveals a white blood cell count of 18,000/μL, hemoglobin of 14 g/dL, hematocrit of 38, ALT of 98 U/L, AST of 88 U/L, GGT of 121 U/L, alkaline phosphatase of 870 U/L, amylase of 332 U/L, and lipase of 650 U/L. Of the following, what is the most likely diagnosis?

A. Acute myocardial infarct

B. Acute cholecystitis

C. Alcoholic hepatitis

D. Acute pancreatitis

E. Splenic sequestration syndrome

Pancreas

3. A 55-year-old African American male presents to his family physician. Over the past few days he has developed yellow discoloration of the whites of his eyes, and over the past week has had abdominal pain, which would sometimes also be present in his back. He has a 50-pack-per-year smoking history and hypertension controlled with medication. His vital signs are a temperature of 98.9°F, pulse of 82 bpm, and blood pressure of 142/84 mm Hg. A physical examination reveals yellow discoloration of the conjunctivae and skin and abdominal pain due to palpation; however, the patient also has a palpable gallbladder. Laboratory testing reveals a direct bilirubin of 2.3 mg/dL and CA 19-9 of 250 U/mL. Of the following, what is the term for the change identified on physical examination of the abdomen?

A. Chvostek's sign

B. Homans' sign

C. Courvoisier's sign

D. Trousseau's sign

E. Sign of Leser-Trélat

Pancreas

4. Given the previous clinical scenario, which of the following is the most likely diagnosis?

A. Aortic dissection

B. Acute cholecystitis

C. Viral hepatitis

D. Pancreatic carcinoma

E. Acute myocardial infarct

Pancreas

5. Given the previous clinical scenario, of the following, what condition is this individual at risk for because of his presenting condition?

A. An acute myocardial infarct

B. An aortic dissection

C. Pulmonary thromboembolus

D. Acute pyelonephritis

E. Prostatic adenocarcinoma

Pancreas

14.2 Diseases of the Pancreas–Answers and Explanations

1. Correct: Head of the pancreas (A)

Pancreatic adenocarcinoma has a poor prognosis. The sooner a patient presents with a neoplasm, the earlier in its course it can be resected and treated. Pancreatic adenocarcinoma can often be asymptomatic for a long period of time; however, a small neoplasm in the head of the pancreas can still potentially obstruct the common bile duct, leading to jaundice and early discovery and treatment of the tumor (**A**). If the tumor is in any of the locations listed (**B-E**), the time when it produces symptoms will most likely be later in the course of the disease process, and thus, the chances of survival are less.

2. Correct: Acute pancreatitis (D)

The signs and symptoms are consistent with acute pancreatitis (**D**). While many conditions, including hepatitis, can cause an increase in amylase, lipase is more specific (**A-C, E**).

3. Correct: Courvoisier's sign (C)

A palpable gallbladder associated with obstructive jaundice is Courvoisier's sign (**C**). Trousseau's syndrome is migratory thrombophlebitis (**D**), Chvostek's sign is twitching of facial muscles produced by light tapping of the facial nerve and is associated with hypocalcemia (**A**), and Homans' sign is calf pain produced by dorsiflexion of the foot and is associated with deep venous thrombi (**B**). The sign of Leser-Trelat is the acute onset of multiple seborrheic keratoses, which is associated with an internal malignancy (**E**).

Pancreas

4. Correct: Pancreatic carcinoma (D)

The palpable gallbladder associated with jaundice is termed Courvoisier's sign and is associated with pancreatic carcinoma; African American males have a higher risk of the neoplasm, and the tumor is associated with cigarette smoking. The elevated direct bilirubin indicates conjugated bilirubin. The elevated CA19-9 is not diagnostic of pancreatic carcinoma but supports the diagnosis (**D**). Given the time course and symptomatology, an aortic dissection and acute myocardial infarct are not likely and would not explain the jaundice (**A, E**). A viral hepatitis would not explain the palpable gallbladder (**C**). Given that the patient is afebrile, has an elevated CA 19-9, and has no risk factors for the condition, acute cholecystitis is not likely (**B**).

5. Correct: Pulmonary thromboembolus (C)

Based on the signs, symptoms, and laboratory testing, the patient has pancreatic carcinoma. Patients with pancreatic syndrome can develop migratory thrombophlebitis (i.e., Trousseau's syndrome), which puts them at risk for a pulmonary thromboembolus (**C**). Pancreatic carcinoma does not markedly increase the risk for the other conditions (**A-B, D-E**).

Chapter 15

Diseases of the Male and Female Genital Tract

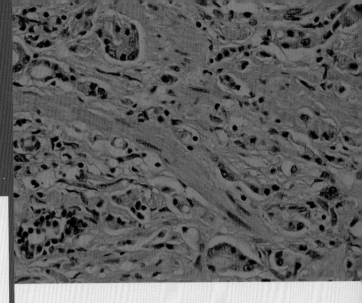

LEARNING OBJECTIVES

15.1 Diseases of the Testes

- List the types of testicular tumors, including both germ cell and non–germ cell tumors
- Describe the clinical presentation for a testicular lymphoma
- Diagnose testicular torsion
- Describe the appearance of germ cell tumors of the testicle
- Describe the histologic features of germ cell tumors of the testicle
- List the age range for germ cell tumors of the testicle
- List the cytogenetic abnormalities associated with testicular tumors and their mechanism of action

15.2 Diseases of the Uterus

- List the types of human papillomavirus associated with low-grade and high-grade dysplasia, respectively
- Describe the risk factors for cervical dysplasia and carcinoma
- List the causes of abnormal uterine bleeding, including the most common cause
- Describe the mechanism of dysfunctional uterine bleeding
- Describe the histologic features of endometrial hyperplasia; list the risk factors associated with its development, and its risk for progression to carcinoma
- Describe the histologic appearance of endometrial carcinoma; list the molecular changes associated with the neoplasm
- Diagnose endometrial carcinoma
- List the differential diagnosis and determine appropriate testing when there is vaginal bleeding in a reproductive-age female
- List the risk factors and etiologic agents of and diagnose pelvic inflammatory disease
- Describe the histologic viral changes associated with HPV infection
- Describe the various types of cervical dysplasia; list the types of HPV associated with low- and high-grade cervical dysplasia
- Name the risk factor for clear cell adenocarcinoma of the cervix
- Describe the clinical presentation of adenomyosis

- Describe the clinical presentation of acute endometritis
- Describe the histologic features of chronic endometritis; list the causes of chronic endometritis
- Describe the clinical presentation of endometriosis
- Diagnose endometriosis
- Describe the histologic features of endometriosis
- Given the signs, symptoms, and gross and histologic description, diagnose adenomyosis

15.3 Diseases of the Ovaries

- Diagnose and list the complications of pelvic inflammatory disease

15.4 Diseases of the Prostate, Penis, and Pregnancy

- Diagnose and list the complications of benign prostatic hyperplasia
- Describe the histologic features of benign prostatic hyperplasia
- Diagnose prostatic adenocarcinoma
- Describe the appearance of metastatic prostatic adenocarcinoma
- List the etiologic agents of and diagnose acute prostatitis
- List the risk factors for squamous cell carcinoma of the penis
- Describe the bony metastases produced by and diagnose metastatic prostatic adenocarcinoma
- List the risk factor of development for and diagnose a urinary tract infection
- Diagnose an ectopic pregnancy
- Diagnose endometriosis

15.1 Diseases of the Testes— Questions

Easy	Medium	Hard

1. A 62-year-old male presents to his family physician. Over the past 3 months, he has noted a painless enlargement of both testicles. An ultrasound does not reveal a fluid-filled cavity in either testicle. Of the following, what is the most likely diagnosis?

A. Seminoma

B. Embryonal carcinoma

C. Choriocarcinoma

D. Teratoma

E. Lymphoma

Testis

2. A 16-year-old male presents to the emergency room with his parents. He developed a sudden pain in his right testicle 3 hours ago and feels that it is swollen. He is also nauseated. His vital signs are a temperature of 99.4°F, pulse of 113 bpm, and blood pressure of 145/86 mm Hg. A physical examination reveals a right testicle that is firm and more superiorly located than the left testicle but is smooth in texture. Of the following, what is the most likely diagnosis?

A. Incarcerated hernia

B. Testicular torsion

C. Hemorrhage into a choriocarcinoma

D. Hydrocele

E. Varicocele

Testis

3. A 34-year-old male is having a yearly physical examination. His family physician performing the physical palpates a mass in his right testis, which is confirmed by ultrasound to be solid and not a fluid collection. Laboratory testing reveals human chorionic gonadotropin in the blood. The mass is resected by a surgeon. When the pathologist examines the testicular mass, he notes that it is solid and has a fairly homogenous tan appearance. Of the following, what is the most likely diagnosis?

A. Seminoma

B. Embryonal carcinoma

C. Choriocarcinoma

D. Lymphoma

E. Teratoma

Testis

4. A pathologist is examining a microscopic section taken from a testicular tumor. In the microscopic section she sees a pure tumor, and not a mixed germ cell neoplasm. Within the neoplasm are eosinophilic globules, and in other areas are structures that resemble primitive glomeruli. Of the following, what is the most likely age of this patient?

A. 1 year

B. 20 years

C. 40 years

D. 60 years

E. 80 years

Testis

5. A 23-year-old male presents to his family physician because he has developed a painless swelling of his left testicle. After workup, a resection is performed. The pathology report returns with a diagnosis of mixed germ cell tumor of the testicle, 50% seminoma, 35% choriocarcinoma, and 15% yolk sac tumor. Of the following, which genetic abnormality is most likely to be present?

A. Isochromosome 10p

B. Isochromosome 11p

C. Isochromosome 12p

D. Isochromosome 13p

E. Isochromosome 14p

Testicle

15.2 Diseases of the Uterus—Questions

Easy	Medium	Hard

6. A 32-year-old female has her yearly physical examination, which includes a Pap smear. The pathologist interprets the Pap smear as high-grade dysplasia (HSIL), which is confirmed by subsequent cervical biopsy. Of the following, what is the most likely cause?

A. HPV type 6

B. HPV type 16

C. CMV

D. HHV6

E. HHV8

Cervix

7. Given the previous clinical scenario, which of the following is the most significant risk factor for her disease process?

A. Chronic alcoholism

B. Precocious puberty

C. Multiple sexual partners

D. Thalidomide exposure

E. Congenital adrenal hyperplasia

Cervix

8. A 17-year-old thin female presents to her gynecologist. She states that her menstrual period has lasted longer than normal in 5 of the last 6 months, and at times, was excessive. She is G0P0, has a long-term boyfriend, and they use condoms for birth control. She has no other significant past medical history, other than fracturing her left radius during a fall while skiing when she was 15 years old. Her physical examination, including pelvic examination, is unremarkable. An hCG is 2.3 IU/L. Of the following, what is the most likely diagnosis?

A. A uterine fibroid

B. Invasive squamous cell carcinoma of the cervix

C. Endometriosis

D. Dysfunctional uterine bleeding

E. Polycystic ovarian syndrome

Uterus

9. Given the previous clinical scenario, which of the following is the most likely mechanism for her menstrual abnormalities?

A. Excess estrogen compared to progesterone

B. Excess progesterone compared to estrogen

C. Compressive atrophy of endometrium

D. Lodged foreign body

E. Polypoid proliferation of endometrium

Uterus

10. A 66-year-old female presents to her gynecologist, reporting that she has been having vaginal bleeding intermittently for the last 3 months. Her vital signs are a temperature of 98.6°F, pulse of 82 bpm, and blood pressure of 120/76 mm Hg. A physical examination, including a pelvic examination, identifies no significant abnormalities. An endometrial biopsy is scheduled and performed. In the biopsy, the pathologist sees back-to-back glands without atypia. Of the following, which is true regarding this condition?

A. A hysterectomy is required soon to prevent metastatic disease.

B. High levels of progesterone are a risk factor.

C. Molecular analysis would reveal HPV viral DNA.

D. Obesity is a risk factor.

E. Nuclear pleomorphism and atypical mitotic figures are present throughout the biopsy.

Uterus

11. A 68-year-old female presents to her gynecologist, reporting that she has been having vaginal bleeding intermittently for the last 4 months. Her vital signs are a temperature of 98.8°F, pulse of 77 bpm, and blood pressure of 122/75 mm Hg. Physical examination, including pelvic examination, identifies no significant abnormalities. An endometrial biopsy is scheduled and performed. In the biopsy, the pathologist identifies back-to-back glands with nuclear pleomorphism and abnormal mitotic figures. There is no papilla formation, and the amount of nuclear atypia is not marked. Evidence of invasion is present. Of the following, which would molecular analysis most likely reveal?

A. *RB*

B. *TP53*

C. *PTEN*

D. t(14;18)

E. *BRCA2*

Uterus

12. A 68-year-old female presents to her gynecologist, reporting that she has been having vaginal bleeding intermittently for the last 3 months. Her vital signs are a temperature of 98.6°F, pulse of 82 bpm, and blood pressure of 120/76 mm Hg. A physical examination, including a pelvic examination, identifies no significant abnormalities. An endometrial biopsy is scheduled and performed. The pathologist identifies papillae and not discrete glands. The neoplastic cells have marked variation in nuclear cell size and shape, and there are abnormal mitotic figures. Of the following, what is molecular analysis most likely to reveal?

A. *RB*

B. *TP53*

C. *PTEN*

D. t(14;18)

E. *BRCA2*

Uterus

13. A 63-year-old postmenopausal female presents to her family physician. She has not seen a doctor in five years. Over the past year and a half, she has had intermittent vaginal bleeding and sometimes a thick white, mucus-like discharge from her vagina. She has also felt a fullness in her pelvic region. Her vital signs are a temperature of 99.1°F, pulse of 88 bpm, and blood pressure of 104/65 mm Hg. Pelvic examination reveals an enlarged uterus that is fixed and does not move with palpation. Of the following, what is the most likely diagnosis?

A. Multiple uterine fibroids

B. Metastatic ovarian carcinoma

C. Endometrial carcinoma

D. Age-related changes

E. Polycystic uterus

Uterus

203

14. A 22-year-old college female presents to an acute care clinic with vaginal bleeding. She reports that her last menstrual period was 2 months ago. Of the following, what is the most likely test to have a positive result?

A. An endometrial biopsy

B. PT and PTT

C. Pap smear

D. hCG

E. Factor V Leiden

Uterus

15. A 19-year-old female presents to an acute care clinic, complaining of vaginal discharge. She reports that her menstrual period has been regular for the last year. Her vital signs are a temperature of 100.6°F, pulse of 98 bpm, and blood pressure of 103/72 mm Hg. On physical examination she is ill-appearing and uncomfortable. Auscultation of the chest and abdomen reveals no abnormalities. Palpation of the abdomen produces some tenderness. Pelvic examination reveals a purulent cervical discharge. Laboratory testing reveals a white blood cell count of 16,000 cells/μL, hemoglobin of 12 g/dL. Of the following, what was the most significant risk factor in the development of her condition?

A. Cigarette use

B. Intravenous drug use

C. Unprotected sex

D. Abdominal trauma

E. Impacted fecolith

Cervix

16. A pathologist is examining a cervical biopsy from a 27-year-old female who had an acetowhite lesion noted on colposcopic examination following an abnormal Pap smear. The Pap smear was interpreted as low-grade dysplasia. Of the following, which microscopic finding is most likely to be present?

A. Schistocytes

B. Koilocytes

C. Dacryocytes

D. Poikilocyte

E. Acanthocyte

Cervix

17. A pathologist is examining a cervical biopsy from a 25-year-old female who has had multiple sexual partners. The pathologist identifies dysplastic changes affecting essentially the entire thickness of the cervical mucosa. No invasion is present. Of the following, which one most likely caused the histologic changes?

A. HPV, type 6

B. HPV, type 11

C. HPV, type 18

D. HSV

E. Syphilis

Cervix

18. A 27-year-old female presents to her family physician with complaints of vaginal bleeding. She has no other symptoms. Her vital signs are a temperature of 98.7°F, pulse of 83 bpm, and blood pressure of 101/72 mm Hg. Pelvic examination reveals an ulcerated mass of the cervix. Biopsy provides the diagnosis of clear cell adenocarcinoma. Of the following, what was the most significant risk factor for the development of this tumor?

A. Cigarette use

B. Infection with HPV type 18

C. Maternal use of diethylstilbestrol

D. Maternal use of Thalidomide

E. Previous pelvic irradiation

Cervix

19. A 33-year-old female presents to her family physician. She reports that she has pain on intercourse, and occasional heavy menstrual bleeding. She has been married for 10 years and has had two sexual partners, including her husband. She has three children. Her vital signs are temperature of 98.5°F, pulse of 85 bpm, and blood pressure of 103/73 mm Hg. Physical examination reveals no abnormalities with the exception of a pelvic examination that reveals the possibility of a slightly enlarged uterus. A β-hCG is negative. Of the following, what is the most likely diagnosis?

A. Pelvic inflammatory disease

B. Polycystic ovarian syndrome

C. Acute endometritis

D. Adenomyosis

E. Endometrial adenocarcinoma

Uterus

20. A 24-year-old female presents to an acute care clinic. Over the past two days, she has developed a fever and foul-smelling vaginal discharge. Her vital signs are a temperature of 100.1°F, pulse of 95 bpm, and blood pressure of 120/79 mm Hg. Physical examination reveals no significant findings other than uterine tenderness on palpation during the pelvic examination. She has been married for 3 years. A culture of the discharge grows Group B streptococcus. Of the following, what was her risk factor for the presenting condition?

A. Unfaithful husband

B. Cigarette smoking

C. Cesarean section just prior to onset

D. Congenital hypoplasia of cervix

E. Endometriosis

Uterus

21. A pathologist is examining an endometrial biopsy, which was performed to evaluate infertility. The patient had previously been able to conceive but, on subsequent attempts, was unable to. During his microscopic examination of the tissue, the pathologist identified plasma cells in the endometrium. Of the following, what is the underlying cause of the presenting condition?

A. Obesity

B. Anorexia

C. Retained placental tissue

D. Endometrial hyperplasia

E. Endometriosis

Uterus

22. A 36-year-old female presents to her family physician with complaints of abdominal pain. She says that the pain has been ongoing for multiple months now, and that occasionally it occurs when she has a bowel movement. She also says that the pain is worse when she is having her menstrual period, and lessens in intensity following her menstrual period. She also reports pain with sexual intercourse. Her vital signs are a temperature of 98.6°F, pulse of 81 bpm, and blood pressure of 101/65 mm Hg. A physical examination is unrevealing except the pelvic exam portion, in which an enlarged uterus is identified and a possible right adnexal mass is palpated. No cervical or vaginal discharge is identified. Of the following, what is the most likely diagnosis?

A. Adenomyosis

B. Endometriosis

C. Pelvic inflammatory disease

D. Metastatic ovarian carcinoma

E. Acute intermittent porphyria

Uterus

23. A 36-year-old female presents to her obstetrician with complaints of blood in her urine. She also has occasional episodes of abdominal pain. Both symptoms occur during her menstrual period. She does not use cigarettes and has never traveled outside the United States. Of the following, what would histologic examination of the causative lesion reveal?

A. Glands, stroma, and hemosiderin

B. Interlocking fascicles of smooth muscle

C. Polyps lined with neoplastic cells

D. *Schistosoma haematobium*

E. Dysplastic calcification

Uterus, bladder

24. A 46-year-old female presents to her family physician because of complaints of vaginal bleeding and some vague lower abdominal pain, both of which are intermittent. An hCG is negative. She had three children, the last one being delivered 15 years ago. After evaluation, she decides to undergo a hysterectomy. The uterus is diffusely enlarged. The endometrium is not thickened. Histologic examination reveals endometrial glands and stroma in the myometrium. Of the following, what is the most likely diagnosis?

A. Leiomyoma

B. Adenomyosis

C. Endometrial carcinoma

D. Gestational trophoblastic disease

E. Endometrial stromal sarcoma

Uterus

15.3 Diseases of the Ovaries—Questions

Easy	Medium	Hard

25. A 19-year-old female presents to an acute care clinic, complaining of vaginal discharge. She reports that her menstrual period is regular and that she has not missed in the last year. Her vital signs are a temperature of 100.6°F, pulse of 98 bpm, and blood pressure of 103/72 mm Hg. On physical examination she is ill-appearing and uncomfortable. Auscultation of the chest and abdomen reveals no abnormalities. Palpation of the abdomen produces some tenderness. A pelvic examination reveals a purulent cervical discharge. Laboratory testing reveals a white blood cell count of 16,000 cells/µL, hemoglobin of 12 g/dL. Of the following, what is the most likely diagnosis?

A. Acute appendicitis

B. Squamous cell carcinoma of the cervix

C. Pelvic inflammatory disease

D. Acute vaginitis

E. Ovarian torsion

Cervix

26. Given the previous clinical scenario, which of the following is a possible complication in the future that she may develop?

A. Primary amenorrhea

B. Secondary amenorrhea

C. Squamous cell carcinoma of the cervix

D. Infertility

E. Uterine hypoplasia

Cervix

27. A third-year medical student is watching a laparoscopic tubal ligation. During the procedure, the attending ob/gyn directs the camera more superior and identifies fibrous adhesions between the diaphragm and liver, which remind the medical student of violin strings. Of the following, what is the patient most at risk for, which is in association with the disease process producing the changes noted around the liver?

A. Hepatocellular carcinoma

B. Small bowel obstruction

C. Acute appendicitis

D. Intracerebral hemorrhage

E. Acute cholecystitis

Liver

28. A 24-year-old female presents to the emergency room in acute distress. She describes abdominal pain that recently developed and has gotten progressively worse. Her vital signs are a temperature of 101°F, pulse of 107 bpm, and blood pressure of 132/84 mm Hg. A physical examination of the abdomen reveals rebound tenderness and guarding. A pelvic examination reveals malodorous vaginal discharge and a palpably enlarged left ovary. She reports that she is frequently sexually active, and often practices unprotected sex. Of the following, what is the most likely diagnosis?

A. Acute appendicitis

B. Acute endometritis

C. Ruptured tubo-ovarian abscess

D. Metastatic malignant surface epithelial carcinoma

E. Adenomyosis

Ovary

15.4 Diseases of the Prostate, Penis, and Pregnancy—Questions

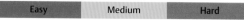

29. A 62-year-old male presents to his family physician. He reports that over the past year he has had to urinate more often, including having to get up at night, and that when he urinates his urine stream is slow and he always feels like his bladder does not empty completely. His vital signs are a temperature of 98.5°F, pulse of 82 bpm, and blood pressure of 145/84 mm Hg. Physical examination reveals an enlarged, but non-nodular, prostate with no tenderness. His PSA is 2 ng/mL. Of the following, what is the most likely diagnosis?

A. Prostatic adenocarcinoma

B. Chronic urinary tract infection

C. Benign prostatic hyperplasia

D. Strangulated hernia

E. Testicular lymphoma

Prostate

30. Given the previous clinical scenario, of the following, what condition is he most at risk for?

A. Prostatic adenocarcinoma

B. Hydronephrosis

C. Testicular lymphoma

D. Testicular feminization

E. Bladder carcinoma

Prostate

31. Given the previous clinical scenario, if the gland is removed at surgery, of the following, which is most likely to be identified within the parenchyma?

A. Widespread invasive glandular epithelium

B. Squamous metaplasia

C. Glandular metaplasia

D. Ectopic Sertoli cells

E. Schiller-Duval bodies

Prostate

32. A 64-year-old African American male presents to an acute care clinic complaining of back pain. He has not seen a physician in 20 years. A review of the symptoms reveals that over the past two years, he has had difficulty urinating and often has to urinate at night. His vital signs are temperature of 98.7°F, pulse of 87 bpm, and blood pressure of 157/91 mm Hg. A physical examination reveals a nodular prostate and a negative fecal occult blood test. Laboratory testing reveals a PSA of 230 ng/mL. Of the following, what is the most likely cause of the back pain?

A. Osteoblastic metastatic adenocarcinoma

B. Osteolytic metastatic adenocarcinoma

C. Osteoblastic metastatic sarcoma

D. Osteolytic metastatic sarcoma

E. Osteoblastic metastatic germ cell tumor

F. Osteolytic metastatic germ cell tumor

Prostate

33. A 26-year-old male presents to his family physician with complaints of difficulty urinating, increased frequency with urinating, lower back pain, and chills. He has no significant past medical history and has never had a urinary tract infection. He smokes cigarettes, consumes about 1 to 2 beers per day, more on the weekends, and is not married, but dates frequently. His vital signs are a temperature of 101°F, pulse of 109 bpm, and blood pressure of 132/76 mm Hg. A physical examination reveals a normal abdominal examination, and on rectal examination, he has a soft boggy prostate, which is tender to palpation. Laboratory testing reveals a PSA of 10 ng/mL. Of the following, what is the most likely diagnosis?

A. Acute prostatitis

B. Chronic prostatitis

C. Early-onset benign prostatic hyperplasia

D. Prostatic adenocarcinoma

E. Urinary tract infection

Prostate

34. Given the previous clinical scenario, which of the following is the most likely etiologic agent for his condition?

A. *Escherichia coli*

B. *Staphylococcus aureus*

C. *Neisseria gonorrheae*

D. *Klebsiella pneumoniae*

E. *Pseudomonas aeruginosa*

Prostate

35. A 56-year-old male presents to his family physician, who he has not seen in several years. He is obviously embarrassed and tentative about allowing an examination. He finally says that over the past 8 months he has had a mass growing on the tip of his penis, which has begun to bleed, prompting him to seek a doctor. Examination reveals a 1.1-cm ulcerated firm mass on the glans of the penis. Of the following, which is most directly a risk factor for this condition?

A. Infection with HPV type 6

B. HIV infection

C. Presence of foreskin

D. Prostatic adenocarcinoma

E. Cirrhosis of the liver

Penis

36. A 67-year-old male presents to his family physician, whom he has not seen in several years, with complaints of back pain and left thigh pain. Other than mild hypertension controlled with a β-blocker, he has no other significant past medical history. Vital signs are a temperature of 98.9°F, pulse of 81 bpm, and blood pressure of 129/71 mm Hg. Laboratory testing reveals ALT of 23 U/L, AST of 31 U/L, GGT of 21 U/L, alkaline phosphatase of 223 U/L, TSH of 1.0 mIU/L, and PSA of 53 ng/mL. His physician is concerned for metastatic disease. Of the following, what would be the most likely cause of the elevated alkaline phosphatase?

A. Undiagnosed inflammatory bowel disease

B. Osteoblastic metastases

C. Osteolytic metastases

D. Occult rib fractures

E. Hyperparathyroidism

Prostate, bone

37. A 67-year-old male presents to his physician with complaints of dysuria, frequency, and urgency. His vital signs are a temperature of 99.1°F, pulse of 85 bpm, and blood pressure of 131/87 mm Hg. A physical examination reveals a mild suprapubic discomfort on palpation. A urinalysis reveals positivity for leukocyte esterase, hemoglobin, and nitrites. The pH is 8.1. Of the following, what other abnormality that is a direct cause of the patient's presenting condition may be identified on physical examination?

A. A positive fecal occult blood test

B. A systolic ejection murmur

C. Decreased bowel sounds

D. Nodular prostate

E. Inguinal hernia

Prostate, bladder

38. A 27-year-old female is brought to the emergency room by her husband. She had been complaining of abdominal pain earlier in the day, but thought it was a bad reaction to her breakfast. However, the abdominal pain continued, and she wanted to go to the hospital as she was beginning to feel lightheaded. Her vital signs are a temperature of 98.9°F, pulse of 121 bpm, blood pressure of 85/65 mm Hg. History reveals that she has missed her last two menstrual periods. A pelvic exam reveals a closed cervical os and a right adnexal mass. The uterus is not enlarged. A urine screen for hCG is negative; however, a serum β-hCG is positive. A complete blood count reveals a hemoglobin of 9.1 mg/dL. Of the following, what is the most likely diagnosis?

A. Serous cystadenoma of the ovary
B. Inevitable abortion
C. Gestational trophoblastic disease
D. Ectopic pregnancy
E. Placenta previa

Uterus

39. Given the previous clinical scenario, of the following, what is a risk factor for this condition?

A. Previous history of *Streptococcus* pharyngitis
B. Fecolith
C. Chronic constipation
D. Previous history of a *Neisseria gonorrheae* infection
E. *BRCA1* mutation

Uterus

40. A 32-year-old female presents to her gynecologist with complaints of pain during her menstrual periods, which is occasionally associated with headaches and intermittent nausea. Physical examination reveals induration of the cul-de-sac and nodularity of the uterosacral ligament. Of the following, what is the most likely diagnosis?

A. Polycystic ovarian syndrome
B. Endometriosis
C. Uterine leiomyoma
D. Metastatic ovarian carcinoma
E. Colloid carcinoma of the appendix

Uterus

15.5 Diseases of the Testes—Answers and Explanations

Easy	Medium	Hard

1. Correct: Lymphoma (E)
A lymphoma is the most common testicular tumor in men over the age of 60 years, and is usually bilateral (**E**). The remainder of the tumors listed most commonly present in younger males (**A-D**).

2. Correct: Testicular torsion (B)
The signs and symptoms, the sudden onset of testicular pain and swelling of the testicle, are consistent with a testicular torsion (**B**). A varicocele can present as sudden pain in the testes, but the texture is like a bag of worms, because it is dilated veins (**E**). A hydrocele would not likely present suddenly and with pain (**D**). Choriocarcinoma is known to hemorrhage but only rarely presents in the described clinical manner (**C**). Given the physical examination findings, a testicular torsion is more likely than an incarcerated hernia (**A**).

3. Correct: Seminoma (A)
Seminoma is the most common germ cell tumor of the testis and normally appears as a homogeneous tan mass (**A**). Embryonal and choriocarcinoma frequently have hemorrhage within the mass (**B, C**). Teratomas are often nonhomogeneous in appearance, and tissue such as cartilage can be identified (**E**). Lymphomas can appear as a homogeneous tan mass, but are commonly bilateral and found in older men (**D**). Seminomas can have syncytiotrophoblasts, and therefore, the patient can have an elevated beta-hCG.

4. Correct: 1 year (A)
The description fits that of a pure yolk sac tumor. Although yolk sac tumors can occur at many ages when they are part of a mixed germ cell tumor, pure yolk sac tumors occur predominantly in children under the age of 2 years, and are the most common tumor of children (**A-E**). The characteristic histologic features are collections of α-fetoprotein and Schiller-Duval bodies, which are neoplastic cells that form a ring around a blood vessel and can look similar to a primitive glomerulus.

5. Correct: Isochromosome 12p (C)
Isochromosome 12p is the genetic abnormality associated with testicular tumors, being found in most seminomas and commonly in mixed germ cell tumors (**C**). The other genetic abnormalities listed are not commonly associated with germ cell tumors (**A-B, D-E**).

15.6 Diseases of the Uterus—Answers and Explanations

Easy	Medium	Hard

6. Correct: HPV type 16 (B)

High-grade cervical dysplasia is associated with human papillomavirus types 16, 18, 31, 33, 35 (**B**), and low-grade dysplasia is associated with HPV types 6 and 11 (**A**). HHV8 is associated with Kaposi sarcoma and primary effusion lymphoma (**E**). HHV6 is associated with encephalitis and a variety of other conditions but not cervical dysplasia (**D**). Cytomegalovirus is associated with a variety of conditions, but not with cervical dysplasia (**C**).

7. Correct: Multiple sexual partners (C)

The description is consistent with cervical dysplasia. Cervical dysplasia is caused by human papillomavirus, which is a sexually transmitted disease (**C**). The other conditions listed (**A-B, D-E**) are not, by themselves, a risk factor for cervical dysplasia.

8. Correct: Dysfunctional uterine bleeding (D)

Although all of the possible answers could cause abnormal uterine bleeding, given the negative physical examination, lack of other supporting features for an alternative diagnosis, and the fact that it is the most common cause of abnormal uterine bleeding, the most likely diagnosis is dysfunctional uterine bleeding (**A-E**).

9. Correct: Excess estrogen compared to progesterone (A)

Estrogen causes proliferation of endometrial glands; however, they do not enter the secretory phase, and without progesterone the stroma does not grow, making it easier for the endometrium to breakdown and for bleeding to occur (**A**). As the most likely diagnosis is dysfunctional uterine bleeding, the other mechanisms listed are incorrect (**B-E**)

10. Correct: Obesity is a risk factor. (D)

The women has complex hyperplasia without atypia, indicating there is little nuclear pleomorphism, and essentially no atypical mitotic figures (**E**), the risk for progression to carcinoma is low (**A**), high levels of estrogen are a risk factor (**B**), HPV is not a causative agent (**C**), and obesity, diabetes mellitus, hypertension, and infertility are risk factors (**D**).

11. Correct: PTEN (C)

The histologic description is consistent with endometrial carcinoma. Of the following, *PTEN* is most commonly associated with endometrial carcinoma (**C**). It is a tumor suppressor gene functioning in the PI-3kinase/AKT signaling. Mutation of *TP53* is uncommon in endometrial carcinoma (**B**). Mutations of *RB* or *BRCA2* or t(14;18) are not commonly associated with endometrial carcinoma (**A, D-E**).

12. Correct: TP53 (B)

The pathologic description fits serous endometrial carcinoma, which has papillae instead of glands, and marked atypia. It is most commonly associated with *TP53* mutations (**B**), a tumor suppressor gene, and rarely with *PTEN* (**C**). It is not associated with *RB*, t(14;18), or *BRCA2* (**A, D-E**).

13. Correct: Endometrial carcinoma (C)

The symptoms, vaginal bleeding and leukorrhea, in combination with the pelvic examination revealing an enlarged and fixed uterus, are most consistent with endometrial carcinoma (**C**). Uterine fibroids can cause an enlarged uterus and can cause vaginal bleeding but would not cause the uterus to be fixed in place (**A**). Metastatic ovarian carcinoma to the uterus, the serosal surface, would not cause vaginal bleeding (**B**). The changes are not age-related, which would be an atrophic uterus (**D**), and the uterus is not normally associated with any form of cystic change (**E**).

14. Correct: hCG (D)

In a young reproductive-age female who presents with missed menstrual periods and vaginal bleeding, a pregnancy and possible spontaneous abortion must be ruled out, as it would be the most common cause, other than dysfunctional uterine bleeding. An hCG is the necessary test (**D**). While the patient could have many other diseases that could potentially present with that clinical scenario, and for which the other testing listed may prove useful (**A-C, E**), the most likely diagnosis is pregnancy.

15. Correct: Unprotected sex (C)

She has the clinical features of pelvic inflammatory disease (fever, elevated white blood cell count, and purulent cervical discharge). In this age group, the disease is most commonly due to *Chlamydia trachomatis* or *Neisseria gonorrheae*, which she would have contracted through unprotected sex (**C**). Her presentation is not a consequence of trauma (**D**), and it is not most consistent with acute appendicitis, which can be caused by an impacted fecolith (**E**). While cigarette use and intravenous drug use may be indirectly associated with the circumstances leading to unprotected sex, the use of these substances is not a direct risk factor for the development of pelvic inflammatory disease (**A, B**).

16. Correct: Koilocytes (B)

Given the patient's history, she is most likely infected with a human papillomavirus, and the characteristic cell type associated with low-grade dysplasia is the koilocyte, which has a wrinkled nucleus (**B**). Schisto-cytes and dacryocytes are morphologic types of red blood cells, associated with intravascular hemolysis and bone marrow fibrosis respectively (**A, C**). Poikilo-cytosis is a variation in red blood cell size (**D**). Acanthocytes have small spurs projecting outward from the surface of the red blood cell (**E**).

17. Correct: HPV, type 18 (C)

Cervical dysplasia and neoplasia are due to infection with human papillomavirus. The description fits a high-grade dysplasia, or CIN III. High-grade lesions are associated with HPV types 16, 18, 31, 33, 35, 39, and 45 (**C**), and low-grade lesions are associated with HPV type 6, 11, 42, and 44 (**A, B**). HSV and syphilis, while sexually transmitted, are not associated with cervical dysplasia/neoplasia (**D, E**).

18. Correct: Maternal use of diethylstilbestrol (C)

Clear cell adenocarcinoma of the cervix is a rare condition, strongly associated with maternal use of diethylstilbestrol during pregnancy (**C**). Thalidomide is associated with birth defects (**D**). HPV type 18 is associated with squamous cell carcinoma of the cervix (**B**), and cigarette use can contribute to its development (**A**). Pelvic irradiation is not commonly associated with clear cell adenocarcinoma of the cervix (**E**).

19. Correct: Adenomyosis (D)

Adenomyosis, which is the presence of endometrium in the myometrium, can be asymptomatic but can also cause pain, dyspareunia, abnormal bleeding, and infertility (**D**). Given her past history, PID is unlikely; also, she has no fever or cervical discharge (**A**). Acute endometritis would have a fever and foul-smelling discharge and would either occur after pregnancy or be associated with PID (**C**). Endometrial adenocarcinoma would most commonly occur in an older individual (**E**). Given the fact that she has three children, polycystic ovarian syndrome is less likely, and it would not normally present with pain on intercourse (**B**).

20. Correct: Cesarean section just prior to onset (C)

The patient has acute endometritis, which is the most common cause of a postpartum fever, frequently occurring in association with a Cesarean section (**C**). Given her past history and the organism cultured, PID is not the cause (**A**). Cigarette smoking, congenital hypoplasia of the cervix, and endometriosis would be insignificant risk factors compared to the history of Cesarean section just prior to presentation (**B, D-E**).

21. Correct: Retained placental tissue (C)

Although all of those conditions could result in infertility, the finding of plasma cells in the endometrium indicates a chronic endometritis. Chronic endometritis is caused by pelvic inflammatory disease, retained placental tissue, intrauterine devices, and

tuberculosis, among other conditions (**C**). The other entities listed would not commonly be associated with a plasma cell infiltrate (**A-B, D-E**).

22. Correct: Endometriosis (B)

Cyclical variation in pelvic pain is characteristic of endometriosis (**B**). Also, the uterus can be enlarged and adnexal masses (chocolate cysts) can be present. Without a fever or cervical discharge, PID is unlikely (**C**). Acute intermittent porphyria can present with abdominal pain, but the abnormal pelvic exam is not consistent with the diagnosis (**E**). Adenomyosis would not as likely produce pain with a bowel movement, and the condition is not associated with adnexal masses (**A**). Metastatic ovarian carcinoma would be less likely in a younger patient; also, the pain would not vary in time with her menstrual cycle (**D**).

23. Correct: Glands, stroma, and hemosiderin (A)

When hematuria occurs at the same time as the menstrual period, a strong possibility is endometriosis. Endometriosis can also cause abdominal pain, which develops during menstrual periods. The symptoms are due to sloughing of endometrial tissue, which is located in an abnormal location (**A**). Interlocking fascicles of smooth muscle describes a smooth muscle tumor, which would be an uncommon tumor of the bladder (**B**). Neoplasia is unlikely (**C**). While *Schistosoma* infections can be associated with hematuria, given that she has no travel outside the United States, it would be highly unlikely (**D**). While both metastatic and dystrophic calcification are recognized pathologic processes, dysplastic calcification is not (**E**).

24. Correct: Adenomyosis (B)

The finding of endometrial glands located within the myometrium is consistent with the diagnosis of adenomyosis (**B**). As the endometrium is not thickened, and as both endometrial glands and stroma are present in the myometrium, endometrial carcinoma is not the diagnosis (**C**). Neither gestational trophoblastic disease nor endometrial stromal sarcoma fit the clinical scenario and histologic examination (**D, E**). A leiomyoma is composed of interlocking fascicles of smooth muscle and not glands (**A**).

15.7 Diseases of the Ovaries—Answers and Explanations

Easy	Medium	Hard

25. Correct: Pelvic inflammatory disease (C)

The findings of fever, elevated white blood cell count, and a purulent cervical discharge are characteristic of pelvic inflammatory disease (**C**). Abdominal pain can be present and can be localized to the right upper quadrant. Acute appendicitis would not produce a purulent cervical discharge (**A**). While possible, squamous cell carcinoma of the cervix in a 19-year-old would be much less likely, and also, not commonly would it present acutely as an infectious process (**B**). Acute vaginitis would not produce cervical discharge (**D**). Ovarian torsion would not likely cause a purulent cervical discharge (**E**).

26. Correct: Infertility (D)

She has the clinical features of pelvic inflammatory disease (fever, elevated white blood cell count, and purulent cervical discharge). Due to the adhesions that can result from this condition, infertility is a complication (other complications due to adhesions include ectopic pregnancy and intestinal obstruction) (**A**). The condition should not cause amenorrhea, either primary or secondary (**A, B**), and it is not, by itself, associated with squamous cell carcinoma of the cervix (**C**), although both are due to a sexually transmitted disease. Uterine hypoplasia would be present from birth and would not be a major risk factor for pelvic inflammatory disease (**E**).

27. Correct: Small bowel obstruction (B)

The fibrous adhesions between the liver and the diaphragm is perihepatitis, i.e., Fitz-Hugh-Curtis syndrome, which is a manifestation of pelvic inflammatory disease. With pelvic inflammatory disease, the patient can develop tubo-ovarian adhesions, which are a risk factor for the development of a small bowel obstruction (**B**). None of the other conditions are related to pelvic inflammatory disease (**A, C-E**).

28. Correct: Ruptured tubo-ovarian abscess (C)

The clinical findings are consistent with an acute abdomen. Given the history of a fever and purulent discharge, followed shortly by the identification of an adnexal mass, a tubo-ovarian abscess as the result of pelvic inflammatory disease is a very likely diagnosis, and, given that the patient is presenting with an acute abdomen, a ruptured tubo-ovarian abscess is most likely (**C**). An acute appendicitis would not produce the vaginal discharge (**A**). Acute endometritis would not be associated with an enlarged left ovary (**B**). A metastatic malignant surface epithelial carcinoma would be less likely in a younger patient, and also would be less likely to present acutely as an infectious process (**D**). Adenomyosis would not cause a fever, the acute abdomen, or the vaginal discharge (**E**).

15.8 Diseases of the Prostate, Penis, and Pregnancy— Answers and Explanations

Easy	Medium	Hard

29. Correct: Benign prostatic hyperplasia (C)

The most common reason for enlargement of the prostate, and blockage of urine flow, is benign prostatic hyperplasia (**C**). A chronic urinary tract infection would not cause such symptoms (**B**). Early in its course, prostatic adenocarcinoma does not obstruct the urinary tract, and with the negative PSA, this is less likely (**A**). Given his extended period of symptoms and without an acute change in symptomatology, a strangulated hernia is unlikely (**D**). Although testicular lymphoma is most commonly present in older males, the clinical scenario does not otherwise support this diagnosis (**E**).

30. Correct: Hydronephrosis (B)

The most common reason for enlargement of the prostate and blockage of urine flow is benign prostatic hyperplasia. BPH is not a risk factor for prostatic adenocarcinoma, testicular lymphoma, bladder carcinoma, or testicular feminization (**A, C-E**). BPH, by obstructing urine, can lead to hydronephrosis, due to increased pressure in the renal pelvis (**B**).

31. Correct: Squamous metaplasia (B)

The most common reason for enlargement of the prostate and blockage of urine flow is benign prostatic hyperplasia, and BPH is not a risk factor for prostatic adenocarcinoma; also, given the normal PSA, the likelihood of a widespread neoplasm is less likely (**A**). Common microscopic findings in benign prostatic hyperplasia include glandular proliferations; however, infarcts can occur in enlarged prostate glands, and at their periphery is squamous metaplasia (**B**). Schiller-Duval bodies are found in yolk sac tumors of the testis (**E**). Neither glandular metaplasia nor ectopic Sertoli cells are commonly associated with benign prostatic hyperplasia (**C, D**).

32. Correct: Osteoblastic metastatic adenocarcinoma (A)

The signs, symptoms, and laboratory testing are consistent with prostatic adenocarcinoma. Prostatic adenocarcinoma commonly metastasizes to bone, and most often produces an osteoblastic response (**A, B**). While a sarcoma or metastatic germ cell tumor is always possible, given the clinical scenario, the most likely diagnosis is prostatic adenocarcinoma (**C-F**).

33. Correct: Acute prostatitis (A)

The patient has the clinical features of acute prostatitis, with urinary abnormalities, lower back pain, fever and chills, and a boggy enlarged prostate on examination, which is tender to palpation (**A**). The PSA can be elevated in acute prostatitis. Prostatic adenocarcinoma and benign prostatic hyperplasia would be exceptionally rare in a young patient, and would not be tender to palpation or cause fever (**C, D**). The urinary tract infection by itself would not cause the changes in the prostate (**E**). Given his age and presentation, he most likely has an acute process, instead of a chronic process (**B**).

34. Correct: *Neisseria gonorrheae* (C)

In a young adult, acute bacterial prostatitis is uncommon. Although acute prostatitis in older males is most often due to urinary tract pathogens and often occurs in association with a urinary tract infection, in a younger male, *Neisseria gonorrheae* or *Chlamydia trachomatis* as the underlying etiology is the more common scenario (**C**). Answers (**A-B, D-E**) do not best fit the clinical scenario.

35. Correct: Presence of foreskin (C)

The patient has squamous cell carcinoma of the penis. While circumcised males can develop squamous cell carcinoma of the penis, the disease most frequently occurs in noncircumcised males (**C**). Other risk factors include HPV, phimosis, balanitis, and smoking (**A**). An HIV infection, prostatic adenocarcinoma, and cirrhosis of the liver are not independent risk factors for the development of squamous cell carcinoma of the penis (**B, D-E**).

36. Correct: Osteoblastic metastases (B)

Although all of the possible answers could be associated with an elevated alkaline phosphatase, the patient also has an elevated PSA, and, given that the PSA is elevated well above the reference range, the cause of the osteoblastic metastases is most likely prostatic adenocarcinoma, which most commonly produces osteoblastic metastases (**A-E**).

37. Correct: Nodular prostate (D)

The patient has the signs, symptoms, and laboratory testing consistent with a urinary tract infection, a condition that is less common in males than females. Benign prostatic hyperplasia can, by obstructing the flow of urine, predispose an individual to the development of a urinary tract infection. Palpation of the prostate would reveal it to be nodular (**D**). The other conditions listed would not be direct causes of a urinary tract infection or be indicative of a condition that is normally a cause of a urinary tract infection (**A-C, E**).

38. Correct: Ectopic pregnancy (D)

The clinical scenario is consistent with a patient who is bleeding. Given the positive serum β-hCG and the palpable adnexal mass, of the choices, the most likely diagnosis is an ectopic pregnancy (**D**). Although an ovarian tumor can bleed, the serum β-hCG would not be positive (**A**). With an inevitable abortion, the cervical os would be open (**B**). Gestational trophoblastic disease results in an enlarged uterus, and patients usually have vomiting, and can pass grape-like structures, which are the villi (**C**). Placenta previa usually presents later in the gestation and the patient would be having vaginal bleeding (**E**).

39. Correct: Previous history of *Neisseria gonorrheae* infection (D)

Based on the clinical scenario, the most likely diagnosis is an ectopic pregnancy, which has ruptured causing internal bleeding. Risk factors for ectopic pregnancy include a past history of *Neisseria gonorrheae* or *Chlamydia trachomatis* causing pelvic inflammatory disease, with the scarring contributing to the possibility of ectopic implantation (**D**). Other risk factors for ectopic pregnancy include intrauterine devices, previous abdominal surgery, and previous ectopic pregnancy. Streptococcal pharyngitis, a fecolith, chronic constipation, and a *BRCA1* mutation are not risk factors for an ectopic pregnancy (**A-C, E**).

40. Correct: Endometriosis (B)

Given that endometriosis is abnormally located endometrial tissue, including both stroma and glands, and that it can function as normal endometrial tissue (i.e., undergoing changes according to hormone stimulation), having pain corresponding to the menstrual period reflects this. Endometriosis can form small nodules of tissue and thus cause the described physical examination findings (**B**). Polycystic ovarian syndrome and uterine leiomyoma would not produce such physical changes, and a uterine leiomyoma may present as a palpable mass (**A, C**). Metastatic breast carcinoma could cause studding of the peritoneal cavity and mimic the physical findings of endometriosis, but the symptoms would not vary with the menstrual period (**D**). A colloid carcinoma of the appendix can present as a pseudomyxoma peritonei, but not as described (**E**).

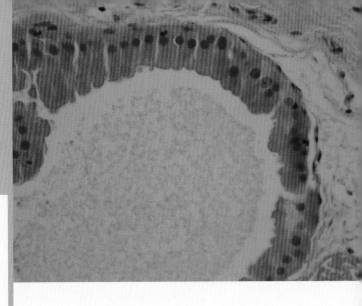

Chapter 16

Diseases of the Breast

LEARNING OBJECTIVES

16.1 Diseases of the Breast

► List the indicators of prognosis for breast carcinoma

► Diagnose acute mastitis

► Describe the histologic appearance of various benign and malignant lesions of the breast

► List the relative increased risk for breast cancer associated with various benign and premalignant lesions of the breast

► Diagnose a fibroadenoma

► Diagnose an intraductal papilloma

► Diagnose breast carcinoma

► Describe the relative frequency of various malignant forms of breast carcinoma

► Describe ductal and lobular carcinoma in situ

► Describe Paget's disease of the nipple and list its associations

► List the prognostic factors for breast carcinoma

16.1 Diseases of the Breast—Questions

Easy	Medium	Hard

1. A 43-year-old woman, during a breast self-examination, identifies a nodule in her left breast. She subsequently undergoes a lumpectomy. A pathologist determines that the malignant tumor is of glandular origin. Which of the following is true?

A. A colloid carcinoma would have a worse prognosis than ductal carcinoma.

B. She most likely has a *BRCA1* or *BRCA2* mutation.

C. Skin involvement is a good sign.

D. If the tumor is ER/PR positive, it has a better prognosis.

E. A tubular carcinoma would have a worse prognosis than a ductal carcinoma.

Breast

2. A 21-year-old female presents to her family physician with complaints of pain in her left breast. Her vital signs are a temperature of 99.5°F, pulse of 98 bpm, and blood pressure of 101/68 mm Hg. Physical examination reveals focal erythema of the left breast centered on the nipple. There is no retraction of the skin or nipple. Of the following, what activity or condition most likely led to her presenting state?

A. Trauma to the left breast

B. Breastfeeding

C. An underlying neoplasm

D. An autoimmune disorder

E. Bullous pemphigoid

Breast

3. A 45-year-old female is having her yearly examination by her gynecologist because she has noticed that her breasts have developed an ill-defined lumpy texture in a few areas when she performs a monthly breast self-examination. Her mother had breast cancer diagnosed at age 55 years, and she is concerned. She does get a yearly mammogram. A subsequent biopsy reveals moderate focal epithelial hyperplasia, fibrosis, and some cysts. Compared to the normal population, of the following, what is her risk of developing carcinoma of the breast, based only on the lesion diagnosed by the pathologist?

A. Less than the normal population

B. The same chance as the normal population

C. 1 to 2× the normal population

D. 5 to 10× the normal population

E. 25 to 50× the normal population

Breast

4. A 21-year-old female presents to her ob/gyn because during a breast self-examination, she identified a mass in her left breast. A physical examination reveals a painless and mobile nodule that has a rubbery texture in the lower quadrant of her left breast. A surgical excision is scheduled, and, at surgery, the mass literally pops out of the normal breast tissue and can be removed without a rim of surrounding fat. Of the following, what is the most likely diagnosis?

A. Proliferative fibrocystic disease

B. Fibroadenoma

C. Ductal carcinoma in situ

D. Invasive ductal carcinoma

E. Benign teratoma

Breast

5. A 37-year-old female presents to her gynecologist. Over the past 6 months, she has had occasionally nonmilky discharge from her left nipple; however, two days ago, she had bloody discharge. She has no history of breast cancer in her family but is still concerned by the symptoms. Physical examination reveals no masses in the left or right breast; however, compression of the left areola does express a small amount of slightly blood-tinged fluid, and a small nodule is palpable in the areola. The overlying skin has no changes. Of the following, what is the most likely diagnosis?

A. Paget's disease of the nipple

B. Invasive ductal carcinoma

C. Leiomyoma of the nipple

D. Phylloides tumor

E. Intraductal papilloma

Breast

6. A 61-year-old female presents to an acute care clinic. She has not seen a physician in 5 years because of lack of financial resources. Over the last year, she has noticed a lump in her left breast, which has grown in size. Her sister died from breast cancer at the age of 62 years. Physical examination reveals a firm mass in the left breast. The mass in nontender, nonmobile, and somewhat ill-defined as to its boundaries. The overlying skin is retracted but otherwise unremarkable. Of the following, what is the most likely diagnosis?

A. Proliferative fibrocystic disease

B. Fibroadenoma

C. Malignant phylloides tumor

D. Invasive ductal adenocarcinoma

E. Medullary carcinoma of the breast

Breast

7. A 44-year-old female is having her yearly examination by her gynecologist because she has noticed that her breasts have developed an ill-defined lumpy texture in a few areas when she performs a monthly breast self-examination. Her mother had breast cancer diagnosed at age 56 years, and she is concerned about her chances. She does get a yearly mammogram, and this year, some linear calcification was noted. A breast biopsy was scheduled. The pathologist identified ducts distended by atypical cells with necrosis in the center. No infiltrating tumor cells are present. Compared to the normal population, which of the following is her risk of developing carcinoma of the breast, based only on the lesion diagnosed by the pathologist?

A. Less than the normal population

B. The same as the normal population

C. 1 to 2× the normal population

D. 4 to 6× the normal population

E. 10 to 15× the normal population

Breast

8. Given the previous clinical scenario, based on the pathologic description of the breast lesion, of the following, what condition is this patient most directly at risk for?

A. Lymphedema of her left upper extremity

B. Metastases to the brain

C. Paget's disease of the nipple

D. Lobular carcinoma in situ

E. Multifocal fibroadenoma

Breast

9. A 61-year-old female suffers a seizure while having lunch with her friends. She is taken to the emergency room, where a CT scan identifies a mass in her left cerebral hemisphere. A biopsy is performed, and is read as metastatic ductal carcinoma of the breast. Among only the following choices, which one is most likely to be a feature of the primary tumor in the breast?

A. It is less than 1.0 cm in size.

B. It is both ER and PR positive.

C. It is a tubular carcinoma.

D. The pathologist did not identify lymphovascular invasion.

E. It has a high proliferative rate.

Breast

16.2 Diseases of the Breast—Answers and Explanations

Easy	Medium	Hard

1. Correct: If the tumor is ER/PR positive, it has a better prognosis. (D)

Colloid, medullar, and tubular carcinomas have a better prognosis than invasive ductal or invasive lobular carcinoma (**A, E**). Although women having *BRCA1* or *BRCA2* mutations are at greatly increased risk for breast carcinoma, most breast carcinomas occur in women without these mutations (**B**). Skin involvement, ER/PR negativity, and the presence of Her-2-Neu are all indicative of a worse prognosis (**C, D**).

2. Correct: Breastfeeding (B)

The patient's symptoms—painful and erythematous breast—are consistent with acute mastitis, which most commonly occurs due to a bacterial infection (commonly *Staphylococcus aureus*), due to breast feeding (**B**). Trauma to the breast is associated with fat necrosis (**A**). The condition does not represent inflammatory carcinoma (**C**), an autoimmune disorder (**D**), or a bullous skin disease (**E**).

3. Correct: 1 to 2× the normal population (C)

She has a proliferative form of fibrocystic disease, which has a slightly increased risk for the future development of breast carcinoma, around 1 to 2× (**C**). The other choices are incorrect, as proliferative breast disease has an increased risk over the normal population (**A, B**), but it is relatively small (**D, E**).

4. Correct: Fibroadenoma (B)

Given the age of the patient, a neoplasm would be more rare, and neoplasms are infiltrative and would not be so easily removed without a surrounding rim of tissue (**D**). The patient is young for proliferative fibrocystic disease, and proliferative fibrocystic disease does not normally form well-defined masses but instead produces a lumpy breast (**A**). A benign teratoma of the breast would be exceedingly rare (**E**). In this age group, and given the description, the most likely diagnosis is a fibroadenoma (**B**). Ductal carcinoma in situ, while not an invasive neoplasm, would not likely shell out from the surrounding breast tissue (**C**).

5. Correct: Intraductal papilloma (E)

Intraductal papillomas can cause obstruction of a duct and produce a nonmilky, sometimes bloody, nipple discharge (**E**). Although most intraductal papillomas are benign, some can be malignant. Bloody nipple discharge can also result from an invasive neoplasm, but this is a less common cause (**B**). A phylloides tumor is a rare neoplasm of the breast, and a leiomyoma would be a very rare neoplasm of the breast, neither likely to cause a bloody nipple discharge (**C, D**). Paget's disease affects the skin and does not usually cause a bloody nipple discharge (**A**).

6. Correct: Invasive ductal adenocarcinoma (D)

Given that the mass is nontender, nonmobile, and has ill-defined borders (i.e., indicating that it is infiltrating into the surrounding breast parenchyma), the most likely diagnosis is a malignant neoplasm, and not proliferative fibrocystic disease or a fibroadenoma (**A-B, D**). Also, given her age, a fibroadenoma would be very unlikely (**B**). Of the choices, invasive ductal adenocarcinoma is the most common of the tumor types, and a malignant phylloides tumor and medullary carcinoma would be much less common (**C, E**).

7. Correct: 4 to 6× the normal population (D)

The patient has ductal carcinoma in situ, which is characterized by atypical cells distending the duct, producing lumens with a punched-out appearance, and not slitlike as can be seen with ductal hyperplasia, and with the neoplastic cells not piling on top of each other as can be seen with ductal hyperplasia. Central necrosis (comedo necrosis) indicates a high-grade ductal carcinoma in situ. There is a greatly increased risk for the future development of carcinoma at the site, around 4 to 6× (**D**). The other answers are incorrect (**A–C, E**).

8. Correct: Paget's disease of the nipple (C)

The pathologist's description is that of a ductal carcinoma in situ (DCIS). DCIS is, while a strong risk factor for future development of invasive carcinoma of the breast, not itself invasive (although DCIS and an invasive carcinoma can both be present in a biopsy), and therefore, not by itself a risk factor for lymphedema of the upper extremity or metastases (**A, B**). However, the neoplastic cells can extend along ducts to the nipple and produce Paget's disease of the nipple (**C**). DCIS is not by itself an independent risk factor for lobular carcinoma in situ or multiple fibroadenomas (**D, E**).

9. Correct: It has a high proliferative rate. (E)

The choices are various tumor traits that have prognostic significance. As the patient presented with a metastatic lesion, the tumor has a poor prognosis. Of the choices, tumors with a high proliferative rate are associated with a poorer prognosis (**E**). Tumors less than 1.0 cm in size, and those that are ER/PR positive and without lymphovascular invasion, have a better prognosis (**A-B, D**). The subtypes colloid, tubular, and medullary have a better prognosis than a typical ductal carcinoma (**C**).

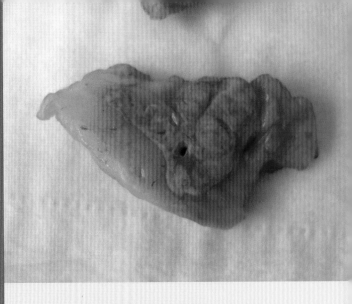

Chapter 17

Diseases of the Endocrine System

LEARNING OBJECTIVES

17.1 Diseases of the Pituitary Gland

- ▶ Diagnose and list the causes of hyperprolactinemia
- ▶ Diagnose acromegaly; list the causes of acromegaly
- ▶ Diagnose Sheehan's syndrome
- ▶ Diagnose and list the common causes of acute hypopituitarism and list common causes
- ▶ Provide a description of the clinical scenario for common cause of acute hypopituitarism
- ▶ Identify mass effects in the region of the pituitary gland
- ▶ Diagnose multiple endocrine neoplasia
- ▶ Diagnose and list all the causes of Cushing's disease
- ▶ Describe complications of the Cushing's disease process
- ▶ Describe the use of the low-dose and high-dose dexamethasone suppression tests to identify the source of elevated cortisol in the blood in Cushing's disease
- ▶ Diagnose and determine the underlying cause of hyponatremia
- ▶ List the causes of SIADH
- ▶ Describe the histologic appearance of lung tumors
- ▶ Describe the stalk effect in relation to prolactin concentrations in the blood
- ▶ List the causes of bitemporal hemianopia
- ▶ Diagnose and list the causes of diabetes insipidus
- ▶ Compare and contrast central and nephrogenic diabetes insipidus

17.2 Diseases of the Thyroid Gland and Parathyroid Glands

- ▶ List the causes of and diagnose hypothyroidism
- ▶ Describe the laboratory evaluation of hypothyroidism
- ▶ Describe the histologic appearance of Hashimoto's thyroiditis
- ▶ Diagnose thyroid storm
- ▶ Describe the testing methods to diagnose Graves' disease
- ▶ Describe the physical findings in Graves' disease
- ▶ Discuss the causes of an elevated TSH
- ▶ List causes of secondary hyperthyroidism
- ▶ Diagnose hypothyroidism
- ▶ Describe the laboratory abnormalities associated with hypothyroidism
- ▶ List the causes of hyperthyroidism and describe their histologic appearance

- ▶ Describe the histologic features of papillary thyroid carcinoma
- ▶ Diagnose hypoparathyroidism
- ▶ Diagnose hypocalcemia
- ▶ Describe the mechanism of hypocalcemia
- ▶ Compare and contrast the signs and symptoms of hyperthyroidism and hypothyroidism
- ▶ Describe the clinical scenario for subacute thyroiditis, including physical findings
- ▶ Describe the histology appearance of subacute thyroiditis
- ▶ Describe the relationship between MALTomas and autoimmune disorders, including Hashimoto's thyroiditis
- ▶ Determine the cause of hypercalcemia and increased parathyroid gland hormone

17.3 Diseases of the Adrenal Glands

- ▶ Diagnose primary chronic hypoadrenalism
- ▶ Diagnose Addison's disease
- ▶ List the laboratory abnormalities associated with Addison's disease
- ▶ List the autoantibody associated with the Addison's disease process
- ▶ Describe the clinical presentation and the laboratory testing used to diagnose a patient with a pheochromocytoma
- ▶ Diagnose a pheochromocytoma
- ▶ List the tumor types associated with the various types of MEN syndromes
- ▶ Describe the histologic features of thyroid gland tumors
- ▶ Describe the effect of negative feedback on the pituitary gland
- ▶ Describe the morphologic changes associated with a decreased amount of ACTH, TSH, GH, and PTH
- ▶ Describe the gross features, laboratory findings and clinical presentation of secreting tumors of the adrenal gland, specifically cortisol-secreting, aldosterone-secreting, and catecholamine-secreting tumors

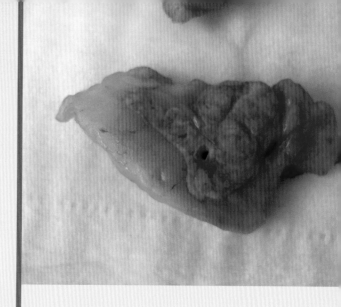

▶ Diagnose renal artery stenosis; describe the laboratory abnormalities associated with secondary hyperaldosteronism

▶ Diagnose congenital adrenal hyperplasia

▶ Compare and contrast congenital adrenal hyperplasia and polycystic ovarian syndrome

▶ Describe the clinical presentation and list the causes of an acute primary adrenocortical insufficiency

▶ Diagnose acute primary adrenocortical insufficiency

▶ List the common tumors of the adrenal gland, comparing adults versus children

▶ Describe the histologic, genetic, and laboratory study features of a neuroblastoma

17.4 Diseases of the Endocrine Pancreas

▶ Diagnose diabetic ketoacidosis

▶ Describe the laboratory testing used in the evaluation of diabetic ketoacidosis

▶ Describe the histologic changes associated with diabetes mellitus

▶ Compare and contrast hypertonic, isotonic, and hypotonic hyponatremia, and list causes of each

▶ Diagnose diabetes mellitus

▶ Describe laboratory testing used in the diagnosis and treatment of diabetes mellitus

17.1 Diseases of the Pituitary Gland—Questions

1. A 25-year-old female presents to her obstetrician. She says that for the past 4 months, she has not had a menstrual period, and several home pregnancy tests have all indicated negative results. She also states that she occasionally has had milky discharge from her nipples. She is concerned the home pregnancy test is incorrect. An hCG is 2.8 IU/L. Of the following, what is the most likely diagnosis?

A. Ectopic pregnancy

B. Choriocarcinoma

C. Pituitary adenoma

D. Graves' disease

E. Primary hyperadrenalism

Pituitary gland

2. A 42-year-old male presents to a family physician. He has not seen a physician in 5 years, but he reports that slowly, over the past two years, he has noticed a gradual increase in the size of his hands and feet, and his wife says that his face has become more rough. His vital signs are a temperature of 98.7°F, pulse of 83 bpm, and blood pressure of 131/85 mm Hg. A physical examination reveals a slightly displaced PMI and hepatomegaly. Laboratory testing reveals a glucose of 220 mg/dL. Of the following, what is the most likely source of his condition?

A. Adrenal adenoma

B. Multinodular goiter

C. Pituitary adenoma

D. Muscular dystrophy

E. A cerebral neoplasm

Pituitary adenoma

3. Given the previous clinical scenario, of the following, what mutation does this individual most likely possess that is the cause of his condition?

A. Mutation of *GNAS1* gene

B. Mutation of *GSNA1* gene

C. Mutation of *GNSA1* gene

D. Mutation of *GRSA1* gene

E. Mutation of *GSRA1* gene

Pituitary adenoma

4. Given the previous clinical scenario, of the following, what is the patient most at risk for?

A. Acute cerebral infarct

B. Cirrhosis of the liver

C. Chronic pancreatitis

D. Congestive heart failure

E. Pulmonary thromboembolus

Pituitary gland

5. A 21-year-old female who is at 36-weeks EGA presents to the emergency room with vaginal bleeding. Her vital signs are a temperature of 98.5°F, pulse of 130 bpm, and blood pressure of 60/palpable. She undergoes an emergent cesarean section and has a diagnosis of placenta previa. Following the surgery, she develops excessive thirst and frequent urination, constipation, intolerance to cold, nausea, vomiting, and increased sleepiness. Laboratory testing reveals a TSH of 0.1 mIU/L. Of the following, what is the most likely diagnosis?

A. Waterhouse-Friderichsen syndrome

B. Postpartum depression

C. Nephrogenic diabetes insipidus

D. Sheehan's syndrome

E. Thyroid storm

Pituitary gland

6. A 46-year-old female presents to the emergency room because of sudden onset of a headache and double vision. She is admitted to the hospital. In the subsequent few days, she develops excessive thirst and frequent urination. She also suffers from nausea, and has vomiting and constipation. On the 3rd day, she is found dead in her hospital bed. An autopsy is performed. Which of the following is most likely to be found?

A. *Neisseria meningitidis*

B. A glioblastoma multiforme

C. Hemorrhage into a pituitary gland adenoma

D. Ruptured berry aneurysm and subarachnoid hemorrhage

E. Colloid cyst of the 3rd ventricle

Pituitary gland

7. A 6-year-old child is brought to the emergency room by his parents. Over the past few days, he has been drinking water excessively and going to the bathroom often. This morning he started to say that he was having problems seeing, and also complained of nausea. He vomited three times, and has a headache. A physical examination reveals no tenderness of the neck. The function of the extraocular muscles is abnormal, with his lateral gaze impaired. Of the following, what is the most likely diagnosis?

A. Subarachnoid hemorrhage due to ruptured berry aneurysm

B. *Neisseria meningitidis*

C. Craniopharyngioma

D. Pituitary adenoma

E. Posterior fossa medulloblastoma

Pituitary gland

219

8. A 34-year-old female presents to her family physician with complaints of having missed her last several menstrual periods and apparent breast milk production. Several home pregnancy tests have been negative. An hCG test at the clinic is also negative. She subsequently undergoes a CT scan of the head and body. The scan reveals masses in the pituitary gland, parathyroid gland, and the pancreas. Of the following, what gene is most likely mutated?

A. *MEN1*

B. *BRCA*

C. *APC*

D. *RET*

E. *GNAS1*

Parathyroid

9. A 47-year-old female is being seen by her family physician. Over the past year, she has gained 50 lbs., which is concentrated mostly in her abdominal region. She states that she does not have much energy, and often feels that the muscles in her arms and thighs are weak. Her vital signs are a temperature of 98.8°F, pulse of 85 bpm, and blood pressure of 153/91 mm Hg. A physical examination reveals the patient to have a rounded facial profile, comparatively small arms and thighs, abdominal striae, and hair on her upper lip. Laboratory testing reveals a blood glucose concentration of 167 mg/dL. Of the following, what is the most likely cause of her condition?

A. A pituitary adenoma

B. Excessive consumption of food

C. Hyperplasia of the adrenal glands

D. Filariasis

E. Diabetes mellitus, type 2

Pituitary gland

10. Given the previous clinical scenario, of the following, which condition is she most directly at risk for?

A. Breast carcinoma

B. Cholelithiasis

C. Fractures

D. Cirrhosis of the liver

E. Emphysema

Pituitary gland

11. A 52-year-old female is being seen by her family physician. Over the past year, she has gained 45 lbs., which is concentrated mostly in her abdominal region. She also complains of fatigue and weakness in her arms. Her vital signs are a temperature of 98.7°F, pulse of 89 bpm, and blood pressure of 157/93 mm Hg. A physical examination reveals the patient to have comparatively small arms and thighs,

abdominal striae, and hair on her upper lip. Laboratory testing reveals a blood glucose concentration of 173 mg/dL. Her serum cortisol concentration, drawn at 3:00 pm, is 44 µg/dL. A low-dose dexamethasone test does not elicit a change in the cortisol concentration, but after a high-dose dexamethasone suppression test, the cortisol concentration decreases to 21 µg/dL. Of the following, what is the most likely source of her elevated cortisol?

A. Small-cell lung carcinoma

B. An adrenal adenoma

C. A pituitary adenoma

D. Carcinoid tumor

E. Exogenous use of steroids

Pituitary gland

12. A 63-year-old male with a 70-pack-per-year smoking history is brought to the emergency room by his wife. Over the past three days, he has not eaten, has had occasional vomiting, and complained of a headache, but today he began to act confused, trying to take a footstool for a walk instead of the dog. His vital signs are a temperature of 99.1°F, pulse rate of 85 bpm, and blood pressure of 130/72 mm Hg. His past medical history is significant for hypertension. A physical examination reveals his mucous membranes to be moist. He has no peripheral edema. Routine laboratory testing reveals a sodium level of 115 mEq/L, a serum osmolality of 263 mOsm/kg, a urine osmolality of 289 mOsm/kg, and urine sodium of 56 Eq/L. An X-ray reveals hilar lymphadenopathy. Of the following, what is the most likely diagnosis for his presenting condition?

A. Congestive heart failure due to hypertensive heart disease

B. Syndrome of inappropriate antidiuretic hormone

C. Excessive ingestion of water

D. Sarcoidosis

E. Acute renal failure

Kidney

13. Given the previous clinical scenario, of the following, what would a biopsy of the lymph nodes most likely reveal?

A. Neoplastic squamous cells associated with keratin pearls

B. Neoplastic glands

C. Neoplastic cells with a high nuclear:cytoplasm ratio and with nuclear molding

D. Caseating granulomas

E. Noncaseating granulomas

Lung

14. A 48-year-old female presents to her family physician because of complaints of loss of vision. A review of systems reveals only occasional headaches. She is referred to an ophthalmologist, who determines that the patient has decreased visual acuity in both of her temporal fields. Her prolactin is 61 ng/mL. She has no significant past medical history. Of the following, what is the most likely diagnosis?

A. Osteosarcoma

B. Prolactin-secreting pituitary adenoma

C. Arachnoid cyst

D. Multiple sclerosis

E. Acromegaly

Pituitary gland

15. A 29-year-old male falls while rock climbing, striking his head and causing a small basilar skull fracture. Several months after the accident he presents to his primary care physician, telling him that since the accident he has been very thirsty and has been urinating excessively. He always drinks a lot of water. A urinalysis reveals a specific gravity of 1.001 and a serum osmolality is 331 mOsm/L. Of the following, what is the most likely diagnosis?

A. Delayed subdural hemorrhage

B. Nephrogenic diabetes insipidus

C. Central diabetes insipidus

D. ADH-secreting pituitary adenoma

E. SIADH due to head trauma

Pituitary gland

16. Laboratory analysis of a patient reveals a sodium level of 151 mEq/L, a urine sodium level of < 20 mEq/L, and a urine osmolality of 280 mOsm/kg. A physical examination does not reveal edema of the lower extremities or an elevated jugular pressure. Of the following, what is the most likely diagnosis?

A. Acute tubular necrosis

B. Cushing's syndrome

C. Syndrome of an inappropriate antidiuretic hormone

D. Excessive sweating

E. Central diabetes insipidus

Pituitary gland

17. A 13-year-old Caucasian child is brought to an acute care clinic by her parents because she is urinating excessively. Her parents saved her urine so they could measure it, and they noted that she produced about 6 L of urine in one day. Associated with the polyuria, she has been drinking a lot of water. Her vital signs are a temperature of 98.6°F, pulse of 105 bpm, and blood pressure of 95/70 mm Hg. Laboratory testing reveals a serum glucose concentration of 83 mg/dL. Additional laboratory testing reveals a sodium of 148 mEq/L, and a urine osmolality of 210 mOsm/kg. Of the following, what is the most likely diagnosis?

A. Craniopharyngioma

B. Medulloblastoma

C. Sickle cell anemia

D. Streptococcal meningitis

E. Primary polydipsia

Pituitary gland

17.2 Diseases of the Thyroid Gland and Parathyroid Glands—Questions

Easy	Medium	Hard

18. A 53-year-old female presents to her family physician in Nebraska with complaints of fatigue and constipation. The fatigue has been increasing over the past several months. She has otherwise felt healthy. Her family history includes a mother with breast cancer and systemic lupus erythematosus and a father with colon cancer. A physical examination reveals coarse hair, a doughy skin texture, and myoclonic reflexes. Auscultation of the heart, lungs, and abdomen reveals no significant findings. Laboratory testing reveals a hemoglobin of 13 g/dL and normal electrolytes. Of the following, which is the most likely diagnosis?

A. Multinodular goiter

B. Hashimoto's thyroiditis

C. Graves' disease

D. Subacute granulomatous thyroiditis

E. Papillary thyroid carcinoma

Thyroid gland

19. Given the previous clinical scenario, of the following, what would additional laboratory testing most likely reveal?

A. Increased TSH, increased total T4, increased T3

B. Increased TSH, decreased total T4, decreased T3

C. Decreased TSH, decreased total T4, decreased T3

D. Decreased TSH, increased total T4, increased T3

E. Decreased TSH, increased total T4, decreased T3

Thyroid gland

20. Given the previous clinical scenario, of the following, which antibody would most likely be identified during additional laboratory testing?

A. Anti-dsDNA

B. Antithyroid peroxidase

C. Anti-TSH receptor

D. Anti-Jo-1

E. Anti-topoisomerase-1

Thyroid gland

221

21. Given the previous clinical scenario, of the following, which would histologic examination of the thyroid gland most likely reveal?

A. Granulomas and giant cells

B. Clear nuclei and psamomma bodies

C. Lymphocytic infiltrate and oncocytic change

D. Papillae without fibrovascular cores

E. Abscesses and fibrosis

Thyroid gland

22. A 33-year-old female presents to her family physician with complaints of fatigue and diarrhea, which have been ongoing for about a month. She also reports that she has been losing weight despite an increased appetite. Vital signs are a temperature of 99.0°F, pulse of 108 bpm, respiratory rate of 18 breaths per minute, and blood pressure of 110/70 mm Hg. A physical examination reveals fine hair. Auscultation of the heart, lungs, and abdomen reveals no significant findings. She reports no travel outside the country. Other than the fatigue and diarrhea, she reports no other symptoms and otherwise feels healthy. Of the following, what is the most likely diagnosis?

A. Multinodular goiter

B. Hashimoto's thyroiditis

C. Graves' disease

D. Subacute granulomatous thyroiditis

E. Papillary thyroid carcinoma

Thyroid gland

23. Given the previous clinical scenario, of the following, which antibody would most likely be identified during additional laboratory testing?

A. Anti-dsDNA

B. Antithyroid peroxidase

C. Anti-TSH receptor

D. Anti-Jo-1

E. Anti-topoisomerase-1

Thyroid gland

24. A 28-year-old female undergoes an emergency cesarean section because of vaginal bleeding determined to be caused by placenta previa. Very shortly after the surgery, she develops a fever to 104°F, shows marked diaphoresis, and becomes agitated. On questioning, she is not oriented to place or time. A physical examination reveals a pulse of 115 bpm. Of the following, what is the most likely cause?

A. Postsurgical sepsis

B. Undiagnosed placental abruption

C. Undiagnosed cocaine toxicity

D. Thyroid storm

E. Postsurgical acute myocardial infarction

Thyroid gland

25. A 36-year-old female presents to her family physician with complaints of weight loss and diarrhea. She says she has lost 30 lbs. in the last 6 months despite having a good appetite. During her review of symptoms, she says that she has felt more warm lately, often sweating when normally she wouldn't. Her vital signs are a temperature of 99.0°F, pulse of 104 bpm, and blood pressure of 110/76 mm Hg. Her doctor also notes that his patient appears anxious. Of the following, what is the most likely diagnosis?

A. Hyperthyroidism

B. Hypothyroidism

C. Hyperadrenalism

D. Hypoadrenalism

E. Hyperparathyroidism

F. Hypoparathyroidism

Thyroid gland

26. Given the previous clinical scenario, of the following, what is the most likely diagnosis?

A. Hashimoto's thyroiditis

B. Papillary thyroid carcinoma

C. Graves' disease

D. TSH-secreting pituitary adenoma

E. Goiter

Thyroid gland

27. A 38-year-old female presents to her family physician with complaints of weight loss and diarrhea. She says she has lost 28 lbs. in the last 5 months despite having a good appetite. She complains of sweating when normally she wouldn't. Her vital signs are a temperature of 99.1°F, pulse of 108 bpm, and blood pressure of 112/74 mm Hg. Her doctor also notes that his patient appears anxious. Laboratory testing reveals a TSH of 0.1 mIU/L, and free thyroxine is 7.7 ng/dL. Of the following, which would most likely identify the cause of her symptoms?

A. CT scan of the head

B. Uptake of radioactive iodine by the thyroid gland

C. Chest X-ray

D. CT scan of the pelvis

E. Assay for antithyroglobulin antibodies

Thyroid gland

28. A 38-year-old female presents to her family physician with multiple complaints, including weight loss despite increased appetite, diarrhea, and palpitations. A physical examination reveals scaly and thickened skin on the anterior surface of her legs. Of the following, which sign might also be present?

A. Exophthalmos

B. Pinpoint pupils

C. Ulcers on the lower extremities and decreased pulses

D. Moon-like facies

E. Delayed deep tendon reflexes

Thyroid gland

29. A 47-year-old male presents to his family physician. Over the past year, he has lost about 40 lbs., despite having a good appetite. He also feels as though he is very intolerant to the heat, and sweats at times when no one else does. Many times, he has also had diarrhea. His vital signs are a temperature of 98.6°F, pulse of 103 bpm, and blood pressure of 119/74 mm Hg. A physical examination reveals no significant abnormalities. Laboratory testing reveals a TSH of 14.3 mIU/L and a free thyroxine of 5.6 ng/dL. Of the following, what is the most likely diagnosis?

A. Hashimoto's thyroiditis

B. Graves' disease

C. Papillary thyroid carcinoma

D. Pituitary adenoma

E. Goiter

Thyroid gland

30. A 36-year-old female presents to her family physician because over the past year she has gained 30 lbs., despite a poor appetite, the cold of her native Minnesota bothers her much more lately, and she frequently has constipation. Her vital signs are a temperature of 98.8°F, pulse of 73 bpm, and blood pressure of 110/90 mm Hg. She has delayed relaxation of deep tendon reflexes. Which of the following laboratory values might be expected to be elevated in this patient?

A. Alanine aminotransferase

B. Alkaline phosphatase

C. Prolactin

D. Adrenocorticotropic hormone

E. Uric acid

Thyroid gland

31. A 33-year-old female presents to an acute care clinic. She appears quite anxious. She describes that over the past several months, she has lost about 25 lbs., despite a good appetite. Also, she feels that her scalp hair has changed, becoming much thinner. Review of systems indicates that she sweats more frequently than normal and has intermittent diarrhea. Physical examination reveals no exophthalmos or pretibial myxedema, and the thyroid gland is unremarkable to palpation, with nodules or diffuse enlargement appreciated. Her vital signs are a temperature of 98.9°F, pulse of 108 bpm, and blood pressure of 110/79 mm Hg. Laboratory testing reveals a TSH of 0.01 mIU/L and free thyroxine of 10.1 ng/dL. The patient has never had a history of a thyroid gland

malignancy. Ultimately, a pathologist examines the organ causing her symptoms and identifies essentially normal-appearing thyroid parenchyma. Of the following, what is the most likely source?

A. Thyroid gland

B. Lung

C. Liver

D. Ovary

E. Colon

Thyroid gland

32. A 33-year-old female is having her yearly examination when her primary care physician palpates a nodule in her thyroid gland. A subsequent fine needle aspiration reveals cells with grooved nuclei and occasional psammoma bodies. Of the following, what is the most likely diagnosis?

A. Follicular carcinoma

B. Subacute thyroiditis

C. Anaplastic carcinoma

D. Papillary thyroid carcinoma

E. Medullary thyroid carcinoma

Thyroid gland

33. A 47-year-old female presents to her family physician a few days after a surgical procedure with complaints of a tingling feeling in her muscles. When the doctor inflates the cuff to take her blood pressure, he notices a contraction of the muscles in her forearm. Following this observation, he taps the skin over the facial nerve and produces twitching of the facial muscles. Of the following, what surgical procedure did she have?

A. A thyroidectomy

B. An adrenalectomy

C. A cervical laminectomy

D. Nephrectomy

E. Cholecystectomy

Parathyroid gland

34. A patient examined by a doctor has a positive Trousseau's sign and a positive Chvostek's sign. Of the following, what is the mechanism of action of their disease process?

A. Increased potential difference at the neuromuscular junction

B. Decreased potential difference at the neuromuscular junction

C. Increased release of epinephrine at the neuromuscular junction

D. Decreased release of epinephrine at the neuromuscular junction

E. Antibodies against the neuromuscular junction

Parathyroid gland

223

35. A 40-year-old female presents to her family physician. Several weeks ago, she had a runny nose and cough, after which, for a short period of time, she felt hyperactive, had a few episodes of diarrhea, and could feel her heartbeats. However, now she feels more fatigued and has been suffering from constipation. A physical examination reveals a tender thyroid gland. Laboratory testing reveals a TSH of 12 mIU/L and an ESR of 84 mm/hr. Of the following, what would a histologic examination of the thyroid gland reveal?

A. Papillae

B. Markedly atypical cells

C. Granulomas

D. Foreign material

E. Enlarged cells with large intranuclear inclusions

Thyroid gland

36. A 63-year-old female is having her yearly physical examination when her physician notes an enlargement of the thyroid gland. A subsequent fine-needle aspiration of the gland reveals lymphocytes. She undergoes a thyroidectomy, and the pathologic diagnosis is marginal zone lymphoma. Of the following, which condition would be listed in her medical history?

A. Papillary thyroid carcinoma

B. Graves' disease receiving radiation therapy

C. Myasthenia gravis

D. Hashimoto's thyroiditis

E. Small-cell carcinoma of the lung

Thyroid gland

37. A 43-year-old female presents for her yearly physical examination; her only complaint on review of her systems is intermittent constipation. Laboratory testing indicates alkaline phosphatase of 213 U/L, total calcium of 11.6 mg/dL, a phosphorus of 1.4 mg/dL, and PTH of 127 pg/mL. Of the following, what is the most likely diagnosis?

A. Chronic renal disease

B. Recent surgical removal of thyroid gland

C. Bone metastases from undiagnosed breast cancer

D. Parathyroid gland adenoma

E. Sarcoidosis

Parathyroid gland

38. A 46-year-old male presents to his family physician with complaints of intermittent abdominal pain and intermittent constipation. A review of his systems highlights some muscle weakness. Laboratory testing indicates alkaline phosphatase of 221 U/L, total calcium of 12.1 mg/dL, a phosphorus of 1.3 mg/dL, and PTH of 131 pg/mL. Of the following, which bony abnormality is this patient at risk for?

A. Aneurysmal bone cyst

B. Osteitis fibrosa cystica

C. Osteosarcoma

D. Paget's disease

E. Fibrous dysplasia

Parathyroid gland, bone

17.3 Diseases of the Adrenal Glands—Questions

Easy	Medium	Hard

39. Over a 1-year period, a 37-year-old male has developed weakness, nausea and vomiting, intermittent diarrhea and constipation, and a 25 lb. weight loss. He reports that he occasionally passes out. Also, he feels that his mouth has become darker. His vital signs, when first examined, are temperature of 98.6°F, pulse of 105 bpm, and blood pressure of 91/65 mm Hg. A physical examination reveals darkening of the skin of his elbows, knees, and buttocks. Laboratory testing reveals a sodium of 129 mEq/L, potassium of 5.7 mEq/L, and glucose of 65 mg/dL. Of the following, what is the most likely diagnosis?

A. Tuberculosis

B. Waterhouse-Friderichsen syndrome

C. Secondary hypoadrenalism

D. Addison's disease

E. Cushing's syndrome

Adrenal gland

40. Given the previous clinical scenario, of the following, what is the most likely mechanism of his disease process?

A. Antibody against acetylcholine receptor

B. Antibody against 21-hydroxylase or 17-hydroxylase

C. Antibody against endomysial protein

D. Antibody against cyclic citrullinated peptide

E. Antibody against nuclear cytoplasmic antigen

Adrenal gland

41. A 36-year-old female presents to her family physician stating that she has episodes where her heart races, and at these times, she sweats and has a bad headache. She is raising two children on her own, and the episodes often coincide with stressful periods. She is concerned she is having anxiety attacks. Her vital signs are a temperature of 98.7°F, pulse of 82 bpm, and blood pressure of 107/71 mm Hg. Which of the following tests would be most useful for establishing her diagnosis?

A. Measurement of plasma free metanephrines

B. Measurement of plasma catecholamines

C. Serial blood pressures

D. Blood culture

E. CT scan of the head

Adrenal gland

42. A 37-year-old female presents to her family physician stating that she has episodes where her heart races, and at these times, she sweats and has a bad headache. A stressful event often induces these episodes. Her vital signs are a temperature of 98.9°F, pulse of 82 bpm, and blood pressure of 107/71 mm Hg. During his physical examination, the physician palpates a nodule in the thyroid gland. Given that the patient's symptoms and thyroid nodule are related, of the following, what would histologic examination of the thyroid nodule most likely reveal?

A. Psammoma bodies

B. Granulomas

C. Amyloid

D. Neutrophils

E. Colloid

Adrenal gland, thyroid gland

43. A 52-year-old male undergoes a right nephrectomy and adrenalectomy for a renal cell carcinoma. When the pathologist is dissecting the specimen, she identifies an incidental neoplasm in the adrenal gland; the neoplasm is yellow and located in the cortex. Of the following, which would indicate the neoplasm was secreting cortisol?

A. Focal hemorrhage within the nodule

B. Atrophy of the surrounding nonneoplastic adrenal cortex

C. Infiltration into the surrounding soft tissue

D. Granular cortical surface of the kidney

E. Hyperplasia of the surrounding nonneoplastic adrenal cortex

Adrenal gland

44. A 24-year-old Caucasian male with a history of hypertension undergoes an adrenalectomy, with the right adrenal gland being removed. The pathologist examining the adrenal gland identifies a yellow nodule in the cortex. The nodule weighs 7 grams. The patient weighs 163 lbs. and has never been diagnosed with hyperglycemia or presented with muscle weakness. Of the following, what would laboratory testing most likely have revealed prior to the adrenalectomy?

A. Elevated concentration of catecholamines

B. Decreased concentration of catecholamines

C. Elevated plasma renin activity level

D. Decreased plasma renin activity level

E. Elevated concentration of cortisol

F. Decreased concentration of cortisol

Adrenal gland

45. A 33-year-old female presents to her family physician for an annual examination. She reports no specific complaints. Her vital signs are a temperature of 98.7°F, pulse of 82 bpm, and blood pressure of 148/91 mm Hg. A physical examination reveals no abnormalities other than a bruit on the left side of the back. Of the following, which may laboratory testing reveal?

A. Decreased aldosterone concentration and decreased plasma renin activity

B. Decreased aldosterone concentration and increased plasma renin activity

C. Increased aldosterone concentration and decreased plasma renin activity

D. Increased aldosterone concentration and increased plasma renin activity

Kidney

46. A 17-year-old female presents to her family physician with her parents. She has yet to have a menstrual period, and she is embarrassed about hair growth on her upper lip. Laboratory testing reveals an FSH of 7.1 IU/L, LH of 6.2 IU/L, and 17-hydroxy-progesterone of 7.3 ng/mL. Of the following, what is the most likely diagnosis?

A. Polycystic ovarian syndrome

B. Cushing's disease

C. Congenital adrenal hyperplasia

D. Addison's disease

E. Granulosa cell tumor

Adrenal gland

47. A 37-year-old male is brought to the emergency room by his wife. Over the past several days, he has complained of abdominal pain and nausea, which has been associated with occasional vomiting. During the past two days, he has been much more sleepy than normal. His vital signs are a temperature of 99.0°F, pulse of 113 bpm, and blood pressure of 91/61 mm Hg. His ACTH is 121 ng/L, and his cortisol is 1 microg/dL. Of the following, what is the most likely diagnosis?

A. Infarction of the pituitary gland

B. Waterhouse-Friderichsen syndrome

C. Cushing's disease

D. Congenital adrenal hyperplasia

E. Pheochromocytoma

Adrenal gland

48. A 57-year-old female is brought to the emergency room by her husband. Over the past several days, she has complained of abdominal pain and nausea, which has been associated with occasional vomiting. During the past two days, she has been much more sleepy than normal. She has no significant past medical history, other than temporal arteritis. Her vital signs are a temperature of 99.0°F, pulse of 113 bpm, and blood pressure of 91/61 mm Hg. Her ACTH is 4 pg/mL, and her cortisol is 1 µg/dL. Despite treatment, she goes into cardiac arrest and cannot be resuscitated. An autopsy reveals atrophic adrenal glands. Of the following, what was the most likely mechanism of her disease process?

A. Infection with *Neisseria meningitidis*

B. Use of anticoagulants

C. Rapid withdrawal of exogenous steroids

D. Neoplastic infiltration of adrenal gland

E. Antimitochondrial antibodies

Adrenal gland

49. A 34-year-old male is being followed by his family physician for about 1 year. In this time, he has developed weakness and weight loss, losing about 30 lbs. Despite occasional diarrhea, he still eats, and craves canned soup. On this visit his physician orders an electrolyte panel, which indicates sodium of 128 mEq/L, potassium of 5.6 mEq/L, and glucose of 54 mg/dL. His vital signs are a temperature of 98.9°F, pulse of 112 bpm, and blood pressure of 91/65 mm Hg. His morning cortisol is 2 µg/dL. Of the following, what is his most likely diagnosis?

A. Waterhouse-Friderichsen syndrome

B. Addison's disease

C. Cushing's disease

D. Hyperthyroidism

E. Central pontine myelinolysis

Adrenal gland

50. Given the previous clinical scenario, additional laboratory testing would most likely reveal which of the following?

A. Elevated ACTH; elevated aldosterone

B. Elevated ACTH; decreased aldosterone

C. Decreased ACTH and elevated aldosterone

D. Decreased ACTH and decreased aldosterone

E. Normal ACTH and elevated aldosterone

F. Normal ACTH and decreased aldosterone

Adrenal gland

51. A 3-year-old male walks too close to an embankment and tumbles about 30 feet down it. In the emergency room, a CT scan of the head and body reveals a 3.0-cm mass in the left adrenal gland. Of the following, what is true regarding this lesion?

A. Urinalysis would reveal a decreased concentration of homovanillic acid.

B. The most likely genetic abnormality is a t(9;22).

C. Microscopic examination would reveal Schiller-Duval bodies.

D. It is associated with MEN syndromes.

E. In lesions of this type, in some cases, mature ganglion cells can develop.

Adrenal gland

17.4 Diseases of the Endocrine Pancreas— Questions

Easy	Medium	Hard

52. A 17-year-old male is brought to the emergency room by his parents. Over the past two days, he has developed nausea and vomiting, weakness and fatigue, abdominal pain, and has had an incessant thirst. His vital signs are a temperature of 99.4°F, pulse of 110 bpm, and blood pressure of 112/71 mm Hg. His body weight is 137 lbs. His parents report that recently he has also been eating more than normal but has not gained weight. He has no past medical history. A physical examination reveals the patient to have warm and dry skin and poor skin turgor. Laboratory testing reveals a blood glucose of 556 mg/dL. Of the following, what is the most likely diagnosis?

A. Acute anxiety attack

B. Diabetic ketoacidosis

C. Von Gierke's disease

D. Primary hyperadrenalism

E. Primary hypoadrenalism

Endocrine pancreas

53. A 21-year-old male is brought to the emergency room by EMS services after his parents found him unresponsive in his bedroom in the midmorning. He had been complaining of nausea and abdominal pain the last time they saw him, but he had thought he had a virus and went to bed early the night before. For the last two days he has had a cough, which was sometimes productive, and a slight fever. Laboratory testing reveals a glucose of 501 mg/dL, serum bicarbonate of 8 mEq/L, sodium of 130 mEq/L, chloride of 95 mEq/L, creatinine of 2.1 mg/dL, and amylase of 141 mg/dL. Blood gases reveal a pH of 6.92. A chest X-ray reveals an infiltrate in the left lower lobe of the lung. Of the following, what would urinalysis most likely reveal?

A. Methamphetamine positive urine drug screen

B. Red blood cell casts

C. Ketones

D. Urobilinogen

E. Positivity for leukocyte esterase

Endocrine pancreas

54. A pathology resident is examining glass slides of organs from an autopsy. In the kidney, she identifies smaller blood vessels with a thick, acellular, eosinophilic wall, and in the pancreas, she notes that the islets have collections of acellular pink material, which stains red with a Congo red stain and has apple-green birefringence when polarized. Which of the following conditions does this individual have?

A. Systemic hypertension

B. Polyarteritis nodosa

C. Diabetes mellitus

D. Chronic pancreatitis

E. Zollinger-Ellison syndrome

Pancreas, kidney

55. Laboratory testing of a patient indicates a sodium concentration of 126 mEq/L. The serum osmolality is measured at 285 mOsm/L. Of the following, what is the patient's most likely diagnosis?

A. Central pontine myelinolysis

B. Syndrome of inappropriate antidiuretic hormone

C. Hereditary mixed hyperlipidemia

D. Diabetic ketoacidosis

E. Dehydration

Kidney

56. A 53-year-old obese female presents to her family physician. Over the last 6 months, she has lost 30 lbs. despite a good appetite and diet, has been thirsty, and has been urinating more frequently than usual. Her urine specific gravity is elevated at 1.042. Of the following, which test is most likely to be elevated?

A. Alkaline phosphatase

B. Hemoglobin A1C

C. ADH

D. Hemoglobin F

E. Urine ketones

Pancreas

57. A 21-year-old male is found down in his apartment by a friend who has come to visit. He is lying on the bed, breathing rapidly and deep. The day before he had told his friend that he had been having abdominal pain along with nausea and vomiting for two days. In the emergency room, an arterial blood gas test reveals a pH of 7.13, HCO_3^- of 10 mEq/L, and CO^2 of 25 mm Hg. The sodium is 122 mEq/L and the serum osmolality is 305 mOsm/kg. Of the following, what is the most likely diagnosis?

A. Pulmonary thromboembolus

B. Diabetes insipidus

C. Diabetic ketoacidosis

D. Prolonged vomiting

E. Cerebrovascular accident

Pancreas

17.5 Diseases of the Pituitary Gland—Answers and Explanations

Easy	Medium	Hard

1. Correct: Pituitary adenoma (C)

The features of amenorrhea, infertility, and galactorrhea are consistent with a prolactinoma, the most common form of pituitary adenoma (**C**). An ectopic pregnancy and choriocarcinoma would have an elevated hCG (**A, B**). While hypothyroidism can cause elevated levels of prolactin, as TRH stimulates the release of prolactin, this would not occur in Graves' disease (**D**). Hyperadrenalism would not produce the symptoms she presented with (**E**).

2. Correct: Pituitary adenoma (C)

With increased size of the hands and feet (acral enlargement), coarse facial features, enlargement of the liver, and hyperglucosemia, the features are consistent with acromegaly. Acromegaly is due to a pituitary adenoma that is secreting growth hormone (**C**). The other conditions listed would not produce the symptoms described (**A-B, D-E**).

3. Correct: Mutation of *GNAS1* gene (A)

With increased size of the hands and feet (acral enlargement), coarse facial features, enlargement of the liver, and hyperglucosemia, the features are consistent with acromegaly. Acromegaly is due to a pituitary adenoma that is secreting growth hormone. Around 40% of GH-secreting adenomas are due to the mutation of the *GNAS1* gene, which is on chromosome 20q13 and results in activation of a G protein (**A**). The other choices are incorrect (**B-E**).

4. Correct: Congestive heart failure (D)

With increased size of the hands and feet (acral enlargement), coarse facial features, enlargement of the liver, and hyperglycemia, the features are consistent with acromegaly. Acromegaly is due to a pituitary adenoma that is secreting growth hormone. Individuals with acromegaly can develop hypertension and ultimately congestive heart failure (**D**). They are also at risk for arthritis, osteoporosis, and muscle weakness. The other conditions listed are not directly associated with acromegaly (**A-C, E**).

5. Correct: Sheehan's syndrome (D)

During pregnancy, the pituitary gland will increase in size, due to the increased production of prolactin. However, the blood supply does not also increase, and, therefore, the pituitary gland is sensitive to blood loss and resultant ischemic injury, such as could occur with placenta previa. The patient has features of diabetes insipidus, hypothyroidism, and hypoadrenalism, such as would occur with damage to the pituitary gland. This condition is termed Sheehan's syndrome (**D**). The other choices do not best fit the clinical scenario (**A-C, E**).

6. Correct: Hemorrhage into a pituitary gland adenoma (C)

The sudden onset of a headache and diplopia, followed by signs of hypopituitarism, including the polyuria and polydipsia, nausea, vomiting, and constipation, is consistent with pituitary apoplexy, which is often due to hemorrhage into an adenoma. The condition can lead to death (**C**). The other conditions listed would not best fit the clinical scenario (**A-B, D-E**).

7. Correct: Craniopharyngioma (C)

The patient has features of a mass lesion at the sella turcica, with damage to the posterior pituitary gland (polyuria and polydipsia), headache, and visual disturbances (bitemporal hemianopia, and impaired function of cranial nerves). Although a pituitary adenoma could produce the same symptoms, in children the most common lesion at this site is a craniopharyngioma (**C**), and pituitary adenomas usually occur in an older population (**D**). A tumor in the posterior fossa would not produce such symptoms (**E**), and while subarachnoid hemorrhage and meningitis can produce headache and potentially cranial nerve abnormalities, they are not normally associated with posterior pituitary abnormalities (**A, B**).

8. Correct: MEN1 (A)

The finding of neoplasms of the pituitary gland, parathyroid gland, and pancreas would be consistent with Wermer syndrome (MEN I). The gene mutation is *MEN1*, which is at 11q13 and involves the protein menin (**A**). *BRCA* mutations are associated with breast cancer (**B**), *APC* mutations with familial adenomatous polyposis (**C**), *RET* mutations with MENIIa (**D**), and *GNAS1* with thyroid follicular adenomas (**E**).

9. Correct: A pituitary adenoma (A)

The patient has characteristic features of Cushing's disease (hypertension, fatigue, muscle weakness, truncal obesity, moonfacies, hirsutism, hyperglycemia). Other than exogenous use of steroids, the most common cause of Cushing's disease/syndrome is a pituitary adenoma (**A**). The other choices would not best fit the clinical scenario (**B-E**).

10. Correct: Fractures (C)

The patient has characteristic features of Cushing's disease (hypertension, fatigue, muscle weakness, truncal obesity, moonfacies, hirsutism, hyperglycemia). Cushing's disease causes resorption of bone, leading to osteoporosis and thus the increased risk of fractures (**C**). Cushing's syndrome is not directly related to the development of any of the other listed conditions (**A-B, D-E**).

11. Correct: A pituitary adenoma (C)

A low-dose dexamethasone test should inhibit cortisol production if the source of the increased cortisol is exogenous steroids. The remaining choices all could produce Cushing's syndrome/disease and cause an elevated cortisol concentration; however, the concentration of cortisol will decrease with a high-dose dexamethasone suppression test when the source is a pituitary adenoma secreting ACTH (**C**); however, with the other conditions listed, suppression will not occur, even with a high dose (**A-B, D-E**).

12. Correct: Syndrome of inappropriate antidiuretic hormone (B)

The anorexia, vomiting, headache, and confusion are consistent with symptomatic hyponatremia. As the serum osmolality is < 275 mOsm/kg, the patient has a hypotonic hyponatremia. The moist mucous membranes and lack of edema indicate that the patient is neither hypovolemic or hypervolemic (ruling out acute renal failure and congestive heart failure) (**A, E**). With a urine osmolality of > 100 mOsm/kg, excessive ingestion of water is not the diagnosis (as that would have a urine osmolality of < 100 mOsm/kg) (**C**). Of the choices remaining, SIADH would be a hypotonic hyponatremia, where patients are euvolemic and have a urine osmolality of > 100 mOsm/kg, due to concentration of the urine. Although people with SIADH retain water due to the effects of ADH, they have a normal extracellular fluid volume and will not exhibit edema (**B**). Sarcoidosis most commonly presents in a younger person (40 years of age or less) and is only very rarely associated with SIADH (**D**).

13. Correct: Neoplastic cells with a high nuclear:cytoplasm ratio and with nuclear molding (C)

The anorexia, vomiting, headache, and confusion are consistent with hyponatremia. As the serum osmolality is < 275 mOsm/kg, the patient has a hypotonic hyponatremia. The moist mucous membranes and lack of edema indicate that the patient is neither hypovolemic or hypervolemic. SIADH would be a hypotonic hyponatremia, where patients are euvolemic and have a urine osmolality of > 100 mOsm/kg, due to concentration of the urine. Although people with SIADH retain water due to the effects of ADH, they have a normal extracellular fluid volume and will not exhibit edema. Sarcoidosis most commonly presents in a younger person (40 years of age or less) and is only very rarely associated with SIADH (**E**). A common cause of SIADH is small-cell carcinoma of the lung, which was previously described (**C**). Neither squamous cell carcinoma or adenocarcinoma are commonly associated with SIADH (**A, B**), nor is *Mycobacterium tuberculosis* (**D**).

14. Correct: Arachnoid cyst (C)

The findings of bitemporal hemianopia associated with a headache is consistent with a suprasellar mass. Often pituitary adenomas will present due to the effects of the secreted hormone, and not mass effect, with nonfunctioning tumors presenting with mass effect (**B**). Although the prolactin concentration is elevated, it is only mildly elevated and would not be consistent with a prolactin-secreting pituitary adenoma but would be associated with stalk effect, a mass compressing the pituitary stalk, blocking the flow of dopamine, which normally inhibits the production of prolactin. Multiple sclerosis can present with visual abnormalities but would not be associated with a mildly elevated prolactin (**D**). The sella turcica would be a rare location for an osteosarcoma, and the age of the patient would most likely be lower (**A**). The patient does not have clinical features of acromegaly (**E**). Of the choices, an arachnoid cyst is the best, as these lesions can occur at the base of the brain and could produce a stalk effect (**C**).

15. Correct: Central diabetes insipidus (C)

Diabetes insipidus is due to a lack of ADH (central diabetes insipidus) due to damage to the pituitary gland, such as could occur during head trauma with a basilar skull fracture (**C**) or due to lack of kidney response to response to ADH (nephrogenic diabetes insipidus) (**B**). Given the low specific gravity and increased serum osmolality, ADH production is not likely, considering this would cause concentration of the urine (**D, E**). A chronic subdural hemorrhage is not likely and would not normally present in this manner (**A**).

16. Correct: Central diabetes insipidus (E)

The low urine sodium indicates the cause of fluid loss is not the kidney, and thus acute tubular necrosis is not likely (**A**). Cushing's syndrome can cause hypernatremia, but the patient should be volume overloaded, which this patient is not (**B**). SIADH would cause retention of water and lead to hyponatremia (**C**). With excessive sweating, the patient should try to retain water, and the urine would be concentrated and have a much higher urine osmolality (**D**). With central diabetes insipidus, the lack of ADH leads to water loss, causing hypernatremia. The urine osmo-

lality will be low, because the patient is producing dilute urine (**E**).

17. Correct: Craniopharyngioma (A)

Polyuria and polydipsia can indicate diabetes mellitus; however, the normal serum glucose concentration rules out this diagnosis. The hypernatremia combined with an inappropriately low urine osmolality indicates that the patient is not able to concentrate her urine. The most likely diagnosis is diabetes insipidus; a craniopharyngioma is a tumor that occurs in the region of the pituitary gland and can cause diabetes insipidus (**A**). Sickle cell anemia would be very rare in a Caucasian (**C**), and the normal temperature is inconsistent with streptococcal meningitis (**D**). A patient with primary polydipsia would manifest with hyponatremia rather than hypernatremia (**E**). Although a tumor could cause diabetes insipidus, a CNS tumor in this age group is more likely to be infratentorial (**B**).

17.6 Diseases of the Thyroid Gland and Parathyroid Glands—Answers and Explanations

Easy	Medium	Hard

18. Correct: Hashimoto's thyroiditis (B)

This patient has clinical signs consistent with hypothyroidism (fatigue, coarse hair, decreased reflexes). Of the conditions listed, the most common cause of hypothyroidism would be Hashimoto's thyroiditis (**B**). Graves' disease causes hyperthyroidism (**C**). Subacute granulomatous thyroiditis can cause a transient hypothyroidism but is much less common than Hashimoto's thyroiditis (**D**). Patients with multinodular goiter and papillary thyroid carcinoma are commonly euthyroid (**A, E**).

19. Correct: Increased TSH, decreased total T4, decreased T3 (B)

The patient has the signs and symptoms of hypothyroidism. In primary hypothyroidism, which would be most common, there will be an increased TSH and decreased total T4 and T3 (**B**). Secondary hypothyroidism would have a decreased TSH, total T4 and T3, but this is due to a pituitary abnormality and would be less common than a primary hypothyroidism (**C**). Hyperthyroidism due to a TRH-producing pituitary adenoma would produce an elevated TSH and increased total T4 and T3 (**A**), and hyperthyroidism originating in the thyroid gland (e.g., Graves' disease) would cause a decreased TSH and increased total T4 and T3 (**D**). (**E**) is also incorrect.

20. Correct: Antithyroid peroxidase (B)

The patient has the signs and symptoms of hypothyroidism. The most common cause of primary hypothyroidism is Hashimoto's thyroiditis, which is associated with antithyroid peroxidase antibodies (**B**). Anti-dsDNA antibodies are associated with SLE (**A**), anti-TSH receptor antibodies with Graves' disease (**C**), Anti-Jo-1 with polymyositis/dermatomyositis (**D**), and anti-topoisomerase-1 with systemic sclerosis (**E**).

21. Correct: Lymphocytic infiltrate and oncocytic change. (C)

The patient has the signs and symptoms of hypothyroidism. The most common cause of primary hypothyroidism is Hashimoto's thyroiditis, which histologically is characterized by a lymphocytic infiltrate and oncocytic change (**C**). The other choices (**A-B, D-E**) are not characteristic features of Hashimoto's thyroiditis.

22. Correct: Graves' disease (C)

This patient has clinical signs consistent with hyperthyroidism. Of the choices, Graves' disease is consistently associated with hyperthyroidism (**C**). Although Hashimoto's thyroiditis can cause an initial transient hyperthyroidism, it most commonly causes hypothyroidism (**B**). Subacute granulomatous thyroiditis can cause a transient hypothyroidism but is usually preceded by an upper respiratory tract infection (**D**). Patients with multinodular goiter and papillary thyroid carcinoma are commonly euthyroid. (**A, E**)

23. Correct: Anti-TSH receptor (C)

The patient has the signs and symptoms of hyperthyroidism. The most common cause of primary hyperthyroidism is Graves' disease, which is associated with anti-TSH receptor antibodies (**C**). Anti-dsDNA antibodies are associated with SLE (**A**), antithyroid peroxidase antibodies with Hashimoto thyroidits (**B**), Anti-Jo-1 with polymyositis/dermatomyositis (**D**), and anti-topoisomerase-1 with systemic sclerosis (**E**).

24. Correct: Thyroid storm (D)

The patient has signs and symptoms consistent with a thyroid storm (**D**). Thyroid storm can occur in patients with Graves' disease following surgery or acute infections due to increased catecholamines associated with these two conditions. Given the short time frame, sepsis is not likely (**A**), and with no risk factors, an acute myocardial infarction is unlikely (**E**). Although a cocaine toxicity could present as such, given the circumstances, it is less likely (**C**). Given the clinical diagnosis, absence of a history of hypertension, and the remainder of the presentation, an undiagnosed placental abruption is not likely (**B**).

25. Correct: Hyperthyroidism (A)

The patient has features of thyrotoxicosis, which include heat intolerance, weight loss even with an increased appetite, diarrhea, tachycardia, and anxiety. Hyperthyroidism would present in this manner (**A**). The other endocrine disorders do not present in this manner. (**B-F**) Hyperthyroidism increases the body's metabolic rate. The tachycardia and heat intolerance are due to sensitivity to catecholamines. The best answer of the choices is hyperthyroidism; however, thyrotoxicosis can occur due to diseases other than those originating in the thyroid gland, such as struma ovarii.

26. Correct: Graves' disease (C)

The patient has features of hyperthyroidism. The most common cause of hyperthyroidism is Graves' disease (**C**). Goiters most commonly are not hyperfunctioning (**E**). Hashimoto's thyroiditis most commonly is associated with hypothyroidism; however, early on a transient hyperthyroidism can be seen (**A**). A TSH-secreting pituitary adenoma would be uncommon compared to the incidence of Graves' disease (**D**). Papillary thyroid carcinoma is not a cause of hyperthyroidism (**B**).

27. Correct: Uptake of radioactive iodine by the thyroid gland (B)

The patient has features of hyperthyroidism, which include heat intolerance, weight loss even with an increased appetite, diarrhea, tachycardia, and anxiety. The most common cause of hyperthyroidism is Graves' disease. Individuals with Graves' disease have increased uptake of radioactive iodine by the thyroid gland. Anti-thyroglobulin antibodies are found in Hashimoto's thyroiditis; anti-TSH receptor antibodies are found in Graves' disease (**E**). A CT scan of the head (**A**), chest X-ray (**C**), and CT scan of the pelvis would not be useful, unless a struma ovarii was suspected (**D**).

28. Correct: Exophthalmos (A)

The symptoms of weight loss despite increased appetite, diarrhea, and palpitations are found in hyperthyroidism. Two features of hyperthyroidism are pretibial myxedema and exophthalmos (**A**). The other features are not found with hyperthyroidism (**B-E**). Moon-like facies is found in hyperadrenalism (**D**), and delayed deep tendon reflexes are found in hypothyroidism (**E**).

29. Correct: Pituitary adenoma (D)

An elevated TSH and an elevated free thyroxine are consistent with secondary hyperthyroidism. While Graves' disease and a toxic goiter could produce hyperthyroidism, the high levels of thyroid hormone they produce would feed back on the pituitary and cause a decreased TSH (**B, E**). If a papillary thyroid carcinoma were to be functional, it would also exert a negative feedback on the pituitary gland (**C**). Although Hashimoto's thyroiditis can have a transient hyperthyroidism, this patient's symptoms have been going on for a year, and the TSH would be expected to be low, due to feedback inhibition (**A**). A TSH-secreting pituitary adenoma is a cause of secondary hyperthyroidism (**D**).

30. Correct: Prolactin (C)

The patient has features of hypothyroidism (weight gain, cold intolerance, constipation, increased diastolic blood pressure, delayed relaxation of deep tendon reflexes). TRH, which will be elevated in primary hypothyroidism, also stimulates release of prolactin (**C**). Hypothyroidism is associated with lower than normal concentrations of alkaline phosphatase (**B**) and does not normally affect concentrations of the ALT, adrenocorticotropic hormone, or uric acid (**A, D, E**).

31. Correct: Ovary (D)

Based on the signs, symptoms, and laboratory analysis, the patient has hyperthyroidism. Struma ovarii is an ovarian teratoma with thyroid tissue. These can secrete thyroid hormone and cause hyperthyroidism. The thyroid tissue appears as essentially normal tissue (**D**). Although lesions within the thyroid gland are the main causes of hyperthyroidism, in all conditions, the thyroid parenchyma would not appear histologically normal (**A**). Also, given the lack of history of a thyroid gland malignancy, and the lack of nodules in the thyroid gland, metastatic well-differentiated thyroid carcinoma as a cause of the hyperthyroidism is not very likely. The other choices are incorrect (**B-C, E**).

32. Correct: Papillary thyroid carcinoma (D)

The most common neoplasm of the thyroid gland is papillary thyroid carcinoma. Papillary thyroid carcinoma cells have cleared-out nuclei on histologic section, grooved nuclei, and psammoma bodies. The latter two can be seen in a smear (**D**). Medullary thyroid carcinoma has amyloid (**E**). Anaplastic carcinoma is an aggressive neoplasm (**C**), whereas papillary thyroid carcinoma has a more benign clinical course. Neither follicular carcinoma or subacute thyroiditis is associated with nuclear grooves or psammoma bodies (**A, B**).

33. Correct: A thyroidectomy (A)

The patient has features of hypocalcemia, which can be due to hypoparathyroidism, tingling in the muscles, a positive Trousseau's sign (contraction of muscles in the forearm when inflating the blood pressure cuff), and positive Chvostek's sign (twitching of the facial muscles when the facial nerve is tapped), and, the most common cause of hypoparathyroidism, iatrogenic, with accidental removal of parathyroid glands during a thyroidectomy (**A**). The other choices are not a routine cause of hypocalcemia (**B-E**).

34. Correct: Decreased potential difference at the neuromuscular junction (B)

A positive Chvostek's sign and positive Trousseau's sign indicate hypoparathyroidism. Hypoparathyroidism causes hypocalcemia, and hypocalcemia causes a reduction in the potential difference at the neuromuscular junction (**B**). The other choices are incorrect (**A, C-E**).

35. Correct: Granulomas (C)

The clinical scenario is consistent with hypothyroidism (elevated TSH associated with fatigue and constipation) following a period of hyperthyroidism (diarrhea, hyperactivity, and palpitations) following a flu-like illness, which is consistent with subacute thyroiditis, or de Quervain's thyroiditis (**C**). In this condition, the thyroid gland will be tender. Papillae are found in Graves' disease (**A**), marked atypical cells in an anaplastic carcinoma (**B**), and enlarged cells with large intranuclear inclusions are consistent with CMV (**E**). Foreign material could be found after a fine-needle aspiration of a thyroid nodule or another surgical procedure (**D**).

36. Correct: Hashimoto's thyroiditis (D)

A marginal zone lymphoma is a lymphoma arising from the mucosa-associated lymphoid tissue (hence, they are also referred to as MALTomas) and can present as symptomatic enlargement of the thyroid gland. Marginal zone lymphomas of the thyroid gland are strongly associated with Hashimoto's thyroiditis (**D**). The other conditions listed are not strongly associated with the development of a marginal zone lymphoma in the thyroid gland (**A-C, E**).

37. Correct: Parathyroid gland adenoma (D)

In patients with elevated PTH and chronic renal disease, the calcium is low and the phosphorus is high (**A**). Recent surgical removal of the thyroid gland can cause hypoparathyroidism (due to inadvertent removal of parathyroid glands, and the PTH would be low) (**B**). In patients with hypercalcemia due to bone metastases, the PTH, by feedback from the high calcium, would be low (**C**). Sarcoidosis is not a routine cause of increased PTH (**E**). With a parathyroid gland adenoma, there is increased PTH, leading to increased calcium and decreased phosphorus, and, because of the bone activity, the alkaline phosphatase can be elevated (**D**).

38. Correct: Osteitis fibrosa cystica (B)

The laboratory findings of elevated PTH, elevated calcium, and decreased phosphorus is consistent with a primary hyperparathyroidism, which, because of bony activity, can have an elevated alkaline phosphatase. The symptoms are consistent with hypercalcemia, with the elevated calcium affecting muscle contraction, leading to muscle weakness and constipation. Primary hyperparathyroidism is a cause of osteitis fibrosa cystica (**B**). The other conditions are not commonly associated with primary hyperparathyroidism (**A, C-E**).

17.7 Diseases of the Adrenal Glands—Answers and Explanations

Easy	Medium	Hard

39. Correct: Addison's disease (D)

Features of Addison's disease include weakness, diarrhea and constipation, weight loss, salt craving, hyponatremia, hyperkalemia, hypoglycemia, and hypotension. Increased pigmentation is seen only with primary hypoadrenalism (Addison's disease), due to melanocyte-stimulating hormone being produced along with ACTH (**D**), and would not be seen in secondary adrenalism (**C**). Waterhouse-Friderichsen's syndrome causes acute hypoadrenalism (**B**). Cushing's syndrome is hyperadrenalism (**E**), and there would be weight gain. Tuberculosis is a cause of hypoadrenalism, and, technically, a cause of Addison's disease, however, most cases of Addison's disease in the United States now are due to an autoimmune disorder and not tuberculosis (**A**).

40. Correct: Antibody against 21-hydroxylase or 17-hydroxylase (B)

The mechanism of autoimmune Addison's disease is antibody against 21-hydroxylase or 17-hydroxylase (**B**). Myasthenia gravis has an antibody against the acetylcholine receptor (**A**), celiac disease has antibody against endomysial protein (**C**), rheumatoid arthritis has antibody against cyclic citrullinated peptide (**D**), and various vasculitides have antibody against nuclear cytoplasmic antigen (**E**).

41. Correct: Measurement of plasma free metanephrines (A)

Given the episodic nature of the patient's complaints, and the history of tachycardia/palpitations, diaphoresis, and headache, with symptoms correlating with times of stress, the patient may have a pheochromocytoma. While both plasma free metanephrines and plasma catecholamines can be measured and detected in patients with a pheochromocytoma, plasma free metanephrines are more sensitive and specific (**A, B**). The other tests listed would not be useful (**C-E**).

42. Correct: Amyloid (C)

The signs and symptoms are suggestive of a pheochromocytoma, episodic tachycardia/palpitations, diaphoresis and headache, induced by stressful events. The finding of a thyroid nodule indicates the possibility of MEN syndrome. MENIIa and IIb patients have pheochromocytomas, parathyroid gland hyperplasia, and medullary thyroid carcinoma. Medullary thyroid carcinoma contains amyloid (**C**). The other choices are incorrect (**A-B, D-E**).

43. Correct: Atrophy of the surrounding non-neoplastic adrenal cortex (B)

If the adrenal adenoma was functioning, and secreting cortisol, that cortisol would feedback on the pituitary gland, causing a decrease in the amount of ACTH secreted. If the concentration of ACTH in the body falls, there is no positive stimulus on the non-neoplastic adrenal cortex to produce cortisol, and it will subsequently atrophy (**B**). The other choices are incorrect (**A, C-E**).

44. Correct: Decreased plasma renin activity level (D)

Given the history, the patient most likely has an adrenal adenoma that is secreting aldosterone, causing his hypertension. The size of the nodule indicates that it is not very likely to be a carcinoma; thus, the tumor was not removed because it was a neoplasm, but would have been removed to treat the hypertension. Pheochromocytomas are tumors of the medulla and would secrete catecholamines (**A, B**). Cushing's syndrome can be due to an adrenal adenoma secreting cortisol, but the patient has no features of the disease (which would include weight gain, muscle weakness, hyperglycemia, and thinning of the skin on top of the hands) (**E, F**). People with Cushing's syndrome can have hypertension. Secretion of aldosterone should feedback and inhibit release of renin (**C, D**).

45. Correct: Increased aldosterone concentration and increased plasma renin activity (D)

The finding of hypertension and a bruit is consistent with renal artery stenosis. Renal artery stenosis, due to decreased perfusion of the kidney, can lead to secondary aldosteronism, with decreased renal perfusion stimulating increased release of renin and subsequently increased plasma concentrations of aldosterone (**D**). The other choices are incorrect (**A-C**).

46. Correct: Congenital adrenal hyperplasia (C)

Three causes of hirsutism in this clinical scenario are polycystic ovarian syndrome, congenital adrenal hyperplasia, and Cushing's disease. In congenital adrenal hyperplasia and polycystic ovarian syndrome, the 17-hydroxyprogesterone concentration can be elevated; however, in polycystic ovarian syndrome, the LH will be elevated, and the LH:FSH ratio would be around 2.5 (**A, C**). Cushing's disease would not be associated with changes in LH or FSH (**B**). Addison's disease is not associated with amenorrhea (**D**), and with a granulosa cell tumor the concentration of 17-hydroxyprogesterone would be not affected (**E**).

47. Correct: Waterhouse-Friderichsen's syndrome (B)

The signs and symptoms are consistent with an acute primary adrenocortical insufficiency. One cause of this condition is Waterhouse-Friderichsen's syndrome, which is associated with *Neisseria meningitidis* and *Pseudomonas aeruginosa* infections (**B**). Congenital adrenal hyperplasia can result in increased ACTH and decreased cortisol concentrations; however, the onset is not usually acute, it is often diagnosed around the time of puberty, and patients have hirsutism and other signs of virilization (**D**). Cushing's disease would have an elevated cortisol (**C**). An infarction of the pituitary gland would have a decreased cortisol but also a decreased ACTH (**A**). The clinical history is not consistent with a pheochromocytoma (**E**).

48. Correct: Rapid withdrawal of exogenous steroids (C)

The patient has signs and symptoms consistent with acute primary adrenocortical insufficiency, being abdominal pain, nausea, vomiting, somnolence, and hypertension. Causes of this include rapid withdrawal of exogenous steroids, which, given her history of temporal arteritis, is more likely (**C**). The atrophy of the adrenal glands would occur because of the use of exogenous steroids, causing decreased ACTH and, thus, atrophy of the adrenal glands. Although infection with *Neisseria meningitidis* and the use of anticoagulants are associated with acute primary adrenocortical insufficiency, the expected pathologic finding would be hemorrhage in the adrenal glands (**A, B**). Neoplastic infiltration of the adrenal gland could cause adrenal cortical insufficiency, but the appearance of the glands would be different and the time course would probably not be acute (**D**). Antimitochondrial antibodies are not associated with hypoadrenalism (**E**).

49. Correct: Addison's disease (B)

The patient has signs and symptoms consistent with Addison's disease, including weakness, GI disturbances, weight loss, salt craving, hyponatremia, hyperkalemia, hypoglycemia, and hypotension (**B**). Although Waterhouse-Friderichsen's syndrome is a cause of hypoadrenalism, the presentation is more acute (**A**). Cushing's disease would have elevated cortisol, hypertension, and weight gain (**C**). Hyperthyroidism would not likely have the electrolyte abnormalities (**D**). Also, central pontine myelinolysis results from rapid correction of hyponatremia (**E**).

50. Correct: Elevated ACTH and decreased aldosterone (B)

The patient has signs and symptoms consistent with Addison's disease, including weakness, GI disturbances, weight loss, salt craving, hyponatremia, hyperkalemia, hypoglycemia, and hypotension. As the defect is in the adrenal gland, the cortisol concentration will be low, the concentration of aldosterone will be low (thus, the hyponatremia), and the concentration of ACTH will be high (**B**). The other choices are incorrect (**A, C-F**).

51. Correct: In lesions of this type, in some cases, mature ganglion cells can develop. (E)

In this age group, the most common adrenal gland tumor would be a neuroblastoma. Neuroblastomas can be asymptomatic. In neuroblastomas, urinalysis would reveal increased concentrations of homovanillic acid and vanillylmandelic acid (**A**); t(9;22) is not an associated genetic abnormality (**B**); however, N-MYC can be amplified and if so is a poor prognostic indicator, and neuroblastomas are not associated with MEN (**D**). Schiller-Duval bodies are a feature of yolksac tumors (**C**). Neuroblastomas have Homer-Wright rosettes. Neuroblastomas can spontaneously mature to ganglioneuroblastomas and ganglioneuromas (**E**).

17.8 Diseases of the Endocrine Pancreas— Answers and Explanations

Easy	Medium	Hard

52. Correct: Diabetic ketoacidosis (B)

The features of nausea and vomiting, weakness and fatigue, abdominal pain, and thirst, coupled with an increased blood glucose concentration are consistent with diabetic ketoacidosis (**B**). Primary hyperadrenalism can have hyperglycemia but also has hypertension, weight gain, and other features (**D**). Primary hypoadrenalism would have hypoglucosemia (**E**). The features are not consistent with an acute anxiety attack or von Gierke's disease (**A, C**).

53. Correct: Ketones (C)

The elevated glucose, low bicarbonate, low sodium, elevated creatinine, low pH, and elevated anion gap of 27, combined with the previous history of nausea and abdominal pain, are consistent with diabetic ketoacidosis. The urinalysis would reveal ketones (**C**). The other answers are incorrect (**A-B, D-E**).

54. Correct: Diabetes mellitus (C)

The vascular change in the kidney is hyaline arteriolosclerosis, which is found in both hypertension and diabetes mellitus (**A**). The change in the pancreas is amyloidosis of the islets, which is a feature of diabetes mellitus (**C**). Polyarteritis nodosa would have a segmental, necrotizing inflammation of the vessels, and segmental fibrosis of the vessels (**B**). Chronic pancreatitis would have fibrosis and calcification and usually spares the islets (**D**). Zollinger-Ellison syndrome is associated with a gastrin-secreting neoplasm, which can occur in the pancreas but has none of the previously listed features (**E**).

55. Correct: Hereditary mixed hyperlipidemia (C)

The laboratory tests indicate an isotonic hyponatremia, the two main causes of which are hyperlipidemia and hyperproteinemia. With hyperglycemia, there is a resultant hyponatremia. For every 100 mg/dL increase in glucose, the measured sodium concentration decreases by 2.4 mEq/L, and even more when the glucose concentration is above 400 mg/dL. However, the serum osmolality will be elevated in hyperglycemia (**C, D**). Central pontine myelinolysis is due to the rapid correction of hyponatremia (**C**). SIADH would produce a hypotonic hyponatremia (**B**), and dehydration would produce a hypertonic hypernatremia (**E**).

56. Correct: Hemoglobin A1C (B)

Given the history of polyuria, polyphagia, and polydipsia, with weight loss, in an obese patient, the most likely diagnosis is diabetes mellitus (adult-onset type), although with type 2 diabetes mellitus, those symptoms are not always present. Although not used for diagnosis, the hemoglobin A1C would be elevated, as it reflects the level of hyperglycemia for the last 2 to 3 months (**B**). Ketosis is not usual for type 2 diabetes mellitus (**E**). Diabetes mellitus does not specifically affect alkaline phosphatase, ADH, or hemoglobin F (**A, C, D**).

57. Correct: Diabetic ketoacidosis (C)

The rapid and deep breathing is Kussmaul respiration, and, in association with the presenting symptoms of nausea and vomiting and abdominal pain, is consistent with diabetic ketoacidosis. The laboratory findings indicate a metabolic acidosis, which is also consistent with diabetic ketoacidosis, as is hyponatremia with an increased serum osmolality (**C**). Diabetes insipidus would have hypernatremia, and, with treatment (drinking adequate water) is manageable (**B**). Prolonged vomiting can produce hyponatremia, but the patient would be hypotonic (**D**). Nothing in the clinical scenario strongly supports a pulmonary thromboembolus or cerebrovascular accident (**A, E**).

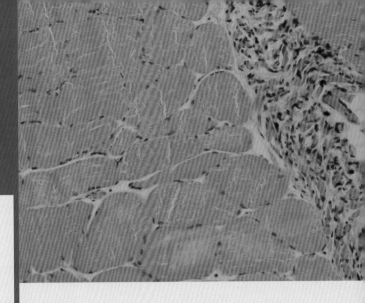

Chapter 18

Diseases of the Musculoskeletal System

LEARNING OBJECTIVES

18.1 Non-Neoplastic Diseases of the Bone

► Describe the clinical features of and list the genetic abnormality associated with osteogenesis imperfecta

► Diagnose osteopetrosis

► Describe the microscopic features of osteopetrosis

► List the causes of fractures in older patients

► List the risk factors for osteoporosis

► List the secondary causes of osteoporosis

► Describe the laboratory abnormalities associated with parathyroid gland hyperplasia

► Diagnose osteonecrosis

► Diagnose reactive arthritis

► Diagnose septic arthritis

► Diagnose and list the autoantibody associated with juvenile rheumatoid arthritis

► Diagnose calcium pyrophosphate disease

► Diagnose a synovial cyst

► Diagnose Lyme disease

18.2 Neoplastic Bone Disease

► Compare the different types of bone tumors

► Diagnose a giant cell tumor

► Describe the mechanism of formation, prognosis, and epidemiology of giant cell tumor

18.1 Non-Neoplastic Diseases of the Bone— Questions

Easy	Medium	Hard

1. A 23-year-old male is being examined by a physician. In his past, the patient has sustained fractures of his right radius, ribs on his left side, and his left tibia. On examination, the doctor notes that the sclerae are blue. Of the following, which is the underlying abnormality leading to his physical and historical findings?

A. Vitamin C deficiency

B. Vitamin D deficiency

C. Mutation of a1 chains of type I collagen

D. Mutation of b1 chains of type I collagen

E. Mutation of FGF receptor 3 (p arm of chromosome 4)

Bone

2. A 23-year-old male is being seen by a physician. He has a history of a fractured left ulna, fractured ribs, and a fractured left tibia, all occurring after relatively minor accidents. Over the past years, he has also frequently had a normocytic and normochromic anemia. He presents today because of ringing in his ears and balance problems. His father has similar conditions, although he sustained episodes of diplopia and weakness of facial muscles prior to his diagnosis. Of the following, what is the most likely diagnosis?

A. Vitamin C deficiency

B. Paget's disease

C. Osteopetrosis

D. Chronic osteomyelitis

E. Chronic lymphocytic leukemia

Bone

3. Given the previous clinical scenario, of the following, what would microscopic examination of the bone reveal?

A. Aplasia of bone marrow elements

B. A mosaic pattern of the bone

C. Obliteration of the marrow cavity with woven bone

D. Infiltration of the bone marrow with neoplastic cells

E. Extensive granulomatous inflammation

Bone

4. A 76-year-old female presents to the emergency room after a fall at home. An X-ray reveals a fracture of the neck of the left femur. Additional X-rays reveal three healing compression fractures of her thoracic vertebral column, involving T4–T6. Of the following, what is a risk factor for her underlying disease process?

A. Increased estrogen exposure

B. High body mass index

C. High-calcium diet

D. Lack of weight-bearing exercise

E. Metastatic tumor

Bone

5. A 47-year-old female presents to the emergency room after a fall at home. An X-ray reveals a fracture of the neck of the right femur. An X-ray of the chest reveals healing compression fractures of the T3-T5 and T8 vertebrae. A physical examination reveals some curvature of the upper back. Of the following, what might laboratory testing reveal?

A. Elevated serum calcium

B. Elevated serum phosphorus

C. Decreased alkaline phosphatase

D. Decreased 1,25-dihydroxyvitamin D

E. Elevated angiotensin-converting enzyme

Bone

6. A 36-year-old female with systemic lupus erythematosus is evaluated by her primary care doctor for pain in the left groin. The pain is constant, began three weeks prior to her visit, and is worse with bearing weight. After imaging is performed, the patient is referred to orthopedic surgery and undergoes left total hip arthroplasty. The surgical specimen shows a pale yellow wedge-shaped area of bone below the cartilage with separation of the bone and cartilage with empty lacunae microscopically. What is the diagnosis?

A. Osteoarthritis

B. Osteonecrosis

C. Osteomyelitis

D. Hyperparathyroidism

E. Osteosarcoma

Bone, joint

7. A 22-year-old male is evaluated by his primary care physician for dysuria. A urethral swab is positive for *Chlamydia trachomatis*. He receives appropriate antibiotic treatment. He returns to the clinic four weeks later complaining of pain in the knees, ankles, and lower back. Repeat testing is negative for both *Chlamydia* and *Neisseria gonorrheae*. Which additional finding might be expected on examination?

A. Right upper quadrant pain and hepatomegaly

B. Scleral icterus

C. Conjunctival injection

D. Nontender subcutaneous nodules over several large joints

E. Crackles in both lung fields

Bone, joint

8. A 43-year-old male with uncontrolled type 2 diabetes is brought to the emergency room for fever and pain in the right knee. His temperature is 101.2°F, pulse is 113/min, and blood pressure is 148/92 mm Hg. An examination of the right knee reveals limited range of motion, a moderate joint effusion, and severe tenderness to palpation. Which of the following tests should be ordered next?

A. Plain radiographs of the right knee

B. MRI of the right knee

C. CT of the right knee

D. Synovial fluid analysis and culture

E. Arthrogram

Bone, joint

9. An 11-year-old girl with no past medical history is evaluated by her pediatrician for pain in the bilateral hands, wrists, and feet that began 3 weeks earlier. Her physical examination is normal except for tenderness in the aforementioned joints. Her pediatrician orders plain films of the hands and wrists, which are normal, as well as a complete blood count, which showed a slightly decreased hemoglobin, and an erythrocyte sedimentation rate of 55 mm/hr. Which of the following additional tests would likely be positive?

A. Anti-dsDNA

B. Anti-Sm

C. Antinuclear antibody (ANA)

D. Rheumatoid factor

E. Anti-CCP IgG

Bone, joint

10. A 63-year-old male with well-controlled hypertension and dyslipidemia presents to his family physician for right knee pain. He denies any preceding factors. The pain started three days prior to his visit and is severe and constant. On examination there is tenderness to palpation, mild decreased range of motion, and no overlying erythema. Provocative testing (anterior and posterior drawer tests, McMurray test, and varus and valgus stress tests) are normal. Plain radiographs of the right knee show extensive chondrocalcinosis. Synovial fluid analysis shows multiple rhomboidal and square-shaped crystals. What is the diagnosis?

A. Osteomyelitis

B. Gout

C. Calcium pyrophosphate deposition disease

D. Rheumatoid arthritis

E. Osteoarthritis

Bone, joint

11. A 46-year-old female presents to her internist for evaluation of a "nodule" on her wrist. She first noticed the nodule a month ago. She denies any pain and has no other complaints. On examination there is a rubbery, somewhat mobile 1.5 cm nodule on the radial aspect of the dorsal wrist, which transilluminates. What is the most likely diagnosis?

A. Rheumatoid nodule

B. Tenosynovial giant cell tumor

C. Volar lymphadenopathy

D. Tendon xanthoma

E. Synovial cyst

Bone, joint

12. A 48-year-old male presents to his primary care physician for a rash that started 1 week prior to his visit. The rash is erythematous, is located on the right lower leg, and has an area of central clearing with a small necrotic center. He is treated with a 10-day course of clindamycin. The rash resolves; however, two months later he presents, complaining of new intermittent pain in both knee joints. On examination there is slight right hemifacial weakness, which involves the forehead. What is the most likely diagnosis?

A. Osteomyelitis with brain abscess

B. Osteosarcoma with metastasis

C. Gaucher's disease

D. Lyme disease

E. Whipple's disease

Bone

18.2 Neoplastic Bone Disease—Questions

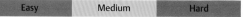

13. A 25-year-old male presents complaining of pain and swelling at the proximal lower leg. On examination the proximal anterior tibia is tender to palpation, and swelling is noted without overlying erythema. The patient is afebrile. Plain X-rays show an expansile mass of the epiphysis. Surgical resection is performed, and microscopic examination reveals sheets of ovoid mononuclear cells with many osteoclast-type multinucleated cells. Which of the following statements are true regarding this disease?

A. The osteoclasts are malignant cells.

B. The osteoclasts express high levels of RANK-L.

C. Chemotherapy is the treatment of choice.

D. 5-year survival is less than 10%.

E. Lung metastases do not affect long-term survival.

Bone, joint

18.3 Non-Neoplastic Diseases of the Bone— Answers and Explanations

1. Correct: Mutation of a1 chains of type I collagen (C)

Multiple fractures and blue sclerae are features of osteogenesis imperfecta, which is due to decreased synthesis of, or production of abnormal, a1 or a2 chains of type I collagen (**C**). Vitamin D deficiency and vitamin C deficiency cause osteomalacia (in adults) and scurvy, respectively, but are not associated with blue sclerae (**A, B**). The blue sclerae are from thin collagen that allows the choroid to be visible. A mutation of the FGF receptor 3 is found in achondroplasia (**E**).

2. Correct: Osteopetrosis (C)

Osteopetrosis is a hereditary bone disease that has both autosomal recessive and autosomal dominant forms. The autosomal dominant form can cause fractures, anemia (due to bone marrow obliteration), and cranial nerve defects due to impingement on foramina (**C**). The other conditions would not address the familial component of the disease (**A-B, D-E**).

3. Correct: Obliteration of the marrow cavity with woven bone (C)

The patient has features consistent with osteopetrosis. Osteopetrosis is a hereditary bone disease that has both autosomal recessive and autosomal dominant forms. The autosomal dominant form can cause fractures, anemia (due to bone marrow obliteration), and cranial nerve defects due to impingement on foramina. The microscopic feature of the disease is obliteration of marrow cavities by woven bone (**C**). The other choices are incorrect (**A-B, D-E**).

4. Correct: Lack of weight-bearing exercise (D)

The patient has features consistent with osteoporosis. The risk factors for osteoporosis include decreased estrogen (**A**), low body mass index (**B**), low-calcium diet (**C**), and lack of weight-bearing exercise (**D**). Also, advanced age, family history, smoking, and alcoholism are risk factors for the disease. Although metastatic disease can cause pathologic fractures, the most likely cause of the fractures in this clinical scenario is osteoporosis (**E**).

5. Correct: Elevated serum calcium (A)

The patient has features consistent with osteoporosis—fractures, compression fractures, and kyphosis. Given her young age, a secondary osteoporosis should be considered. A parathyroid adenoma or parathyroid gland hyperplasia would produce elevated serum calcium (**A**), decreased serum phosphorus (**B**), increased alkaline phosphatase (**C**), and increased 1,25-dihydroxyvitamin D (**D**). An elevated angiotensin-converting enzyme would be indicative of sarcoidosis (**E**). Vitamin D deficiency would not commonly be associated with multiple fractures of this severity.

6. Correct: Osteonecrosis (B)

The gross description is classic for osteonecrosis (avascular necrosis) (**B**). Conditions predisposing to osteonecrosis include long-term corticosteroid use, sickle cell anemia, decompression sickness, and trauma. Osteoarthritis may produce subchondral cysts and loss of cartilage (**A**). Osteosarcoma would cause infiltration of the bone and formation of bone by tumor cells (**E**). Hyperparathyroidism causes osteitis fibrosa cystica, brown tumor, and osteroporosis (**D**).

7. Correct: Conjunctival injection (C)

The history of polyarthritis of the lower extremities four weeks after nongonococcal urethritis is highly suggestive of reactive arthritis. This condition is more common in men and is usually preceded by infection. 80% of patients with reactive arthritis are

HLA-B27 positive. Common manifestations include arthritis, synovitis, and conjunctivitis (**C**). Right upper quadrant pain and tenderness can be seen in Fitz-Hugh-Curtis syndrome. However, the repeat testing was negative for *Chlamydia* and gonorrhea (**A**). None of the other answer choices are commonly seen in reactive arthritis (**B, D-E**).

8. Correct: Synovial fluid analysis and culture (D)

This patient has multiple signs and symptoms of septic arthritis. The best next test to order is arthrocentesis with synovial fluid analysis and culture, since this is ideally performed prior to the initiation of antibiotics (**D**). Plain radiographs would likely also be obtained since, in rare cases, there may be concomitant osteomyelitis; however, these can be done after arthrocentesis so as not to delay appropriate treatment (**A**). The other choices are not the next best step (**B, C, E**)

9. Correct: Antinuclear antibody (ANA) (C)

The clinical scenario is consistent with juvenile rheumatoid arthritis (JRA). Positive antinuclear antibodies are common in JRA (**C**); however, the other autoantibodies listed are rarely present in these patients (**A-B, D-E**). A positive rheumatoid factor in a patient with polyarticular arthritis should prompt consideration of a diagnosis other than JRA (**D**).

10. Correct: Calcium pyrophosphate deposition disease (C)

The finding of square and rhomboid-shaped crystals in the synovial fluid is diagnostic of calcium pyrophosphate disease. Crystals in gout are typically needle-shaped and negatively birefringent (**B**), whereas the crystals seen in calcium phosphate disease are typically weakly positively birefringent (**C**). One would not expect to find crystals in synovial fluid in patients with rheumatoid arthritis, osteoarthritis, or osteomyelitis (**A, D-E**).

11. Correct: Synovial cyst (E)

A synovial cyst is the most common soft tissue mass of the wrist. A synovial cyst would transilluminate (**E**), whereas the other possible answer choices listed would not be expected to transilluminate (**A-D**).

12. Correct: Lyme disease (D)

The skin lesion described is classic for erythema migrans. Erythematous lesions with necrotic centers can be seen in cellulitis; however, central clearing of the lesion would never be seen in cellulitis. The late manifestation of arthritis and cranial nerve palsy are extremely suggestive of Lyme disease (**D**). Neither a brain abscess nor a brain metastasis would cause cranial nerve VII palsy (**A, B**). With no other systemic symptoms, and given the fact that Lyme disease is much more common than Whipple's disease, (**D**) is incorrect. Such skin changes are not usually associated with Gaucher's disease (**C**).

18.4 Neoplastic Bone Disease—Answers and Explanations

Easy	Medium	Hard

13. Correct: Lung metastases do not affect long-term survival. (E)

The clinical and pathologic description is that of a giant cell tumor. This low-grade malignancy is most common in young adults and rarely occurs before skeletal maturity. Up to 4% of cases result in metastasis to the lungs; however, the clinical behavior is benign (**E**). Such metastases are frequently referred to as "benign pulmonary implants." The actual malignant cell, thought to be an osteoblast precursor, expresses high levels of RANK-L, which bind to the RANK on osteoclast precursors, triggering proliferation (**A, B**). Surgery is still the mainstay of treatment, though the rate of local recurrence is high (**C**). Long-term prognosis, except in the case of true malignant transformation, is excellent (**D**).

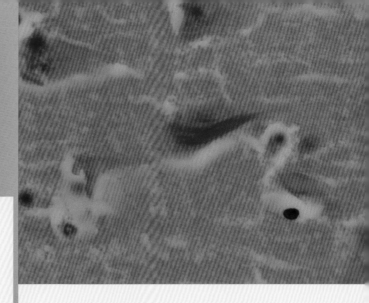

Chapter 19
Diseases of the Peripheral and Central Nervous Systems

LEARNING OBJECTIVES

19.1 Ischemic and Hypertensive Diseases of the Brain

- ▶ Diagnose Broca's aphasia
- ▶ Identify the location of Broca's area
- ▶ Diagnose Wernicke's aphasia
- ▶ Identify the site of an ischemic lesion
- ▶ Correlate the pathologic finding of red neurons, indicative of ischemic injury, to the appropriate clinical scenario in which it would occur
- ▶ Locate lesions of the cerebellum
- ▶ Describe the neurologic defect caused by injury to the subthalamic nucleus
- ▶ Diagnose and describe the risk factors for a stroke
- ▶ Describe the morphologic changes present during the evolution of a cerebral infarct
- ▶ Describe the appearance and mechanism of formation of a venous infarct
- ▶ Describe the vascular supply of border zone regions of the cerebral hemispheres
- ▶ Describe the appearance of an acute infarct
- ▶ List the cause of border zone infarcts
- ▶ Identify a lacunar infarct
- ▶ Diagnose an acute intracerebral hemorrhage
- ▶ List the risk factors for and diagnose an intracerebral hemorrhage
- ▶ Describe the complications and clinical features of cerebral edema

19.2 Traumatic Injuries of the Brain

- ▶ List the types of herniations due to cerebral edema and describe their effects
- ▶ Describe the pathways for pain, temperature, touch, and proprioception
- ▶ Identify the site of a central nervous system lesion
- ▶ Describe the mechanism by which head trauma causes an epidural hemorrhage
- ▶ Diagnose chronic subdural hemorrhage
- ▶ Describe the etiology of a subdural hemorrhage
- ▶ Diagnose a vertebral artery dissection
- ▶ Describe the clinical features of the various types of herniation
- ▶ Describe the clinical features of epidural, subdural, and subarachnoid hemorrhage

19.3 CNS Infections and Aneurysms

- ▶ Diagnose a subarachnoid hemorrhage; describe the common locations for a berry aneurysm to occur
- ▶ Diagnose and list the complications of a subarachnoid hemorrhage
- ▶ List the risk factors for development and rupture of a berry aneurysm
- ▶ Diagnose bacterial meningitis
- ▶ Discuss the physical examination findings associated with meningitis
- ▶ List the risk factors for development of acute bacterial meningitis
- ▶ Diagnose acute bacterial meningitis
- ▶ List the common bacteria causing acute bacterial meningitis
- ▶ Discuss when bacterial meningitis should be considered in the differential diagnosis; describe the use of cerebrospinal fluid analysis to determine the cause of meningitis
- ▶ Diagnose *Mycobacterium tuberculosis* meningitis
- ▶ Describe complications of a basilar meningitis
- ▶ Describe the histologic features of an HIV infection in the brain

19.4 Demyelinating, Alcohol-Related Disease, and Miscellaneous Diseases

- ▶ Diagnose and list the etiology of Korsakoff's syndrome
- ▶ Describe the mechanism of formation of central pontine myelinolysis
- ▶ Diagnose multiple sclerosis
- ▶ Describe the mechanism by which multiple sclerosis affects signaling in the nervous system
- ▶ Describe the relative distribution pattern for multiple sclerosis in the United States
- ▶ Describe the gross and microscopic features of multiple sclerosis
- ▶ Diagnose central pontine myelinolysis
- ▶ Describe the pathologic changes in central pontine myelinolysis

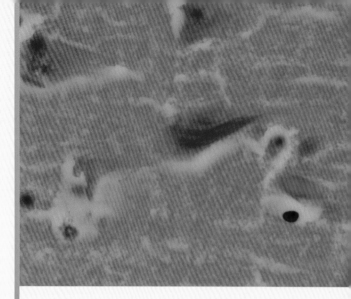

19 Diseases of the Peripheral and Central Nervous Systems

▶ Describe the causes of and diagnose Horner's syndrome

▶ Describe the laboratory testing abnormalities associated with multiple sclerosis

▶ Describe the underlying pathophysiologic process for multiple sclerosis

▶ Diagnose Guillain-Barré syndrome

▶ Describe the mechanism for and diagnose Lambert-Eaton syndrome

19.5 Neurodegenerative Diseases, Hydrocephalus, and Motor Neuron Disease

▶ Describe the histologic features of and diagnose Alzheimer's disease

▶ Describe the protein components of the histologic features of Alzheimer's disease

▶ Describe how the diagnosis of Alzheimer's disease is made and confirmed

▶ Identify a hydrocephalus

▶ Describe the complications of a subarachnoid hemorrhage

▶ Compare lower and upper motor neuron disease

▶ List diseases causing lower, upper, or combined lower and upper motor neuron syndromes

▶ Diagnose Duchenne's muscular dystrophy

▶ Diagnose myasthenia gravis

▶ Describe the mechanism by which myasthenia gravis produces its symptoms

▶ List the tumor associated with myasthenia gravis

▶ Diagnose amyotrophic lateral sclerosis

▶ Compare and contrast upper and lower motor neuron signs

▶ Diagnose Pick's disease

▶ Describe the microscopic findings of Pick's disease

▶ Describe the association between Alzheimer's disease and Down's syndrome

▶ Describe the histologic features of and diagnose Creutzfeldt-Jakob disease

▶ Describe the genetic abnormality associated with Huntington's chorea

▶ Diagnose Huntington's chorea

▶ Describe the inheritance pattern associated with Huntington's chorea

19.6 CNS Neoplasms

▶ Compare the location, age range, genetic abnormalities, and gross and microscopic descriptions of cerebral neoplasms

▶ Diagnose a tumor of the sella turcica

▶ Describe the common location and appearance of a craniopharyngioma

▶ Diagnose pilocytic astrocytoma

▶ Describe the prognosis of pilocytic astrocytomas

▶ List tumor types that produce erythropoietin

▶ Describe the clinical presentation of an acoustic schwannoma

▶ Describe the gross and microscopic features, epidemiology, and general location of meningiomas

▶ Describe the mechanism of formation of communicating and noncommunicating hydrocephalus

19.1 Ischemic and Hypertensive Diseases of the Brain—Questions

| Easy | Medium | Hard |

1. A 67-year-old male with a 70-pack-per-year smoking history and hypertension is eating dinner with friends when he suddenly begins to speak in incomplete sentences and with noticeable pauses between small groups of words. His friends call 9-1-1, and he is brought to the emergency room. During his subsequent hospital admission, a follow-up CT scan is performed 24 hours after his arrival at the emergency room. Of the following, which is most likely to be identified?

A. Ischemic injury in the superior left frontal lobe

B. Ischemic injury in the superior right frontal lobe

C. Ischemic injury in the superior left parietal lobe

D. Ischemic injury in the inferior left frontal lobe

E. Ischemic injury in the inferior right frontal lobe

F. Ischemic injury in the inferior left parietal lobe

Brain

2. A 68-year-old female is eating dinner with friends, when she suddenly starts talking in long sentences, such as "My brown dog sat in the kitchen chair in the living room bathtub when I see see over the moon and I want banana." At first her friends thought she was joking, and then tried to get her to stop, but she did not appear to understand what they were asking her to do. They called 9-1-1 and she was brought to the emergency room. Of the following, what is her most likely diagnosis?

A. Subarachnoid hemorrhage due to ruptured berry aneurysm

B. Ischemic stroke causing Wernicke's aphasia

C. Encephalitis due to West Nile virus

D. Hypothyroid-induced metabolic encephalopathy

E. A glioblastoma multiforme

Brain

3. Given the previous clinical scenario, of the following, which is most likely to be identified?

A. Ischemic injury in superior left frontal lobe

B. Ischemic injury in superior right frontal lobe

C. Ischemic injury in inferior left frontal lobe

D. Ischemic injury in inferior right frontal lobe

E. Ischemic injury in the superior left temporal lobe

F. Ischemic injury in the superior right temporal lobe

Brain

4. A 27-year-old male is partying with friends and snorts cocaine. Shortly thereafter, he becomes unresponsive on the couch. Fortunately, his friends call 9-1-1 and EMTs arrive within minutes. Resuscitation is begun, but a pulse is not restored until they arrive at the emergency room, approximately 20 minutes after he went unresponsive. He does not regain consciousness. One day later, he is pronounced brain dead. An autopsy is performed by a forensic pathologist. Of the following, which change would be identified in the hippocampus?

A. Gliosis

B. Red neurons

C. Neurofibrillary tangles

D. Microglial nodules

E. Foamy macrophages

Brain

5. A 68-year-old male with a history of hypertension, diabetes mellitus type 2, and a 60-pack-per-year smoking history is playing cards with friends when he begins to have difficulty speaking. His friends rush him to the hospital, where the emergency room physician identifies nystagmus, an intention tremor in the right upper extremity, and a gait disturbance due to difficulty with the right lower extremity. Of the following, what is the most likely diagnosis?

A. Acute infarct of the left parietal lobe

B. Acute infarct of the right parietal lobe

C. Acute infarct of the corpus callosum

D. Acute infarct of the left cerebellum

E. Acute infarct of the right cerebellum

Brain

6. A 68-year-old male with a history of poorly controlled hypertension suddenly starts flailing his left upper extremity. Of the following, what is the most likely diagnosis?

A. Acute cerebral infarct involving the right red nucleus

B. Acute cerebral infarct involving the right subthalamic nucleus

C. Acute infarct involving the right cerebellar hemisphere

D. Acute cerebral infarct involving the right cingulate gyrus

E. Acute cerebral infarct involving the right internal capsule

Brain

7. A 32-year-old female is having lunch with her father and mother when she suddenly begins to slur her speech and drool. They immediately call 9-1-1 and she is transported to the hospital via ambulance. Her past medical history is significant only for an ankle sprain that occurred 2 weeks ago and required a walking cast. She has no history of alcoholism or intravenous drug abuse. She also has no history of foreign travel. A review of her systems is essentially negative. A physical examination reveals no significant abnormalities other than a neurologic examination consistent with her presenting symptoms. She has no visual field abnormalities or diplopia. If she died and an autopsy was performed, which of the following would most likely be identified?

A. Vertebral artery dissection

B. Endocarditis of the tricuspid valve

C. Patent foramen ovale

D. Temporal arteritis

E. Aortic dissection

Brain

8. A 27-year-old male is hanging out with friends and playing video games, when suddenly his right upper extremity goes numb and he loses muscular control. He is no longer being able to work the game controller. His friends think he is joking and continue playing, until they realize he is not joking and finally call an ambulance. A review of his symptoms, other than the acute changes, is essentially negative. Vital signs are a temperature of 99.3°F, pulse of 110 bpm, and blood pressure of 131/82 mm Hg. A physical examination reveals neurologic changes consistent with his presenting condition and a holosystolic murmur. He has track marks on his forearm. Of the following, what pathologic change in the brain is the source of his condition?

A. Septic embolus

B. Patchy demyelination

C. Ruptured berry aneurysm

D. Microglial nodules in the cerebral parenchyma

E. Astrocytic neoplasm with necrosis and vascular proliferation

Brain

9. A 67-year-old female is playing cards with friends when she suddenly drops her cards, stating that she cannot feel her right arm and that it had suddenly lost all of its strength. Her friends take her to the emergency room. She is admitted to the hospital. One week later, she sustains an acute myocardial infarct and cannot be resuscitated. Of the following, which would an autopsy most likely reveal?

A. Red neurons in the left cerebral hemisphere along the greater longitudinal fissure

B. Red neurons in the left cerebral hemisphere just superior to the sylvian fissure

C. Foamy macrophages in the left cerebral hemisphere along the greater longitudinal fissure

D. Foamy macrophages in the left cerebral hemisphere just superior to the sylvian fissure

E. Gliosis in the left cerebral hemisphere along the greater longitudinal fissure

F. Gliosis in the left cerebral hemisphere just superior to the sylvian fissure

Brain

10. A 62-year-old female is cooking dinner with her husband when she suddenly collapses. She says she feels like her legs gave out. Her husband helps her to the sofa and brings her some water. Over the next few hours, she develops weakness of both lower extremities and he brings her to the emergency room. A CT scan of the head reveals a sagittal sinus thrombus and changes in the cerebral hemispheres. What pathologic finding caused her symptoms?

A. Brainstem infarct

B. Bilateral hemorrhagic infarcts of the cerebral hemispheres

C. Bilateral nonhemorrhagic infarcts of the cerebral hemispheres

D. Acute subdural hemorrhage

E. Huntington's chorea

Brain

11. A pathologist is examining the brain of an individual who died a day after being hospitalized. She identifies an area of dusky discoloration at the depth of the gyri in the left and right cerebral hemispheres at the junction between the anterior cerebral artery distribution and the middle cerebral artery distribution. Of the following, what was the most likely cause of death of the patient?

A. Cardiac arrest two days postop for knee replacement

B. Delayed death following aortic dissection

C. Thrombotic thrombocytopenic purpura

D. Diabetic ketoacidosis

E. Hypertensive intracerebral hemorrhage

Brain

12. A pathologist is examining a brain at autopsy. In the right basal ganglia is a small (< 1.0 cm) cystic space. Of the following, what is the most likely cause of this finding?

A. Septic emboli from endocarditis

B. Hypertension

C. CNS vasculitis

D. Multiple sclerosis

E. *Cryptococcus* meningitis

Brain

13. A 51-year-old male with a history of hypertension complains to his wife of a headache at dinnertime. While they watch television that night, the headache increases in severity, despite his taking acetaminophen. He becomes sleepier as the night goes on, with his wife interpreting it as him having had a long day, until he has a seizure. She calls 9-1-1. At the hospital, his vital signs are a temperature of 98.5°F, pulse of 110 bpm, and blood pressure of 191/101 mm Hg. Of the following, what is the most likely cause of his condition?

A. Acute epidural hemorrhage

B. Acute subdural hemorrhage

C. Intracerebral hemorrhage

D. Bacterial meningitis

E. Cerebral neoplasm

Brain

14. A 55-year-old male complains to his wife of a headache after mowing the yard. She notices that as the night goes on, he becomes drowsier. After witnessing her husband having a seizure and becoming unresponsive, she calls 9-1-1. On presentation to the ER, his wife reports that he has no significant past medical history but has not seen a doctor in 10 years. Despite treatment, he dies. At autopsy, a 4.5-cm hemorrhage within one of the cerebral hemispheres is identified. Of the following, what preexisting medical condition did he most likely have?

A. Diabetes mellitus

B. Cirrhosis of the liver

C. Systemic hypertension

D. Bacterial endocarditis

E. Cerebral neoplasm

Brain

15. A 37-year-old male is involved in a car accident and sustains a closed head injury, for which he is admitted to the ICU. Three days after the injury, his nurse is examining him and notes that both upper eyelids are drooping, and both pupils are dilated. Of the following, what complication is this patient most directly at risk for (i.e., the most immediately related pathologic change producing the pupillary dilation and lid lag will also produce the complication).

A. Kernohan's notch

B. Duret's hemorrhage

C. Bilateral occipital lobe infarcts

D. Bilateral medial frontal lobe infarcts

E. Postconcussive dementia

Brain

19.2 Traumatic Injuries of the Brain—Questions

Easy	Medium	Hard

16. A 26-year-old male is involved in a motorcycle accident and survives, but sustains a subarachnoid hemorrhage and cerebral contusions, most prominently on the right side of the brain, which are diagnosed by a CT scan. Over the next several days, his mental status declines, and on the 3rd day, a physical examination by his nurse reveals dilation of the right pupil and ophthalmoplegia. Which of the following processes is causing this change?

A. An incidental tumor at the optic chiasma

B. Contusions of the right occipital lobe

C. Herniation of the right cingulate gyrus

D. Herniation of the right uncus

E. Herniation of the right cerebellar tonsil

Brain

17. Given the previous clinical scenario, of the following, what other complication is this patient at risk for due to the process causing the change in the eye?

A. Infarct of the left occipital lobe

B. Infarct of the right occipital lobe

C. Infarct of the left temporal lobe

D. Infarct of the right temporal lobe

E. Infarct of the left cerebellar hemisphere

F. Infarct of the right cerebellar hemisphere

Brain

18. A 27-year-old male is involved in a motor vehicle collision and sustains an injury of the central nervous system. Following the injury, he is not paraplegic or quadriplegic but has motor and sensory deficits of the lower extremities. He has weakness of the right lower extremity, decreased touch sensation in the right lower extremity, and movement difficulties with the right lower extremity, and he has loss of pain sensation in the left lower extremity, and loss of temperature sensation in the left lower extremity. Of the following, where was his injury?

A. Left cerebral hemisphere

B. Right cerebral hemisphere

C. Left side of the cervical spinal cord

D. Right side of the cervical spinal cord

E. Left side of the lower thoracic spinal cord

F. Right side of the lower thoracic spinal cord

Central nervous system

19. A 29-year-old male falls while rock climbing, striking his head when he lands. As a result of the fall, the middle meningeal artery is lacerated as a result of a cranial fracture. Of the following, what bone was most likely fractured, and what type of hemorrhage is the likely result?

A. Frontal bone; subdural hemorrhage

B. Frontal bone; epidural hemorrhage

C. Temporal bone; subdural hemorrhage

D. Temporal bone; epidural hemorrhage

E. Occipital bone; subdural hemorrhage

F. Occipital bone; epidural hemorrhage

Brain

20. A 63 year-old female is brought to the emergency room by her family. They say that for the past 5 weeks she has been complaining of headaches that have been increasing in intensity and were described as achy and steady. However, they said that over the past week, she has been much more irritable than usual and much more easily angered than ever before. Today, they noticed that she was having weakness in her right arm when trying to eat breakfast, as she could barely lift the spoon. Of the following, what is the most likely diagnosis?

A. Acute meningitis

B. Alzheimer's dementia

C. Parkinson's disease

D. Chronic subdural hematoma

E. Schizophrenia

Brain

21. Given the previous clinical scenario, which of the following is the most likely pathologic mechanism?

A. Inflammation of the temporal artery

B. Tearing of a bridging vein

C. Rupture of a berry aneurysm

D. Rupture of a Charcot-Bouchard aneurysm

E. Tearing of the middle meningeal artery

Brain

22. A 31year-old male is drinking at a bar with friends. He gets into an argument with another bar patron who is the ex-boyfriend of his current girlfriend, who punches him in the chin, knocking him to the ground. He resumes drinking. Two hours later, he starts to complain of pain in his neck and jaw, following which he becomes confused and shortly thereafter collapses. 9-1-1 is called and he is taken to the hospital, where he becomes unresponsive and cannot be resuscitated. Of the following, which is an autopsy most likely to reveal?

A. Atlanto-occipital dislocation

B. Acute subdural hemorrhage

C. Acute myocardial infarction

D. Vertebral artery dissection

E. Pulmonary thromboembolus

Brain

23. A 47-year-old alcoholic falls while walking out of a bar and strikes his head on the sidewalk, producing a gaping laceration of the occipital region of his scalp. EMTs are called and take him to the hospital for treatment, where the laceration is sutured. A CT scan reveals a fracture of the occipital bone. No neurosurgeon is available, and hours after the event he develops a dilated right pupil. Of the following, what is the most likely diagnosis?

A. Right-sided epidural hemorrhage

B. Left-sided epidural hemorrhage

C. Right-sided subdural hemorrhage

D. Left-sided subdural hemorrhage

E. Right-sided subarachnoid hemorrhage

Brain

19.3 CNS Infections and Aneurysms—Questions

Easy	Medium	Hard

24. A 36-year-old male is playing a game of basketball with friends. Suddenly, he grabs his head and collapses to the ground, complaining of an excruciating headache. His friends try to walk him to their car, but he appears confused, and then becomes nauseated and vomits. They drive him to the emergency room, and on the way he lapses into a coma. In the emergency room, he develops asystole, and despite resuscitative measures, expires. He has no significant past medical history. In the emergency room, they were able to get a temperature of 98.9°F, and perform a lumbar puncture, which reveals blood in the cerebrospinal fluid. An autopsy is performed. Of the following, where is the pathologist most likely to find the lesion that caused his death?

A. Within one of the basal ganglia

B. Circle of Willis

C. Foramen of Munro

D. Pons

E. Sella turcica

Brain

25. Given the previous clinical scenario, of the following, if the patient had survived, what would he be most at risk for in the future?

A. Aggressive meningioma

B. Central pontine myelinolysis

C. Alzheimer's disease

D. Communicating hydrocephalus

E. Glioblastoma multiforme

Brain

26. Given the previous clinical scenario, of the following, what underlying undiagnosed condition might the patient have that contributed to his presenting condition?

A. HIV infection

B. Cirrhosis of the liver

C. Diabetes mellitus

D. Carotid artery atherosclerosis

E. Hypertension

Brain

27. A 43-year-old alcoholic is brought to the emergency room by EMTs, who were called by the patient's family. Over the past two days, he has complained of a headache, which he described as severe and throbbing. Today, they found him unresponsive in his bed, with vomit on the bed. His vital signs are a temperature of 101.3°F, pulse of 108 bpm, and blood pressure of 152/87 mm Hg. Of the following, which physical examination finding is this patient most likely to have?

A. Positive Babinski's sign

B. Positive Brudzinski's sign

C. Positive Levine's sign

D. Positive Courvoisier's sign

E. Positive Lhermitte's sign

Brain

28. Given the previous clinical scenario, of the following, what is the most likely etiology of his condition?

A. *Staphylococcus aureus*

B. *Neisseria meningitidis*

C. *Hemophilus influenzae*

D. *Streptococcus pneumoniae*

E. *Mycobacterium tuberculosis*

Brain

29. Given the previous clinical scenario, of the following, which is this patient most likely to have in his past medical history that is directly related to his presenting condition?

A. Severe abdominal trauma

B. Perforated appendicitis

C. Kidney stones

D. Metastatic colonic adenocarcinoma

E. Coagulation disorder

Brain

30. A 45-year-old alcoholic is brought to the emergency room by EMTs, who were called by the patient's family. He lives by himself in an abandoned house with several other homeless individuals. They found him unresponsive in his bed, with vomit on the floor. In the emergency room, his vital signs are a temperature of 101.5°F, pulse of 111 bpm, and blood pressure of 157/89 mm Hg. A lumbar puncture is performed. The cerebrospinal fluid has a total protein of 198 mg/dL, CSF/serum glucose ratio of 0.27, total white blood cell count of 325 cells/µL, and is 38% neutrophils. Of the following, what is the most likely etiologic agent?

A. *Streptococcus pneumoniae*

B. *Neisseria meningitidis*

C. *Mycobacterium tuberculosis*

D. West Nile virus

E. *Candida albicans*

Brain

247

31. Given the previous clinical scenario, of the following, which physical examination finding is most likely to be identified?

A. Sensory loss in both lower extremities

B. Motor loss in both lower extremities

C. Abnormalities of eye movements

D. Gait disturbance

Brain

32. A neuropathologist is examining the brain from a patient with HIV, and, in the cerebral parenchyma, he identifies multinucleated cells. The virus is inducing a change in what type of cell to produce these giant cells?

A. Neurons

B. Astrocytes

C. Oligodendroglial cells

D. Microglial cells

E. Ependymal cells

Brain

19.4 Demyelinating, Alcohol-Related Disease, and Miscellaneous Diseases—Questions

Easy	Medium	Hard

33. A 43-year-old chronic alcoholic male is brought to the emergency room by his friends. They say that recently he had been falling down much more than usual and they say that he cannot seem to remember things that he did before, even when they were really exciting. During his history and physical examination, the doctor asks him whether he can explain the theory of relativity, and the patient gives a long, but obviously incorrect answer. Physical examination reveals an inability to gaze laterally. Of the following, what is the most likely diagnosis?

A. Basilar subarachnoid hemorrhage due to ruptured berry aneurysm

B. Brainstem hemorrhagic stroke

C. Hypothyroidism-induced metabolic encephalopathy

D. HSV encephalitis

E. Korsakoff's syndrome

Brain

34. Given the previous clinical scenario, of the following, what is the underlying cause of his symptoms?

A. Riboflavin deficiency

B. Thiamine deficiency

C. Viral infection of the temporal lobe

D. Lead toxicity

E. Cocaine toxicity

Brain

35. A 41-year-old alcoholic is brought to the emergency room by his family because of confusion. Laboratory testing reveals a sodium concentration of 119 mEq/L. The emergency room physician prescribes hypertonic saline to be rapidly applied to quickly fix the electrolyte abnormality and correct his confusion. Of the following, what condition does the physician risk causing?

A. A lacunar infarct of the pons

B. A subarachnoid hemorrhage

C. Progressive multifocal leukoencephalopathy

D. Acute disseminated encephalomyelitis

E. Central pontine myelinolysis

Brain

36. A 31-year-old white female develops decreased visual acuity in her left eye, which ultimately resolves. Over the next 10 years, she has intermittent episodes of ataxia, spasticity and weakness, and sensory abnormalities. Each episode usually resolves, and between the episodes, she is relatively symptom free. Which of the following mechanisms plays the most significant role in her disease process?

A. Intermittent compression of structures by a benign mass

B. Inflammation of neurons

C. Loss of saltatory conduction

D. Abnormal Na^+/K^+ conduction

E. Decreased intra-axonal transport

Brain

37. Given the previous clinical scenario, of the following, which state has the highest incidence of her disease process?

A. Hawaii

B. California

C. Montana

D. Texas

E. Florida

Central nervous system

38. A 35-year-old white female develops decreased visual acuity in her right eye that ultimately resolves. Over the next 5 years, she has intermittent episodes of gait difficulties, muscle weakness, and changes in sensation. She dies in a car accident, and an autopsy is performed. Within the brain are gray-white translucent regions in the white matter, some of which are more soft and slightly pink. Histologic examination of these areas reveals well-defined sheets of foamy macrophages. Of the following, what should be found among the macrophages?

A. Neurofibrillary tangles

B. Corpora amylacea

C. Lewy bodies

D. Microthrombi

E. Essentially normal neurons

Central nervous system

39. A 46-year-old male is admitted to the hospital after a sodium concentration of 101 mEq/L is identified during laboratory testing conducted in the emergency room. He is rapidly given hypertonic solutions, which raises his sodium concentration. Five days later, still while in the hospital, he develops an upper gastrointestinal bleed, which, despite treatment, causes his death. An autopsy is performed. Of the following, related to his hospital treatment, which might be identified in the brain?

A. Foamy macrophages in the pons

B. Onion bulbs

C. Myelin ovoids

D. Microglial nodules

E. Mallory's hyaline

Brain

40. A 71-year-old male with a past medical history that includes hypertension, diabetes mellitus type 2, and a 100-pack-per-year smoking history presents to his family physician with complaints that his left upper eyelid is drooping and that his skin is dry on the left side of his face. During the examination, his physician notes that, in his relatively warm exam room, that the left side of the patient's face is not sweating, while the right side is, and the left pupil is constricted compared to the right pupil. If the underlying cause of his symptoms is a neoplasm, of the following, which organ contains the tumor?

A. Left cerebral hemisphere of brain

B. Upper lobe of left lung

C. Left atrium of the heart

D. Pituitary gland

E. Left parotid gland

Brain

41. A 37-year-old first presented to her family physician with loss of vision in her right eye about 7 years ago. Since that time, she has done fairly well, with occasional episodes where she has had a variety of symptoms including weakness of her left lower extremity, loss of sensation in her right upper extremity, and one episode where she had urinary incontinence. Of the following, what would CSF analysis most likely reveal?

A. Tau protein

B. Oligoclonal bands

C. M-spike

D. High concentration of glucose

E. Albuminocytologic dissociation

Brain

42. A 41-year-old female has had recurrent episodes of muscle weakness and loss of sensation in her lower and upper extremities over the course of 10 years, which has left her wheelchair bound. Occasionally she has also had visual changes. She frequently recovers fully from an episode, but not always, leaving her in her current state. Of the following, which cell type in her nervous system was affected by her disease process?

A. Neurons

B. Astrocytes

C. Microglial cells

D. Oligodendroglial cells

E. Schwann cells

Brain

43. A 34-year-old male has a one-week history of cough, congestion, and a slight fever. Following these he develops weakness in his legs, which then progresses to his thighs. He is admitted to the hospital. The weakness continues and involves his abdominal musculature and his diaphragm, necessitating intubation. Ultimately, the weakness passes, he is extubated and able to leave the hospital with no lingering complications. He had no significant past medical history, and, at the time of his weakness, other than the preceding symptoms, no other manifestations. Of the following, what is the most likely diagnosis?

A. Lyme disease

B. Lambert-Eaton syndrome

C. Myasthenia gravis

D. Guillain-Barré syndrome

E. Transient ischemic attack

Muscle, nerves

44. A 71-year-old male who has emphysema and a 60-pack-per-year smoking history presents to his family physician complaining of weakness in his thighs and arms. A CT scan of his chest and abdomen reveal a 3.5 cm left hilar mass and several up to 2.0-cm masses in the liver. If the CT scan findings and presenting complaint are related, what is the most likely diagnosis of the lung mass?

A. Squamous cell carcinoma

B. Adenocarcinoma

C. Large-cell carcinoma

D. Small-cell carcinoma

E. Pulmonary hamartoma

Lung, muscle

45. Given the previous clinical scenario, if the CT scan findings and presenting complaint are related, which of the following is the most likely mechanism for the patient's weakness?

A. Diminished calcium in the sarcoplasmic reticulum

B. Antibody against the sarcoplasmic reticulum

C. Accelerated uptake of the neurotransmitter at the nerve-muscle junction

D. Antibody against presynaptic channels at the nerve-muscle junction

E. Antibody against postsynaptic channels at the nerve-muscle junction

Lung, nerve

19.5 Neurodegenerative Diseases, Hydrocephalus, and Motor Neuron Disease— Questions

Easy	Medium	Hard

46. An 83-year-old male is being seen for a routine examination by his primary care physician at the nursing home where he resides. Over the past 4 years, he has developed progressively worsening memory loss, impaired language function, and altered social skills. A CT scan of the head revealed no anatomic abnormalities. Testing for RPR, B12, folate, and thyroid function were all within normal limits. Of the following, what is the most likely diagnosis?

A. Parkinson's disease

B. Alzheimer's dementia

C. Cerebral infarct involving the left middle cerebral artery distribution

D. Creutzfeldt-Jakob disease

E. Multiple sclerosis

Brain

47. Given the previous clinical scenario, of the following, what feature would be identified on pathologic examination of the brain?

A. Neurofibrillary tangles in the cortex

B. Lewy bodies in the substantial nigra

C. Corpora amylacea in the neocortex

D. Collections of foamy macrophages

E. Microglial nodules

Brain

48. Given the previous clinical scenario, of the following, what are the components of the histologic features associated with the patient's condition?

A. Elastin and tau protein

B. Hyaline and tau protein

C. Amyloid and tau protein

D. Hyaline and α-synuclein protein

E. Amyloid and α-synuclein protein

Brain

49. A 77-year-old male is brought to his primary care physician by his wife, because over the past several years his memory has become worse, and he is beginning to make decisions that exhibit poor judgment and she has noticed a change in his personality, with him becoming more withdrawn and sometimes confrontational, when he used to be very gentle and kind. The doctor suspects Alzheimer's disease. Of the following, which would confirm his diagnosis?

A. A CT scan of the head

B. Analysis of cerebrospinal fluid for tau protein

C. Genetic analysis for mutation of chromosome 19

D. Autopsy examination after death

E. MRI of the brain

Brain

50. A pathologist is performing an autopsy on an individual who died in the hospital. When the brain is removed from the cranium, it essentially collapses. After formalin fixation, the brain is cut, revealing dilated lateral ventricles. The third and fourth ventricles are not dilated. Of the following, what is the diagnosis?

A. Global hypoxic-ischemic encephalopathy

B. Encephalitis

C. Communicating hydrocephalus

D. Noncommunicating hydrocephalus

E. Porencephaly

Nervous system

51. A 26-year-old male has a severe headache and goes to the emergency room. A CT scan of the head reveals a ruptured berry aneurysm. An emergent procedure is performed and the aneurysm is clipped. In the following years, which of the following is he at risk for?

A. Porencephaly

B. Noncommunicating hydrocephalus

C. Communicating hydrocephalus

D. Encephalitis

E. Glioblastoma multiforme

Brain

52. A neurologist is performing an examination on a 47-year-old male who is hospitalized. With stimulation of the sole of the feet, the neurologist elicits dorsiflexion of the great toe. Of the following, which other physical examination finding is he most likely to find?

A. Muscle wasting

B. Fasciculations

C. Reduced resistance to passive stretching

D. Hyperactivity of deep tendon reflexes

Central nervous system

53. A neurologist is performing a physical examination on a patient in the hospital. During the examination, she notes wasting of muscles, fasciculations, reduced resistance to passive stretching, and loss of deep tendon reflexes. Assessment of the cranial nerves reveals no abnormalities. Of the following, which condition is the most likely cause of these symptoms?

A. Werdnig-Hoffman's syndrome

B. Amyotrophic lateral sclerosis

C. Infarct of the pons

D. Hereditary spastic paraplegia

E. Parkinson's disease

Central nervous system

54. A family had four children: two boys and two girls. Both boys developed muscle weakness in their upper and lower extremities around the age of 3 years, and by the age of 11 years, both were wheelchair bound. Both died by the age of 16 years. Of the following, what is the most likely diagnosis?

A. Amyotrophic lateral sclerosis

B. Juvenile Parkinson's syndrome

C. Duchenne's muscular dystrophy

D. Spinal muscular atrophy

E. Chronic meningitis

Skeletal muscles

55. A 46-year-old female presents to her family physician with the complaint of double vision. Physical examination reveals ptosis. The doctor diagnoses Bell's palsy, and tells the patient the condition will most likely pass. Over the next 6 months, she presents to her physician several times, both with similar changes involving her eyes, and also with muscle weakness involving her thighs and arms. No muscle wasting develops. Her symptoms abate with a trial of cholinesterase inhibitor. Of the following, what is the most likely diagnosis?

A. Amyotrophic lateral sclerosis

B. Duchenne's muscular dystrophy

C. Myasthenia gravis

D. Eaton-Lambert syndrome

E. Guillain-Barré syndrome

Brain

56. Given the previous clinical scenario, of the following, what is the mechanism of the disease process?

A. Antibodies to norepinephrine receptors

B. Antibodies to epinephrine receptors

C. Antibodies to acetylcholine receptors

D. Decreased uptake of acetylcholine

E. Decreased uptake of epinephrine

Brain

57. Given the previous clinical scenario, of the following, which tumor is this patient most likely to have?

A. Small-cell carcinoma of the lung

B. Thymoma

C. Diffuse large B cell lymphoma

D. Hodgkin's lymphoma

E. Atrial myxoma

Brain

58. A neurologist is examining a 39-year-old male patient. The patient is alert and oriented to person, place, and time, and has no memory deficits, remembering information from the previous day as well as from his days in college. Neurological examination reveals no deficits of the cranial nerves and no sensory deficits, with both fine touch and pain intact and normal. The patient has weakness of his upper and lower extremities, and occasional fasciculations. He also has an upgoing Babinski. His examinations have been similar in the past. Of the following, what is the most likely diagnosis?

A. Parkinson's disease

B. Multiple sclerosis

C. Amyotrophic lateral sclerosis

D. B12 deficiency

E. Polio

Brain

251

59. A 71-year-old with a several-year history of decreased cognitive function, memory loss, a tremor, and a shuffling gait dies after an episode of bronchopneumonia. The family requests a brain-only autopsy. The neuropathologist identifies atrophy of the frontal and temporal lobes. Of the following, what is the neuropathologist most likely to identify on microscopic examination?

A. Neurofibrillary tangles

B. Lewy bodies

C. Spongiform change

D. Pick bodies

E. Intranuclear inclusions

Brain

60. A 46-year-old male dies and an autopsy is performed. Microscopic examination of the brain reveals an extensive number of neurofibrillary tangles and senile plaques. Of the following, what is the decedent's most likely diagnosis?

A. Creutzfeldt-Jakob disease

B. Multiple sclerosis

C. Down's syndrome

D. Turner's syndrome

E. Viral encephalitis

Brain

61. A 60-year-old male with a past medical history of hypertension treated with a β-blocker develops worsening memory loss over the course of 8 months. Occasionally he has myoclonus. The memory loss is associated with decreased ability to care for himself, mostly in the last two months before his death. At autopsy, which of the following is the most likely to be identified?

A. Neurofibrillary tangles and senile plaques in the hippocampus

B. Spongy changes in the gray matter

C. Intracelluar aggregates of tau protein

D. Lewy bodies

E. Intracytoplasmic inclusions

Brain

62. A 37-year-old first presented to her family physician with loss of vision in her right eye about 7 years ago. Since that time, she has done fairly well, with occasional episodes in which she has had a variety of symptoms including weakness of her left lower extremity, loss of sensation in her right upper extremity, and one episode where she had urinary incontinence. Of the following, what would gross examination of the brain most likely reveal?

A. Normal parenchyma

B. Metastatic carcinoma

C. Plaques

D. Multiple foci of hemorrhage

E. Central pontine myelinolysis

Brain

63. A 41-year-old male commits suicide by shooting himself in the chest. The forensic pathologist who is performing the autopsy examines the brain and notes that both caudate nuclei appear atrophic. Of the following, what molecular abnormality was present in this individual?

A. CAG repeats

B. CGA repeats

C. Mutation of chromosome 1

D. Mutation of chromosome 14

E. Inability to catabolize very-long-chain fatty acids

Nervous system

64. A 42-year-old woman had a history of making sudden moves that had no purpose (e.g., suddenly raising her right hand), and she developed some memory loss. Her condition led to depression, and she committed suicide through a drug overdose. She has one son. Of the following, what is the likelihood that he will develop the condition his mother had?

A. 0

B. 1 to 3

C. 25

D. 50

E. 100

Brain

19.6 CNS Neoplasms—Questions

Easy	Medium	Hard

65. A 12-year-old child is brought to the emergency room by his parents because he is complaining about not being able to see correctly. An examination reveals bilateral temporal defects in his visual field. A CT scan of the head reveals a mass that has some calcification. Of the following, what is the most likely diagnosis?

A. Pilocytic astrocytoma

B. Medulloblastoma

C. Ependymoma

D. Oligodendroglioma

E. Craniopharyngioma

Brain

66. A 13-year-old child is brought to the emergency room by EMTs because he had a seizure during breakfast, which was witnessed and reported by his parents. A CT scan of the head reveals a mass in the left cerebral hemisphere, which is subsequently excised by a neurosurgeon. A pathologist identifies numerous Rosenthal fibers and notes that the tumor is GFAP positive. Of the following, what is another feature of this tumor?

A. It has a poor prognosis.

B. It commonly produces erythropoietin.

C. It is likely to metastasize to the liver.

D. It is derived from astrocytes.

E. Rosettes or pseudo-rosettes are likely to be found microscopically.

Brain

67. A 37-year-old male presents to an acute care clinic. Over the past year, he has developed hearing problems and quite frequently has problems with his balance. The symptoms have progressed to the point that he cannot handle them anymore. Physical examination reveals decreased hearing in his left ear, and balance problems, being unable to stand on one leg unaided. A CT scan of the head reveals a mass. Of the following, what is the most likely diagnosis?

A. Glioblastoma multiforme

B. Meningioma

C. Schwannoma

D. Ependymoma

E. Craniopharyngioma

Brain

68. A pathologist is examining a brain tumor resected from a 63-year-old male. The pathologist identifies psammona bodies in the histologic section. Of the following, what is true of this tumor type?

A. The prognosis is good.

B. The tumor most frequently occurs at the cerebellopontine angle.

C. The tumor derives from Rathke's pouch.

D. The appearance of the tumor cells is sometimes described as a fried egg.

E. The tumor is rare.

Brain

69. A 23-year-old female develops an ependymoma of the third ventricle for which she undergoes surgery. As a result of the surgery, she has scarring of the cerebral aqueduct, leading to stenosis. She develops cerebral swelling and requires the placement of a ventriculostomy drain into her peritoneal cavity. Of the following, which condition did she develop?

A. Hydrocephalus ex vacuo

B. Communicating hydrocephalus

C. Noncommunicating hydrocephalus

D. Subarachnoid hemorrhage

E. Global hypoxic-ischemic encephalopathy

Brain

19.7 Ischemic and Hypertensive Diseases of the Brain—Answers and Explanations

Easy	Medium	Hard

1. Correct: Ischemic injury in the inferior left frontal lobe (D)

The patient is manifesting Broca's aphasia. While he is speaking in broken sentences, his ability to comprehend the physician would not be impaired. Broca's area is in the dominant hemisphere, which is most often the left side, in the inferior portion of the frontal lobe, near the sylvian fissure (**D**). The other choices are incorrect (**A-C, E-F**).

2. Correct: Ischemic stroke causing Wernicke's aphasia (B)

With Wernicke's aphasia, the patient cannot comprehend written or spoken language and will speak in meaningless and wordy sentences (**B**). Although a glioblastoma multiforme could affect the same region of the brain, as the onset was sudden, Wernicke's aphasia is much more likely (**E**). The other conditions listed would produce more of a diffuse neurologic process (e.g., coma), not a focal process (**A, C-D**).

3. Correct: Ischemic injury in the superior left temporal lobe (E)

The patient is manifesting Wernicke's aphasia. With Wernicke's aphasia, the patient cannot comprehend written or spoken language and will speak in meaningless and wordy sentences. Wernicke's area is in the dominant hemisphere, which is most often the left side, in the superior portion of the temporal lobe, near the sylvian fissure (**E**). The other choices are incorrect (**A-D, F**).

4. Correct: Red neurons (B)

Red neurons are neurons with increased eosinophilia of the cytoplasm and a loss of nuclear basophilia. Red neurons are a sign of hypoxic-ischemic injury, which would occur in the described scenario (**B**). Gliosis is microscopic scarring and would not be present at 1 day (**A**). Neurofibrillary tangles are found in Alzheimer's disease (**C**) and microglial nodules in encephalitis (**D**). Foamy macrophages would be expected at a later time, in areas of organizing necrosis, or if there is demyelination (**E**).

5. Correct: Acute infarct of the right cerebellum (E)

Nystagmus (uncoordinated eye movements), dysarthria, intention tremor in the upper limbs, and ataxia (gait disturbance) are consistent with a cerebellar syndrome. The defect producing the abnormalities is on the same side of the cerebellum as the abnormalities occur, in this case, on the patient's right side (**E**). The other choices are incorrect (**A-D**).

6. Correct: Acute cerebral infarct involving the right subthalamic nucleus (B)

The patient has hemiballismus, which is characteristic of a lesion of the contralateral subthalamic nucleus (**B**). The other choices are incorrect (**A, C-E**).

7. Correct: Patent foramen ovale (C)

Given the sudden focal neurological changes, the patient is having a stroke. The history of recent trauma and the relative immobility it would cause can lead to deep venous thrombi. If a deep venous thrombus enters the right atrium, and there is a patent foramen ovale, the thrombus can enter into the left atrium (i.e., a paradoxical embolus) and cause a cerebral infarct (**C**). A vertebral artery dissection is rare and would more likely affect the brainstem and occipital lobes, leading to visual disturbances (**A**). Endocarditis of the tricuspid valve would cause pulmonary septic emboli (**B**). There is no history to suggest aortic dissection (**E**). Given her age alone, temporal arteritis is not the diagnosis; however, the lack of visual changes or headache also does not support the diagnosis of temporal arteritis (**D**).

8. Correct: Septic embolus (A)

The patient is having a stroke, a sudden focal neurological change, causing loss of sensation and motor control of his right upper extremity. Given the findings of fever, a heart murmur, and track marks, his underlying medical condition is most likely endocarditis, with an embolus to the brain (**A**). The sudden onset of symptoms of this type is not as suggestive of a demyelinating disorder (**B**), and both a ruptured berry aneurysm and encephalitis would be more likely to present with diffuse-type symptoms (e.g., coma) and not focal symptoms (**C, D**). In this age group, a high-grade astrocytoma would be rare (**E**).

9. Correct: Foamy macrophages in the left cerebral hemisphere just superior to the sylvian fissure (D)

The patient has a sudden focal neurological change, with loss of sensation and with muscular weakness, which is consistent with a stroke. As the right upper extremity is involved, the damage is in the left cerebral hemisphere. Damage to the cortex along the greater longitudinal fissure would cause neurological deficits in the lower extremities; whereas, the segment of the cerebral hemisphere controlling the upper extremities is nearer the sylvian fissure. As the patient survived one week following the initial insult, the infarct would be organizing and would be characterized by foamy macrophages (**D**). The other choices are incorrect (**A-C, E**).

10. Correct: Bilateral hemorrhagic infarcts of the cerebral hemispheres (B)

Obstruction of the sagittal sinus will cause a backup of blood and lead to a venous infarct. As the sagittal sinus drains blood from both cerebral hemispheres, a sagittal sinus thrombus can produce bilateral infarcts. As blood is still flowing through the arteries, venous infarcts are hemorrhagic (**B, C**). A sagittal sinus thrombus would not cause a brainstem infarct (**A**). An acute subdural hemorrhage would be a very unlikely manifestation of a sagittal sinus thrombus (**D**) and unlikely to present such focal symptoms. Given her age of presentation, lack of family history, and the sudden nature of the symptoms, Huntington's chorea is not the correct choice (**E**).

11. Correct: Delayed death following aortic dissection (B)

The pathologic description is that of a border zone (or watershed) infarct, involving the boundary between the anterior cerebral and middle cerebral arteries. These are most commonly due to hypotension, with low perfusion pressures unable to bring blood to the most distal extents of the distribution of the cerebral arteries—the tissue at the boundaries between the two is then at most risk for ischemic injury. Of the choices, aortic dissection would cause hypotension due to blood loss, and with a delayed death, an infarct could be expected to develop (**B**). The remainder of the conditions are less likely to cause a period of hypotension, and then the patient will survive (**A, C-E**).

12. Correct: Hypertension (B)

The description is that of a lacunar infarct. Although lacunar infarcts can cause symptoms, many are asymptomatic. The most common cause of lacunar infarcts is hypertension (**B**). The other choices are incorrect (**A-C, E**)

13. Correct: Intracerebral hemorrhage (C)

Intracerebral hemorrhage can occur for a variety of reasons, but the most common cause is hypertension (**C**). With an intracerebral hemorrhage, patients can have a headache (with the severity reflective of the severity of the bleed), decreased alertness, and seizures. Given there is no trauma, an acute epidural hemorrhage or subdural hemorrhage is unlikely (although an intracerebral hemorrhage can rupture through the cortical surface of the brain and cause a secondary subdural hemorrhage) (**A, B**). The lack of a fever would not favor bacterial meningitis (**D**), and, although hemorrhage within a cerebral neoplasm could present similarly, this would be much less common than an intracerebral hemorrhage due to hypertension (**E**).

14. Correct: Systemic hypertension (C)

A headache, increasing in severity, progressing to somnolence, and causing a seizure, is consistent with the autopsy finding of an intracerebral hemorrhage. Most intracerebral hemorrhages are due to hypertension (**C**). Other conditions causing intracerebral hemorrhage include amyloid angiopathy, vasculitis, coagulation disorders, and neoplasms, but they are a rarer cause than hypertension (**E**). Bacterial endocarditis, while it could produce septic emboli that can be associated with hemorrhage, would be unlikely in an individual with no risk factors, and progressing from septic emboli to a symptom-causing, space-occupying lesion would not likely occur so quickly (**D**). Diabetes mellitus and cirrhosis of the liver are not, by themselves, a significant contributor to the risk of an intracerebral hemorrhage (**A, B**).

15. Correct: Bilateral occipital lobe infarcts (C)

Ptosis and pupil dilation indicate herniation of the uncus, which can compress CN III, damaging parasympathetics, leading to ptosis and pupillary dilation. At this same location, the uncus can also compress the posterior cerebral artery, which would lead to infarction of the occipital lobe. Given that the changes noted by the nurse are bilateral, both the left and right posterior cerebral arteries could be affected, leading to bilateral infarction (**C**). Kernohan's notch, which is compression of the contralateral crus cerebri, a Duret's hemorrhage, and possible infarction of the medial portion of the frontal lobes (due to compression of the anterior cerebral artery by cingulate gyrus herniation) will also be results of cerebral edema, but not uncal herniation (**A-B, D**). Post-concussive dementia, if it occurred, would be a long-term complication (**E**).

19.8 Traumatic Injuries of the Brain—Answers and Explanations

Easy	Medium	Hard

16. Correct: Herniation of the right uncus (D)

Cerebral edema causes various forms of herniation, including cingulate gyrus (subfalcine herniation), uncal, and cerebellar tonsillar herniations. Herniation of the uncus can impinge on the oculomotor nerve, which carries parasympathetic fibers. Damage of the parasympathetic fibers will cause a dilated pupil and ophthalmoplegia (**D**). The other conditions listed would not cause the changes described in the clinical scenario (**A-C, E**)

17. Correct: Infarct of the right occipital lobe (B)

Adjacent to CN III (oculomotor nerve) is the posterior cerebral artery. The changes in the eye—pupillary dilation and ophthalmoplegia—are due to compression of CN III and damage to the parasympathetic nerve fibers contained within, as would occur with herniation of the uncus. Compression of the posterior cerebral artery can also occur, and the posterior cerebral artery supplies the occipital lobe, and its compression would lead to infarction (**B**). The other changes would not be produced by a herniation of the right uncus (**A, C-F**).

18. Correct: Right side of lower thoracic spinal cord (F)

There is dissociated sensory loss in the lower extremities, with pain and temperature sensation loss on the left side and touch and proprioception loss on the right side. The fibers carrying pain and temperature signals cross over at the point they enter the spinal cord, while the fibers carrying touch and proprioception ascend before crossing over; thus, when there is dissociation between the two sensory types, the lesion is on the same side of the cord as the touch and proprioception loss (**E, F**). As there are no deficits in the upper extremities, the cervical portion of the spinal cord is not likely injured (**C, D**). The symptoms are not due to damage to the cerebral hemispheres (**A, B**).

19. Correct: Temporal bone, epidural hemorrhage (D)

With head trauma that tears the middle meningeal artery, it is usually due to a fracture of the temporal bone, which, of the cranial bones of the vault, is usually the thinnest. The middle meningeal artery runs along the inner surface of the temporal bone, and a fracture of the bone can lacerate the vessel, leading to an epidural hemorrhage (**D**). The other choices are incorrect (**A-C, E-F**).

20. Correct: Chronic subdural hematoma (D)

Given the slow onset, and localizing symptoms (the weakness of the right arm), and lack of other signs of an acute infection, acute meningitis is unlikely (**A**). She does not have the normal motor difficulties described in Parkinson's disease (flat affect, pill-rolling tremor, shuffling gait) (**C**). Any elderly person with late onset of psychiatric-type symptoms should be considered for a chronic subdural hemorrhage (**D**). The clinical scenario is not consistent with Alzheimer's dementia (**B**) or schizophrenia (**E**).

21. Correct: Tearing of a bridging vein (B)

Given the relatively extended course of events, progression of headache, personality changes, and development of weakness on one side of the body, the clinical scenario is consistent with a chronic subdural hemorrhage. Subdural hemorrhage is due to tearing of a bridging vein (**B**). Temporal arteritis can cause headache and visual problems, but is not usually associated with personality change or weakness (**A**). Given the relatively long time course, subarachnoid hemorrhage due to rupture of a berry aneurysm and rupture of a Charcot-Bouchard aneurysm, and resultant intracerebral hemorrhage, are not likely (**C, D**). Given the lack of a history of trauma, tearing of a middle meningeal artery is not likely, and an epidural hemorrhage is not normally associated with the clinical scenario as described (**E**).

22. Correct: Vertebral artery dissection (D)

Trauma to the chin can lacerate the vertebral artery, leading to a dissection, which can cause neck and jaw pain. A vertebral artery dissection can lead to ischemia of the brainstem, which could cause confusion and a coma (**D**). Relatively simple trauma such as a punch and fall would be very unlikely to cause an atlanto-occipital dislocation (**A**), and, the pain in the neck and jaw are not characteristic of subdural hemorrhage (**B**). The overall clinical scenario is

not consistent with an acute myocardial infarction or pulmonary thromboembolus as the most likely cause of death (**C, E**).

23. Correct: Right-sided subdural hemorrhage (C)

The dilated right pupil indicates right uncal herniation, which would occur with a right-sided space-occupying lesion in the head (**C, D**). Epidural hemorrhages most commonly occur due to fractures of the temporal bone and a resultant tear of the middle meningeal artery (**A, B**). A subarachnoid hemorrhage would not lead to a space-occupying lesion, and, if herniation occurred, it would likely be bilateral due to generalized edema (**E, F**).

19.9 CNS Infections and Aneurysms—Answers and Explanations

| Easy | Medium | Hard |

24. Correct: Circle of Willis (B)

Given the symptoms of sudden onset of severe headache, followed by nausea and vomiting, and coma, and with blood in the cerebrospinal fluid, the most likely cause of death is a subarachnoid hemorrhage due to a ruptured berry aneurysm. The berry aneurysm would be found in the circle of Willis, most commonly in the anterior circulation, at a branch point (**B**). The other choices are incorrect (**A, C-E**).

25. Correct: Communicating hydrocephalus (D)

Given the symptoms of sudden onset of severe headache, followed by nausea and vomiting, and coma, and with blood in the cerebrospinal fluid, the most likely diagnosis is a subarachnoid hemorrhage due to a ruptured berry aneurysm. The hemorrhage in the subarachnoid space can induce scarring, which will lead to a communicating hydrocephalus (**D**). Survivors of a ruptured berry aneurysm are not at risk for the development of aggressive meningiomas, central pontine myelinolysis, or Alzheimer's disease, but they are also at risk for seizures (**A-C, E**).

26. Correct: Hypertension (E)

Given the symptoms of sudden onset of severe headache, followed by nausea and vomiting, and coma, and with blood in the cerebrospinal fluid, the most likely diagnosis is a subarachnoid hemorrhage due to a ruptured berry aneurysm. Berry aneurysms are believed to develop from congenital weaknesses in the wall of the circle of Willis; however, hypertension can contribute to their enlargement and rupture (**E**). The other conditions are not directly associated with berry aneurysms or their rupture (**A-D**).

27. Correct: Positive Brudzinski's sign (B)

The patient has signs and symptoms consistent with bacterial meningitis. Brudzinski's sign is positive when, while lying down, the patient's neck is flexed forward, causing the hips and knees to flex in response. This is a sign of meningeal inflammation (**B**). A positive Babinski's sign is dorsiflexion of the great toe with stimulus of the sole of the foot, and is associated with upper motor neuron disease (**A**). A positive Levine's sign is clutching the hand across the chest and is associated with myocardial infarction (**C**). A positive Courvoisier's sign is a palpable gallbladder and is often associated with pancreatic carcinoma, although other causes of biliary obstruction can also produce the sign (**D**). Lhermitte's sign indicates a lesion of the dorsal columns of the spinal cords and can be seen in vitamin B12 deficiency, multiple sclerosis, and transverse myelitis (**E**).

28. Correct: *Streptococcus pneumoniae* (D)

The patient has signs and symptoms consistent with a bacterial meningitis. The most common cause of bacterial meningitis in adults is *Streptococcus pneumoniae* (**D**). The other organisms listed are possible causes of acute bacterial meningitis but are not as common as *S. pneumoniae* (**A-C, E**).

29. Correct: Severe abdominal trauma (A)

The patient has signs and symptoms consistent with bacterial meningitis. In the adult population, the most common cause of bacterial meningitis is *Streptococcus pneumoniae*. Individuals without a spleen, such as abdominal trauma requiring a splenctomy could result in, are at greater risk for infection with encapsulated bacteria, including *S. pneumoniae* (**A**). The other conditions listed would not directly be a risk factor for *S. pneumoniae* meningitis.

30. Correct: *Mycobacterium tuberculosis* (C)

Being that the patient was found unresponsive, having vomited, and with a high fever, a bacterial meningitis should be considered. In bacterial meningitis, other than *Mycobacterium tuberculosis*, the total protein is often 245 to 270 mg/dL, CSF/serum glucose ratio is 0.20 to 0.36, the total white blood cell count is 500 to 2500 cells/μL, and the neutrophils are 80 to 90% (**A, B**). In an aseptic meningitis, such as caused by a virus, the total protein is often around 75 mg/dL, the CSF/serum glucose ratio is around 0.54, the total white blood cell count is around 98 cells/μL,

and the neutrophil count is around 37% (**D**). *Candida albicans* is not commonly a cause of meningitis (**E**). The results of the CSF evaluation are not consistent with a bacterial or viral meningitis, but are consistent with a *M. tuberculosis* meningitis (**C**).

31. Correct: Abnormalities of eye movements (C)

The signs and symptoms are consistent with meningitis. The analysis of the spinal fluid is most consistent with *Mycobacterium tuberculosis*, which tends to have a total protein of between 191 to 314 mg/dL, CSF/serum glucose ratio of 0.27 to 0.28, total white blood cell count of 300 to 375 cells/μL, and neutrophil percentage of around 37%. *Mycobacterium tuberculosis* can often affect the base of the brain, instead of the convexities, and can involve the cranial nerves, thus producing abnormalities of the extra ocular muscle movements (**C**); the other choices are not the best, given the organism identified (**A-B, D**).

32. Correct: Microglial cells (D)

Multinucleated cells in the brain are associated with HIV infection. The multinucleated cells result from the fusion of microglial cells (**D**). The other choices are incorrect (**A-C, E**).

19.10 Demyelinating, Alcohol-Related Disease, and Miscellaneous Diseases—Answers and Explanations

Easy	Medium	Hard

33. Correct: Korsakoff's syndrome (E)

Patients with Korsakoff's syndrome have anterograde amnesia, confabulation, ophthalmoplegia, and ataxia (**E**). Basilar subarachnoid hemorrhage, brainstem hemorrhage, and hypothyroid metabolic encephalopathy would all be expected to produce a decreased level of consciousness or coma (**A-C**). HSV encephalitis typically causes fever with severe headache, lethargy, and delirium, and, frequently, seizures (**D**).

34. Correct: Thiamine deficiency (B)

The patient has the signs and symptoms of Korsakoff's syndrome (anterograde amnesia, confabulation, ophthalmoplegia, and ataxia). Korsakoff's syndrome is due to a thiamine deficiency, and is most commonly found in chronic alcoholics (**B**). The other answers are incorrect (**A, C-E**).

35. Correct: Central pontine myelinolysis (E)

Both rapid correction of hyponatremia and chronic alcoholism itself are associated with central pontine myelinolysis, which is a demyelination of the central portion of the pons (**E**). The effects range from asymptomatic to death. Progressive multifocal leukoencephalopathy is a demyelinating disorder due to infection with the JC virus, and acute disseminated encephalomyelitis is a demyelinating disorder that usually follows a viral illness (**C, D**). A lacunar infarct can result from hypertension, and most are silent (**A**). Hypernatremia has been associated with the development of a subarachnoid hemorrhage by some authors but denied by others (B).

36. Correct: Loss of saltatory conduction (C)

The patient has multiple sclerosis, which is more common in whites, females, and young adults. Often the disease is characterized by neurologic episodes with in-between periods of no symptoms. The symptoms can be motor (spasticity and weakness), sensory, or autonomic (urinary frequency and urgency). The optic nerve is commonly involved. The disease damages oligodendroglial cells, causing loss of myelin. With loss of myelin, saltatory conduction, which normally allows for the rapid transmission of signals down the length of the axon, is no longer possible (**C**). The other choices are incorrect (**A-B, D-E**).

37. Correct: Montana (C)

The patient has multiple sclerosis, which is more common in whites, females, and young adults. Often the disease is characterized by neurologic episodes with in-between periods of no symptoms. The symptoms can be motor (spasticity and weakness), sensory, or autonomic (urinary frequency and urgency). The optic nerve is commonly involved. Multiple sclerosis is most common in the northern states, most specifically from eastern Washington to Minnesota (**C**). The incidence of multiple sclerosis in the other states would be less (**A-B, D-E**), although the absolute number of individuals with multiple sclerosis in the other states may be higher, because the other states have a higher population.

38. Correct: Essentially normal neurons (E)

The patient has multiple sclerosis, which is more common in whites, females, and young adults. Often the disease is characterized by neurologic episodes with in-between periods of no symptoms. The symptoms can be motor (spasticity and weakness), sensory, or autonomic (urinary frequency and urgency). The optic nerve is commonly involved. The disease targets oligodendroglial cells, not neurons. With the breakdown of myelin, foamy macrophages will be formed, but the neurons will be normal (unlike in an organizing cerebral infarct, where neurons will be absent) (**E**). The other features listed are best identified with Alzheimer's disease and normal aging (**A, B**), Parkinson's disease (**C**), and various hematologic conditions (**D**).

39. Correct: Foamy macrophages in the pons (A)

With rapid correction of hyponatremia, patients are predisposed for the development of central pontine myelinolysis, which can also occur in alcoholics. With central pontine myelinolysis, the center of the pons will have foamy macrophages (**A**). Within the clusters of macrophages will be histologically viable neurons, because, as in multiple sclerosis, the disease does not normally cause the death of neurons. Onion bulbs and myelin ovoids are found in nerves, related to axonal injury (**B**). Onion bulbs are concentric layers of Schwann cell cytoplasm around axons, and associated with demyelination. Microglial nodules are found in encephalitis (**D**), and Mallory's hyaline, while associated with alcoholism, is found in the liver (**E**).

40. Correct: Upper lobe of left lung (B)

The patient has Horner's syndrome, which is characterized by ptosis (drooping of the eyelid), anhidrosis (no sweating), and miosis (pupillary constriction). Horner's syndrome is caused by damage to the sympathetic pathway—from the hypothalamus, to the spinal cord at the interomedial column, then to the superior cervical ganglion. A lung tumor eroding through the superior portion of the lung (Pancoast tumor) can damage this pathway (**B**). Of the choices, (**B**) is the best and most likely to produce the clinical scenario presented (**A, C-E**).

41. Correct: Oligoclonal bands (B)

The clinical scenario is consistent with multiple sclerosis. Patients with multiple sclerosis can have a variety of symptoms, depending on where the plaques occur, and can manifest varying degrees of muscle weakness and/or loss of sensation. Visual changes can occur, and sometimes are the initial symptoms. Cerebrospinal fluid analysis in patients with multiple sclerosis typically shows elevated immunoglobulin levels, elevated IgG index, and oligoclonal immunoglobulin bands as well as slightly elevated protein levels (**B**). Albuminocytologic dissociation is characteristic of Guillain-Barré syndrome (**E**). An M-spike on serum electrophoresis is seen in multiple myeloma (**C**). Tau proteins and a high concentration of glucose are not associated with multiple sclerosis (**A, D**).

42. Correct: Oligodendroglial cells (D)

The clinical scenario of neurological changes, involving both the motor and sensory systems, occurring in a younger patient, and with occasional visual disturbances, is consistent with multiple sclerosis. The disease process is due to loss of myelination of nerve fibers because of loss of oligodendroglial cells (**D**). The other choices are incorrect (**A-C, E**).

43.   Correct: Guillain-Barré syndrome (D)

The clinical presentation is classic for Guillain-Barré syndrome, with an ascending paralysis occurring following a respiratory-type infection. The condition has also been associated with CMV and EBV infections (**D**). None of the other conditions listed are characteristically ascending, and none, except TIA, would pass with only symptomatic treatment (**A-C**). Also, a transient ischemic attack would not be bilateral and continuously developing (**E**).

44.   Correct: Small-cell carcinoma (D)

Small-cell carcinoma is associated with a paraneoplastic syndrome referred to as Lambert-Eaton syndrome, which causes weakness in the proximal muscle groups, which include those in the arm and those in the thigh (**D**). The other choices are incorrect (**A-C, E**).

45.   Correct: Antibody against presynaptic channels at the nerve–muscle junction (D)

The clinical scenario, weakness in the proximal muscle groups, associated with a pulmonary neoplasm with metastases, is consistent with Lambert-Eaton syndrome associated with small-cell carcinoma. In Lambert-Eaton syndrome, the tumor causes the production of an antibody directed against the presynaptic calcium channels. The other mechanisms are not correct (**A-C, E**).

19.11 Neurodegenerative Diseases, Hydrocephalus, and Motor Neuron Disease— Answers and Explanations

Easy	Medium	Hard

46.   Correct: Alzheimer's dementia (B)

Individuals with Alzheimer's dementia can have abnormal function in memory, language skills, social skills and personality, or judgment and reasoning (**B**). The disease is usually slowly progressive; whereas Creutzfeldt-Jakob disease causes a rapid onset of dementia (**D**). Parkinson's disease can have dementia as a component; however, the main symptoms are related to motor function, including a shuffling gait and pill-rolling tremor (**A**). A cerebral infarct would not cause global disease (**C**). Multiple sclerosis can affect motor or sensory function, but memory, language skills, and the other areas mentioned would be preserved (**E**).

47.   Correct: Neurofibrillary tangles in the cortex (A)

The signs and symptoms—memory loss, impaired language function, and altered social skills—progressing over years, and with no etiology identi-

fied on imaging or laboratory testing, is consistent with Alzheimer's disease. The histologic feature of Alzheimer's disease is neurofibrillary tangles and senile plaques (**A**). Lewy bodies in the substantia nigra are found in Parkinson's disease (**B**); corpora amylacea are a normal age-related change commonly found in the brain (**C**); collections of foamy macrophages could occur in an organizing infarct (**D**), among other conditions, but are not a feature of Alzheimer's disease; and microglial nodules are associated with encephalitis (**E**).

48.   Correct: Amyloid and tau protein (C)

The signs and symptoms—memory loss, impaired language function, and altered social skills—progressing over years, and with no etiology identified on imaging or laboratory testing, is consistent with Alzheimer's disease. The histologic feature of Alzheimer's disease is neurofibrillary tangles and senile plaques. The neurofibrillary tangles have tau protein, and the senile plaques have amyloid (**C**). α-synuclein is found in Lewy bodies, which are associated with Parkinson's disease (**D, E**). Elastin and hyaline are not significant components, and hyaline is a descriptive term, covering many different underlying compounds (**A, B**).

49.   Correct: Autopsy examination after death (D)

The diagnosis of Alzheimer's disease requires a clinico-pathologic correlation, with the clinical signs of dementia being associated with increased neurofibrillary tangles and senile plaques in the brain. An antemortem definitive diagnosis of Alzheimer's disease is not possible (**A-C, E**). The diagnosis of Alzheimer's disease cannot be made on neuropathologic examination of the brain, as neurofibrillary tangles and senile plaques are age-related changes, and their presence alone, without confirmation of the clinical history, is inadequate for the diagnosis (**D**).

50.   Correct: Noncommunicating hydrocephalus (D)

Hydrocephalus is dilation of the cerebral ventricles. The two forms are communicating and noncommunicating. In communicating hydrocephalus, the blockage to cerebrospinal fluid flow is within the arachnoid granulations (**C**), whereas in noncommunicating hydrocephalus, the blockage is somewhere within the ventricular system. As the lateral ventricles were dilated, but the remainder of the ventricular system was not, the blockage is at the foramen of Munro (**D**). The other conditions listed would not explain the autopsy findings (**A-B, E**).

51.   Correct: Communicating hydrocephalus (C)

As he has blood in the subarachnoid space from the ruptured berry aneurysm, scarring of the arachnoid granulations can occur, blocking cerebrospinal fluid flow. The entire ventricular system would dilate and is termed a communicating hydrocephalus (**C**). The subarachnoid hemorrhage would not put him at risk for any of the other conditions (**A-B, D-E**).

52. Correct: Hyperactivity of deep tendon reflexes (D)

Dorsiflexion of the great toe elicited by stimulation of the sole of the foot, Babinski's reflex, is characteristic of an upper motor neuron disease. The other features are weakness of specific movements (e.g., flexion at the elbow), no muscle wasting (**A**), increased resistance to passive stretching (**C**), and hyperactivity of deep tendon reflexes (**D**). The features of lower motor neuron disease are weakness of individual muscles, wasting of muscles, fasciculations (**B**), reduced resistance to passive stretching, and loss of deep tendon reflexes.

53. Correct: Werdnig-Hoffman syndrome (A)

The patient has the features of a lower motor neuron disease: wasting of muscles, fasciculations, reduced resistance to passive stretching, and loss of deep tendon reflexes. Of the choices, only Werdnig-Hoffman is a pure lower motor neuron disease (**A**). Amytrophic lateral sclerosis is a combined upper and lower motor neuron disease and should show some features of upper motor neuron disease as well (**B**). An infarct of the pons would damage upper motor neurons (**C**). Hereditary spastic paraplegia is a pure upper motor neuron disease (**D**). Parkinson's disease is not usually associated with lower or upper motor neuron changes (**E**).

54. Correct: Duchenne's muscular dystrophy (C)

The early onset of muscular dystrophy, affecting both males in a family, is consistent with an X-linked disorder, and the diagnosis is Duchenne's muscular dystrophy (**C**). Although the two boys have muscle wasting, they have no other signs of upper or lower motor neuron disease, as would be found in amyotrophic lateral sclerosis (upper and lower motor neuron disease) (**A**) and spinal muscular atrophy (lower motor neuron disease) (**D**). Juvenile Parkinson's disease is autosomal recessive, and, given the familial component of this disease, chronic meningitis is not a good choice (**B, E**).

55. Correct: Myasthenia gravis (C)

Weakness of cranial nerve muscles, including causing diplopia and ptosis, and weakness of the proximal muscles of the limbs occurs in patients with myasthenia gravis (**C**). Amyotrophic lateral sclerosis would present with upper and lower motor neuron disease (**A**), Duchenne's muscular dystrophy occurs in a young patient population, (**B**) and Eaton-Lambert syndrome is a paraneoplastic syndrome (**D**) and has similar symptoms as myasthenia gravis, but it does not respond to anticholinesterase. Guillian-Barré is an acute condition that causes ascending paralysis (**E**).

56. Correct: Antibodies to acetylcholine receptors (C)

Weakness of cranial nerve muscles, including causing diplopia and ptosis, and weakness of the proximal muscles of the limbs occurs in patients with myasthenia gravis. The mechanism of action is antibodies to acetylcholine receptors (**C**). The other choices are incorrect (**A-B, D-E**).

57. Correct: Thymoma (B)

Weakness of cranial nerve muscles, including causing diplopia and ptosis, and weakness of the proximal muscles of the limbs occurs in patients with myasthenia gravis. Individuals with myasthenia gravis are at risk for thymic hyperplasia and thymomas (**B**). The other tumors are not usually associated with myasthenia gravis (**A, C-E**).

58. Correct: Amyotrophic lateral sclerosis (C)

The patient has signs of both lower motor neuron damage (fasciculations) and upper motor neuron damage (positive Babinski's sign), associated with no loss of sensation and no cranial nerve defects, which is consistent with amyotrophic lateral sclerosis (**C**). B12 deficiency affects the dorsal columns and would cause defects in proprioception and other senses (**D**). Multiple sclerosis can affect both sensory and motor function, but would not cause an upgoing Babinski's sign (**B**). Polio produces lower motor neuron defects, due to destruction of neurons in the anterior horn (**E**). The signs of Parkinson's disease (pill-rolling tremor and shuffling gait) are not described (**A**).

59. Correct: Pick bodies (D)

Pick's disease is a cause of dementia, and in addition to the dementia, patients also have Parkinson-like symptoms. Grossly, the frontal and temporal regions of the brain are the most affected, and the characteristic microscopic feature is a Pick body (**D**). With the tremor and shuffling gait, it is less likely to be Alzheimer's disease (**A**), and the gross autopsy findings are not those associated with Parkinson's disease, which has pallor of the substantia nigra (**B**). The gross changes and time course are not consistent with Creutzfeldt-Jakob disease (**C**) or HSV encephalitis (**E**).

60. Correct: Down's syndrome (C)

The findings of extensive neurofibrillary tangles and senile plaques is consistent with the diagnosis of Alzheimer's disease. Down's syndrome patients have an increased risk for Alzheimer's disease, and it will develop at a younger age (**C**). With Creutzfeldt-Jakob disease, the patient has spongiosis (**A**). Turner's syndrome is not a risk factor for Alzheimer's disease (**D**). Neither multiple sclerosis or viral encephalitis are associated with neurofibrillary tangles or senile plaques (**B, E**).

61. Correct: Spongy changes in the gray matter (B)

The patient has a rapidly developing dementia associated with myoclonus, which is consistent with Creutzfeldt-Jakob disease. In Creutzfeldt-Jakob disease, the characteristic histologic feature is a spongy change of the gray matter (**B**). Neurofibrillary tangles and senile plaques are found in Alzheimer's disease (**A**), intracellular aggregates of tau protein are found in Pick's disease (**C**), Lewy bodies are associated with Parkinson's disease (when they are in the substantia nigra) (**D**), and Lewy body dementia (when found in the cerebral cortex). Creutzfeldt-Jakob disease is not associated with intranuclear inclusions (**E**).

62. Correct: Plaques (C)

The clinical scenario is consistent with multiple sclerosis. In multiple sclerosis, the characteristic gross features are plaques, which can often occur in a periventricular distribution (**C**). Although it is possible to have neurological changes and no identifiable lesion of the brain (**A**), and to have similar symptoms as this patient has with the other conditions listed as the underlying cause, they would be much less common (**B, D-E**).

63. Correct: CAG repeats (A)

The gross pathologic findings are consistent with Huntington's chorea. Huntington's chorea is associated with CAG repeats (**A**), not CGA repeats (**B**). Mutation of pre-senilin 2 (chromosome 1) and pre-senilin 1 (chromosome 14) are seen in Alzheimer's disease (**C, D**). Patients with adrenoleukodystrophy have an X-linked disorder of very-long-chain fatty acid (LVCFA) catabolism (**E**).

64. Correct: 50% (D)

The patient has a clinical scenario that is consistent with Huntington's chorea, having chorea, depression, and features of dementia (i.e., memory loss), but likely committed suicide before the condition could completely manifest. Huntington's chorea is autosomal dominant, and thus her son has a 50% chance of inheriting the disorder (**D**). The other choices are incorrect (**A-C, E**).

19.12 CNS Neoplasms— Answers and Explanations

Easy	Medium	Hard

65. Correct: Craniopharyngioma (E)

The child is presenting with bitemporal hemianopia, which is most characteristic for a tumor affecting the optic chiasm. In children, the most common tumor at this site is a craniopharyngioma, which can have calcification (**E**). Pilocytic astrocytomas, medulloblastomas,

and ependymomas are common tumors in children, but not at the sella turcica (**A-C**). Oligodendrogliomas would be very rare tumors to find in childhood (**D**).

66. Correct: It is derived from astrocytes. (D)

The tumor is a pilocytic astrocytoma, which is commonly associated with Rosenthal fibers, is GFAP positive, and is derived from astrocytes (**D**). Although these tumors are usually infratentorial, they can occur in a supratentorial location. Pilocytic astrocytomas have a good prognosis (**A**), they do not usually produce erythropoietin (**B**), and rosettes and pseudorosettes are not a microscopic appearance (**E**). Tumors producing erythropoietin include renal cell carcinoma, hemangioblastomas, and hepatocellular carcinoma. No CNS tumor, whether in children or adults, usually metastasizes (**C**). Rosettes are characteristic of medulloblastoma, and pseudorosettes can occur in a variety of tumors.

67. Correct: Schwannoma (C)

Acoustic schwannomas are a common tumor of the brain, most often occur at the cerebellopontine angle, and affect CN VIII, resulting in hearing and balance difficulties (**C**). The other tumors listed are brain tumors; however, they are not commonly found at the location which would produce the previously described clinical scenario (**A-B, D-E**).

68. Correct: The prognosis is good (A)

Among brain tumors, psammoma bodies are most frequently associated with meningiomas. Meningiomas are a common type of brain tumor (**E**), occur at the convexities or in the parasagittal region (**B**), are derived from arachnoidal cells (**C**), and have a good prognosis (**A**). Acoustic schwannomas occur most frequently at the cerebellopontine angle. Cracniopharyngiomas are derived from Rathke's pouch. Oligodendrogliomas have a fried egg appearance (**D**).

69. Correct: Noncommunicating hydrocephalus (C)

With scarring of the cerebral aqueduct, this would cause the flow of cerebrospinal fluid to back up into the third ventricle and lateral ventricles. This dilation of the cerebral ventricles would be hydrocephalus. A noncommunicating hydrocephalus is due to an obstruction somewhere within the ventricular system, such as in the cerebral aqueduct or at the foreman of Munro (**C**). In a communicating hydrocephalus, the blockage is in the subarachnoid space, and this occurs after a scarring process involving the arachnoid, such as a subarachnoid hemorrhage or meningitis (**B**). Hydrocephalus ex vacuo is not actual hydrocephalus; instead, when the brain atrophies due to dementia or another process, the amount of space filled with cerebrospinal fluid increases in compensation (**A**). The history is not consistent with a subarachnoid hemorrhage or global hypoxic ischemic encephalopathy (**D, E**).

Chapter 20

Diseases of the Skin

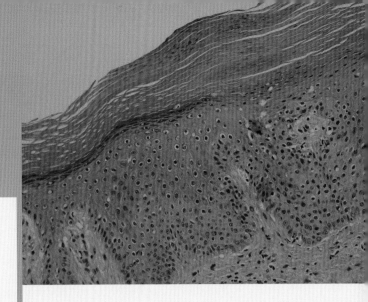

LEARNING OBJECTIVES

20.1 Diseases of the Skin

▸ Diagnose psoriasis

▸ Discuss the epidemiology, affected portions of the body, genetic associations, and histologic features of psoriasis

▸ Diagnosis and list the infectious agent associated with erythema multiforme

▸ List the conditions associated with and diagnose vitiligo; list conditions that vitiligo is associated with

▸ Diagnose a malignant melanoma

▸ Compare the different types of a malignant melanoma

▸ Describe the prognostic factors for a malignant melanoma

▸ Compare junctional, compound, intradermal and dysplastic nevi

▸ Diagnose and describe the histologic features of basal cell carcinoma

▸ Describe the location, metastatic risk, and mutations associated with basal cell carcinoma

▸ Diagnose a type IV hypersensitivity skin reaction

▸ Diagnose and describe the histologic features of rosacea

▸ Diagnose and describe the common locations for lichen planus

▸ Diagnose dermatitis herpetiformis

▸ Describe the relationship between dermatitis herpetiformis, gluten, and foods that contain gluten

▸ Diagnose pemphigus vulgaris

▸ List the immune mechanism that causes pemphigus vulgaris

20.1 Diseases of the Skin—Questions

Easy	Medium	Hard

1. A 41-year-old male is visiting his family physician for his yearly checkup. He is currently being followed for a skin disease, which has produced red plaques covered with silvery-white scales, on his elbows, knees, and scalp. His father had the same condition. If any of the plaques are peeled off his skin, he develops petechial hemorrhages at the site. Of the following, what is the most likely diagnosis?

A. Acute eczematous dermatitis

B. Erythema multiforme

C. Psoriasis

D. Bullous pemphigoid

E. Urticaria

Skin

2. Given the previous clinical scenario, of the following, what is a characteristic of this disease process?

A. It is a rare condition, affecting about 1 in 500,000 people.

B. Arthritis is a rare complication of the disease, affecting about 0.1% of patients.

C. The disease is associated with HLA-Cw*0602.

D. Immunofluorescence staining would reveal a linear pattern at the basement membrane.

E. Oral mucosal involvement is common.

Skin

3. A pathologist is examining a skin biopsy from a patient. She identifies acanthosis, elongation of the dermal papillae, and parakeratosis, and, within the parakeratosis, collections of neutrophils. Of the following, which is most characteristic of the disease process?

A. It commonly presents in elderly patients.

B. Autoantibodies against hemidesmosomes are present.

C. It most commonly affects the antecubital and popliteal fossa.

D. Patients can have pitting of the nails.

E. Nikolsky's sign is positive.

Skin

4. A 35-year-old female presents to an acute care clinic. Over the past three days she has developed a rash on her forearms, palms, and face. Examination of the rash reveals it to be symmetric. The lesions, which are macular, most commonly have a purple center with a pink halo that are separated by a pale ring. The lesions itch somewhat. Of the following, what is the most likely etiology of her rash?

A. Syphilis

B. HSV infection

C. HIV infection

D. *Streptococcus pneumoniae*

E. *Borrelia burgdorferi*

Skin

5. A 35-year-old female is being examined by her dermatologist. Scattered on her hands and around her external genitalia, she has about five up to 3.0 cm patches of white skin. Of the following, what histologic change may be present in her body, which is associated with the skin changes?

A. Invasive glands in the wall of the colon

B. Marked neutrophilic infiltrates in the lung

C. Lymphocytes and oncocytic change in the thyroid gland

D. Zellballen appearance of an adrenal medullary nodule

E. Granulomas in the lung

Skin, gland

6. A 56-year-old male presents to an acute care clinic. For the past year, his wife has been watching a pigmented lesion on his neck expand in size. Now, he can feel a few nodules underneath the skin of his neck. The mass is excised, and the pathologist identifies cytologic atypia, pigment, and numerous mitotic figures. The lesion is HMB-45 positive by immunohistochemical stain. Of the following, which is most characteristic of this lesion?

A. It most commonly occurs on non-sun-exposed skin.

B. The diameter of the lesion in the skin is more prognostically significant than its depth.

C. Mutations in *CDKN2A* contribute to its development.

D. Actinic keratosis is a precursor lesion.

E. It never involves the sole of the foot or palm of the hand.

Skin

7. A 32-year-old female has a brown macule on her left forearm that she asks her dermatologist to remove. The skin lesion is examined by a pathologist who identifies proliferations of bland nevus cells in the dermis. No mitotic figures are identified. Of the following, what is the diagnosis?

A. Malignant melanoma

B. Dysplastic nevus

C. Junctional nevus

D. Compound nevus

E. Intradermal nevus

Skin

8. A 76-year-old male who is a patient of the VA Hospital has had 13 skin lesions removed over the course of 5 years. Each time, the lesion was described as nests of cells in the dermis, with the nests having a peripheral palisading of nuclei. In some biopsies, a connection between the nests of cells in the dermis and the epidermis could be distinguished. Of the following, what is most characteristic of these skin lesions?

A. They grow rapidly.

B. Metastases to the brain are common.

C. Metastases to the lung are common.

D. They commonly occur on non-sun-exposed skin.

E. They are associated with mutations of the PTCH gene.

Skin

9. A 37-year-old male presents to his family physician complaining of skin changes. His family physician biopsies the skin lesion, and the pathologist later determines that there is parakeratosis, acanthosis, and occasional collections of neutrophils in the stratum corneum. In addition, the epidermis overlying the dermal papillae is thin. Of the following, what is most characteristic of the disease?

A. Involvement of the antecubital fossa is common.

B. The likelihood of an underlying malignancy is high.

C. Auspitz's sign is often positive.

D. The condition is rare, involving about 1 in 10,000 people.

E. The condition only occurs in males.

Skin

10. A 76-year-old male is referred to a dermatologist for a 0.5-cm raised, pearly, flesh-colored nodule with telangiectasia 2 cm lateral to the right ala of the nose. The lesion has been slowly increasing in size over the preceding 24 months. An excisional biopsy is performed. Microscopic examination of the surgical specimen will show which of the following?

A. Atypia of the lower layers of the epidermis with basal cell hyperplasia and intercellular bridges

B. Sheets of small cells resembling basal cells containing melanin, with surface hyperkeratosis and sharp demarcation from the surrounding tissues

C. Islands of basaloid cells within the dermis separated from the adjacent stroma by clefts

D. Infiltrates of atypical lymphocytes invading the epidermis in clusters

E. Markedly enlarged melanocytes with irregular borders and chromatin clumping

Skin

11. A 17-year-old girl presents with a circumferential, erythematous, slightly weeping dermatitis around her neck. The rash began 2 weeks ago and has gradually worsened. Three weeks ago, after her 17th birthday, she began taking oral contraceptives for "acne." She describes the rash as intensely itchy. No other skin lesions are present on examination. What is the underlying mechanism causing the dermatitis?

A. Chemical irritation of the skin

B. Mechanical irritation of the skin

C. Type IV hypersensitivity reaction

D. Drug-induced photosensitivity

E. Seborrheic dermatitis

Skin

12. A 68-year-old male is evaluated by his primary care physician for redness and thickening of the skin of the nose with general centrofacial erythema. He also complains of flushing of the face when eating spicy foods or consuming alcohol. Were a biopsy to be performed, what microscopic features would be observed?

A. Sezary cells and Pautrier microabscesses

B. Spongiosis with separation of the keratinocytes in the stratum spinosum and intradermal vesicle formation

C. Epidermal cell proliferation with thinning of the stratum granulosum and parakeratotic scaling

D. Closed comedones with parafollicular inflammatory cell infiltration

E. Lymphocytic infiltration around the follicles with dermal edema and telangiectasia

Skin

13. A 47-year-old male is referred to a dermatologist for further evaluation of a pruritic dermatitis on the volar surfaces of both wrists. On examination, the rash appears as multiple small violaceous papules with a lacelike pattern of fine white lines on the surface. What part of the patient's body would be most likely to also show signs of this disease?

A. The back

B. The external auditory canals

C. The brain

D. The penis

E. The lungs

Skin

14. A 32-year-old male is evaluated for an intensely pruritic erythematous papular and vesicular dermatitis involving the forearms and buttocks bilaterally. His primary care physician treats him with a high-potency topical steroid, which helps with the itching; however, the rash fails to resolve. He is referred to dermatology, and a skin biopsy is performed, which shows granular deposits of IgA within the dermal papillae. Which of the following foods is most likely to cause the patient's dermatitis to worsen?

A. French fries

B. Cheese

C. Beer

D. Corn chips

E. Orange juice

Skin

15. An 18-year-old man is seen by his family physician for a rash on his back. The rash has been present for over a year. On examination there are multiple variably hypopigmented maculae coalescing in patches with a fine overlying scale. What is the underlying mechanism of this patient's dermatitis?

A. Autoimmune destruction of melanocytes

B. Atopic dermatitis

C. Dermatophyte infection

D. Yeast infection

E. Medication effect

Skin

16. A 48-year-old male is evaluated by his internist for sores in his mouth and a rash. His internist notices multiple erosions of the mucosal surface of the oropharynx and identifies multiple flaccid bullous lesions of the arms and lower legs that spare the hands and feet. The bullae appear to be easily ruptured as evidenced by several eroded lesions, which are intensely painful. What is the underlying mechanism of this man's skin condition?

A. IgG autoantibodies against the desmosome

B. IgG autoantibodies against the hemidesmosome

C. IgE mediated type I hypersensitivity reaction

D. Uroporphyrinogen decarboxylase deficiency

E. Gluten sensitivity

Skin

20.2 Diseases of the Skin—Answers and Explanations

| Easy | Medium | Hard |

1. Correct: Psoriasis (C)

Red plaques covered with silvery-white scales occurring on the extensor surfaces of the body, including the elbows, knees, and sacral region, and also the scalp, are consistent with psoriasis (**C**). The production of petechial hemorrhages occurring when a plaque is peeled away from the skin is Auspitz's sign, and occurs because the dermal papillae are elongated and the overlying epidermis is thinning, resulting in dermal capillaries being very close to the surface and easily traumatized, producing the bleeding. The clinical scenario is not consistent with the other conditions (**A-B, D-E**).

2. Correct: The disease is associated with HLA-Cw*0602. (C)

The signs and symptoms are consistent with psoriasis, with the petechial hemorrhages being a positive Auspitz's sign. Psoriasis is common, affecting about 1 to 2% of the population (**A**), and arthritis is present in about 5% of patients (**B**), being associated with HLA-B27 and HLA-Cw*0602 (**C**), and thus, patients can also have spondylosis. Immunofluorescence is not commonly used to evaluate the disease (**D**). Bullous pemphigoid can produce a linear pattern at the basement membrane. Oral mucosal involvement is not associated with psoriasis (**E**).

3. Correct: Patients can have pitting of the nails. (D)

The pathologic description is consistent with psoriasis. The collections of neutrophils in the areas of parakeratosis are Munro's microabscesses. Psoriasis most commonly presents in younger patients, and not the elderly (**A**). Autoantibodies against hemidesmosomes are characteristic of bullous pemphigoid, which most commonly affects elderly men (**B**). Psoriasis involves the extensor surfaces of the body, such as the elbows and knees, and also the scalp (**C**). A positive Nikolsky's sign is seen in pemphigus vulgaris (**E**). Patients with psoriasis can have pitting of the nails (**D**).

4. Correct: HSV infection (B)

The patient has erythema multiforme, which is usually symmetrical, involves the face and distal extremities, and is symmetric. The lesions can be macules, papules, vesicles, or bullae and often have a central pale area, or appearance as previously described, representing a target lesion. The disease is most commonly associated with HSV-1, and may represent a T-cell–mediated reaction to HSV DNA (**B**). The other organisms listed are not as commonly associated with erythema multiforme (**A, C-E**).

5. Correct: Lymphocytic and oncocytic change in the thyroid gland (C)

The patient has vitiligo. Vitiligo is due to damage to and loss of melanocytes, possibly of autoimmune origin, and vitiligo can be found in association with other autoimmune disorders. Lymphocytes and oncocytic change in the thyroid gland is a description that is consistent with Hashimoto's thyroiditis (**C**). Colonic adenocarcinoma may be associated with acanthosis nigricans, but not commonly with vitiligo (**A**). A Zellballen appearance is a histologic description of a pheochromocytoma, which is not associated with vitiligo (**D**). Marked neutrophilic infiltrates (consistent with acute bronchopneumonia), and granulomas, which are found in a variety of disorders, including sarcoidosis and some infections, are also not commonly associated with vitiligo (**B, E**).

6. Correct: Mutations in *CDKN2a* contribute to its development. (C)

Based on the clinical scenario and pathologic examination, the most likely diagnosis is a malignant melanoma. The nodules palpated in the skin are likely lymph nodes with metastatic disease. Malignant melanoma stains with HMB-45 and also S-100 (although many tumors stain with S-100). Malignant melanomas can occur in a variety of locations, including the esophagus and spinal cord, but most commonly occur on sun-exposed skin (**A**). The depth of invasion (Breslow depth) is more important in determining prognosis than the diameter of the lesion in the skin is (**B**). The precursor lesion is a dysplastic nevus; actinic keratosis is a precursor lesion to squamous cell carcinoma of the skin (**D**). Acral lentiginous melanoma, one type of melanoma, can affect the nail bed, and palms and soles (**E**). Mutations of *CDKN2A* occur in malignant melanoma (**C**).

7. Correct: Intradermal nevus (E)

The absence of both cytologic atypia (indicated by "bland cells") and mitotic figures would rule out a malignant melanoma and dysplastic nevus (**A, B**). In junctional nevi, the proliferating cells are located at the basal portion of the epidermis (**C**), and in compound nevi, they are both at the basal portion of the epidermis and within the dermis (**D**). In intradermal nevi, the nevus cells are confined to the dermis. An intradermal nevus is not a significant risk factor for the future development of melanoma (**E**).

8. Correct: They are associated with mutations of the *PTCH* gene. (E)

Given that the patient has had multiple skin lesions over the course of several years, each tumor is most likely of low-grade malignancy. The pathologic description is that of basal cell carcinoma. Basal cell carcinomas growly slowly (**A**), and they rarely metastasize (**B**, **C**), but they are locally aggressive. Basal cell carcinoma commonly occurs on sun-exposed skin (**D**). It is associated with mutations of the *PTCH* gene (**E**).

9. Correct: Auspitz's sign is often positive. (C)

The pathologic description is consistent with psoriasis. The collections of neutrophils in the stratum corneum are Munro's microabscesses, which are characteristic of psoriasis. Psoriasis most characteristically involves the extensor surfaces, thus elbows and knees, and not the flexor surfaces, such as the antecubital fossa (**A**). Psoriasis is not associated with underlying malignancies (**B**), it is a fairly common condition, affecting a few percent of the population (**D**), and it occurs both in males and females (**E**). Auspitz's sign is positive when removal of the plaque causes petechial bleeding. As the epidermis is thin overlying the dermal papillae, which contain capillaries, when the plaque is removed, trauma to these capillaries can occur, which results in petechial bleeding (**C**).

10. Correct: Islands of basaloid cells within the dermis separated from the adjacent stroma by clefts (C)

The gross appearance of the skin lesion is classic for basal cell carcinoma. The thin clefts separating nests of tumor cells from the adjacent stroma (**C**) are a separation artifact that assists in distinguishing basal cell carcinoma from other similarly appearing conditions. (**A**) describes typical findings in actinic keratosis. Intercellular bridges, present in this condition, are not found in basal cell carcinoma. (**B**) describes the microscopic appearance of a seborrheic keratosis. (**D**) describes a cutaneous T-cell lymphoma. (**E**) describes the typical findings in melanoma.

11. Correct: Type IV hypersensitivity reaction (C)

The presentation is highly suggestive of contact dermatitis due to nickel allergy, seen frequently on the neck, wrists, and other places where jewelry is likely to be worn. Contact dermatitis may be either allergic or irritant in nature, with the allergic variety, as in nickel allergy, being a manifestation of T-cell–mediated Type IV hypersensitivity (**C**). Irritant contact dermatitis results from physical, mechanical, or chemical irritation of the skin (**A**, **B**). Oral contraceptives can cause photosensitivity and photo-allergic dermatitis; however, in this case one would not expect the rash to be limited to the neck and spare other commonly sun-exposed parts of the body (**D**). This distribution of the rash would never be seen in seborrheic dermatitis (**E**).

12. Correct: Lymphocytic infiltration around the follicles with dermal edema and telangiectasia (E)

Sezary cells and Pautier microabscesses would be expected in mycosis fungoides (**A**); however, the clinical description of the skin lesion is consistent with rosacea, a much more commonly encountered clinical entity. (**B**) describes microscopic findings seen in eczematous dermatitis. Epidermal cell proliferation with thinning of the stratum granulosum and parakeratotic scaling would be expected in psoriasis (**C**). Lymphocytic infiltration around the follicles with dermal edema and telangiectasia (**E**) is consistent with the clinical diagnosis of rosacea.

13. Correct: The penis (D)

The cause of the patient's dermatitis is lichen planus. Lichen planus is frequently remembered by the four P's (purple, polygonal, pruritic, and papular) and most commonly occurs on the volar surfaces of the wrists. Other commonly involved sites include the oral mucosa and the glans penis (**D**). The other answer choices are not commonly involved (**A-C**, **E**).

14. Correct: Beer (C)

The distribution of the rash, the clinical description, and histopathologic findings all indicate dermatitis herpetiformis due to underlying celiac disease. The most common gluten-containing foods are products made from wheat, barley, and rye. Of the answer choices listed, beer, which is made from malted barley, would be most likely to aggravate the patient's condition (**A-E**).

15. Correct: Yeast infection (D)

The location and description of the rash is most consistent with tinea versicolor, caused by infection with yeast of the genus *Malassezia* (**D**). Of the other alternative answer choices, only vitiligo (autoimmune destruction of melanocytes) is plausible (**B-C, E**); however, in vitiligo, pigmentation is completely absent (as opposed to hypopigmentation) and variable hypopigmentation should prompt consideration of another diagnosis (**A**). Furthermore, vitiligo, compared with tinea versicolor, is less common.

16. Correct: IgG autoantibodies against the desmosome (A)

This patient is suffering from pemphigus vulgaris. The patient's age, the presence of Nikolsky's sign, and the oral mucosal involvement all support the diagnosis of pemphigus vulgaris (caused by autoantibodies against the desmosome) rather than bullous pemphigoid (caused by autoantibodies to the hemidesmosome) (**B**). A type I hypersensitivity reaction (such as in urticaria) does not play a role in the pathogenesis of pemphigus (**C**). Porphyria cutanea tarda, caused most often by acquired deficiency of uroporphyrinogen decarboxylase, presents with skin fragility and bullae on sun-exposed parts of the body, most commonly the hands (**D**). Gluten sensitivity does not cause bullous disease (**E**).

Chapter 21

Mixed Items

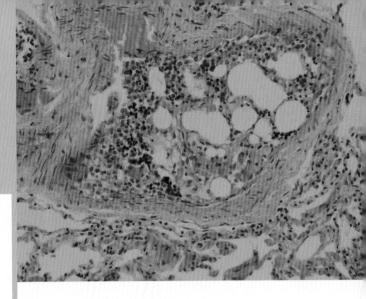

LEARNING OBJECTIVES

21.1 Mixed Items

- List the causes of anemia
- List and describe the complications of an acute myocardial infarct
- Describe the pathologic changes associated with unilateral renal artery stenosis
- Diagnose claudication and describe its underlying cause
- Diagnose a pulmonary thromboembolus
- List the risk factors for pulmonary thromboemboli
- List the pathologic conditions associated with tuberous sclerosis
- Diagnose Marfan's syndrome and list the associated genetic abnormality
- Describe the mechanism of a type II hypersensitivity reaction
- List and describe examples of type II hypersensitivity reactions, including those seen in transfusion reactions
- List and describe the types of hemorrhage
- Describe the various morphologic forms of inflammation and list the conditions associated with each form
- List and describe the forms of cellular accumulations and list the circumstances or conditions under which they are found
- List the forms of cellular accumulations and describe their appearance and the process by which each occurs
- Describe the process of apoptosis, including the cellular mediators involved
- List morphologic features of reversible and irreversible cellular injury and describe the physiologic process by which they occur
- Discuss examples of the gross and microscopic features produced by hypertrophy, hyperplasia, atrophy, and metaplasia
- List and describe the causes of atrophy
- List the various forms of amyloidosis and their associated protein
- Diagnose intralobar pulmonary sequestration
- Compare extralobar and intralobar pulmonary sequestration
- Diagnose Kartagener's syndrome
- Diagnose lobar pneumonia
- List and describe the complications of lobar pneumonia
- Compare lobar pneumonia due to *Streptococcus pneumoniae* and *Klebsiella pneumoniae*
- Diagnose group B streptococcal pneumonia
- List other conditions caused by GBS infection of a neonate
- Diagnose a *Mycobacterium tuberculosis* infection
- Diagnose a lung abscess
- Describe the characteristic histologic findings in and diagnose diffuse alveolar damage
- Diagnose Goodpasture's syndrome
- Diagnose and describe the histologic findings in chronic bronchitis
- Diagnose and describe the pathologic features of emphysema
- Diagnose pulmonary emphysema; describe the pathophysiologic process occurring in emphysema
- Diagnose chronic berylliosis
- Diagnose chronic hypersensitivity pneumonitis
- Diagnose restrictive lung disease
- Compare the histologic features of UIP, NSIP, and DIP
- Diagnose pulmonary hypertension
- Diagnose a tracheoesophageal fistula
- Diagnosis achalasia
- Diagnose and describe the complications of a hiatal hernia
- Compare and contrast a sliding and a paraesophageal hiatal hernia
- Diagnose and describe the complication of gastric reflux
- Diagnose herpes simplex infection of the esophagus
- Diagnose an esophageal carcinoma

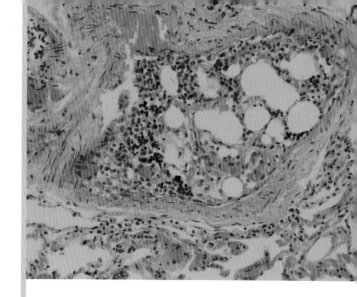

- ▶ Compare squamous cell carcinoma and adenocarcinoma of the esophagus
- ▶ Diagnose congenital pyloric stenosis
- ▶ Diagnose and list the complications of a cerebral edema
- ▶ Compare Curling's, Cushing's, and peptic ulcers
- ▶ Diagnose a diffuse-type gastric carcinoma
- ▶ Describe the development of MALT lymphoma in the stomach, including how to treat the disorder
- ▶ Describe the origin of gastrointestinal stromal tumors
- ▶ List the complications of cystic fibrosis
- ▶ Diagnose celiac disease
- ▶ Describe the epidemiology, serologic testing, and HLA antigen associated with celiac disease
- ▶ List the tumors associated with von Hippel-Lindau syndrome
- ▶ Diagnose and describe the histologic features of Peyronie's disease

21.1 Mixed Items—Questions

| Easy | Medium | Hard |

1. A 46-year-old postmenopausal white female presents to her family physician with complaints of fatigue and dizziness. The fatigue has been increasing in severity for several months. Physical examination reveals a temperature of 98.5°F, pulse of 107 bpm, respiratory rate of 19 breaths per minute, and blood pressure of 98/69 mm Hg. A physical examination is unremarkable other than slight pallor of the conjunctivae. Laboratory testing reveals a hemoglobin of 10.2 g/dL. The MCV is 111 fL. She has no family history of cancer; however, she consumes about 6 beers per day. Of the following, what is the most likely cause of her symptoms?

A. Menstrual blood loss

B. Colonic adenocarcinoma

C. Warm autoimmune hemolytic anemia

D. Vitamin B12 deficiency

E. Sickle cell disease

Hematopoietic

2. A 53-year-old male with a history of high cholesterol, 45-pack-per-year smoking history, and hypertension sustains an acute myocardial infarct while golfing with his friends. In the emergency room, he is found to have sinus tachycardia, but no murmurs are heard on auscultation of the chest. Two days later, he develops a new systolic murmur and shortness of breath and rapidly decompensates. Which of the following complications of his acute myocardial infarct is the cause of this murmur?

A. Pericarditis

B. A cardiac dysrhythmia

C. A mural thrombus

D. Rupture of one of the mitral valve papillary muscles

E. Contractile dysfunction of one of the mitral valve papillary muscles

Cardiovascular

3. At autopsy, a 56-year-old female is found to have a small left kidney (60 grams) and a normal-sized right kidney (120 grams). The left kidney has a smooth cortex and the right kidney has a granular cortex (arteriolar nephrosclerosis). Which of the following other findings at autopsy would explain these findings?

A. Aldosterone-secreting adrenal cortical adenoma

B. Coarctation of the aorta

C. Fibromuscular dysplasia of the left renal artery

D. Cushing's syndrome

E. A renin-producing tumor in the tail of the pancreas

Kidney

4. A 66-year-old male who has a 45-pack-per-year smoking history and has type 2 diabetes mellitus presents to his family physician complaining of pain when he walks. The pain ceases when he stops walking. Of the following, which is the most likely diagnosis?

A. Atherosclerosis of the right and left femoral arteries

B. An abdominal aortic aneurysm

C. Endocarditis, with septic emboli to the legs

D. Polyarteritis nodosa

E. Giant cell arteritis involving the aortic arch

Vessels

5. A 37-year-old male is in a motor vehicle accident and sustains a femoral fracture requiring surgical repair. Several days following the accident, he develops shortness of breath and a sharp pain in his chest. His symptoms resolve. Ten days later, he is released from the hospital, and, while walking into his house, suddenly collapses and cannot be revived. He has no past medical history. Of the following, what would laboratory testing most likely reveal?

A. Decreased C-reactive protein

B. A Factor V Leiden gene mutation

C. An LDL of > 500 mg/dL

D. A β-myosin heavy chain gene mutation

E. An increased antinuclear antibody

Vessels

6. A 21-year-old female has a seizure while playing basketball with her friends. She is taken to the emergency room and a CT scan of the head is performed, revealing a lesion in the right cerebellar hemisphere. A neurosurgeon excises the mass, and a pathologist confirms a diagnosis of subependymal giant cell astrocytoma. When the patient was younger, she had a mass excised from her heart. Of the following, what was the most likely diagnosis of the mass in the heart?

A. Lipoma

B. Atrial myxoma

C. Papillary fibroelastoma

D. Rhabdomyoma

E. Angiosarcoma

Heart

7. A 29-year-old male collapses while playing basketball with friends. An autopsy is performed, which identifies a ruptured thoracic aortic aneurysm. Both the decedent and his father are tall and have long fingers. The decedent's father had open-heart surgery to repair an aortic defect in his early 40s. Of the following, a mutation of which gene is responsible for their condition?

A. β-myosin heavy chain
B. Fibrillin
C. Neurofibromin
D. Merlin
E. *COL3A1*

Cardiovascular

8. A 38-year-old female presents to the emergency room. She has recently been feeling weak and fatigued, unable to workout at the gym as she normally has in the past. Her trip to the emergency room is because she developed double vision today. Physical examination reveals ptosis. A CT scan of her body reveals a mass in the upper portion of the mediastinum. What would a biopsy of the mass most likely reveal?

A. An esophageal cyst
B. Esophageal adenocarcinoma
C. Medullary thyroid carcinoma
D. Thymoma
E. Metastatic ductal carcinoma of the breast

Hematopoietic

9. A 36-year-old female with a history of ventricular dysrhythmias due to her underlying hypertrophic cardiomyopathy is treated with procainamide. Three months after her treatment began, she developed pain in her joints. She presents to the emergency room with complaints of chest pain. Her vital signs are a temperature of 99.2°F, heart rate of 108 bpm, and blood pressure of 121/83 mm Hg, and on physical examination a friction rub is identified. Of the following, which would serologic testing most likely identify?

A. Anti-dsDNA antibodies
B. Antihistone antibodies
C. Anti-SSA antibodies
D. Anticentromere antibodies
E. Anti-scl70 antibodies

Immune

10. Given the previous clinical scenario, of the following, what is the most likely diagnosis?

A. Anti–phospholipid antibody syndrome
B. Drug-induced lupus
C. Type II hypersensitivity reaction to procainamide
D. Autoimmune hemolytic anemia
E. Hypertensive crisis

Immune

11. A 24-year-old female presents to her family physician. She has developed a rash on the bridge of her nose, with extension onto both cheeks. Over the past year, she says that she has developed pain in her joints and occasional muscle aches. A physical examination reveals a temperature of 98.5°F, a blood pressure of 105/75 mm Hg, a pulse of 85 beats per minute, and a respiratory rate of 17 breaths per minute. A urine dipstick analysis reveals proteinuria, but no glucose. Of the following physical examination findings, which, most directly related to her disease process, may be identified?

A. An S3
B. An S4
C. A continuous murmur
D. A rub
E. Paradoxical splitting of S2

Immune

12. Given the previous clinical scenario, of the following, which serologic testing would be most specific for her disease process?

A. Anti-Smith antibody
B. Anti-HCV antibody
C. Antiendothelial antibody
D. Antiendomysial antibody
E. Anti-pANCA

Immune

13. A 47-year-old male with a history of Zollinger-Ellison syndrome presents to the emergency room vomiting bright red blood. He has twice before presented to the emergency room vomiting blood. On arrival, a complete blood cell count is performed, revealing a hemoglobin of 5.6 g/dL. A decision to transfuse is made, and he receives 4 units of blood. His blood type is O-. His bleeding is brought under control, and he is admitted to the hospital. He is scheduled for surgery the next day. Prior to surgery, a complete blood cell count reveals a hemoglobin of 6.2 g/dL. Of the following laboratory tests, which is likely to be detected in the blood?

A. Anti-Kell antibody
B. Antiendothelial antibody
C. Anti-D antibody
D. Anti-A antibody
E. Anti-SSA

Immune

14. A 27-year-old male is shot during a drug deal. He is rushed to the emergency room and is determined to have a hemothorax. A chest tube is placed, and intravenous fluids and blood are given. Immediately after the transfusion, he develops a temperature of 100.8°F and chills. Shortly thereafter, he develops a blood pressure of 68/45 mm Hg. Of the following, laboratory testing would most likely reveal an elevation of which test, which is most directly related to the disease process?

A. Troponin I

B. Serum tryptase

C. Angiotensin-converting enzyme

D. Hemoglobin

E. Alanine aminotransferase

Cardiovascular

15. A 9-year-old girl is stung by a bee while playing at school. About 10 minutes later, she becomes nauseous and vomits twice. Her teacher notices that her face begins to swell and she begins to wheeze. 9-1-1 is called and she is taken to the hospital. Of the following, which laboratory test would most likely yield an elevated concentration?

A. Troponin I

B. Tryptase

C. Angiotensin-converting enzyme

D. Creatinine

E. IgA

Immune

16. A 15-year-old boy is struck on the arm by a thrown baseball while at summer camp. At the site where the ball hits, he develops a 3.0-cm red-purple discoloration. Which of the following terms best describes the color change in the skin?

A. Lividity

B. Petechiae

C. Contusion

D. Congestion

E. Hyperemia

Cardiovascular

17. The hospital laboratory receives a specimen from a clinical physician for analysis. The specimen vial contains a cloudy fluid. Testing indicates a high concentration of protein, and many white blood cells are identified on microscopic examination. Of the following disease types, which is the most likely source of the fluid collection from which this sample was obtained?

A. Congestive heart failure

B. Subdural hematoma

C. Viral pericarditis

D. Gonococcal arthritis

E. Membranous glomerulonephropathy

Cardiovascular

18. A forensic pathologist is examining a section of skin. Just underneath the dermis is a large collection of macrophages, each containing a stippled, or somewhat chunky-appearing yellow-brown pigment. The pathologist orders a Prussian blue stain, which causes the pigment to appear blue. Of the following, what is the pigment?

A. Mallory's hyaline

B. Hemosiderin

C. Lipofuscin

D. Tattoo pigment

E. Melanin

Skin

19. A 27-year-old male is found deceased in his messy apartment during a welfare check initiated by concerned friends. At the time of autopsy, his kidneys are noted to be pale. Vitreous electrolyte analysis indicates a vitreous glucose of 576 mg/dL, and acetone is detected in the blood. Of the following, what is his most likely cause of death?

A. Acute myocardial infarct

B. Diabetic ketoacidosis

C. Cocaine intoxication

D. Acute pancreatitis

E. Aortic dissection

Renal

20. A 40-year-old chronic alcoholic with no other medical history dies after an alcohol-related seizure, in which he fell down the stairs at his house and fractured his neck. An autopsy is performed, revealing a diffusely golden-yellow discolored liver. Microscopic examination of the liver reveals almost every hepatocyte to be filled with one large vacuole or a few smaller vacuoles. Of the following, what is accumulating within the cells?

A. Mitochondria

B. Mallory's hyaline

C. Glucose

D. Triglycerides

E. Water

Hepatobiliary

21. A 46-year-old female receives radiation therapy of the neck for a neoplasm of the thyroid gland. After therapy, it is noted that her thyroid gland has markedly decreased in size, leading to hypothyroidism, and she must be placed on a thyroid replacement therapeutic drug regimen. During the time of decrease in size of the thyroid gland, several biopsies of the parenchyma revealed cells with increased eosinophilia and fragmented nuclei, but essentially no inflammatory reaction. Molecular studies, by a scientist researching a therapy for thyroid neoplasms, found an elevated concentration of activated caspase-9. Which of the following was most directly responsible for the elevated concentration of activated caspase-9?

A. Increased concentration of bcl-2

B. Increased concentration of Bax

C. Decreased concentration of BH3 proteins

D. Decreased concentration of Bcl-xL

E. Increased concentration of cytochrome C

Endocrine

22. A pathologist is examining a section of kidney and notes hydropic change in the proximal convoluted tubule epithelial cells. The change in the kidney was precipitated by a temporary occlusion of the renal artery. Of the following, what is the mechanism of action producing this change?

A. Increased production of fatty acids

B. Decreased production of fatty acids

C. Increased sodium concentration in cell

D. Increased endocytosis

E. Increased phagocytosis

Renal

23. A 37-year-old male with a history of chronic alcohol abuse and gallstones is brought to the emergency room by a friend. The patient has been complaining of severe abdominal pain for 3 days following a bout of increased alcohol consumption. Laboratory testing in the emergency room indicates an elevated amylase and lipase. Despite treatment, the patient dies. An autopsy of the individual most likely will reveal which of the following?

A. Neutrophilic infiltrate in the pancreas

B. Lymphocytic infiltrate in the pancreas

C. Neutrophilic infiltrate in the liver

D. Lymphocytic infiltrate in the liver

E. Caseous necrosis of the pancreas

F. Caseous necrosis of the liver

Pancreas

24. A 62-year-old female is found unresponsive on the couch in her apartment by her husband when he returned home from work. Despite the efforts of emergency responders, she was pronounced dead at the hospital. An autopsy reveals a well-demarcated wedge-shaped yellow lesion in the cortex of the left kidney, with preservation of normal gross architecture. Of the following, what is the diagnosis?

A. Tuberculoma

B. Acute pyelonephritis

C. Renal cell carcinoma

D. Metastatic colonic adenocarcinoma

E. Infarct

Renal

25. A 56-year-old male with a history of smoking and hypertension develops an occlusive thrombus in his left anterior descending coronary artery following rupture of an atherosclerotic plaque. He survives the event, and therapeutic lysis of the thrombus is accomplished within 20 minutes. After his recovery, he is told that subsequent testing indicates no permanent damage to the heart. If a biopsy of the subendocardial myocytes had been performed 20 minutes after the occlusion of the vessel, of the following intracellular changes, which might be identified?

A. Markedly increased eosinophilia of the cardiac myocyte cytoplasm

B. Nuclear pyknosis

C. Nuclear karyolysis

D. Nuclear karyorrhexis

E. Clumping of nuclear chromatin

Cardiovascular

26. A 61-year-old male commits suicide by an intraoral shotgun wound. At autopsy, the heart is found to weigh 535 grams. He has a clinical history of systemic hypertension but no history of heart failure. A section of the myocardium from the left ventricle would reveal which of the following processes?

A. Hypertrophy

B. Hyperplasia

C. Atrophy

D. Metaplasia

E. Reversible cell injury

F. Irreversible cell injury

Cardiovascular

27. The autopsy of a 67-year-old male who died in a motor vehicle accident reveals the left kidney to weigh about 50 grams, and the right kidney to weigh about 210 grams. The pelvis of both kidneys is fairly normal in size and the cortical surface of both kidneys is granular, but otherwise, has no loss of parenchyma. Of the following, given that this man was born with normal size kidneys, which condition best explains the change in the left kidney?

A. Occlusive thrombus of the left renal artery

B. Kimmelstiel-Wilson lesion

C. Renal cell carcinoma

D. Severe stenosis of the left renal artery by atherosclerosis

E. Kidney stone obstructing the left ureter

Kidney

28. A 37-year-old male with MEN II is diagnosed with a thyroid nodule. Surgical resection of the thyroid nodule reveals a neoplasm with interspersed homogenous eosinophilic material that displays apple-green birefringence on Congo red stain. Of the following, what protein is deposited that causes this change in the Congo red stain?

A. Amyloid precursor protein

B. Ig light chains

C. Serum amyloid-associated protein

D. Calcitonin

E. Transthyretin

Thyroid

29. A 78-year-old man with urinary obstruction from an enlarged prostate undergoes a prostate biopsy to exclude cancer. His biopsy results are negative for cancer, and he is started on finasteride, a 5-α-reductase inhibitor which blocks conversion of testosterone to the more potent androgen, dihydrotestosterone. His urinary symptoms resolve after 6 months of treatment. He dies of a cardiac arrest 3 years later. Which of the following changes is likely to be observed to have occurred on microscopic examination of his prostate at autopsy since his previous biopsy?

A. Hyperplasia

B. Hypertrophy

C. Atrophy

D. Dysplasia

E. Metaplasia

Gastrointestinal

30. A 36-year-old man with severe heartburn undergoes an upper endoscopy. A biopsy of abnormal mucosa is taken 4 cm above the gastroesophageal junction, revealing normal-appearing columnar epithelia. Which of the following processes best explains this finding?

A. Dysplasia

B. Metaplasia

C. Hyperplasia

D. Carcinoma

E. Atrophy

Gastrointestinal

31. A 12-year-old male with no past medical history is brought to the emergency room by his parents because of flu-like symptoms, including cough, fever, and general malaise, with the recent development of shortness of breath. During his evaluation, an ultrasound of the chest is performed, revealing fluid around the heart. A pericardiocentesis is performed, removing about 50 mL of a cloudy white fluid from around the heart. A smear of the fluid shows sheets of neutrophils. Which of the following forms of inflammation is present?

A. Serous inflammation

B. Fibrinous inflammation

C. Suppurative inflammation

D. Chronic inflammation

E. Ulcer

Cardiovascular

32. A scientist is studying apoptosis. She wishes to extend the life of the cells in her culture, which were originally derived from human liver cells, after exposure to radiation, by introduction of a naturally occurring chemical. Which of the following effects produced by the chemical would produce her desired outcome?

A. Increased concentration of bcl-2

B. Increased concentration of Bax

C. Increased concentration of Bad

D. Decreased concentration of bcl-xL

E. Decreased concentration of BH3 proteins

N/A

33. A 16-year-old female is brought to an acute care clinic because she has recently developed a fever and productive cough. In the past, she has had three similar episodes, always diagnosed to have pneumonia. A sweat chloride test was negative. An X-ray reveals consolidation of the lower lobe of the right lung. Of the following, what is the most likely diagnosis?

A. Extralobar pulmonary sequestration

B. Intralobar pulmonary sequestration

C. Lobar pneumonia

D. Cystic fibrosis

E. Small-cell carcinoma

Lung

34. A 27-year-old male has had multiple episodes of pneumonia during his lifetime and has developed a chronic cough, which is productive and often causes him to cough up a cup or more of sputum per day. A CT scan of his chest has revealed dilated bronchi. In addition to the pneumonia, his past medical history includes recurrent sinusitis, and, over the course of four years, his wife has been unable to become pregnant. Of the following, what is the most likely diagnosis?

A. Allergic bronchopulmonary aspergillosis

B. Granulomatosis with polyangiitis

C. Kartagener's syndrome

D. Squamous cell carcinoma of the lung

E. Chronic bronchitis

Lung

35. A 17-year-old male is brought to the emergency room by his parents, because just two days ago, he developed a fever to 102°F and shaking chills. Today, he developed a sharp pain in his chest, which they found worrisome. He also has some difficulty breathing. A chest X-ray reveals consolidation of the left lower lobe of the lung. Of the following, which condition is the most likely to develop?

A. Diffuse alveolar damage

B. Pleural plaques

C. Adenocarcinoma of the lung

D. Focal segmental glomerulosclerosis

E. Granulomatosis with polyangiitis

Lung

36. A 53-year-old chronic alcoholic, over the course of one week, has developed worsening fever and chills. He also has a productive cough. His friends bring him to the emergency room, where an X-ray reveals consolidation of the lower lobe of the right lung. He is admitted to the hospital and, despite treatment, dies two days later. An autopsy is performed. Sectioning of the lower lobe of the right lung reveals a mucoid appearance to the cut surface. A culture performed postmortem does not grow *Streptococcus pneumoniae*. Of the following, what is the most likely diagnosis?

A. Influenza A pneumonia

B. *Coccidioides immitis* pneumonia

C. *Staphylococcus aureus* pneumonia

D. *Klebsiella pneumoniae* pneumonia

E. *Pseudomonas aeruginosa* pneumonia

Lung

37. Following discharge from the hospital a 5-day-old infant who was born at 40 weeks gestational age quickly develops a fever to 102°F, a productive cough that is occasionally tinged with blood, and difficulty breathing. The infant is brought to the emergency room by her parents. A pulse oximeter reveals an oxygen saturation of 85%. The mother received no prenatal care. Of the following, what is the most likely diagnosis?

A. Hyaline membrane disease

B. *Streptococcus pneumoniae* pneumonia

C. *Staphylococcus aureus* pneumonia

D. *Streptococcus agalactiae* pneumonia

E. *Streptococcus pyogenes* pneumonia

Lung

38. Given the previous clinical scenario, in addition to the patient's presenting condition, of the following, what condition is this infant most at risk for?

A. Meningitis

B. Pharyngitis

C. Myocarditis

D. Hepatitis

E. Ischemic colitis

Lung, brain

39. At autopsy, a 67-year-old male is found to have a small nodule identifiable at the pleural surface of the upper lobe of the right lung immediately adjacent to the interlobar groove, which is found to be fibrotic and have calcium deposition. Also identified is hilar lymphadenopathy with a similar appearance to the subpleural nodule. Of the following, what other finding, that is related to the changes described, might be identified at autopsy?

A. Pleural plaques

B. Diaphragmatic plaques

C. Scars at the apices of the lungs

D. Squamous cell carcinoma

E. Noncaseating granulomas, with a negative acid-fast bacillus stain

Lung

40. A 53-year-old male with a history of chronic alcoholism for 25 years presents to an acute care clinic with complaints of a productive cough and a sharp pain in his chest. He says that the material he coughs up smells terrible. His vital signs include a fever of 101°F. A chest X-ray reveals an area of consolidation in the lower lobe of the right lung, with a central clearing, which is interpreted as cavitation. A CT-guided biopsy of the right lung reveals only neutrophilic infiltration and no tumor. Other than his alcohol use, he has no significant past medical history. Of the following, what is the most likely diagnosis?

A. Metastatic colonic adenocarcinoma

B. Granulomatosis with polyangiitis

C. Microscopic polyarteritis

D. Lung abscess

E. Pulmonary hamartoma

Lung

41. A 43-year-old male worker at a plant is near a container of chlorine when it ruptures, catching him with a blast of the chemical. He is knocked over by the blast, and two coworkers see the accident happen and call for an ambulance. He is taken to the hospital, where a CT scan of the head reveals no hemorrhage. About six hours after the accident, he develops shortness of breath and has a respiratory rate of 34 breaths per minute. An arterial blood gas reveals PO_2 of 73 mm Hg and PCO_2 of 30 mm Hg. He is admitted to the intensive care unit, but, despite treatment, dies 4 days after the accident. Of the following, what would histologic examination of the lungs most likely reveal?

A. Abundant neutrophilic infiltrate

B. Extensive alveolar hemorrhage

C. Plasma proteins and cellular debris layered on alveolar septa

D. Fat emboli

E. Abundant eosinophilic infiltrate

Lung

42. A 35-year-old male presents to an acute care clinic because of blood in his urine. His vital signs are a temperature of 98.9°F and blood pressure of 141/89 mm Hg. Urinalysis identifies red blood cell casts and 2+ protein. His only significant past medical history is that 4 months ago, he went to the same clinic with complaints of shortness of breath accompanied by a cough that occasionally produced blood. A chest X-ray revealed infiltrates, and he was diagnosed with *Mycoplasma* pneumonia. He has no other significant past medical history. Of the following, what is his most likely diagnosis?

A. *Mycobacterium tuberculosis* infection

B. Pulmonary neoplasm

C. Goodpasture's syndrome

D. Idiopathic pulmonary hemosiderosis

E. Organizing lobar pneumonia with septic emboli to the kidney

Lung

43. A 53-year-old male is being seen by his family physician for a chronic cough, which he describes as having been present for the past several years, usually at least about half of the year. He says that with the cough he produces sputum regularly. With physical exertion, he becomes short of breath. He has a 60-pack-per-year smoking history. Of the following, histologic examination would reveal which findings in the lungs that is most consistent with his clinical presentation?

A. Neoplastic cells with a tiny rim of cytoplasm

B. Eosinophilic infiltrates in the walls of the airways

C. Loss of alveolar septa

D. Thickening of the layer of submucosal glands in the bronchi

E. Extensive hemosiderin deposition

Lung

44. A 62-year-old male with a 75-pack-per-year smoking history has been followed by his family physician for years because of his difficulty breathing when he is exerting himself, which is getting worse. Associated with this symptom, he has an occasional cough that only rarely produces sputum, and he has lost 30 lbs. He has no history of hypertension, diabetes mellitus type 2, or hypercholesterolemia. Of the following, what would examination of his lungs most likely reveal?

A. Lymphocytic interstitial infiltrates

B. Hyperinflation

C. Mucous plugging the airways

D. Honeycomb lung

E. Extensive pulmonary hemosiderosis

Lung

279

45. Given the previous clinical scenario, of the following, what is the most likely mechanism of his disease process?

A. Excess production of α-1-antitrypsin

B. Increased activity of elastase

C. Dysfunction of matrix metalloproteinases

D. Mast cell degranulation

E. Increased hydrostatic pressure

Lung

46. A 61-year-old male who is retired from a job working at a nuclear power plant presented to his physician about 5 years ago with complaints of some difficulty breathing when exerting himself. He has no history of hypertension, diabetes mellitus type 2, or hypercholesterolemia. The dyspnea has worsened over the years, finally prompting his physician to pursue a lung biopsy, which reveals interstitial granulomas that are noncaseating. Of the following, what chemical was he most likely exposed to as his work place, which led to his disease process?

A. Uranium

B. Asbestos

C. Beryllium

D. Silica

E. Iron

Lung

47. A 56-year-old male presents to his family physician, complaining of difficulty breathing when he is working. He says that several times over the past many years, after retrieving hay from his barn to feed his cattle, he has, several hours later, had a cough and difficulty breathing which usually passed within a day or two, which he always just attributed to breathing in the dust. His physician performs pulmonary function tests, which indicate a normal FEV1/FVC ratio, but also a decreased FVC. Of the following, what is the most likely diagnosis for his current complaint?

A. Sarcoidosis

B. Usual interstitial pneumonia

C. Hamon-Rich syndrome

D. Acute hypersensitivity pneumonitis

E. Chronic hypersensitivity pneumonitis

Lung

48. A 52-year-old male has been followed by his family physician for 2 years because of shortness of breath when he is working and a cough, which have been progressively getting worse. On his most recent visit, a pulmonary function test is performed that indicates an essentially normal FEV1/FVC ratio; however, the FVC is decreased. A physical examination reveals fine rales. A lung biopsy is ordered. The biopsy reveals abnormal tissue interspersed among normal tissue. The abnormal tissue includes both honeycomb changes and fibroblastic foci. Of the following, what is the most likely diagnosis?

A. Usual interstitial pneumonia

B. Nonspecific interstitial pneumonia

C. Sarcoidosis

D. Desquamative interstitial pneumonitis

E. Cryptogenic organizing pneumonia

Lung

49. A 26-year-old female has been followed by her family physician for 1 year because of increasing shortness of breath with exertion. A biopsy of her lungs reveals some smaller vessels that have a hypertrophied muscularis. She has no history or family history of excessive clotting, and she is thin. An echocardiogram of her heart reveals no abnormalities. Of the following, what is the most likely diagnosis?

A. Hypertrophic cardiomyopathy

B. Recurrent pulmonary thromboemboli

C. Primary pulmonary hypertension

D. Takayasu's arteritis

E. Lymphangioleiomyomatosis

Lung

50. A 3-day-old infant is found to be choking after feeding. An X-ray is performed that shows an infiltrate in the lower lobe of the right lung. An EGD is performed that reveals the esophagus is blind-ended. Of the following, what is the most likely diagnosis?

A. Zenker's diverticulum

B. Pyloric stenosis

C. Tracheoesophageal fistula

D. Schatzki's ring

E. Achalasia

Esophagus

51. A 46-year-old male has a history of difficulty swallowing both solid and liquid foods. At times when he swallows, he has pain, and occasionally he finds himself regurgitating food and must cough exuberantly to prevent aspiration. The symptoms progress, and ultimately, he undergoes a resection of his lower esophagus that reveals a dilation proximal to the lower esophageal sphincter. Of the following, what is the mechanism of his disease?

A. Antibodies against acetylcholine receptors

B. Antibodies against norepinephrine receptors

C. Loss of inhibitory neurons

D. Hyperplasia of stimulatory neurons

E. Defective calcium transporters

Esophagus

52. A 44-year-old male with recurrent episodes of heartburn undergoes an EGD. At the lower esophagus he is noted to have a small pouch of stomach that extends above the diaphragm alongside the esophagus. Of the following, what is he at greatest risk for?

A. A Zenker's diverticulum

B. Squamous cell carcinoma of the esophagus

C. Focal gastric necrosis

D. Gastrointestinal stromal tumor

E. Superior vena cava syndrome

Stomach

53. A 43-year-old male is being seen by his family physician for recurrent heartburn. On several occasions, he had blood drawn for troponin I testing, which was always normal, and he never developed EKG changes. The heartburn is not associated with exertion. Despite treatment, his symptoms continued. After 5 years of such complaints, his family physician recommended he see a gastroenterologist who recommended an EGD. At EGD, the gastroenterologist saw a red discoloration of the distal esophagus and took biopsies. Of the following, what did the gastroenterologist most want to examine the esophagus for?

A. Eosinophils

B. Fungi

C. Viral inclusions

D. Dysplasia

E. Neutrophils

Esophagus

54. A 34-year-old female undergoes a bone marrow transplantation to treat her acute myelogenous leukemia. Several weeks after her transplant procedure, she develops pain when swallowing foods. An EGD reveals small erosions of the esophageal mucosa. A biopsy of these areas reveals multinucleated cells, some with nuclear inclusions. The cells are not enlarged. Of the following, what is the most likely diagnosis?

A. Adenovirus infection

B. Posttransplant Hodgkin's lymphoma

C. Sarcoidosis

D. Herpes simplex virus infection

E. Cytomegalovirus infection

Esophagus

55. A 63-year-old male presents to an acute care clinic with complaints of difficulty swallowing that first started about 3 months ago and has been slowly getting worse. Sometimes when he swallows, he also feels pain in his throat. In the last 3 months he has lost 35 lbs., which he attributes to not eating as much due to the symptoms. His past medical history includes hypertension. He also has a 50-pack-per-year smoking history and has drunk 6 cans of beer per day for the last 20 years. An EGD reveals a mass in the middle portion of the esophagus. On biopsy, intercellular bridges are identified. Of the following, what is the most likely diagnosis?

A. Squamous cell carcinoma

B. Adenocarcinoma

C. Small-cell carcinoma

D. Leiomyoma

E. Esophageal varix

Esophagus

56. A 5-month-old male is brought to see his pediatrician by his parents. The night before, after eating, their son had an episode of projectile vomiting. Of the following, what is the most likely diagnosis?

A. Zenker's diverticulum

B. Schatzki's ring

C. Pyloric stenosis

D. Tracheoesophageal fistula

E. Gastric aplasia

Stomach

57. A 55-year-old male is brought to the emergency room by an ambulance that his family called after he had been complaining of a headache and became unresponsive. A CT scan in the hospital reveals a large intracerebral hemorrhage. He is stabilized for two days; however, he develops decreased consciousness and ultimately sustains a cardiac arrest and cannot be revived. At autopsy, the pathologist identifies a Duret's hemorrhage in the brainstem. Of the following conditions, which one is most likely to be identified in the stomach?

A. Curling's ulcer

B. Cushing's ulcer

C. Peptic ulcer

D. Gastric carcinoma

E. Varices

Stomach

58. A 53-year-old male presents to his family physician with complaints of heartburn. The typical treatment regimen for *Helicobacter pylori* infection is followed; however, the patient does not improve. An EGD is performed and biopsies are taken. The biopsies reveal scattered neoplastic cells with a signet ring appearance. He undergoes a gastrectomy. The stomach has no obvious mucosal mass; however, the wall of the stomach is diffusely thickened. Of the following, what is the most likely diagnosis?

A. Sarcoidosis

B. Malignant lymphoma

C. Diffuse-type gastric carcinoma

D. Ménétrier's disease

E. Chronic gastritis

Stomach

59. A 53-year-old male with a history of recurrent heartburn that he has chosen not to treat presents to an acute care clinic because he has vomited blood recently. He undergoes an EGD. The biopsies indicate an infiltrate of lymphoid cells, which the pathologist subsequently diagnoses as a MALT lymphoma. No mass is identified. Of the following, what is the best first course of treatment?

A. Gastrectomy

B. Radiation

C. Chemotherapy

D. Antibiotics

E. Gastrostomy

Stomach

60. A 58-year-old male presents to an acute care clinic because he vomited blood. A complete blood count reveals a hemoglobin of 14.0 g/dL. He reports that over the past 6 months he has had a sensation of early fullness after eating a relatively small amount of food. A CT scan of his abdomen reveals a mass in the wall of the stomach. He undergoes a resection. The pathologist notes that the tumor is composed of spindle cells and the cells show positivity for CD117. Of the following, which is most characteristic regarding this tumor?

A. It is easy to distinguish benign and malignant forms.

B. It is derived from interstitial cells of Cajal.

C. The bleeding was most likely due to blood vessel invasion by the tumor.

D. *Helicobacter pylori* infection is a risk factor.

E. The prognosis is poor.

Stomach

61. A one-week old infant is brought to the emergency by her parents because she has not passed feces since she left the hospital. A diagnosis of meconium ileus is made. Of the following, what other condition is she at risk for later in life?

A. Multiple sclerosis

B. Ulcerative colitis

C. Chronic pancreatitis

D. Chronic pyelonephritis

E. Autoimmune hepatitis

Intestine

62. A 31-year-old male presents to an acute care clinic. He reports that for the last 5 months he has had intermittent episodes of abdominal pain and diarrhea. He says that recently the diarrhea has appeared very fatty, and been difficult to flush. He is referred to a gastroenterologist who performs an EGD with biopsies. The biopsy shows absence of villi and a lymphoid infiltrate in the submucosa. Of the following, what is the most likely diagnosis?

A. Whipple's disease

B. Giardiasis

C. Pseudomembranous colitis

D. Celiac disease

E. Ménétrier's disease

Intestine

63. Given the previous clinical scenario, of the following, what is most characteristic of the disease process?

A. It normally affects the elderly.

B. It is associated with HLA-B6.

C. Serologic testing will reveal anti–smooth muscle antibodies.

D. Patients have an increased risk for lymphoma.

E. Patients are at risk for primary sclerosis cholangitis.

Intestine

64. Over the course of 10 years, a 35-year-old male was diagnosed with a cerebellar hemangioblastoma, a pheochromocytoma, and a clear cell renal cell carcinoma. Of the following, what is his most likely diagnosis?

A. Multiple endocrine neoplasia type I

B. Multiple endocrine neoplasia type II

C. VonHippel-Lindau syndrome

D. Cronkite-Canada syndrome

E. Lynch's syndrome

Brain, kidney, adrenal gland

65. A 46-year-old man is referred to urology because of pain during erection. On examination his testis and prostate are normal, he is circumcised, and he has a noticeable palpable plaque at the ventral base of the penis and a slight ventral curvature of the penis. A biopsy of this plaque would show which of the following?

A. Adipocytes with atypical spindle cells

B. Infiltrative fibroblastic proliferation

C. Ferruginous bodies

D. Hyperproliferative epidermis with markedly dysplastic cells

E. Panniculitis

Male genitourinary

21.2 Mixed Items—Answers and Explanations

Easy	Medium	Hard

1. Correct: Vitamin B12 deficiency (D)

The low hemoglobin is consistent with anemia, and anemia can cause fatigue and dizziness. Although all of the diseases listed could produce an anemia (**A-C, E**), given the clinical scenario and laboratory testing, the most likely cause is a B12 deficiency (**D**). A B12 deficiency is the only condition listed that produces a macrocytic anemia. At her young age and with her family history, colonic adenocarcinoma is unlikely (**B**). Because she is white, sickle cell disease is very unlikely (**E**). She has no risk factors for a warm autoimmune hemolytic anemia, including an autoimmune disorder or a white blood cell neoplasm (**C**). Menstrual blood loss (**A**) and colonic adenocarcinoma (**B**) would both cause an iron deficiency anemia, which is microcytic.

2. Correct: Rupture of one of the mitral valve papillary muscles (D)

Because the murmur developed suddenly, two days after the myocardial infarct, it is most likely due to a rupture, as this is the time course for a rupture (**D**). If there had been significant contractile dysfunction, it should have manifested itself immediately after the infarct (**E**). The other conditions listed are not a cause of an acute valvular insufficiency (**A-C**).

3. Correct: Fibromuscular dysplasia of the left renal artery (C)

The left kidney is atrophic, such as would be caused by decreased blood flow to the organ, as would occur with stenosis of the renal artery. The atrophic kidney is receiving less blood flow than normal and at a lower pressure, so it will activate the renin-angiotensin-aldosterone system to try and raise the blood pressure, which the opposite kidney will feel the effects of and thus, have a granular surface. Of the choices, only fibromuscular dysplasia of the left renal artery would produce such changes (**C**). The other conditions listed (**A-B, D-E**) would not.

4. Correct: Atherosclerosis of the right and left femoral arteries (A)

Given the patient's age, sex, and risk factors of smoking and diabetes mellitus, he most likely has atherosclerotic cardiovascular disease. His symptoms are referred to as claudication, which occurs due to atherosclerosis of the arteries supplying the lower extremities. With exertion and increased oxygen demand by the muscles, ischemia occurs (**A**). The other choices are not commonly associated with claudication (**B-E**).

5. Correct: A Factor V Leiden gene mutation (B)

Given the recent trauma, and resultant relative immobility, this patient is a set-up for a pulmonary thromboembolus. The episode of sharp chest pain and dyspnea was likely from a small thrombus that reached the periphery of the lung, whereas his death was caused by a saddle pulmonary thromboembolus. Factor V Leiden is a common mutation (around 5% of the population), which predisposes a patient to thrombosis (**B**). Of the choices, thrombosis is the most likely to be identified (**A, C-E**).

6. Correct: Rhabdomyoma (D)

The presence of seizures and subependymal giant cell astrocytoma in a patient with a prior cardiac tumor is highly suggestive of tuberous sclerosis (TS). The characteristic cardiac tumor in TS is the rhabdomyoma (**D**). The other conditions are not commonly associated with tuberous sclerosis (**A-C, E**).

7. Correct: Fibrillin (B)

This patient suffers from Marfan's disease, an autosomal dominant genetic disorder caused by a defect in the structural protein fibrillin (**B**). The other answer choices are not related to the pathology of Marfan's disease (**A, C-E**).

8. Correct: Thymoma (D)

Myasthenia gravis is due to autoantibodies that block the postsynaptic acetylcholine receptors, causing muscle weakness. Ptosis and diplopia are common symptoms and occur due to weakness of extraocular muscles. The degree of weakness fluctuates and can become severe very quickly. About 20% of patients with myasthenia gravis have a thymoma (**D**), which is the mediastinal mass identified on the CT scan. About 50% of thymomas occur in patients with myasthenia gravis. Thymectomy is beneficial to these patients. The other choices (**A-C,E**) do not apply.

9. Correct: Antihistone antibodies (B)

This patient presents with arthritis and pericarditis after treatment with a medication known to cause drug-induced lupus. Antinuclear and antihistone antibodies are present in 95% of patients with drug-induced lupus (**B**), whereas anti-Sm and anti-dsDNA antibodies are common in systemic lupus erythematosus (**A**) and very rare in drug-induced lupus. The other antibodies listed are associated with other diseases (**C-E**).

10. Correct: Drug-induced lupus (B)

The presence of pericarditis and joint pain in a patient on procainamide is drug-induced lupus until proven otherwise (**B**). Other medications known to cause drug-induced lupus include hydralazaine, penicillamine, isoniazid, and minocycline. (**A, C-E**) are incorrect.

11. Correct: A rub (D)

The clinical scenario (facial rash, with a butterfly pattern, arthralgias and myalgias, and some evidence of renal dysfunction, with protein in the urine) is consistent with SLE. Patients with SLE can develop fibrinous exudates in the body cavities, including the pericardial sac, which would produce a friction rub (**D**). None of the other findings are as directly related to SLE (**A-C, E**).

12. Correct: Anti-Smith antibody (A)

In SLE, many different antibodies can be identified: anti-dsDNA, anti-Sm (i.e., anti-Smith), anti-RNP UI, anti-SS-A, anti-SS-B, and antihistone. However, anti-dsDNA and anti-Sm are more specific for SLE than the others (**A**). Anti-HCV antibody is found in hepatitis C infections (**B**). Antiendothelial antibody is found in Kawasaki's disease (**C**). Antiendomysial antibody is found in celiac disease (**D**). pANCA is found in various vasculitides.

13. Correct: Anti-D antibody (C)

Given that he has most likely had past blood transfusions, and that he is O-, there is a good chance he has been exposed to the D antigen (Rh+), as a majority of the population is Rh+. This antigen is the one that is most likely to produce an immune response against it, with Kell being the next most immunogenic. Testing of his blood would most likely identify an anti-D antibody (**C**). An anti-Kell would be, of the choices, the second most likely (**A**). Anti-A antibodies are IgM and cause an immediate transfusion reaction (**D**). Antiendothelial antibodies are found in Kawasaki's syndrome (**B**) and anti-SSA in Sjögren's syndrome (**E**), which are not relevant in this case.

14. Correct: Hemoglobin (D)

Given that the patient just received blood and immediately afterward developed fever and chills, an immediate transfusion reaction caused by IgM reacting against AB blood antigens is the most likely cause. This is a type II hypersensitivity reaction (**B**). The IgM antibodies against the A or B antigen are naturally occurring and do not require previous sensitization to the antigen. Intravascular hemolysis will occur, causing free hemoglobin to be identified in the blood. This type of transfusion reaction can be fatal. (**A, C-E**) are not the best choices.

15. Correct: Tryptase (B)

The laboratory test that is most commonly used to diagnose an allergic reaction is a mast cell tryptase (**B**). Tryptase is a component of mast cell granules, which is fairly specific for anaphylaxis and can help confirm anaphylaxis in the postreaction or even postmortem setting. Given the clinical scenario, (**A, C-E**) would not be of use.

16. Correct: Contusion (C)

The red-purple discoloration of the skin is due to leakage of red blood cells from damaged blood vessels, a contusion (**C**). Hyperemia is a sign of acute inflammation and occurs due to dilation of blood vessels, an active process (**E**). Congestion is passive and results from impaired venous return (**D**). Lividity is the postmortem pooling of blood in the skin due to gravity (**A**). A contusion (i.e., bruise) is due to extravasation of red blood cells into the tissue as a result of trauma (**C**). Petechiae are small, pinpoint hemorrhages that occur due to a variety of processes (**B**).

17. Correct: Gonococcal arthritis (D)

The fluid described is an exudate (**D**). Transudates are produced by either high intravascular pressures, such as would occur with congestive heart failure (**A**), or with low oncotic pressure (as seen in hypoalbuminemia) (**E**). A subdural hematoma would have a high concentration of red blood cells (**B**), and a viral pericarditis can produce a watery or fibrinous pericarditis, but white blood cells would be unlikely (**C**)

18. Correct: Hemosiderin (B)

The pigment being described is hemosiderin. Hemosiderin contains iron, which will stain blue with a Prussian blue stain. Hemosiderin results from the breakdown of red blood cells (**B**). None of the other pigments listed are described as such, nor stain as such (**A, C-E**).

19. Correct: Diabetic ketoacidosis (B)

The findings of an elevated glucose concentration and acetone in the blood are consistent with diabetic ketoacidosis, which can be fatal (**B**). The clinical scenario does not provide evidence for any of the other listed causes of death (**A, C-E**).

20. Correct: Triglycerides (D)

The intracellular accumulation is fat (triglycerides), caused by abnormal metabolism (**D**). Mallory's hyaline, resulting from the accumulation of proteins associated with alcoholism, does not appear as described (**B**). The accumulations are not glucose, water, or mitochondria (**A, C, E**).

21. Correct: Increased concentration of cytochrome C (E)

The thyroid gland is undergoing apoptosis following radiation exposure. Increased concentrations of bcl-2 and decreased concentrations of BH3 proteins would inhibit apoptosis (**A, C**). Increased concentrations of Bax and decreased concentrations of Bcl-xL would promote apoptosis, but the result of Bax or Bak acting on the mitochondria is the release of cytochrome C, which in turn, activates caspases (**B, D, E**).

22. Correct: Retention of sodium in the cells (C)

Hydropic change, cellular swelling, is a sign of reversible cellular injury. The sodium-potassium pump pumps sodium out of the cell and potassium into the cell. With ischemia, one cause of reversible cellular injury, the amount of ATP produced is reduced, and without ATP, the sodium-potassium pump will not function, allowing sodium to enter the cell. Water follows sodium into the cell, causing the cell to swell and producing hydropic change (**C**). (**A-B, D-E**) are incorrect.

23. Correct: Neutrophilic infiltrate in the pancreas (A)

The individual most likely has acute pancreatitis, with alcohol use and gallstones being two risk factors for this condition, and with the symptomatology and laboratory testing supporting this diagnosis. Microscopic examination of the pancreas would reveal a neutrophilic infiltrate (**A**). (**B-F**) are incorrect.

24. Correct: Infarct (E)

The description is that of an infarct (**E**). Preservation of architecture does not occur with liquefactive necrosis (as can be seen with a bacterial pyelonephritis) or caseous necrosis (as can be seen with a tuberculosis infection), and by their nature, tumors do not have preservation of architecture within their boundaries (**A-D**).

25. Correct: Clumping of nuclear chromatin (E)

With an occlusive thrombus of the coronary artery, ischemic injury of the affected cardiac myocytes would occur; however, given that the thrombus was lysed within 20 minutes, any damage to the cardiac myocytes would have been reversible. Of the choices, only clumping of nuclear chromatin is a feature of reversible cellular injury (**E**); all other choices are signs of necrosis, which is irreversible cellular injury (**A-D**).

26. Correct: Hypertrophy (A)

Because of the systemic hypertension, increased pressure is placed on the left ventricular myocardium, which responds by increasing the size of the cells (**A**). The myocardium would be adapting to the increased pressure, and, since there is no failure, there is no reversible or irreversible cell injury (**E, F**). The cardiac myocytes are not capable of division and are increasing in size, not decreasing (**B, C**), and there is no switch in type of cell (e.g., cardiac) muscle to another form of mesenchymal tissue (**D**).

27. Correct: Severe stenosis of left renal artery by atherosclerosis (D)

The left kidney is decreased in size (and the right kidney is increased in size), which is consistent with atrophy. Atrophy occurs due to decreased blood flow, loss of innervation, increased pressure, and decreased hormonal stimulation. Stenosis of the left renal artery by atherosclerosis would cause decreased blood flow and resultant atrophy (**D**). An occlusive thrombus of the left renal artery would cause an infarct (**A**). A kidney stone would increase pressure, which can cause atrophy, but with blockage of urine flow, the renal pelvis would be dilated (**E**). The other choices would not lead to generalized atrophy of the kidney of the degree that the patient has (**B, C**).

28.   Correct: Calcitonin (D)

The eosinophilic material in the tumor is amyloid. Amyloid can be derived from multiple sources including Ig light chains (in multiple myeloma) (**B**), serum amyloid-associated protein (**C**), transthyretin (**E**), amylin, calcitonin (**D**), and amyloid precursor protein (**A**).

29.   Correct: Atrophy (C)

The man in this case suffered from benign prostatic hyperplasia. Blocking conversion of testosterone to its more potent form removed an important growth factor for prostate tissue. This resulted in atrophy of the prostate, which resolved his obstructive symptoms (**C**). The other choices are incorrect (**A-B, D-E**).

30.   Correct: Metaplasia (B)

This finding of normal-appearing tissue in an abnormal location is an example of metaplasia (**B**). In both dysplasia and carcinoma the cells would be abnormal in appearance (**A, D**). Hyperplasia is an increase in the number of cells from the normal state (**C**). Atrophy, on the other hand, would be a decrease in cell size (**E**).

31.   Correct: Suppurative inflammation (C)

The presence of neutrophils in the fluid would indicate pus, a feature of suppurative inflammation (**C**). If such fluid is well-contained to a certain region, it can be termed an abscess. Serous inflammation is watery, with little protein and few cells (**A**). Fibrinous inflammation has more protein than serous inflammation (**B**), but not an extensive amount of neutrophils, and chronic inflammation would have lymphocytes (**D**). An ulcer affects a mucosal surface (**E**).

32.   Correct: Increased concentration of bcl-2 (A)

Bcl-2 inhibits apoptosis, and therefore, increasing its concentration would lengthen the life of the cell (**A**). Bcl-xL also inhibits apoptosis, and decreasing its concentration would allow apoptosis to progress more quickly and shorten the life of the cell (**D**), and similarly, Bax and Bad promote apoptosis, and increasing their concentrations would promote apoptosis and shorten the life of the cells (**B, C**). BH3 proteins normally detect damaged DNA or increased misfolded proteins and promote the activation of Bax and Bad, which are proapoptotic mediators. In decreasing the concentration of BH3 proteins, apoptosis would be inhibited, but the life expectancy of the cell would be less when exposed to radiation (**E**).

33.   Correct: Intralobar pulmonary sequestration (B)

Having multiple episodes of pneumonia for an adolescent is unusual, and must be explained. The likelihood of an underlying anatomic abnormality contributing to the development of pneumonia is a strong possibility. Extralobar pulmonary sequestra-tion is a mass outside of the lung not connected to the bronchi. However, the condition usually presents early in life, even at the age of one day, because of difficulty breathing (**A**). Intralobar sequestration is a mass of pulmonary parenchyma, also not connected to the bronchi, which is most commonly found in the lower lobes and causes recurring episodes of pneumonia. The X-ray supports an intralobar pulmonary sequestration (**B**). Given the past history of episodes of pneumonia, a simple lobar pneumonia is unlikely (**C**). The negative sweat chloride test, and absence of other manifestations of cystic fibrosis, rule out that diagnosis (**D**). Small-cell carcinoma of the lung is highly correlated with tobacco use and would be rare in a child (**E**).

34.   Correct: Kartagener's syndrome (C)

The history of a chronic productive cough, with evidence of dilated airways on CT scan, is consistent with bronchiectasis. Bronchiectasis can occur due to a variety of underlying conditions, including those causing obstruction (e.g., foreign bodies, tumors such as squamous cell carcinoma) and infection. Individuals with respiratory symptoms and recurrent sinusitis can have granulomatosis with polyangiitis (**B**); however, there is no known kidney involvement, and the infertility is not usually associated with granulomatosis with polyangiitis. Chronic bronchitis is associated with a chronic productive cough but not with dilated airways or infertility (**E**). Kartagener's syndrome is an inherited disorder of cilia, and patients develop bronchiectasis, sinusitis, and dextrocardia and can be sterile due to immotile sperm (**C**). Given his age, with no family history, a squamous cell carcinoma of the lung would be very unlikely and would not explain the clinical scenario (**D**). Allergic bronchopulmonary aspergillosis would not explain the infertility (**A**).

35.   Correct: Diffuse alveolar damage (A)

The patient has features consistent with lobar pneumonia—fever, chills, pleuritic chest pain, dyspnea, and consolidation. The most likely causative organism is *Streptococcus pneumoniae*. One common complication of pneumonia is sepsis. Sepsis can lead to acute respiratory distress syndrome, for which the pathologic term is diffuse alveolar damage, which is characterized by the formation of hyaline membranes (**A**). Lobar pneumonia is not a significant risk factor for the remainder of the diagnoses (**B-E**).

36.   Correct: *Klebsiella pneumoniae* pneumonia (D)

The patient has a lobar pneumonia, as revealed by the X-ray, and the clinical signs of fever, chills and productive cough are consistent with the diagnosis. The most common cause of lobar pneumonia is *Streptococcus pneumoniae*. However, *Klebsiella pneumoniae* is the second most common agent, and because of its gelatinous capsule on cut surface the pneumonia associated with it will have a mucoid appearance (**D**). *Klebsiella* is also more common in older males and alcoholics. The other organisms listed cause pneumonia but are not usually causes of a lobar pneumonia (**A-C, E**).

37. Correct: *Streptococcus agalactiae* pneumonia (D)

The history of fever, productive cough, and dyspnea is consistent with pneumonia. As the infant is full term, hyaline membrane disease would not be a consideration (**A**). In the neonate, the most likely cause of pneumonia, especially in a mother who received no prenatal care, is *Streptococcus agalactiae* (Group B streptococcus), which is a bacterium found as part of some women's normal flora, and its presence or absence is usually tested for in the prenatal period (**D**). The other organisms listed would be much less likely to be the cause (**B-C, E**).

38. Correct: Meningitis (A)

Given the clinical scenario—rapid onset of fever, chills, and dyspnea, following very shortly after delivery, the patient most likely has a Group B streptococcal pneumonia. GBS is acquired during passage through the birth canal, and, in addition to pneumonia, is also a cause of meningitis in the neonatal period (**A**). The other conditions are not associated with a group B streptococcal infection in a neonate (**B-E**).

39. Correct: Scars at the apices of the lungs (C)

The described pathology is consistent with a Ghon complex—the Ghon focus is the subpleural nodule near the interlobar groove and, combined with the hilar lymph node changes, is a Ghon complex, which is characteristic of the *Mycobacterium tuberculosis* infection. Tuberculosis, being aerophilic, is also well-known for involvement of the apices of the lungs, which will, with survival, result in apical scarring (**C**). Noncaseating granulomas, with a negative acid-fast bacillus stain, would be consistent with sarcoidosis, which does not produce a Ghon complex (**E**). The dimorphic fungi—*Coccidioides immitis*, *Blastomyces dermatitidis*, and *Histoplasma capsulatum*—can produce similar gross pathologic findings as does tuberculosis. The other findings listed are not associated with a *Mycobacterium tuberculosis* infection (**A, B, D**).

40. Correct: Lung abscess (D)

The presenting symptoms are consistent with a pulmonary abscess—productive cough with foul-smelling sputum, fever, and pleuritic chest pain. The X-ray indicates a cavitary lesion, which could be an abscess or carcinoma; however, the biopsy is consistent with an abscess (**A, D**). While both granulomatosis with polyangiitis and microscopic polyarteritis can affect the lung, the lack of other findings, the lack of granulomas on biopsy, and the relatively rarity of those two conditions make them

much less likely (**B, C**). The most common cause of a lung abscess is aspiration, for which alcoholics are at a significant risk. The other diagnoses are not supported by the findings (**E**).

41. Correct: Plasma proteins and cellular debris layered on alveolar septa (C)

Given the history, diffuse alveolar damage (the pathologic correlate of acute respiratory distress syndrome) is the most likely diagnosis. The inhalation of the chlorine gas would damage the alveolar epithelial cells, allowing proteins from the capillaries to leak into the alveolar airspace. This material, along with damaged epithelial cells, layers on the alveolar septa, producing hyaline membranes, which are most prominent around 3-5 days following the accident (**C**). The amount of inflammation associated with such a change is usually minimal (**A, E**). Given no history of long bone fracture, fat emboli are not consistent with the clinical scenario (**D**). Extensive alveolar hemorrhage is not a necessary component of diffuse alveolar damage (**B**).

42. Correct: Goodpasture's syndrome (C)

The presenting symptoms are consistent with nephritic syndrome—hematuria (with red blood cell casts), hypertension, and proteinuria. The presentation earlier would be consistent with several diagnoses (infection, neoplasm, hemorrhage); however, given the involvement of both the kidney and the lung in a young male, of the choices, Goodpasture's syndrome is the best choice (**C**). *Mycobacterium tuberculosis* (**A**), a pulmonary neoplasm (**B**), idiopathic pulmonary hemosiderosis (**D**), and septic emboli (**E**) are not associated with nephritic syndrome, although infection of or metastases to the kidney could result in hematuria.

43. Correct: Thickening of the layer of submucosal glands in the bronchi (D)

The clinical scenario—a productive cough, occurring for a majority of days in two or more consecutive years—in combination with a history of tobacco use is consistent with the diagnosis of chronic bronchitis. The histologic finding is a thickened submucosal gland layer (**D**). The Reid index is the ratio of the thickness of the submucosal gland layer to the thickness of the bronchial wall from lumen to cartilage. The Reid index will be increased in people with chronic bronchitis. Although tobacco use is a risk factor for small-cell carcinoma and emphysema, the clinical history does not suggest either (**A, C**). The clinical history is not consistent with asthma or an extensive pulmonary hemorrhage (**B, E**).

44. Correct: Hyperinflation (B)

Given his extensive smoking history, the worsening exertional dyspnea not associated with a cough and associated weight loss are most likely due to emphysema. Histologically emphysema is characterized by the loss of pulmonary parenchyma, and grossly, there is hyperinflation of the lungs (**B**). Asthmatics can also, with an acute episode, have hyperinflation of the lungs, but a cough would be expected. Mucous plugging of the airways is seen in asthma (**C**). A variety of conditions are associated with lymphocytic interstitial infiltrates (**A**), honeycomb lung (**D**), and pulmonary hemosiderosis (**E**), but with no history or risk factors for congestive heart failure, recurrent pneumonia, or idiopathic interstitial lung disease, they are very unlikely.

45. Correct: Increased activity of elastase (B)

The chemicals in cigarette smoke impair the function of α-1-antitrypsin, which leads to increased activity of elastase (**B**). Elastase causes destruction of pulmonary parenchyma leading to a loss of elastic recoil and, hence, an obstructive lung disease. Mast cell activity and release of mediators is related to certain types of asthma (**D**). The other mechanisms are not relevant (**A, C, E**).

46. Correct: Beryllium (C)

Workers in the nuclear field can be exposed to beryllium. Exposure to beryllium can cause an acute illness, which manifests histologically as diffuse alveolar damage, and a chronic illness, which manifests as noncaseating granulomas (**C**). The appearance is similar to a hypersensitivity pneumonitis and may indicate that the disease process is due to a hypersensitivity mechanism. The other conditions listed are not normally associated with noncaseating granulomas (**A-B, D-E**).

47. Correct: Chronic hypersensitivity pneumonitis (E)

Given the clinical scenario, the most likely diagnosis is chronic hypersensitivity pneumonitis. The pulmonary function test is consistent with a restrictive lung disease. A common form of hypersensitivity pneumonitis occurs in farmers when they are exposed to moldy hay. His earlier episodes represent acute hypersensitivity pneumonitis (**D**), but, over time, damage has occurred and he now has chronic hypersensitivity pneumonitis (**E**). Although sarcoidosis and usual interstitial pneumonia cause a restrictive lung disease, the historical information better supports a hypersensitivity pneumonitis (**A, B**). Hamon-Rich syndrome is diffuse alveolar damage of undetermined etiology, and would present acutely, not over time (**C**).

48. Correct: Usual interstitial pneumonia (A)

The clinical history of worsening dyspnea associated with a cough and the pulmonary function testing is consistent with a restrictive lung disease. All of the listed diseases can present as a restrictive lung disease; however, cryptogenic organizing pneumonia would have an acute onset (**E**). Usual interstitial pneumonia is characterized by patch involvement of the lung, and both acute and chronic changes, fibroblastic foci and honey comb change, respectively; a heterogenous appearance (**A**). Non-specific interstitial pneumonitis is diffuse and homogenous (**B**). Sarcoidosis has non-caseating granulomas (**C**), and desquamative interstitial pneumonitis has alveolar airspaces filled with pigmented macrophages (**D**).

49. Correct: Primary pulmonary hypertension (C)

The pathologic finding of hypertrophied vessels in some of the smaller vessels supports a diagnosis of pulmonary hypertension. Recurrent pulmonary thromboemboli would produce pulmonary hypertension; however, she has no risk factors for deep venous thrombi (**B**). Primary pulmonary hypertension occurs in young women and has a poor prognosis (**C**). The normal echocardiogram does not favor a hypertrophic cardiomyopathy (**A**), and the lack of widespread smooth muscle proliferation in the biopsy would not favor lymphangioleiomyomatosis (**E**). Takayasu's arteritis with involvement of the lung would be rare (**D**); and the lack of granulomatous inflammation does not favor this diagnosis.

50. Correct: Tracheoesophageal fistula (C)

The most common form of a tracheoesophageal fistula is that where the esophagus is a blind-ended pouch and the distal esophagus connects to the trachea. When the blind-end pouch fills, the infant can aspirate the material into his lungs (**C**). None of the other conditions would cause the esophagus to have a blind-ended pouch. Zenker's diverticulum is a pouch off the esophagus and occurs in adults (**A**). Pyloric stenosis affects the stomach (**B**). A Schatzki's ring causes stenosis of the esophagus to a variable degree, varying from being asymptomatic to causing severe dyspepsia, and is present in the distal esophagus near the junction (**D**). Achalasia produces a dilation of the esophagus proximal to the defect (**E**).

51. Correct: Loss of inhibitory neurons (C)

The findings of dysphagia to both liquids and solids, associated with odynophagia and regurgitation of ingested food, is consistent with the diagnosis of achalasia. Achalasia is a disease process that affects the lower esophageal sphincter, causing it to fail to relax, leading to dilation of the esophagus proximal to this site. Inflammation leads to damage to ganglion cells in the myenteric plexus and loss of inhibition, leading to continued contraction (**C**). Achalasia can be primary, but it can also occur secondary to infiltration by amyloidosis, sarcoidosis, or other similar processes. The other mechanisms are incorrect (**A-B, D-E**).

52. Correct: Focal gastric necrosis (C)

The patient has a paraesophageal hiatal hernia, which is a cause of recurrent dyspepsia. When the stomach prolapses above the diaphragm, it is in danger of being pinched and losing its vascular supply, leading to ischemic necrosis (**C**). A paraesophageal hiatal hernia is not characteristically associated with any of the other listed conditions (**A-B, D-E**). A paraesophageal hiatal hernia could lead to Barrett's esophagus because of the reflux, and the patient would be at risk for the development of glandular metaplasia and subsequently an adenocarcinoma.

53. Correct: Dysplasia (D)

The patient has recurrent heartburn, with a negative workup for cardiac disease. Recurrent heartburn is most often due to the reflux of gastric contents into the esophagus. This exposure causes the esophageal mucosa to transition into glandular epithelium, a form of metaplasia; however, if the abnormal stimulation continues, dysplasia can develop, which can lead to neoplasia (**D**). Given the clinical scenario, this is the best answer. Any of the other choices can also appear in esophageal biopsies, but for different clinical scenarios (e.g., fungi and viral inclusions in immunosuppressed patients, including chronic alcoholics) (**A-C, E**).

54. Correct: Herpes simplex virus infection (D)

Individuals who are immunosuppressed are at risk for developing various infections, but the three most commonly described in the esophagus are *Candida*, herpes simplex virus, and cytomegalovirus infection. Herpes simplex virus produces multinucleated cells and cells with intranuclear inclusions (**D**). Cytomegalovirus produces intranuclear inclusions, but the infected cells are enlarged, and multinucleation is not associated with cytomegalovirus infections (**E**). Sarcoidosis produces noncaseating granulomas (**C**), and an adenovirus infection, which can produce intranuclear inclusions, of a smudged variety, and a posttransplant Hodgkin's lymphoma would be very rare (**A, B**).

55. Correct: Squamous cell carcinoma (A)

The clinical history—worsening dysphagia, odynophagia, and weight loss in an older male with a history of tobacco and alcohol use—favors an esophageal carcinoma. The ulcerated mass confirms this diagnosis. The two most common tumors of the esophagus are squamous cell carcinoma and adenocarcinoma. The location favors squamous cell carcinoma, as adenocarcinomas are almost always located distally and associated with Barrett's esophagus (**B**). Adenocarcinoma of submucosal glands can occur in other locations, but this is very rare. Intracellular bridges are a feature of squamous cell carcinoma (**A**). A small-cell carcinoma or leiomyoma would be rare (**C, D**). Esophageal vari-

ces occur in the distal segment of the esophagus and would not normally appear as a mass (**E**).

56. Correct: Pyloric stenosis (C)

The history of projectile vomiting occurring in an infant prior to the age of 6 months is characteristic of pylori stenosis, a hypertrophy of the smooth muscle at this site (**C**). Zenker's diverticulum and Schatzki's ring are conditions that most frequently present in adults and are not associated with projectile vomiting (**A, B**). Gastric aplasia would be very rare and would present sooner (**E**). A tracheoesophageal fistula would also most likely present sooner and does not cause projectile vomiting (**D**).

57. Correct: Cushing's ulcer (B)

With an intracerebral hemorrhage, a patient is at risk for developing cerebral edema. The finding of a Duret's hemorrhage confirms that the patient did develop and did die from the complications of cerebral edema developing in the background of the intracerebral hemorrhage. Cerebral edema causes increased intracranial pressure, and increased intracranial pressure is associated with Cushing's ulcers (**B**). Curling's ulcers are associated with burns (**A**). The patient's clinical scenario is not consistent with the other three diagnoses (**C-E**).

58. Correct: Diffuse-type gastric carcinoma (C)

The histologic and gross descriptions of the stomach are consistent with a diffuse-type gastric carcinoma. The tumor cells infiltrate singly and induce a marked desmoplastic reaction, which leads to the diffuse thickening of the wall of the stomach. The tumors have a poor prognosis (**C**). The gross description of the stomach, combined with the microscopic description, is not consistent with the other choices (**A-B, D-E**).

59. Correct: Antibiotics (D)

MALT lymphomas occur in the background of chronic gastritis, which is most commonly due to *Helicobacter pylori* infection. Unlike any other neoplasm, the tumor can regress if the underlying cause of its development is eradicated. In the case of a MALT lymphoma of the stomach, eradication of the *H. pylori* infection will usually cure the lymphoma (**D**). The other choices are not as good (**A-C, E**).

60. Correct: It is derived from interstitial cells of Cajal. (B)

The patient has a gastrointestinal stromal tumor. GISTs arise within the wall of the stomach and were originally diagnosed as a leiomyoma or leiomyosarcoma. They are derived from interstitial cells of Cajal and stain with CD117 (**B**). The bleeding that the patient experienced was most likely due to erosion of the mucosa that overlies the tumor, and not blood vessel invasion (**C**). Both benign and malignant versions exist (**A**). however, distinguishing between the two is difficult, and most are not aggressive (**E**). *Helicobacter pylori* infection is not a risk factor (**D**).

61. Correct: Chronic pancreatitis (C)

A meconium ileus is characteristic of cystic fibrosis, due to intestinal obstruction by the thick secretions that result from cystic fibrosis. Patients with cystic fibrosis are at risk for recurrent pneumonia and resultant bronchiectasis, secondary biliary cirrhosis, infertility, and chronic pancreatitis (**C**). Cystic fibrosis is not commonly associated with an increased risk of the other listed conditions (**A-B, D-E**).

62. Correct: Celiac disease (D)

The clinical presentation (diarrhea, abdominal pain, and ultimately steatorrhea) and the biopsy results are consistent with celiac disease (**D**). In Whipple's disease, there are collections of macrophages (**A**). *Giardia* is more commonly associated with watery diarrhea and less commonly malabsorption, and would not have loss of villi on biopsy (**B**). Pseudomembranous colitis affects the colon (**C**), and Ménétrier's disease affects the stomach (**E**).

63. Correct: Patients have an increased risk for lymphoma (D)

The clinical history and biopsy results are consistent with a diagnosis of celiac disease. Patients with celiac disease often have antitransglutaminase antibodies and antiendomysial antibodies (**C**).

Anti–smooth muscle antibodies are associated with autoimmune hepatitis. Celiac disease is common in younger adults (**A**), and it is associated with HLA-B8, -DR3, and DQW2 (**B**). Primary sclerosing cholangitis is not associated with celiac disease (**E**) and instead is associated with ulcerative colitis. Patients with celiac disease are at an increased risk for lymphoma (**D**).

64. Correct: Von Hippel-Lindau syndrome (C)

Von Hippel-Lindau syndrome is an autosomal dominant syndrome in which patients can develop cerebellar hemangioblastomas, clear cell renal cell carcinoma, pheochromocytomas, retinal angiomas, and cysts in different organs (**C**). MEN I is not associated with any of these tumors (**A**), and MEN II is associated with pheochromocytomas, but not the other tumors (**B**). Lynch's syndrome is associated with tumors of the colon, endometrium, bladder, and ovary (**E**), and Cronkite-Canada syndrome is associated with hamartomatous polyps in the GI tract (**D**).

65. Correct: Infiltrative fibroblastic proliferation (B)

The history and examination findings are consistent with Peyronie's disease. Of the answer choices, only infiltrative fibroblastic proliferation would be expected (**B**). Adipocytes with atypical spindle cells would be expected in liposarcoma (**A**), and ferruginous bodies are seen in asbestosis (**C**). Answer (**D**) would be expected in cancer or a premalignant lesion (such as Bowen's disease). Peyronie's disease is not a type of panniculitis (**E**).

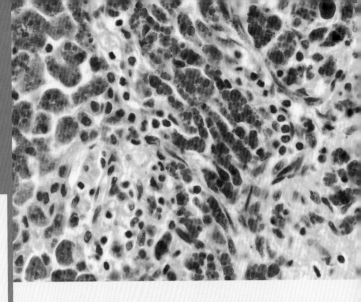

Chapter 22

Images

LEARNING OBJECTIVES

22.1 Images

- ▶ Describe the histologic changes in asthma
- ▶ Describe the gross features of and underlying etiologies for the various forms of pericarditis
- ▶ Describe the histologic features of sarcoidosis
- ▶ Identify a granuloma
- ▶ Describe the gross appearance of complications of an acute myocardial infarction, including rupture
- ▶ Determine the relative length of time since an acute myocardial infarct occurred
- ▶ Diagnose an abdominal aortic aneurysm
- ▶ Describe apoptosis
- ▶ Diagnose an adrenal adenoma
- ▶ Describe the relative incidence of nonfunctioning versus functioning adenomas
- ▶ Describe the types of secretion occurring with adrenal adenomas
- ▶ Describe the appearance of adrenal gland hyperplasia
- ▶ Describe the laboratory changes associated with Cushing's disease and Cushing's syndrome, and the effects of a dexamethasone suppression test
- ▶ Identify Auer rods
- ▶ List the chromosomal translocations associated with the various forms of leukemia and lymphoma
- ▶ Identify anthracotic pigment and list the causes for its accumulation
- ▶ List the disease processes associated with cigarette smoking
- ▶ Describe the gross appearance of an aortic dissection, a bicuspid aortic valve, and ventricular dilation
- ▶ Discuss the physiologic effects and the underlying causes of a hemopericardium
- ▶ Describe the gross and microscopic pathologic features of an aortic dissection
- ▶ Describe the gross appearance of acute appendicitis
- ▶ Describe the gross and microscopic findings of asbestos exposure
- ▶ Diagnose acute rheumatic fever
- ▶ Describe an asteroid body
- ▶ Describe the extrapulmonary manifestations of sarcoidosis
- ▶ Describe the complications arising from an atrial septal defect

- ▶ Compare the histologic features of coronary artery atherosclerosis in relation to stable and unstable plaques
- ▶ Describe the concept of collateral circulation and obstructive coronary artery atherosclerosis
- ▶ Describe the gross appearance of atherosclerosis
- ▶ List the modifiable and nonmodifiable risk factors for the development of atherosclerosis
- ▶ Describe the histologic appearance of adenocarcinoma in situ
- ▶ Identify Barrett's esophagus
- ▶ Distinguish between squamous epithelium and metaplastic glandular epithelium both grossly and microscopically
- ▶ Identify and describe the etiology of a bicuspid aortic valve
- ▶ Describe other causes of aortic stenosis and their gross appearance
- ▶ Identify BOOP/COP
- ▶ Identify axonal spheroids
- ▶ Identify and list the etiologic agents for acute bronchopneumonia
- ▶ Identify Burkitt's lymphoma
- ▶ List the CD markers, etiologic agent, and common locations for Burkitt's lymphoma
- ▶ Identify adenocarcinoma of the lung
- ▶ Compare the location and gross appearance of adenocarcinoma and squamous cell carcinoma
- ▶ Identify and list the most common etiology for caseating granulomas
- ▶ Identify contraction band necrosis
- ▶ Identify a cerebral edema
- ▶ List and describe the complications of a cerebral edema
- ▶ Identify cholesterol-type gallstones
- ▶ Identify and list the common causes of chronic pancreatitis
- ▶ Identify and describe the mechanism of the formation of chronic passive congestion of the lungs
- ▶ Identify chronic rheumatic mitral valvulitis

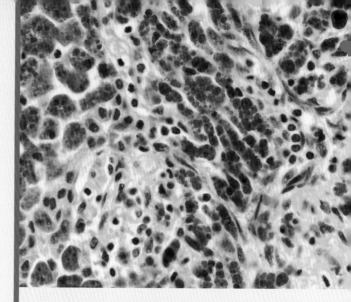

- ▶ Describe the immunologic mechanism of acute rheumatic fever
- ▶ Identify cirrhosis
- ▶ List and describe the complications of cirrhosis
- ▶ Identify chronic lymphocytic leukemia
- ▶ Describe the immune markers, prognosis, and epidemiology of chronic lymphocytic leukemia
- ▶ Identify chronic myelogenous leukemia
- ▶ Describe the epidemiology, prognostic factors, and molecular genetics of chronic myelogenous leukemia
- ▶ Identify cytomegalovirus
- ▶ Identify and discuss the etiologies of an acute myocardial infarct
- ▶ Identify condyloma
- ▶ Identify and describe the common locations for cryptococcal infection
- ▶ Identify cystic medial degeneration
- ▶ Describe the underlying causes of an aortic dissection
- ▶ Identify and describe the etiologies of diffuse alveolar damage (ARDS)
- ▶ Identify a dilated cardiomyopathy
- ▶ Identify steatosis of the liver
- ▶ List the causes of hepatic steatosis
- ▶ identify diverticulosis
- ▶ Identify diffuse large B-cell lymphoma
- ▶ Identify Fitz-Hugh–Curtis syndrome
- ▶ Describe the association between Fitz-Hugh–Curtis syndrome and pelvic inflammatory disease
- ▶ List and describe the complications of pelvic inflammatory disease
- ▶ Identify and describe the underlying causes of a pleural effusion
- ▶ Identify emphysema
- ▶ Describe the pulmonary function test, localization of disease, microscopic features, and epidemiology of emphysema
- ▶ Identify bacterial endocarditis
- ▶ List and describe complications and the common etiologic agents of bacterial endocarditis
- ▶ Identify esophageal varices
- ▶ Describe the mechanism by which esophageal varices are formed
- ▶ Identify and describe the risk factors for fatty emboli syndrome
- ▶ Describe the epidemiology, complications, microscopic appearance, and risk factors for cirrhosis
- ▶ Identify fatty streaks
- ▶ Identify follicular lymphoma

- ▶ Describe the epidemiology, prognosis, and molecular changes associated with follicular lymphoma
- ▶ Identify a nodular goiter
- ▶ Describe the mechanism of goiter formation
- ▶ Identify a granuloma
- ▶ Identify Hashimoto's thyroiditis
- ▶ Describe the laboratory abnormalities associated with Hashimoto's thyroiditis
- ▶ List the autoantibodies associated with Hashimoto's thyroiditis
- ▶ Identify Mallory's hyaline and fat accumulation
- ▶ Identify hairy cell leukemia
- ▶ List the laboratory abnormalities associated with hairy cell leukemia
- ▶ Identify hypertrophic cardiomyopathy
- ▶ Identify a cavernous hemangioma
- ▶ Describe the locations of occurrence and disease associations of cavernous hemangioma
- ▶ Identify hemochromatosis
- ▶ Identify hemosiderin
- ▶ Identify Hodgkin's lymphoma
- ▶ Identify hyaline arteriolosclerosis
- ▶ Describe the mechanisms by which hyaline arteriolosclerosis forms
- ▶ Identify and list the causes of cardiac hypertrophy
- ▶ Identify an acute myocardial infarct and determine the time since the infarct occurred
- ▶ Describe the regions of the heart perfused by each coronary artery
- ▶ Identify squamous cell carcinoma
- ▶ Identify a keratin pearl
- ▶ Identify and describe the cause of red neurons
- ▶ Identify an ulcer of the lower extremity
- ▶ Describe the mechanism underlying nonhealing ulcers of the extremities in people with diabetes mellitus
- ▶ Identify a Kimmelstiel-Wilson lesion

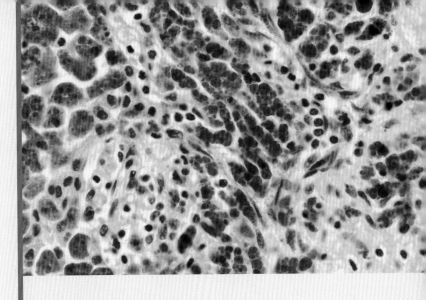

- ▶ Describe the underlying etiology of a Kimmelstiel-Wilson lesion
- ▶ Identify pancreatitis
- ▶ Identify and list the causes of lymphocytic myocarditis
- ▶ Identify steatohepatitis
- ▶ Identify the lines of Zahn
- ▶ Describe the formation of the lines of Zahn and the context of their identification
- ▶ identify pseudomembranous colitis
- ▶ Describe the relationship between antibiotic use and *Clostridium difficile* colitis
- ▶ Identify lipofuscin; describe the mechanism by which lipofuscin accumulates
- ▶ Identify a pitting edema
- ▶ Describe the conditions associated with pitting edema
- ▶ Identify a pleural plaque
- ▶ List the pathologic findings associated with asbestos exposure
- ▶ Identify sickle cell anemia in an organ
- ▶ Describe the complications of sickle cell anemia
- ▶ Identify jaundice
- ▶ List the causes of jaundice
- ▶ Differentiate between hemolytic, hepatic, and cholestatic processes causing jaundice
- ▶ Identify a pulmonary thromboembolus
- ▶ Describe the physical findings associated with deep venous thrombi
- ▶ Diagnose multiple myeloma
- ▶ Describe the serologic features of multiple myeloma
- ▶ Identify papillary thyroid carcinoma
- ▶ Identify centrilobular necrosis
- ▶ Describe the mechanism of formation of centrilobular necrosis
- ▶ Identify squamous metaplasia
- ▶ Describe how squamous metaplasia can develop
- ▶ List conditions of the lung associated with cigarette use
- ▶ Identify the histologic features consistent with Sjögren's syndrome
- ▶ Identify aspiration pneumonia
- ▶ Identify a pheochromocytoma
- ▶ Identify ischemic bowel
- ▶ Identify a Meckel's diverticulum
- ▶ Identify hyaline membranes
- ▶ Identify schistocytes
- ▶ Diagnose TTP
- ▶ List the underlying enzyme deficiency in TTP

- ▶ Identify psammoma bodies
- ▶ Identify acute plaque change
- ▶ Compare stable and unstable anginas
- ▶ Identify a myxomatous mitral valve
- ▶ Identify small-cell carcinoma
- ▶ Identify *Helicobacter pylori*
- ▶ Diagnose Kawasaki's disease
- ▶ Identify hypersegmented neutrophil
- ▶ Compare B12 and folate deficiencies
- ▶ Describe the mechanism by which red neurons form
- ▶ Identify neurofibrillary tangles
- ▶ Describe the histologic features of Alzheimer's disease
- ▶ Identify basal cell carcinoma
- ▶ Identify a berry aneurysm
- ▶ Describe the complications of a berry aneurysm
- ▶ Identify benign prostatic hyperplasia
- ▶ Identify capillary hemangioma
- ▶ Describe the treatment of, epidemiology, and complications of a capillary hemangioma
- ▶ Describe the histologic appearance of squamous cell carcinoma
- ▶ Identify dysplasia
- ▶ Identify a glioblastoma multiforme
- ▶ Identify a leiomyoma of the uterus
- ▶ Describe the gross and microscopic appearance, complications and sensitivity to estrogen of a uterine leiomyoma
- ▶ Identify a meningioma
- ▶ Describe the epidemiology, gross and microscopic appearance, prognosis, and common locations of meningiomas
- ▶ Identify phimosis
- ▶ Identify prostatic adenocarcinoma
- ▶ Describe the microscopic features, epidemiology, prognosis, appearance of bony metastases, and mutations associated with prostatic adenocarcinoma

293

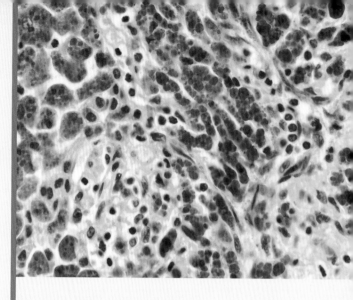

- ▶ Identify hyperplastic arteriolosclerosis
- ▶ Identify cervical intraepithelial neoplasia
- ▶ Compare low- and high-grade cervical intraepithelial neoplasia, and the underlying etiologic agent
- ▶ List the underlying cause of Fitz-Hugh–Curtis syndrome
- ▶ Identify a mucinous cyst adenoma
- ▶ Compare serous and mucinous tumors of the ovary and benign and malignant versions
- ▶ Identify and list the causative agents of meningitis
- ▶ Identify and describe the cause and complications of pelvic inflammatory disease
- ▶ Identify Lewy bodies
- ▶ Describe the disease association with Lewy bodies
- ▶ List the diseases associated with Lewy bodies
- ▶ List the symptoms of Parkinson's disease
- ▶ Identify and list the causes of a subarachnoid hemorrhage
- ▶ Identify crescentic glomerulonephritis
- ▶ Identify a cerebral edema
- ▶ Identify a seborrheic keratosis
- ▶ Identify a subdural hemorrhage
- ▶ Identify vitiligo
- ▶ Describe the association between vitiligo and autoimmune disease
- ▶ Identify and list the causes of intracerebral hemorrhage
- ▶ Identify histologic features of malignancy
- ▶ Identify a meningioma
- ▶ Identify and list the causes of acute tubular necrosis
- ▶ Identify and describe the causes of a cerebral abscess
- ▶ Identify contre-coup contusions
- ▶ Compare coup and contre-coup contusions
- ▶ Identify ductal carcinoma in situ and comedo necrosis
- ▶ Identify an acute cerebral infarct
- ▶ Describe the distribution of blood flow to the brain
- ▶ Describe the neurologic changes that would occur in the distributions of the major vessels with a cerebral infarct
- ▶ Identify an organizing cerebral infarct
- ▶ Describe the cause of cerebral infarction
- ▶ Identify colonic adenocarcinoma
- ▶ Describe prognostic features of colonic adenocarcinoma
- ▶ Identify alveolar proteinosis
- ▶ Diagnosis coal worker's pneumoconiosis
- ▶ Identify adenocarcinoma in situ
- ▶ Identify miliary tuberculosis
- ▶ Identify a molar pregnancy
- ▶ Compare complete and partial hydatidiform moles
- ▶ Identify multiple sclerosis
- ▶ Describe the appearance, etiology, and presenting symptoms of multiple sclerosis
- ▶ Identify axonal spheroids
- ▶ Describe the etiology and staining characteristics of axonal spheroids
- ▶ Identify papillary necrosis
- ▶ Identify AD polycystic kidney disease
- ▶ Describe the pathogenesis, genetic abnormalities, and associated findings of AD polycystic kidney disease
- ▶ Identify acute pyelonephritis
- ▶ Describe the mechanism by which acute pyelonephritis occurs
- ▶ Identify clear cell renal cell carcinoma
- ▶ Identify renal cell carcinoma
- ▶ Describe the risk factors, prognostic indicators, and mutations associated with renal cell carcinoma
- ▶ Identify renal stones; compare and contrast calcium, staghorn, uric acid, and cystine renal stones
- ▶ Identify α-1-antitrypsin deficiency
- ▶ List diseases associated with α-1-antitrypsin deficiency
- ▶ Identify adenomyosis
- ▶ Identify autosomal recessive polycystic kidney disease
- ▶ Describe the disease associations, epidemiology, genetic mutation, and complications of autosomal recessive polycystic kidney disease
- ▶ Identify a myxoma

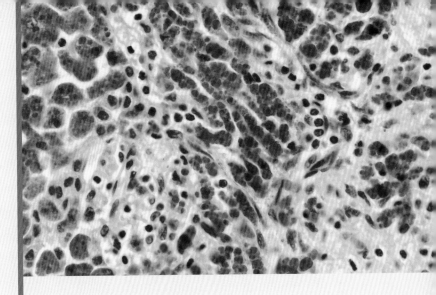

- ▶ Describe the most common location where a myxoma of the heart is likely to occur
- ▶ Identify Barrett's esophagus
- ▶ Identify dysplasia
- ▶ Identify basal cell carcinoma
- ▶ Describe the neoplastic process initiated by HPV infection
- ▶ Identify CIN
- ▶ Identify CMV infection
- ▶ Identify DCIS
- ▶ Compare low- and high-grade DCIS
- ▶ Identify a compound nevus
- ▶ Discuss the prognosis of DCIS and LCIS
- ▶ Identify a tubular adenoma
- ▶ Describe syndromes, prognosis, epidemiology, and risk factors associated with hereditary colon cancer
- ▶ Identify fibrocystic disease
- ▶ Identify a tophus
- ▶ Describe the cause and epidemiology of gout
- ▶ Identify Graves' disease
- ▶ Identify invasive lobular carcinoma
- ▶ Identify primary sclerosing cholangitis
- ▶ List the diseases most commonly associated with primary sclerosing cholangitis
- ▶ Identify seminoma
- ▶ Identify medullary thyroid carcinoma
- ▶ Compare the neoplastic potential of adenomatous polyps
- ▶ Identify Wilms' tumors
- ▶ Describe the genetic characteristics, epidemiology, and prognostic factors of Wilms' tumor
- ▶ Identify *Trichinella*
- ▶ Describe the risk factors associated with trichinosis infections
- ▶ Identify temporal arteritis
- ▶ Identify papillary urothelial carcinoma
- ▶ Describe the histologic features of a papillary urothelial carcinoma
- ▶ Identify Negri bodies
- ▶ Identify Reye's syndrome
- ▶ Describe the clinical scenario in which Reye's syndrome develops
- ▶ Identify complete hydatidiform mole
- ▶ Compare complete and incomplete hydatidiform moles
- ▶ Identify molluscum contagiosum
- ▶ Identify Riedel's thyroiditis
- ▶ Identify encephalitis

- ▶ Identify Brenner's tumor
- ▶ Identify apocrine metaplasia
- ▶ Identify adenocarcinoma
- ▶ Identify chronic pancreatitis
- ▶ List the causes of pancreatitis
- ▶ Identify the histologic features of Alzheimer's disease
- ▶ Identify *Mycobacterium tuberculosis*
- ▶ Describe the type of inflammatory process associated with *M. tuberculosis*
- ▶ Identify angiomyolipoma
- ▶ List the hereditary syndrome associated with angiomyolipoma
- ▶ Identify dysgerminoma
- ▶ Identify neurofibromatosis
- ▶ List the features characteristic of neurofibromatosis 1 and 2
- ▶ List the neoplasms associated with NF1 and NF2
- ▶ Identify thyroidization of the kidney
- ▶ Describe the gross and microscopic features of chronic pyelonephritis
- ▶ Identify synovial sarcoma
- ▶ Identify and describe the causes of dacrocytes
- ▶ Identify small-cell carcinoma
- ▶ List the mutations associated with small cell and non–small-cell lung carcinoma
- ▶ Identify lymphocytic myocarditis; list the organisms commonly causing lymphocytic myocarditis
- ▶ Identify red infarcts; given the clinical scenario, diagnose
- ▶ Identify varicose veins
- ▶ Describe the mechanism of formation of varicose veins
- ▶ Identify decubitus ulcer
- ▶ Identify serous pericardial effusion
- ▶ List the causes of cardiac effusions, and the form of effusion they are most frequently associated with

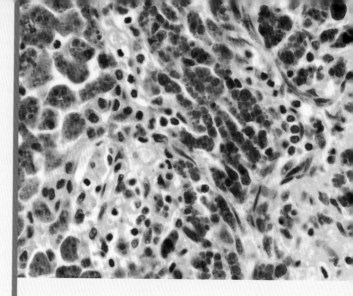

- ▶ Identify Russell bodies
- ▶ Identify hyperplastic polyp
- ▶ Identify hyaline arteriolosclerosis
- ▶ List the disease processes with which hyaline arteriolosclerosis is associated and describe the mechanism of its formation
- ▶ Identify an atypical lymphocyte
- ▶ Describe the diseases with which an atypical lymphocyte is associated
- ▶ Diagnose infectious mononucleosis
- ▶ Describe the testing methods used to diagnose infectious mononucleosis
- ▶ Identify meningitis
- ▶ List the common causes of and the clinical scenario associated with meningitis
- ▶ Identify pituitary adenoma
- ▶ Compare the forms of functioning and nonfunctioning adenomas as to effects and relative frequency
- ▶ Identify squamous cell carcinoma
- ▶ Identify nephrogenic rests
- ▶ Describe the association between nephrogenic rests and Wilms' tumor
- ▶ Identify an endometrial carcinoma
- ▶ Describe the association between a granulosa cell tumor and an endometrial carcinoma
- ▶ Identify a metastatic tumor in the liver
- ▶ List the common sites of metastatic spread for common types of tumors
- ▶ Identify coronary artery atherosclerosis
- ▶ Compare stable and unstable anginas
- ▶ Identify right ventricular dilation and hypertrophy
- ▶ Describe the four general categories of disease causing right ventricular dilation and hypertrophy
- ▶ Identify acute plaque change
- ▶ Describe the gross appearance of the heart due to coronary artery thrombosis, both occlusive and nonocclusive
- ▶ Identify spherocytes
- ▶ Describe the effects of parvovirus B19 infection on individuals with hereditary spherocytosis
- ▶ Identify myeloblasts
- ▶ Identify CLL
- ▶ Identify CML
- ▶ Identify iron deficiency anemia
- ▶ Identify bullous emphysema
- ▶ Identify desquamative interstitial pneumonitis

- ▶ Identify acute pyelonephritis
- ▶ Identify interstitial nephritis
- ▶ Identify oxalic acid
- ▶ Describe the conversion of ethylene glycol to oxalic acid
- ▶ Identify hyperplastic arteriolosclerosis
- ▶ Describe the clinical signs and symptoms of malignant hypertension
- ▶ Identify papillary fibroelastoma
- ▶ Describe the location, malignant potential, and complications of a papillary fibroelastoma
- ▶ Identify pleomorphic adenoma
- ▶ Identify chronic gastritis
- ▶ Identify coagulative necrosis
- ▶ Identify Mallory's hyaline
- ▶ Identify chronic hepatitis
- ▶ Compare hepatitis B and hepatitis C infections
- ▶ Identify a hemangioma
- ▶ Diagnosis hemochromatosis
- ▶ List the stain used to highlight iron
- ▶ Identify hemochromatosis; describe the epidemiology, genetic, and clinical features of hemochromatosis
- ▶ Identify cholesterolosis
- ▶ Identify cholangitis
- ▶ Identify gallstones
- ▶ Discuss the epidemiology and risk factors for gallstones, and compare cholesterol and pigment stones
- ▶ Identify reflux esophagitis
- ▶ Identify pancreatic pseudocyst
- ▶ Identify acute pancreatitis
- ▶ Identify prostatic adenocarcinoma
- ▶ Identify endometrial polyps
- ▶ Identify phylloides tumor

22.1 Images—Questions

Easy	Medium	Hard

1. A 27-year-old male dies suddenly while at home. An autopsy reveals hyperinflated lungs and the histologic findings in the figure. Of the following, what is the diagnosis?

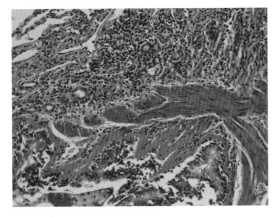

A. Emphysema

B. Bronchiectasis

C. Polyarteritis nodosa

D. Asthma

E. Bronchopneumonia

Lung

2. A 34-year-old female complains of chest pain and her physician auscultates a friction rub. Of the following, what is the diagnosis (see figure)?

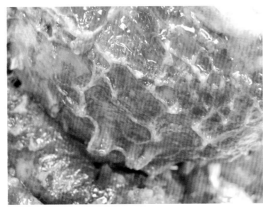

Consider this figure for questions 2 and 3

A. Serous pericarditis

B. Fibrinous pericarditis

C. Purulent pericarditis

D. Hemorrhagic pericarditis

E. Fibrous pericarditis

Heart

3. Given the gross appearance in the previous figure, of the following, what underlying disease process did this individual have that led to the changes on the epicardial surface?

A. Coxsackievirus A infection

B. Metastatic tumor

C. Bacterial infection

D. Uremia

E. Tuberculosis

Heart

4. A 41-year-old male has a chest X-ray for a work-related physical examination. Hilar lymphadenopathy is noted. The figure is the histologic appearance of the adenopathy. He has no respiratory-type symptoms. Stains of the lesion for acid-fast bacilli are negative. Of the following, what is the most likely diagnosis?

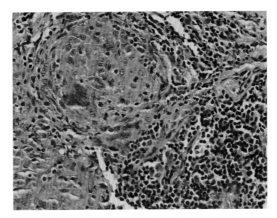

Consider this figure for questions 4 and 5

A. Small-cell lung carcinoma

B. Squamous cell carcinoma

C. *Mycobacterium tuberculosis*

D. Sarcoidosis

E. *Streptococcus pneumoniae*

Lung

5. Although not present in the figure above, of the following histologic findings, which was identified in a pulmonary hilar lymph node, which would be most likely to be identified in adjacent tissue?

A. Asteroid bodies

B. Ferruginous bodies

C. Keratin pearls

D. Fibroblastic foci

E. Charcot-Leyden crystals

Lung

6. A 52-year-old is found dead in bed by a friend who goes to check on him. At autopsy, the pathologic condition in the figure is identified. Of the following, what was the most specific mechanism of his death?

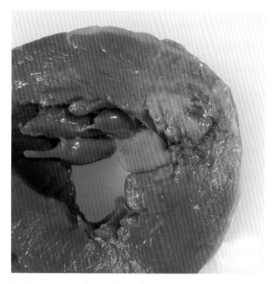

A. Pulmonary thromboembolism

B. Sudden cardiac arrest

C. Cardiac tamponade

D. Acute mitral insufficiency

E. Cerebral infarction due to thromboembolus

Heart

7. A 43-year-old sustains an episode of chest pain and subsequently dies. An autopsy is performed, revealing an acute myocardial infarct. Based on the histologic changes in the figure, of the following, which best describes the time interval between the chest pain and death?

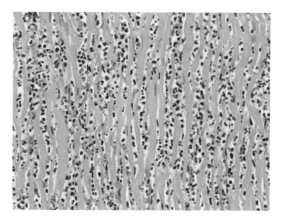

A. 1 minute

B. 1 day

C. 4 days

D. 10 days

E. 2 months

Heart

8. A 60-year-old male presented with abdominal pain and subsequently went into shock, followed by cardiac arrest and death. Autopsy revealed the pathologic lesion in the figure. Of the following, what is the most likely diagnosis?

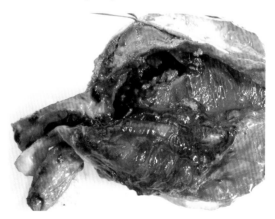

A. Ruptured syphilitic aneurysm

B. Ruptured aneurysm due to giant cell arteritis

C. Aortic dissection

D. Ruptured abdominal aortic aneurysm

E. Vascular angiosarcoma

Aorta

9. A 32-year-old male with mild elevations of his AST and ALT underwent a liver biopsy. Of the following, what pathologic process is occurring in the figure?

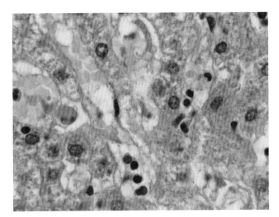

A. Coagulative necrosis

B. Liquefactive necrosis

C. Apoptosis

D. Metaplasia

E. Dysplasia

Liver

10. An autopsy of a 42-year-old female revealed the following pathologic lesion (see figure). Of the following, what abnormality would laboratory testing most likely reveal?

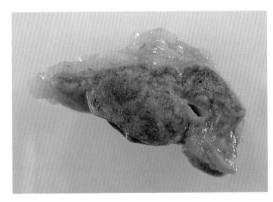

A. Elevated ACTH

B. Elevated cortisol

C. Urinary metanephrines

D. Low plasma renin activity

E. No abnormality

Adrenal gland

11. A 39-year-old obese female with hypertension and osteoporosis has the adrenal glands illustrated in the figure. If these adrenal glands represent the primary source of her obesity, hypertension, and osteoporosis, which of the following findings is most likely?

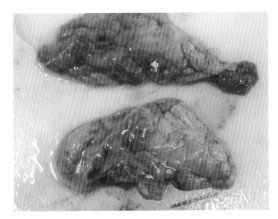

A. Elevated serum ACTH

B. Decreased serum ACTH

C. Suppression of cortisol with low-dose dexamethasone

D. Suppression of cortisol with high-dose dexamethasone

E. Elevated urinary metanephrines

Adrenal gland

12. A 39-year-old female presents to the hospital with complaints of a severe headache, and is ultimately diagnosed with an intracerebral hemorrhage. Shortly thereafter, she begins bleeding from her intravenous access points. Of the following, what translocation/genetic abnormality is associated with the pathologic finding illustrated in the figure?

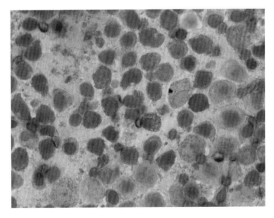

A. t(8;21)

B. inv(16)

C. t(15;17)

D. t(1;14)

E. t(11;14)

Heme

299

13. At autopsy a 34-year-old male was found to have the pathologic change illustrated in the figure. If he had not died, of the following, in future years, what disease process is he most at risk for developing?

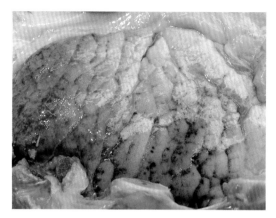

A. Asthma

B. Emphysema

C. Sarcoidosis

D. Asbestosis

E. Usual interstitial pneumonitis

Lung

14. A 46-year-old male presented to the emergency room with complaints of sharp back pain. During evaluation he became unresponsive, and subsequently expired. Autopsy revealed a hemopericardium. Based on the image, of the following, what is the underlying disease process that best explains all pathologic findings in the figure?

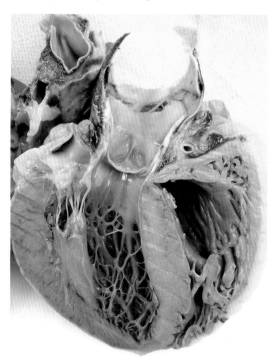

A. Dilated cardiomyopathy

B. Aortic dissection

C. Ruptured aortic aneurysm

D. Bicuspid aortic valve

E. Myocarditis

Heart

15. Of the following, what is the most likely underlying etiology of the pathologic condition illustrated in the figure?

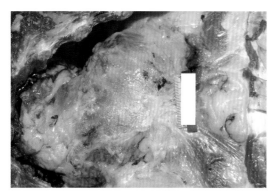

Consider this figure for questions 15 and 16

A. Ruptured abdominal aortic aneurysm

B. Aortic dissection

C. Acute myocardial infarct with rupture of inter ventricular septum

D. Rupture of coronary artery aneurysm

E. Pulmonary thromboembolus

Heart

16. If this lesion causes death, of the following, what is the most likely mechanism?

A. Disruption of electrical system

B. Contractile dysfunction

C. Diastolic dysfunction

D. Aortic insufficiency

E. Thrombus and resultant embolus

Heart

17. A 51-year-old male with a history of hypertension presents with chest pain, which just began. He subsequently becomes unresponsive and cannot be resuscitated. An autopsy reveals the lethal lesion. Of the following, what would microscopic examination (see figure) of the affected organ most likely reveal?

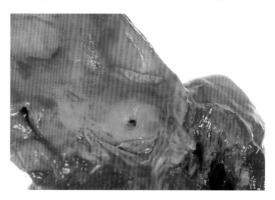

A. Granulomatous inflammation

B. Hemosiderin deposits

C. Cystic medial degeneration

D. Neutrophilic infiltrate and bacterial cocci

E. Infiltrating neoplastic cells

Heart

18. A 16-year-old female presents to the emergency room with her parents because she has been having abdominal pain. The abdominal pain began around her bellybutton and now is mostly in the lower right side of her abdomen. Of the following, what is the most likely diagnosis?

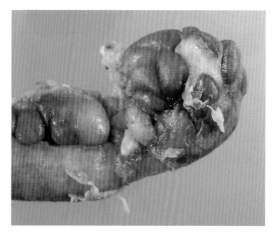

A. Diverticulitis

B. Ectopic pregnancy

C. Ulcerative colitis

D. Acute appendicitis

E. Peptic ulcer

Appendix

19. A 56-year-old male presents with slow onset of dyspnea on exertion, which is getting worse as time progresses. A lung biopsy reveals the pathologic finding in the figure. Of the following, what other pathologic finding is most likely to be identified?

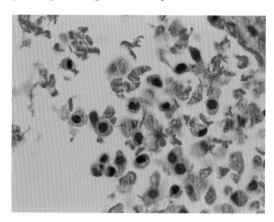

A. Progressive massive fibrosis

B. Schaumann bodies

C. Mesothelioma

D. Bilateral apical scars

E. Caseating granulomas

Lung

20. A 14-year-old boy presents to an acute care clinic with his parents because of a rash, pain in his joints, and dyspnea. Several weeks ago, he had an upper respiratory tract infection for which his parents did not seek medical care. The figure represents a pathologic finding in his heart. Of the following, what is the diagnosis?

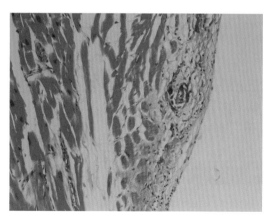

A. Lymphocytic myocarditis

B. Acute rheumatic fever

C. Sarcoidosis of the heart

D. Giant cell myocarditis

E. Rhabdomyoma

Heart

21. A 37-year-old male has hilar lymphadenopathy on chest X-ray. Based on the disease represented by the figure, of the following, which condition is he at risk for developing in the future?

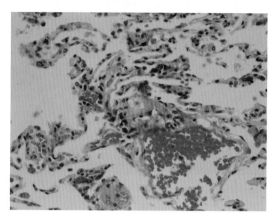

A. Primary sclerosing cholangitis

B. Acute pancreatitis

C. Cardiac dysrhythmia

D. Intracerebral hemorrhage

E. Cirrhosis of the liver

Lung

22. A 4-month-old female infant is asymptomatic and has the lesion illustrated in the figure. Of the following, which condition is she most at risk for the development of in the future?

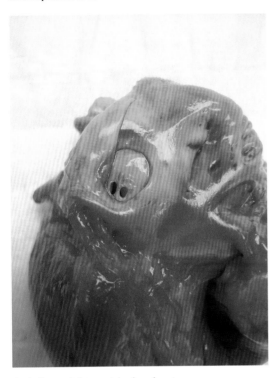

A. Left-to-right ventricular shunt

B. Deep venous thrombus embolizing to the brain

C. Atrial myxoma

D. Myocarditis

E. Kawasaki's syndrome

Heart

23. A 52-year-old male with a past history of hypertension has the pathologic lesion illustrated in the figure. Based only on the image, and not the pathologic process as a whole, of the following, what condition is he most at risk for?

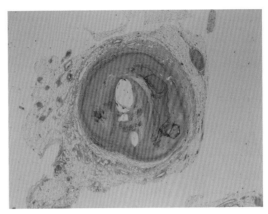

A. Stable angina

B. Unstable angina

C. ST-elevation myocardial infarct

D. Non–ST-elevation myocardial infarct

E. Coronary artery dissection

Heart

24. A 62-year-old male died from blunt force injuries sustained in a car accident. The figure illustrates a lesion in his left anterior descending coronary artery; however, the myocardium had no focal lesions. Of the following, what best explains this apparent discrepancy?

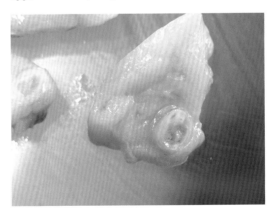

A. Complete resolution of an acute myocardial infarct

B. Protective effects of diabetes mellitus

C. Collateral circulation

D. Paired left anterior descending coronary arteries

E. Adequate diffusion of oxygen from the ventricular blood

Heart

25. A 67-year-old male died as the result of blunt force injuries sustained in a car accident. The lesion in the figure was identified in the aorta. Of the following, what is a nonmodifiable risk factor for its formation?

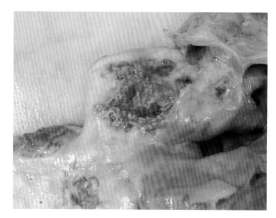

A. Hypertension

B. Diabetes mellitus

C. Gout

D. Sex of the patient

E. Cigarette use

Aorta

26. A 57-year-old male presented to an acute care clinic with complaints of a cough and some difficulty breathing. A chest X-ray (see figure) revealed an infiltrate. He did not respond to antibiotics, and a lung biopsy was performed. Of the following, what is the most likely diagnosis?

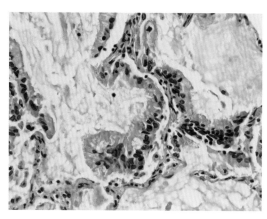

A. Sarcoidosis

B. Usual interstitial pneumonitis

C. Adenocarcinoma in situ

D. Type II pneumocyte hyperplasia

E. Acute bronchopneumonia

Lung

27. A 41-year-old had a recurrent history of dyspepsia. The figure shows his esophagus and stomach. Of the following, what is the most likely diagnosis?

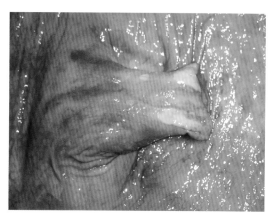

Consider this figure for questions 27 and 28

A. Achalasia

B. Adenocarcinoma

C. Esophageal varices

D. Barrett's esophagus

E. Erosive esophagitis

Esophagus, stomach

28. Of the following, what do the small white areas in the figure above represent?

A. Normal squamous epithelium

B. Normal gastric mucosa

C. Metaplastic squamous epithelium

D. Metaplastic glandular epithelium

E. Dysplasia

Esophagus, stomach

29. A 42-year-old male died as the result of blunt force injuries sustained in a car accident. The pathologic condition illustrated in the figure was identified at autopsy. Of the following, what was the most likely etiology for the lesion?

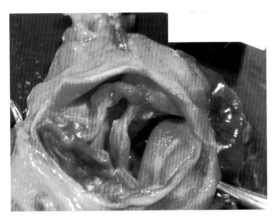

A. Wear and tear

B. Congenital

C. Rheumatic fever

D. Myxomatous degeneration

E. Neoplastic

Heart

30. A 34-year-old male survives a near fatal overdose of oxycodone. A biopsy of his lung several weeks later reveals the pathologic lesion illustrated in the figure. Of the following, what is the most likely diagnosis?

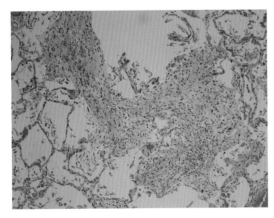

A. Diffuse alveolar damage

B. Bronchiolitis obliterans–organizing pneumonia

C. Cryptogenic organizing pneumonia

D. Usual interstitial pneumonia

E. Desquamative interstitial pneumonia

Lung

31. A 37-year-old male presents with a recent head injury. Of the following, what does the figure illustrate?

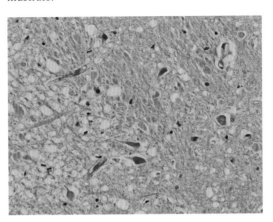

A. Lewy bodies

B. Negri bodies

C. Axonal spheroids

D. Red neurons

E. Rosenthal fibers

Brain

32. A 68-year-old male with a history of congestive heart failure was brought to the emergency room by his family because of his difficulty in breathing. He also was coughing up yellow-green mucus, and had a fever. Of the following, what is the most likely etiologic agent?

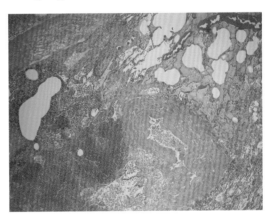

A. Influenza A, with no bacterial superinfection

B. *Mycobacterium tuberculosis*

C. *Coccidioides immitis*

D. *Staphylococcus aureus*

E. *Pneumocystis jiroveci*

Lung

33. A mass is removed from a child. Its histologic appearance is illustrated in the figure. Of the following, what is the most likely translocation associated with this neoplasm?

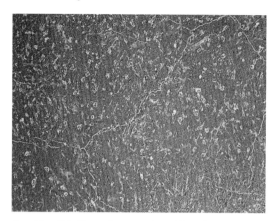

Consider this figure for questions 33 and 34

A. t(14;18)

B. t(11;14)

C. t(9;22)

D. t(15;17)

E. t(8;14)

Heme

34. Of the following, what is the most common characteristic of this lesion?

A. It is commonly associated with HSV type 1 infection.

B. Tumor lysis syndrome is rare.

C. A common location is near the ileocecal valve.

D. The neoplastic cells are CD5 and CD7 positive.

E. It is commonly associated with CMV infection.

Heme

35. A 61-year-old female has a pulmonary mass (see figure). Of the following, what is the most likely diagnosis?

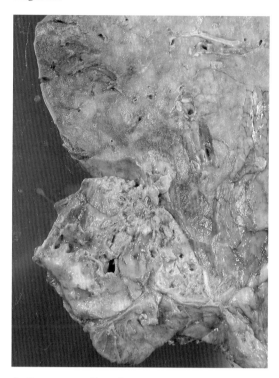

A. Squamous cell carcinoma

B. Adenocarcinoma

C. Pulmonary hamartoma

D. Adenocarcinoma in situ

E. Pulmonary abscess

Lung

36. A 43-year-old man has multiple ill-defined nodules throughout the lung, but concentrated in the apices. Their histologic appearance is illustrated in the figure. Of the following, what is the most likely diagnosis?

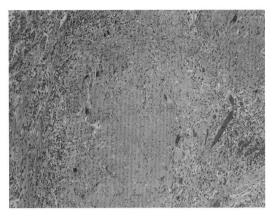

A. Sarcoidosis

B. Chronic hypersensitivity pneumonitis

C. Squamous cell carcinoma

D. Metastatic prostate carcinoma

E. Pulmonary tuberculosis

Lung

37. A 28-year-old male died as the result of the toxic effects of cocaine. Histologic examination of the heart identified the lesion in the figure. Of the following, what is the most likely diagnosis?

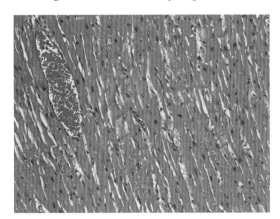

A. Cystic medial degeneration

B. Liquefactive necrosis

C. Contraction band necrosis

D. Normal intercalated disks

E. Myocarditis

Heart

38. A 53-year-old male is involved in a motor vehicle accident, and, several days after the crash, develops the pathologic lesion illustrated in the figure. Of the following, what is the most likely complication of this lesion?

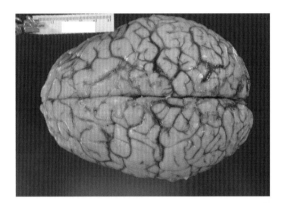

A. Subarachnoid hemorrhage

B. Meningitis

C. Astrocytoma

D. Brainstem hemorrhage

E. Loss of motor function and sensation in the left lower extremity

Brain

39. The stones in the figure were removed from a 43-year-old female with abdominal pain. Of the following, what was the most likely underlying mechanism for their formation?

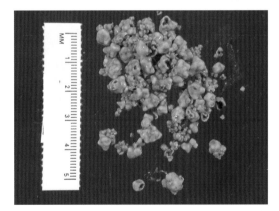

Consider this figure for questions 39 and 40

A. Increased uric acid concentration in the blood

B. Hemolysis

C. Supersaturation of bile with cholesterol

D. Conversion of ethylene glycol to oxalic acid

E. Increased cystine concentration in the blood

Liver, gallbladder

40. A 43-year-old female with a history of intermittent right upper quadrant pain underwent a cholecystectomy. The previous figure illustrates the contents of her gallbladder. Of the following, which statement is most characteristic of her disease process?

A. Almost all patients with the disease are symptomatic.

B. An X-ray of her abdomen would have identified the stones.

C. The stones are the result of increased breakdown of red blood cells.

D. In some patients, the stones can cause obstruction of the small intestine.

E. Her age and sex were not a risk factor.

Pancreas

41. A 37-year-old male is admitted to the hospital with complaints of abdominal pain. The two sections at the top of the figure represent a normal organ, while the two sections at the bottom of the image represent the appearance of his organ. Of the following, what is the most likely cause of the changes in this organ?

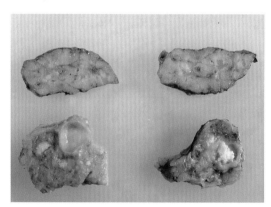

A. Benign neoplasm

B. Bacterial infection

C. Alcohol use

D. Autoimmune disease

E. Blunt force trauma

Lung

42. A 71-year-old male has a history of repeat hospital admissions due to dyspnea from pleural effusions, which were subsequently treated. The figure is a representative section of his lungs. Of the following, what is his most likely underlying diagnosis?

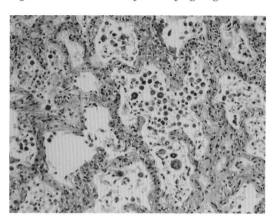

A. Systemic lupus erythematosus

B. Usual interstitial pneumonia

C. Asbestosis

D. Congestive heart failure

E. *Legionella* pneumonia

Heart

43. A 52-year-old female presents to her family physician with complaints of increasing shortness of breath with exertion. Of the following, what was the mechanism for the changes in the valve shown in the figure?

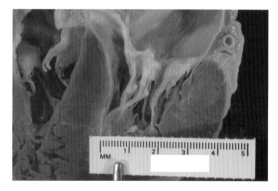

A. Bacterial infection of the leaflets

B. Amyloid deposition

C. Serotonin-producing carcinoid tumor

D. Autoantibodies directed at cardiac antigens

E. Eosinophilic infiltrate

Liver

44. A 44-year-old male with a past history of intravenous drug abuse is found to have increased AST and ALT on routine examination. A subsequent biopsy of his liver identifies the condition illustrated in the figure. Of the following, what is a complication of this disease process?

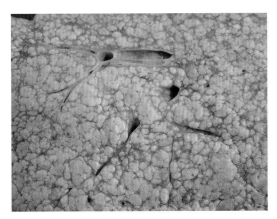

A. Primary sclerosing cholangitis
B. Acute pancreatitis
C. Hepatic hemangioma
D. Hemorrhoids
E. Hiatal hernia

Liver

45. A 41-year-old chronic alcoholic is found dead in his house by a friend who had come to visit. An autopsy reveals the condition illustrated in the figure. Of the following, what is the most likely diagnosis?

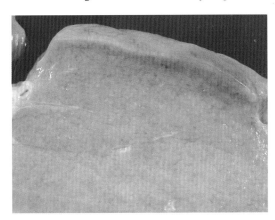

A. Miliary tuberculosis
B. Follicular lymphoma
C. Micronodular cirrhosis of the liver
D. Diffuse fatty liver
E. Metastatic colonic adenocarcinoma

Heme

46. A 56-year-old female presents to her family physician because of fatigue. A complete blood cell count reveals a white blood cell count of 85,000 cells/µL. The blood smear is illustrated in the figure. Of the following, what is the most likely diagnosis?

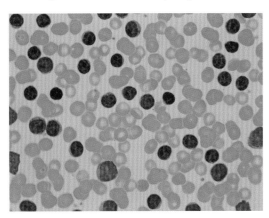

Consider this figure for questions 46 and 47

A. Acute myelogenous leukemia
B. Acute lymphoblastic leukemia
C. Chronic myelogenous leukemia
D. Chronic lymphocytic leukemia
E. Hairy cell leukemia

Heme

47. Of the following, which feature is characteristic of the pathologic condition illustrated in the figure above?

A. Cells are CD5 negative.
B. There is a short survival period after diagnosis.
C. The condition is most common in children.
D. Patients can have a hypogammaglobulinemia.
E. The neoplasm is derived from T cells.

Heme

48. A 55-year-old male presents to his family physician complaining of fatigue and early fullness after eating. A complete blood cell count reveals a white blood cell count of 200,000 cells/μL. A blood smear is illustrated in the figure. Of the following, what is the most likely diagnosis?

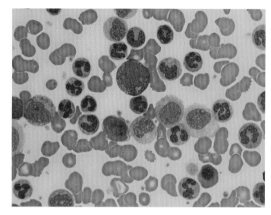

Consider this figure for questions 48 and 49

A. Acute myelogenous leukemia

B. Acute lymphoblastic leukemia

C. Chronic myelogenous leukemia

D. Chronic lymphocytic leukemia

E. Hairy cell leukemia

Heme

49. Of the following, which feature is most characteristic of the pathologic condition illustrated in the figure above?

A. It most commonly affects children.

B. If patients enter a blast crisis, they have a good prognosis.

C. It is a rare form of leukemia.

D. The early satiety is most likely caused by splenomegaly.

E. A t(9;22), juxtaposing the *BCL2* and *ABL* genes, is commonly present.

Heme

50. A 53-year-old male develops a gastrointestinal hemorrhage following a cardiac bypass grafting procedure. The figure, a histologic examination of the wall of the stomach, illustrates the underlying pathologic condition. Of the following, what is the most likely diagnosis?

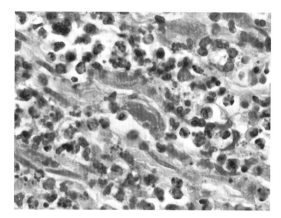

A. Gastric signet ring cell adenocarcinoma

B. Peptic ulcer

C. Cytomegalovirus infection

D. Hodgkin's lymphoma

E. Eosinophilic gastritis

Stomach

51. A 54-year-old male presents to the emergency room with chest pain. Based on the figure, of the following, what is the most likely underlying cause of his chest pain?

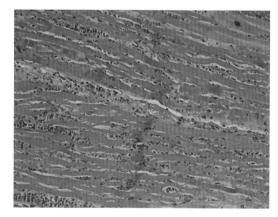

A. Coxsackievirus A infection

B. Sarcoidosis

C. Coronary artery atherosclerosis

D. Coronary artery dissection

E. Endocarditis and septic emboli

Heart

52. A 45-year-old male presented to his family physician with complaints of a mass at his anus. Subsequent excision of the mass was performed by a general surgeon. The mass is illustrated in the figure. Of the following, what was the most likely etiology of his mass?

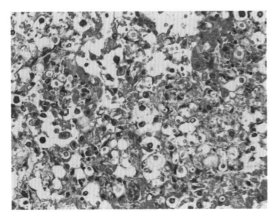

A. Chemical carcinogens in his diet

B. Ulcerative colitis

C. Unprotected anal intercourse

D. Quadriplegia

E. Cirrhosis of the liver

Rectum

53. A 41-year-old male with a history of HIV infection presents to an acute care clinic with complaints of shortness of breath. The figure illustrates the process in his lung. Although the organism present in the lungs most commonly begins in the lungs, it is best known for its involvement of another organ. Of the following, with which organ is the organism found in this lung most commonly identified?

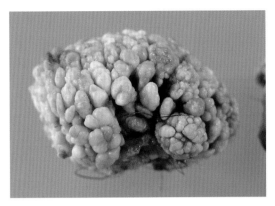

A. Brain

B. Heart

C. Liver

D. Spleen

E. Kidney

Brain, lung

54. An autopsy is performed on a 51-year-old male who was found dead in his house. Based on the histologic changes illustrated in the figure, of the following, what was the most likely cause of his death?

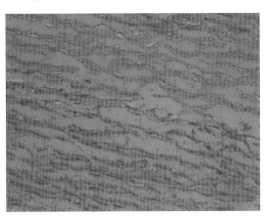

A. Cirrhosis of the liver

B. Parasitic infection

C. Aortic dissection

D. Acute pyelonephritis

E. Metastatic colonic adenocarcinoma

Aorta

55. A 47-year-old male presented to the hospital in shock due to an unidentified etiology. He survived for three days in the hospital prior to his ultimate death. An autopsy is performed. The figure illustrates findings in the lung. Of the following, what is the most likely diagnosis?

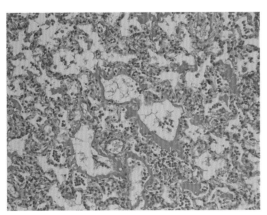

A. Pulmonary edema

B. Usual interstitial pneumonitis

C. Acute respiratory distress syndrome

D. Bacterial pneumonia

E. Influenza A

Lung

56. A 52-year-old male presents to his family physician because of difficulty breathing. A chest X-ray reveals bilateral pleural effusions. The figure illustrates the external appearance of his heart. Of the following, what diagnosis can be made?

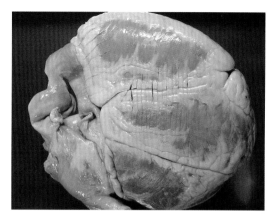

A. Acute myocardial infarct
B. Myocarditis
C. Tricuspid valve endocarditis
D. Dilated cardiomyopathy
E. Aortic dissection

Heart

57. A 41-year-old male has an elevation of AST and ALT and undergoes a liver biopsy. The figure illustrates the pathologic changes in his liver. Of the following, what is the most likely underlying etiology of the observed changes?

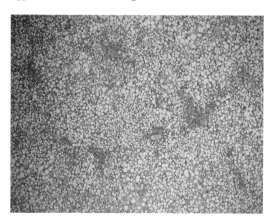

A. Hepatitis B infection
B. Iron deposition
C. Accumulation of α-1-antitrypsin
D. Exposure to alcohol
E. Bile duct obstruction

Liver

58. A 55-year-old male presents to his family physician because he has had some episodes of bleeding while having a bowel movement. The figure illustrates his underlying pathology. Of the following, what is his most likely diagnosis?

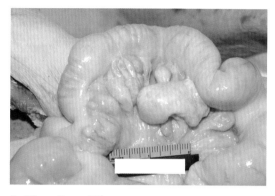

A. Ulcerative colitis
B. Rectal adenocarcinoma
C. Diverticulosis
D. Familial polyposis
E. Multiple Meckel's diverticula

Colon

59. A 63-year-old male was brought to the emergency room by EMTs after he had a seizure while with his friends. He has no history of epilepsy. A CT scan of the head revealed a mass. A biopsy of the mass revealed the neoplasm in the figure. Immunohistochemical staining revealed that the tumor was CD20+. Of the following, what is the most likely diagnosis?

A. Follicular lymphoma
B. Burkitt's lymphoma
C. Diffuse large B-cell lymphoma
D. Plasmacytoma
E. Mixed cellularity Hodgkin's lymphoma

Brain, heme

60. A 35-year-old female undergoes a laparoscopic cholecystectomy because of recurrent right upper quadrant pain. The surgeon identifies the pathologic lesion in the figure. Of the following, what condition is this individual at most risk for?

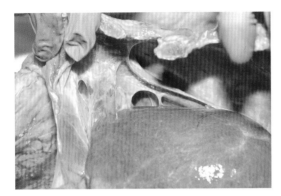

A. Cirrhosis of the liver

B. Adenocarcinoma of the gallbladder

C. Ectopic pregnancy

D. Ovarian neoplasm

E. Acute pancreatitis

Liver, genitourinary

61. A 67-year-old male with a history of hypertension, diabetes mellitus, and chronic alcoholism, presented to the emergency room with complaints of difficulty breathing. In the past two years, he has had six similar visits to the emergency room. Of the following, what is the most likely source of his presenting condition?

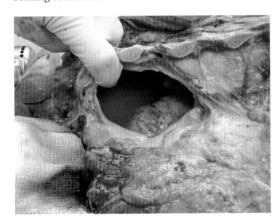

A. Empyema due to bronchopneumonia

B. Chylothorax

C. Congestive heart failure

D. Pulmonary neoplasm

E. Autoimmune disease

Lung, heart

62. A 63-year-old male dies as the result of an acute myocardial infarction. At autopsy, the pathologic condition illustrated in the figure is identified. Of the following, which feature is most characteristic of the disease process?

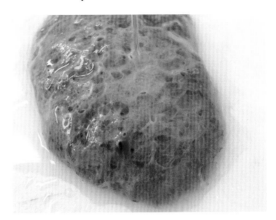

A. Patients have a normal FEV1/FVC ratio.

B. It normally occurs in much younger individuals.

C. Cigarette use contributes to a minority of cases.

D. The lesion is most common in the apices of the lungs.

E. Microscopic examination would reveal fibrosis of the alveolar septa.

Lung

63. A 27-year-old presents to an acute care clinic complaining of dyspnea. The lesion causing his symptoms is illustrated in the figure. Of the following, which is characteristic of this condition?

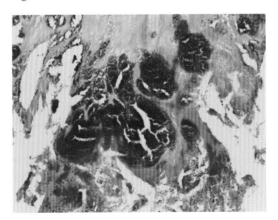

A. It most commonly occurs in the left atrium, adjacent to the fossa ovalis.

B. It most commonly occurs on the pulmonary valve.

C. The causative agent is usually *Pseudomonas aeruginosa*.

D. It is a precursor of papillary fibroelastoma.

E. Raised tender lesions on the fingers can occur.

Heart

313

64. A 47-year-old male presents to the emergency room after vomiting a large amount of blood twice. When he arrives, he is pale, his pulse is 130 bpm, and his blood pressure is 91/60 mm Hg. The figure illustrates the cause of his presenting symptom. Of the following, what is the underlying cause of the pathologic change illustrated in the image?

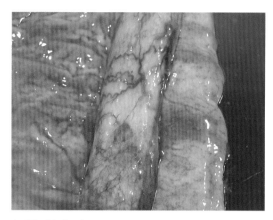

A. Viral infection

B. Gastroesophageal reflux

C. Cirrhosis of the liver

D. Prolonged vomiting

E. Ingestion of lye

Liver

65. A 61-year-old female develops acute dyspnea, mental status changes, and petechial hemorrhages in her axillae. The figure illustrates the cause of her symptoms. Of the following, which condition is the most likely to have led to the development of the changes in her lung?

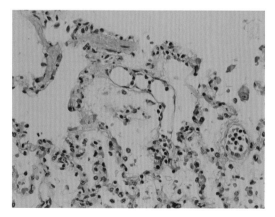

A. Disseminated intravascular coagulation

B. Cerebral infarct

C. Acute myocardial infarct

D. Long bone fracture

E. *Mycoplasma pneumoniae* infection

System

66. A 49-year-old male with a history of chronic alcoholism presents with an upper GI bleed. A physical examination reveals an enlarged liver, which is illustrated in the figure. Of the following, which is most characteristic of his condition?

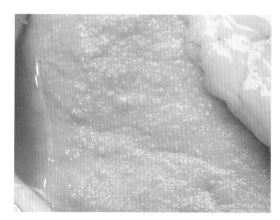

A. Infections with hepatitis A commonly cause this condition.

B. It most commonly affects children.

C. It is a risk factor for acute myocardial infarcts.

D. Males with the condition can have gynecomastia and testicular atrophy.

E. Microscopic examination will reveal granulomatous inflammation.

Liver

67. A 19-year-old male dies in a motor vehicle accident. An autopsy reveals the following lesions in the aorta. Of the following, what is the most likely diagnosis?

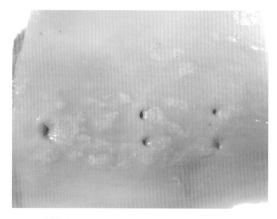

A. Syphilitic aortitis

B. Polyarteritis nodosa

C. Tears due to hypertension

D. Fatty streaks

E. Takayasu's arteritis

Aorta

68. A 61-year-old male presents to his family physician because he can feel a small bump on one side of his neck. Review of systems reveals that he occasionally has night sweats and intermittent fatigue. A biopsy of the nodule reveals the pathologic condition illustrated in the figure. Of the following, which is most characteristic of this condition?

A. It more commonly occurs in children.

B. Following diagnosis, patients usually only survive 1 to 2 years.

C. Most cases have a t(14;18), which involves the *BCL2* gene and the Ig lambda light chain gene.

D. The neoplastic cells frequently stain with CD20.

E. Confusion with an infectious process never occurs.

Lung

69. A 39-year-old female developed a painless enlargement of her neck. The pathologic condition responsible is illustrated in the figure. Of the following, what is the most likely mechanism of development?

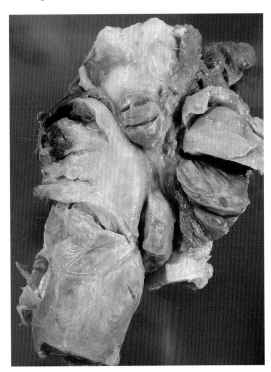

A. A highly malignant tumor

B. An autoimmune disorder

C. A nutrient deficiency

D. An infection

E. Trauma

Thyroid gland

70. A 45-year-old male has a chest X-ray during evaluation of a persistent cough. On the X-ray hilar lymphadenopathy is identified. The figure illustrates the pathologic change in the lymph nodes. Of the following, what is the pathologic lesion?

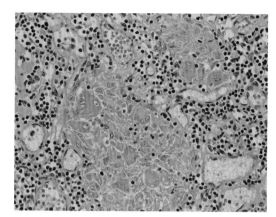

A. Squamous cell carcinoma
B. Caseating granuloma
C. Noncaseating granuloma
D. Neutrophilic infiltration
E. Amyloidosis

Lung

71. A 42-year-old female presents to her family physician because of a weight gain of over 30 lbs over the last 6 months. The responsible disease is represented in the figure. Of the following, what laboratory abnormality would this patient have?

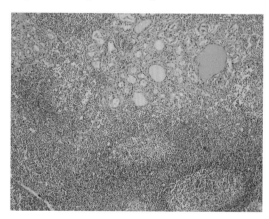

A. Increased TSH
B. Decreased TSH
C. Increased ACTH
D. Decreased ACTH
E. Increased PTH
F. Decreased PTH

Thyroid gland

72. Of the following, what would serologic analysis of the preceding patient's blood most likely identify?

A. Anti-TSH receptor antibodies
B. Antithyroglobulin antibodies
C. Anti-21-hydroxylase antibodies
D. Antimitochondrial antibodies
E. Anti–smooth muscle antibodies

Thyroid gland

73. A 47-year-old with a history of chronic alcoholism and hepatitis C presented to an acute care clinic with complaints of abdominal pain. An ultrasound of the abdomen revealed cirrhosis of the liver and a large 4.5-cm mass in the right lobe. The figure illustrates the histologic features of the tumor. Of the following, what is the most likely diagnosis?

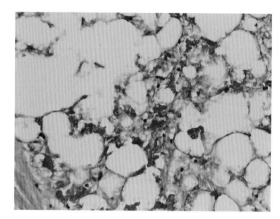

A. Metastatic colonic adenocarcinoma
B. Metastatic melanoma
C. Metastatic liposarcoma
D. Cavernous hemangioma
E. Hepatocellular carcinoma

Lung

74. A 65-year-old male presents to the emergency room with complaints of dyspnea and a productive cough. His vital signs are a temperature of 101°F, pulse of 106 bpm, and blood pressure of 137/87 mm Hg. Laboratory testing reveals a hemoglobin of 11.1 mg/dL, a white blood cell count of 900 cells/μL, and platelet count of 87,000 cells/μL. A physical examination reveals a palpable spleen, and rales on the right side. Of the following, what would further laboratory testing most likely identify?

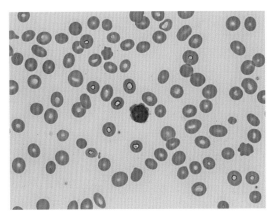

A. A t(9;22)

B. A t(11;14)

C. Positive test for tartrate-resistant acid phosphatase

D. Antibodies directed against the A blood group antigen

E. Positive monospot test

Heme

75. A 29-year-old male collapses while playing basketball with friends, and, despite resuscitative attempts, dies. An autopsy is performed. Histologic examination of the heart reveals the histologic features illustrated in the figure. Of the following, what is the most likely diagnosis?

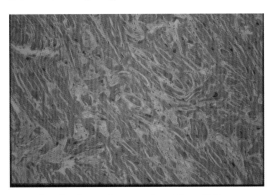

Consider this figure for questions 75 and 76

A. Dilated cardiomyopathy

B. Restrictive cardiomyopathy

C. Hypertrophic cardiomyopathy

D. Acute myocardial infarction

E. Lymphocytic myocarditis

Heart

76. Of the following, what gross feature is most likely to be identified at autopsy?

A. Myxomatous change in the mitral valve

B. Severe coronary artery atherosclerosis

C. Endocardial fibrosis of the left ventricular outflow tract

D. Dilation of all four chambers of the heart

E. Stenosis of the mitral valve

Heart

77. A 46-year-old female is having a laparoscopic cholecystectomy when the surgeon identifies a mass in the liver, which is illustrated in the figure. Which of the following features is most characteristic of the pathologic condition?

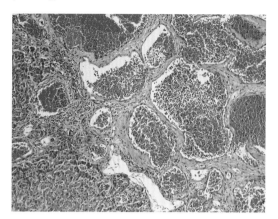

A. It most commonly occurs in the skin.

B. It is likely to regress.

C. Malignant transformation is common.

D. The lesion can cause death.

E. Patients with the mass usually also have neurofibromatosis.

Liver

78. A 37-year-old male with diabetes mellitus undergoes a liver biopsy as part of the workup for abnormal liver function. A biopsy of the liver has the histologic features illustrated in the figure. Of the following, what is the diagnosis?

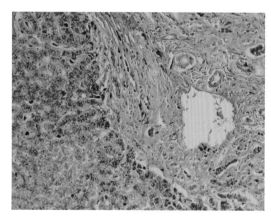

A. Primary biliary cirrhosis

B. Primary sclerosing cholangitis

C. Hemochromatosis

D. α-1-antitrypsin deficiency

E. Sarcoidosis

Liver

79. Histologic examination of a soft tissue lesion in the right lower extremity is illustrated in the figure. Of the following, what was the most likely etiology of the changes?

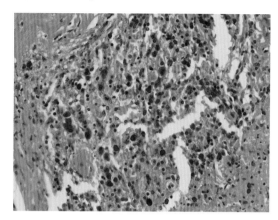

A. Infection

B. Neoplasm

C. Trauma

D. Autoimmune disorder

E. Chemical exposure

Soft tissue

80. A 35-year-old female with a history of fever and night sweats has an X-ray of the chest that reveals a mass in the mediastinum. The histologic features of the mass are illustrated in the figure. Of the following, what is the most likely diagnosis?

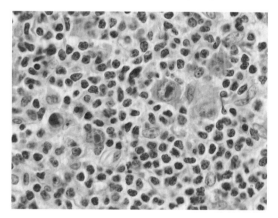

A. Follicular lymphoma

B. Diffuse large B-cell lymphoma

C. Hodgkin's lymphoma

D. Small-cell carcinoma

E. Squamous cell carcinoma

Lymph node

81. A 62-year-old female told her husband she was having chest pain, and then shortly thereafter collapsed. An autopsy was performed, and the pathologic lesion illustrated in the figure was identified in the kidney. Of the following, which disease, which caused the pathologic change illustrated in the figure, did this individual most likely have?

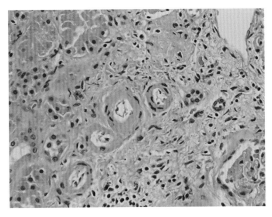

A. Systemic hypertension
B. Hypercholesterolemia
C. Polyarteritis nodosa
D. Acute glomerulonephritis
E. Systemic lupus erythematosus

Heart

82. A 52-year-old male sustained lethal head injuries during a motor vehicle accident and died. At autopsy, his heart was found to weigh 510 grams. Microscopic examination of his heart revealed the finding illustrated in the figure. Of the following, what disease process most likely caused this change?

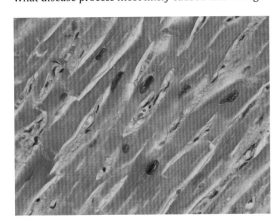

A. Hypertrophic cardiomyopathy
B. Coxsackievirus A infection
C. Amyloidosis
D. Hypertension
E. Cytomegalovirus infection

Heart

83. A 51-year-old male presents to an acute care clinic with complaints of chest pain. During his evaluation, he sustains a cardiac arrest and cannot be resuscitated. An autopsy is performed, which reveals the finding illustrated in the figure. Of the following, what is the most likely diagnosis?

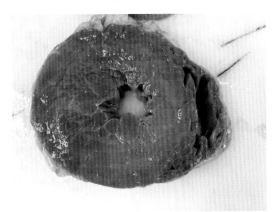

Consider this figure for questions 83, 84, and 85

A. Hypertrophic cardiomyopathy
B. Myocarditis
C. Acute myocardial infarct
D. Cardiac amyloidosis
E. Dilated cardiomyopathy

Heart

84. Of the following, for how long has he most likely been having chest pain?

A. 15 minutes
B. 2 hours
C. 1 day
D. 5 days
E. 10 days

Heart

85. Of the following, assuming the man is right dominant, in the distribution of what vessel are the pathologic changes occurring?

A. Left main
B. Left anterior descending
C. Circumflex
D. First diagonal
E. Right

Heart

86. A 67-year-old male is diagnosed with a tumor of his lung. The mass is resected by a surgeon and examined by a pathologist. Histologic examination of the mass reveals the findings illustrated in the figure. Of the following, what type of tumor is this?

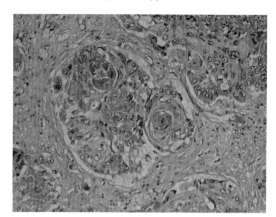

A. Squamous cell carcinoma
B. Adenocarcinoma
C. Small-cell carcinoma
D. Sarcoma
E. Teratoma

Lung

87. Histologic examination of the brain of a 67-year-old male who was autopsied after death reveals the finding illustrated in the figure. Of the following, what was the most likely etiology for the pathologic change?

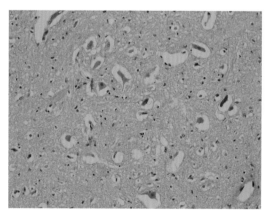

A. Neoplasm
B. Trauma
C. Metabolic abnormality
D. Hypoxia-ischemia
E. Infection

Brain

88. A 43-year-old male undergoes amputation of his right foot because he has developed a chronic non-healing ulcer that has been resistant to all therapy. Of the following, what is his most likely underlying medical condition?

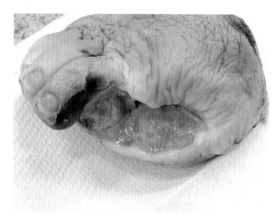

A. Congestive heart failure
B. Diabetes mellitus
C. Thromboangiitis obliterans
D. Amyloidosis
E. Trauma

Soft tissue

89. A 47-year-old male undergoes a kidney biopsy that reveals the finding illustrated in the figure. Of the following, what is the most likely diagnosis?

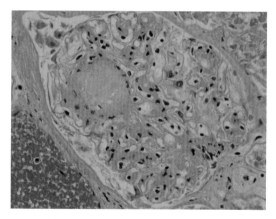

A. Focal segmental glomerulosclerosis
B. Membranous glomerulonephropathy
C. Diabetic nephropathy
D. Crescentic glomerulonephritis
E. Minimal change disease

Kidney

90. A 37-year-old male presents to an acute care clinic with complaints of severe abdominal pain. Laboratory testing reveals an amylase of 1,210 U/L and a lipase of 1,556 U/L. Of the following, what is the diagnosis?

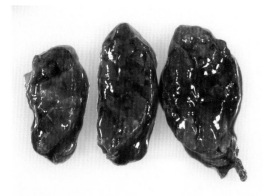

A. Pancreatic adenocarcinoma

B. Acute pancreatitis

C. Chronic pancreatitis

D. Abdominal trauma

E. Waterhouse-Friderichsen syndrome

Pancreas

91. A 36-year-old male presents to an acute care clinic with complaints of chest pain. A biopsy of his heart would reveal the findings illustrated in the figure. Of the following, what is the most likely etiology for his condition?

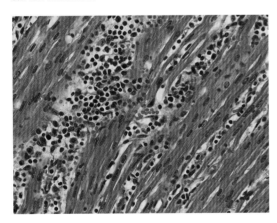

A. Coronary artery atherosclerosis

B. Recent medication change

C. Coxsackievirus A infection

D. Hypertrophic cardiomyopathy

E. Sarcoidosis

Heart

92. A 43-year-old obese male with diabetes mellitus is found to have an elevated AST and ALT. A liver biopsy identifies the pathologic condition illustrated in the figure. Of the following, what is the most likely diagnosis?

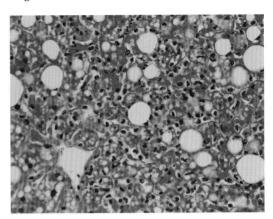

A. Hepatitis C infection

B. Steatohepatitis

C. Hereditary hemochromatosis

D. Gaucher's disease

E. Hepatocellular carcinoma

Liver

93. A 53-year-old dies suddenly five days after surgery. An autopsy is performed and identifies the pathologic lesion illustrated in the figure. Of the following, what is the most likely diagnosis?

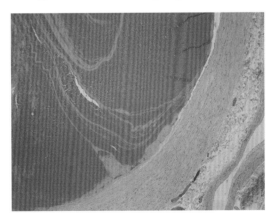

A. Acute myocardial infarct

B. Fatty emboli

C. Vasculitis

D. Pulmonary thromboembolus

E. Ruptured hemangioma

Lung

94. A 46-year-old male develops diarrhea. The figure illustrates the pathology causing his diarrhea. Of the following, which scenario best describes how the condition arose?

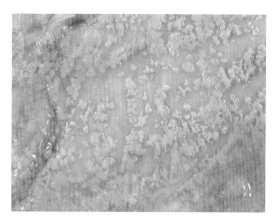

A. Drinking water from a stream
B. Sensitivity to gluten
C. Inheritance of *NOD2* gene
D. Recent use of antibiotics
E. Weakness in the colonic wall

Colon

95. A 71-year-old male dies as the result of an intracerebral hemorrhage. At autopsy, the pathologic change in the figure is identified in the heart. Of the following, what is the most likely diagnosis?

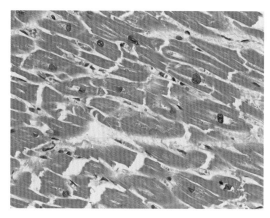

A. Hemochromatosis
B. Age-related changes
C. Myocarditis
D. Acute liver failure
E. Cigarette abuse

Heart

96. A 72-year-old male presents to the emergency room with complaints of shortness of breath. A physical examination reveals the pathologic finding illustrated in the figure. Of the following, what is the most likely diagnosis?

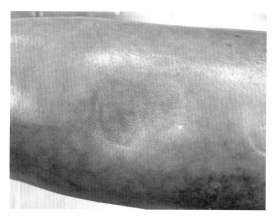

A. Pulmonary thromboembolus
B. Cirrhosis of the liver
C. Metastatic carcinoma
D. Congestive heart failure
E. Peripheral vascular disease

Heart

97. Following autopsy, the pathologist identifies the lesion illustrated in the figure. Of the following, what other condition is this individual most likely to have?

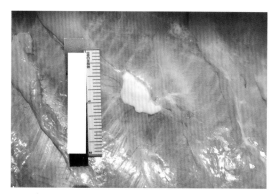

A. Allergic bronchopulmonary aspergillosis
B. Multiple meningiomas
C. Kimmelstiel-Wilson lesions in the kidney
D. Interstitial lung disease
E. Tension pneumothorax

Lung

98. A pathologist is performing an autopsy on a 23-year-old black female who died of an opioid overdose at home. She had been admitted to the hospital several times in her life for severe pain. The autopsy identifies the lesion illustrated in the figure. Of the following, what other finding is most characteristic of her underlying disease process?

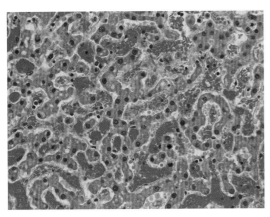

A. Acute pancreatitis
B. Peptic ulcer
C. Renal cell carcinoma
D. Small spleen
E. Ovarian cysts

Liver

99. A 38-year-old male presents to the emergency room, with skin changes as illustrated in the figure. Laboratory testing reveals a haptoglobin of 175 mg/dL, AST of 531 U/L, and alkaline phosphatase of 71 U/L. Of the following, what is the most likely cause of the pathologic change in the image?

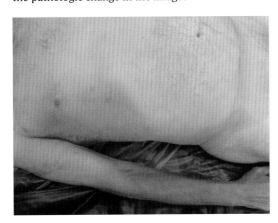

A. Thrombotic thrombocytopenic purpura
B. Hepatitis A infection
C. Ascending cholangitis
D. Excessive ingestion of carrots
E. Betadine staining

Liver

100. A 47-year-old obese female develops shortness of breath while talking with her husband, and shortly thereafter collapses. He calls an ambulance, but she is pronounced dead and an autopsy is performed. The figure illustrates the autopsy finding. If this woman would have had a physical examination the day prior, of the following, what would her physician have identified?

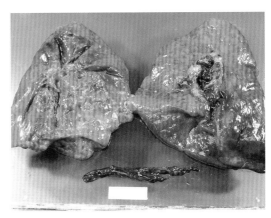

A. A positive Homans' sign
B. A positive Babinski's sign
C. A positive Auspitz's sign
D. A positive Nikolsky's sign
E. A positive Kernig's sign

Lung

101. A 59-year-old male presents to his family physician because of headaches. An X-ray of the skull reveals numerous lytic lesions. A bone marrow biopsy is performed. A counted 53% of the cells in the bone marrow biopsy have a morphology like those illustrated in the figure. Of the following choices, which is most characteristic regarding the patient's condition?

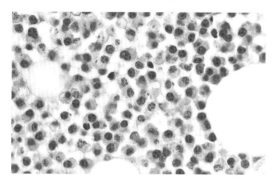

A. A serum electrophoresis is unlikely to have a prominent peak in the γ globulin region.
B. Serologic testing is likely to reveal an increased amount of IgA rather than IgG.
C. Risk of infection is low.
D. Most patients with this condition are normally much younger.
E. Patients can develop a restrictive cardiomyopathy.

Bone marrow, heart

102. During a routine physical examination, a 45-year-old female is found by her family physician to have a nodule in the right lobe of her thyroid gland. The nodule is removed and examined by a pathologist. The neoplasm is illustrated in the figure. Of the following, what is the most likely diagnosis?

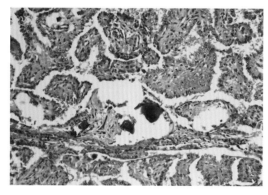

A. Papillary carcinoma
B. Follicular carcinoma
C. Medullary carcinoma
D. Anaplastic carcinoma
E. Marginal zone lymphoma

Thyroid gland

103. A pathologist is performing an autopsy on a 66-year-old male. Examination of the liver reveals the finding illustrated in the figure. Of the following, what was the man's most likely cause of death?

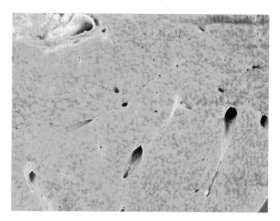

A. Metastatic Kaposi sarcoma
B. Disseminated intravascular coagulation
C. Congestive heart failure
D. Cirrhosis of the liver
E. Acute myelogenous leukemia

Liver, heart

104. A pathologist is performing an autopsy on a 62-year-old male. Histologic examination of the lungs reveals the finding illustrated in the figure. Of the following, what other condition, related to the finding in the image, is the pathologist most likely to find?

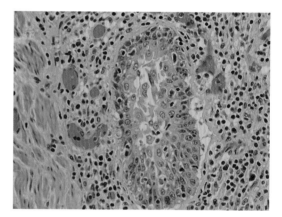

A. Eosinophilic infiltrate in the wall of airways
B. Pleural plaques
C. Pulmonary anthracosis
D. Usual interstitial pneumonia
E. Sarcoidosis

Lung

105. A 41-year-old female presents to her family physician. The figure illustrates the underlying condition causing her disease process. Of the following, which antibody would serologic testing most likely reveal that is most specific for this disease process?

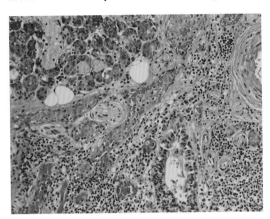

A. Antinuclear antibodies

B. Anti-dsDNA antibodies

C. Anti-Smith antibodies

D. Anti-SSA or anti-SSB

E. Anti-U1 RNP antibodies

Salivary gland

106. A 37-year-old male is found unconscious on the couch by a friend who comes to visit. A chest X-ray reveals an infiltrate in the right lung. The figure illustrates the pathologic process in the lung. Of the following, what is the most likely etiology?

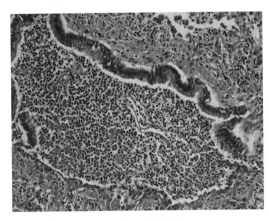

A. *Pseudomonas aeruginosa* infection

B. *Strongyloides stercoralis*

C. Acute alcohol intoxication

D. Chloride inhalation

E. Squamous cell carcinoma

Lung

107. A 43-year-old male is being evaluated for hypertension, which his family physician feels is secondary to another disease process. As part of the workup, he has a CT scan of the trunk, which identifies the mass illustrated in the figure. Of the following, what is his most likely diagnosis?

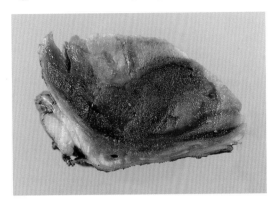

A. Metastatic melanoma

B. Pheochromocytoma

C. Myelolipoma

D. Sarcoidosis

E. Hemangioma

Adrenal gland

108. At autopsy, a 57-year-old male is found to have the condition illustrated in the figure. Of the following, what was the most likely mechanism of its development?

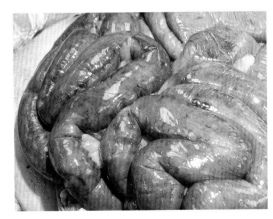

A. Hemorrhage from peptic ulcer

B. Recent antibiotic use

C. Hypotension

D. *Vibrio cholerae* infection

E. Trauma

Gastrointestinal

109. At autopsy, the pathologic condition illustrated in the figure was found incidentally and has no relation to the cause of death. Of the following, what is the most likely diagnosis?

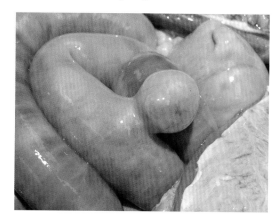

A. Aneurysm

B. Colonic diverticulum

C. Zenker's diverticulum

D. Hiatal hernia

E. Meckel's diverticulum

Small intestine

110. A 63 year-old male develops sepsis as a result of a urinary tract infection, which ascended into his right kidney, causing pyelonephritis. He acutely develops shortness of breath, and despite treatment, dies. An autopsy is performed and identifies the lesion illustrated in the figure. Of the following, what is the most likely diagnosis?

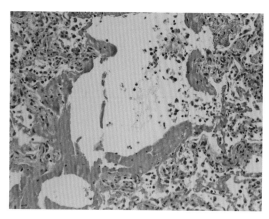

A. Pulmonary sarcoidosis

B. Amyloidosis of the lungs

C. Hyaline membranes

D. Disseminated intravascular coagulation

E. Desquamative interstitial pneumonitis

Lung

111. A 38-year-old male is brought to the emergency room by his wife. Over the past two days, he has had a fever, and just today, he forgot what day it was and where he was. His vital signs are a temperature of 99.9°F, pulse of 112 bpm, and blood pressure of 131/89 mm Hg. Laboratory testing reveals a hemoglobin of 11.8 g/dL, white blood cell count of 5,700 cells/μL and platelet count of 67,000 cells/μL, blood urea nitrogen of 37 mg/dL, and creatinine of 2.4 mg/dL. PT is 19 sec (SI units) and PTT is 71 sec (SI units). His blood smear is illustrated in the figure. Of the following, what is the most likely diagnosis?

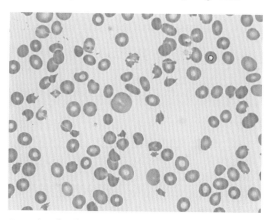

Consider this figure for questions 111 and 112

A. Disseminated intravascular coagulation

B. Idiopathic thrombocytopenic purpura

C. Thrombotic thrombocytopenic purpura

D. von Willebrand's disease

E. Essential thrombocythemia

Heme

112. Given the previous clinical scenario, of the following, what enzyme is deficient?

A. G6PD

B. ADAMTS-13

C. Hexokinase

D. Glucose phosphate isomerase

E. Enolase

Heme

113. A 51-year-old female undergoes a routine physical examination by her family physician, who identifies a nodule in the left lobe of her thyroid gland. Of the following, which characteristic histologic finding is illustrated in the figure?

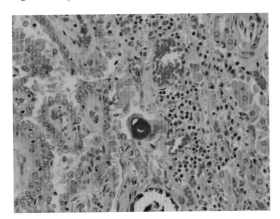

A. Asteroid body

B. Schaumann body

C. Psammoma body

D. Schiller-Duval body

E. Michaelis-Gutmann body

Thyroid gland

114. A 56-year-old male presents to an acute care clinic complaining of chest pain, which he describes as a sensation of pressure on his chest. Laboratory testing reveals no elevation of troponin I. The figure illustrates the pathologic process. Of the following, what is the most likely diagnosis?

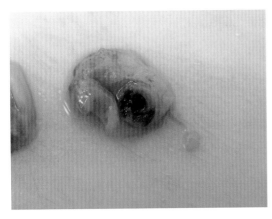

A. Stable angina

B. Coronary artery dissection

C. Coronary artery hemangioma

D. Coronary artery plaque hemorrhage

E. Kawasaki's disease

Heart

115. A 48-year-old female presents to her family physician complaining of some shortness of breath with exertion and some fatigue. The underlying cause of her symptoms is illustrated in the figure. Of the following, what is the most likely diagnosis?

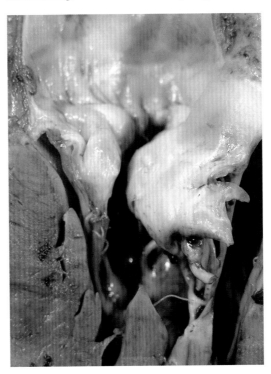

Consider this figure for questions 115 and 116

A. Aortic stenosis

B. Endocarditis

C. Carcinoid syndrome

D. Myxomatous mitral valve

E. Mitral annular calcification

Heart

116. Of the following, what is most characteristic of the preceding condition?

A. It is rare.

B. Patients are not at risk for the development of endocarditis.

C. Sudden death can result.

D. It occurs in females only.

E. It is due to infiltration of the leaflets with adipose tissue.

Heart

117. A 63-year-old male with a 70-pack-per-year smoking history presents to his family physician with complaints of a chronic cough, with occasional blood in the scant amount of sputum that comes up. A CT scan of his chest reveals a mass in the left lung. The histologic appearance of the mass is illustrated in the figure. Of the following, which is most characteristic of this neoplasm?

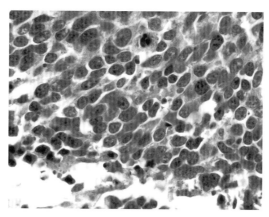

A. This type is usually peripherally located.

B. Asbestos exposure is a major risk factor.

C. Production of a parathyroid-like hormone is common.

D. The prognosis is excellent.

E. He may develop neuromuscular complaints related to the tumor.

Lung

118. A 41-year-old male with current heartburn undergoes an EGD and biopsy of his stomach. The biopsy is illustrated in the figure. Of the following, what is this patient most at risk for?

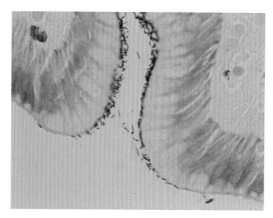

A. Gastrointestinal stromal tumor

B. Autoimmune gastritis

C. Zollinger-Ellison syndrome

D. Peptic ulcer

E. Celiac disease

Stomach

119. A 23-year-old male sustains blunt force injuries in a car accident. When he was a young child, he had one episode where he had a fever of 105°F and palpable nodules in his neck. He does not smoke. Histologic examination of the heart identifies the lesion illustrated in the figure. Of the following, what is the most likely cause of the pathologic change in the image?

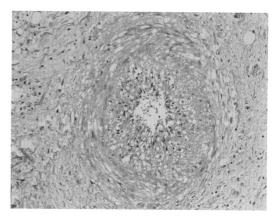

A. Hypertension

B. Chronic rheumatic fever

C. Kawasaki's disease

D. Polyarteritis nodosa

E. Thromboangiitis obliterans

Heart

120. A 54-year-old male who had a gastrectomy for treatment of a signet ring cell adenocarcinoma presents to his physician with complaints of fatigue. A blood smear reveals the pathologic finding illustrated in the figure. Of the following, what condition is this patient most at risk for?

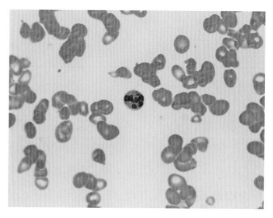

A. Central pontine myelinolysis

B. Descending Wallerian degeneration

C. Subacute combined degeneration of the spinal cord

D. Multiple sclerosis

E. Brainstem astrocytoma

Brain

121. A 28-year-old female with a history of depression is found deceased in her house. At autopsy, the brain is edematous, and histologic examination of the hippocampi reveal the pathologic change illustrated in the figure. Of the following, what is the most likely diagnosis?

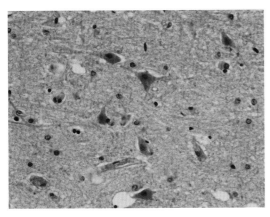

A. Hypoxic injury

B. Encephalitis

C. Organizing cerebral infarct

D. Low-grade astrocytoma

E. Head trauma

Brain

122. A 78-year-old male has had memory loss and changes in his personality and cognitive abilities over the last 10 years, to the point where he can no longer care for himself. Of the following, what is the most likely diagnosis?

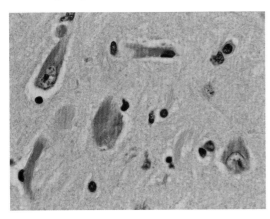

A. Pick's disease

B. Multi-infarct dementia

C. Parkinson's disease associated with dementia

D. Alzheimer's disease

E. Chronic subdural hemorrhage

Brain

123. A 71-year-old male has a small growth on his left ear that is excised by his family physician and examined by a pathologist. Of the following, what is the most likely diagnosis?

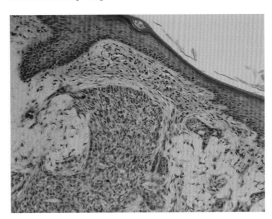

A. Compound nevus

B. Intradermal nevus

C. Basal cell carcinoma

D. Squamous cell carcinoma

E. Malignant melanoma

Skin

124. A 53-year-old male was found at autopsy to have the incidental lesion illustrated in the figure. Of the following, which had he been at most risk for during his life?

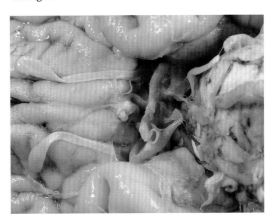

A. Brainstem glioma

B. Noncommunicating hydrocephalus

C. Balance disorders

D. Subarachnoid hemorrhage

E. Subdural hemorrhage

Brain

125. A 71-year-old male presents to his family care physician with the complaint of having difficulty urinating, often having to go during the night, and being unable to produce a strong urine stream. The symptoms have developed over the course of two years. The figure illustrates the underlying pathologic condition. Of the following, what is the most likely diagnosis?

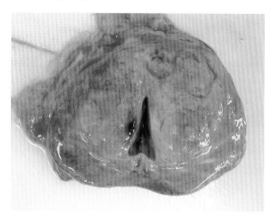

A. Acute prostatitis

B. Benign prostatic hyperplasia

C. Prostatic adenocarcinoma

D. Leiomyoma

E. Transitional cell carcinoma

Prostate

126. A red lesion was present on the skin of the forearm of a 3-year-old girl. The figure illustrates the microscopic appearance of the lesion. Of the following, which is most characteristic of the condition?

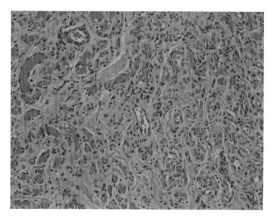

A. It was most likely caused by exposure to HHV8 in utero.

B. It is unlikely to regress.

C. Most likely the girl has a malignant tumor of the liver.

D. Surgical resection is not curative.

E. Thrombocytopenia can occur.

Skin

127. A 61-year-old male is found to have a mass. The mass is resected, and histologic examination of the tumor reveals the features illustrated in the figure. Assuming the mass is primary and not a metastasis, from which of the following organs did the mass originate?

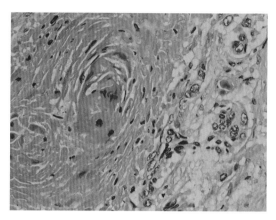

A. Brain

B. Thyroid gland

C. Liver

D. Adrenal gland

E. Bladder

Bladder

128. A 53-year-old male has a colonic polyp removed during his annual colonoscopy. The figure illustrates the histologic features of the polyp. What process is occurring at the top of the image?

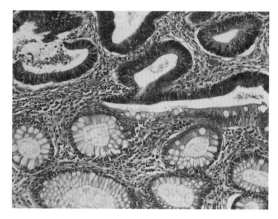

A. Hyperplasia

B. Metaplasia

C. Dysplasia

D. Neoplasia

E. Atrophy

Colon

129. A 65-year-old male has a seizure while golfing with friends. He is taken to the emergency room, where a CT scan reveals a mass in the right cerebral hemisphere. The mass is resected, and histologic examination of the tumor reveals findings illustrated in the figure. Of the following, what is the most likely diagnosis?

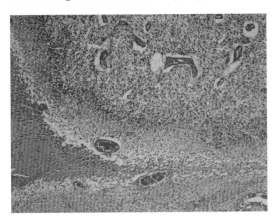

A. Low-grade astrocytoma

B. Pilocytic astrocytoma

C. Oligodendroglioma

D. Glioblastoma multiforme

E. Metastatic melanoma

Brain

130. A 52-year-old female is having her annual physical examination. Her only complaint is occasional heavy menstrual periods. Her gynecologist palpated a mass in the uterus. She underwent a hysterectomy. Examination of the resected uterus revealed the pathologic lesion illustrated in the figure. Of the following, which is most characteristic of this condition?

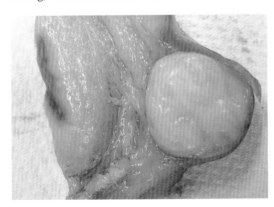

A. Malignant degeneration is common.

B. It is a very rare cause of infertility.

C. Microscopic examination would reveal interlocking fascicles of skeletal muscle.

D. The condition is estrogen sensitive.

E. The condition almost exclusively is present in white females.

Uterus

131. During an autopsy of a 57-year-old male who died as the result of an acute myocardial infarct, a neoplasm is identified in the cranial cavity. The tumor is centered on the dura mater. Of the following, which is most characteristic of this neoplasm?

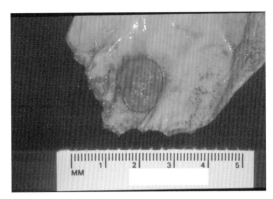

A. It is associated with neurofibromatosis 1.

B. It is highly aggressive and most often invades the brain.

C. The most common location is on the floor of the middle cranial fossa.

D. Microscopic examination will reveal Schaumann bodies.

E. They commonly have progesterone receptors.

Brain

132. A 27-year-old male was found to have the pathologic condition illustrated in the figure. Of the following, what is the most likely diagnosis?

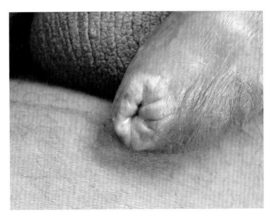

A. Epispadias

B. Hypospadias

C. Penile carcinoma

D. Phimosis

E. Condyloma

Penis

133. A 62-year-old male has a digital rectal examination during his annual physical and his physician palpates some nodularity. A subsequent biopsy reveals the pathologic condition illustrated in the figure. Of the following, what is the most likely diagnosis?

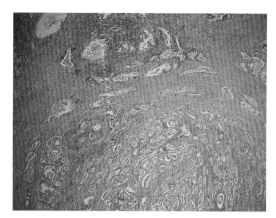

Consider this figure for questions 133 and 134

A. Benign prostatic hyperplasia
B. Acute prostatitis
C. Prostatic infarct
D. Prostatic adenocarcinoma
E. Pelvic intraepithelial neoplasia

Prostate

134. Of the following, what is most characteristic of this disease process?

A. Bony metastases are most commonly osteolytic.
B. Mutation of the glutathione S-transferase gene promoter is often present.
C. High-power examination will reveal two cell layers in the neoplastic glands.
D. Laboratory testing rarely reveals elevated alkaline phosphatase.
E. It rarely causes death.

Prostate

135. The pathologic lesion illustrated in the figure was identified in the kidney of a 53-year-old male. Of the following, what is the most likely diagnosis?

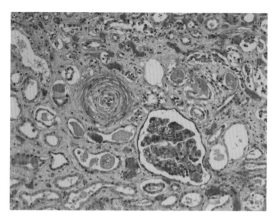

A. Crescentic glomerulonephritis
B. Hyaline arteriolosclerosis
C. Hyperplastic arteriolosclerosis
D. Polyarteritis nodosa
E. Microscopic polyarteritis

Kidney

136. A 28-year-old female has her annual physical examination, and her doctor identifies an aceto-white lesion, which is biopsied. The microscopic appearance of the lesion is illustrated in the figure. Of the following, what is the most likely etiologic agent of the pathologic change?

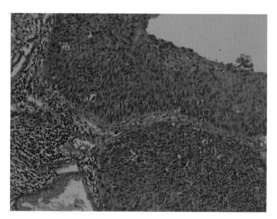

A. HPV11
B. HPV33
C. *Neisseria*
D. Syphilis
E. HSV

Cervix

137. A gynecologist performs a laparoscopic cystectomy and identifies the pathologic condition illustrated in the figure on the liver. Of the following, which infection is the most likely cause of this change?

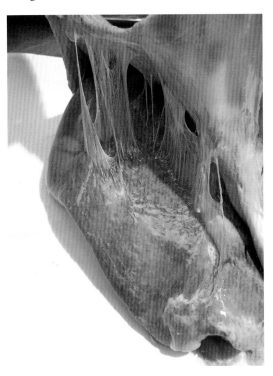

A. Hepatitis A
B. Hepatitis C
C. *Staphylococcus aureus*
D. *Clostridium difficile*
E. *Neisseria gonorrheae*

Liver

138. During her annual physical examination, a patient had a mass palpated in her left ovary by her gynecologist. A cystectomy was scheduled and performed, revealing the mass illustrated in the figure. Of the following, what is the most likely diagnosis?

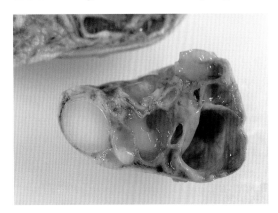

A. Serous cystadenoma
B. Mucinous cystadenoma
C. Serous cystadenocarcinoma
D. Mucinous cystadenocarcinoma
E. Mature cystic teratoma

Ovary

139. A 53-year-old chronic alcoholic develops a fever and headache. His friends bring him to the emergency room. The figure illustrates the pathologic condition causing his symptoms? Of the following, what is the most likely cause?

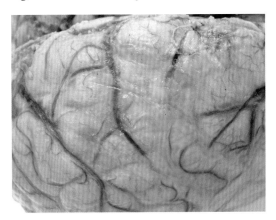

A. *Neisseria meningitidis*
B. *Streptococcus pneumoniae*
C. *Cryptococcus neoformans*
D. *Aspergillus flavus*
E. *Naegleria fowleri*

Brain

140. A 31-year-old female sustains blunt force injuries in a motor vehicle accident and dies. During the autopsy, the pathologic condition illustrated in the figure was identified. Of the following, what is most characteristic of this lesion?

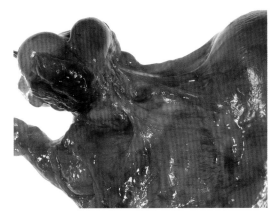

A. It is a significant risk factor for ovarian carcinoma.

B. Microscopic examination would reveal all three: glands, hemosiderin, and stroma.

C. It does not cause infertility.

D. The causative agent is often *Neisseria meningitidis.*

E. It can lead to high-pitched bowel sounds and tympany to percussion.

Ovary

141. The pathologic findings illustrated in the figure are identified in a 67-year-old male. Of the following, what is the most likely diagnosis?

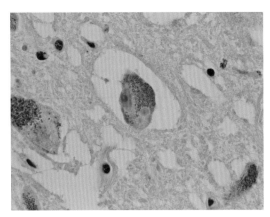

Consider this figure for questions 141 and 142

A. Alzheimer's dementia

B. Huntington's chorea

C. Parkinson's disease

D. Acute disseminated encephalomyelitis

E. Rabies

Brain

142. Of the following, what would be a common presenting symptom for the disease process most commonly associated with the histologic findings?

A. Chorea

B. Memory loss and diminished cognitive function

C. Cogwheel rigidity and flat affect

D. Aphasia

E. Cranial nerve palsies

Brain

143. A 27-year-old male is brought to the emergency room by his friend because of a severe headache, unlike any he has had before. He has no significant past medical history. A lumbar puncture is performed, which reveals blood. He is taken to surgery but becomes unresponsive before he can be treated. An autopsy is performed. One finding at autopsy is illustrated in the figure. Of the following, what is the most likely underlying cause of this autopsy finding?

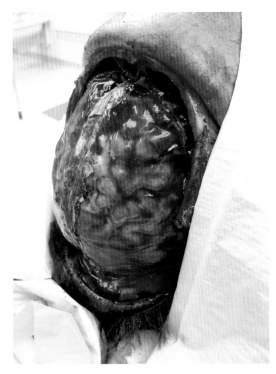

A. Acute myelogenous leukemia

B. An intracerebral hemorrhage

C. Hemorrhagic meningitis

D. Ruptured berry aneurysm

E. Ruptured brain tumor

Brain

144. A 43-year-old male presents to an acute care clinic with complaints of blood in his urine and fatigue. His blood pressure is 148/86 mm Hg. The figure illustrates the pathologic process responsible for his symptoms. Of the following, what is the diagnosis?

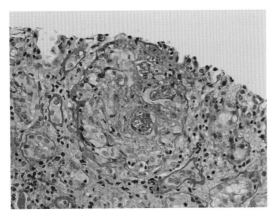

A. Focal segmental glomerulosclerosis
B. Membranous glomerulonephropathy
C. Postinfectious glomerulonephritis
D. Rapidly progressing glomerulonephritis
E. Membranoproliferative glomerulonephritis

Kidney

145. A 36-year-old male is found by his wife to be unresponsive. Lying on the floor next to him is a container with three oxycodone tablets. The prescription was filled two days earlier for 30 tablets. He is pronounced dead and an autopsy is performed. The figure illustrates a pathologic lesion of the brain. Of the following, what is the diagnosis?

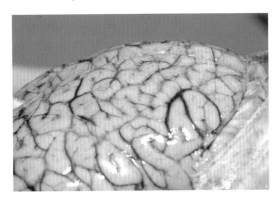

A. Polymicrogyria
B. Pachencephaly
C. Cerebral edema
D. Meningitis
E. Subarachnoid hemorrhage

Brain

146. A 63-year-old male is found by his family physician to have the skin lesion illustrated in the figure. The lesion was relatively slow growing, and there are several other similar lesions at various points around his body. Of the following, what is the most likely diagnosis?

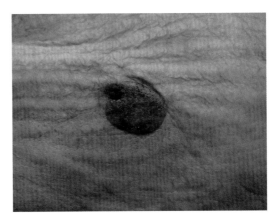

A. Compound nevus
B. Intradermal nevus
C. Nodular malignant melanoma
D. Actinic keratosis
E. Seborrheic keratosis

Skin

147. A 53-year-old alcoholic stumbles out of a bar, falls, and strikes his head. He stumbles home and the next day is found unresponsive on his bed. He is pronounced dead and an autopsy is performed. Representation of the main finding at autopsy is illustrated in the figure. Of the following, what was the most likely cause of this man's death?

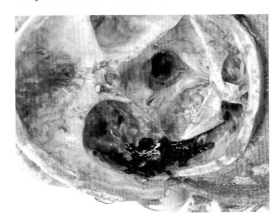

A. An epidural hemorrhage
B. A subdural hemorrhage
C. A subarachnoid hemorrhage
D. An intracerebral hemorrhage
E. Meningitis

Brain

335

148. A 37-year-old male is being seen by his family physician. He has some complaints of weight gain and decreased energy levels. Physical examination reveals scattered patches of skin appearing as illustrated in the figure. Of the following, what condition is this man most likely to have?

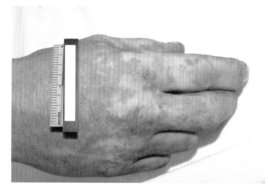

A. Cirrhosis of the liver due to hepatitis C infection

B. Colonic adenocarcinoma

C. Severe coronary artery atherosclerosis

D. Hashimoto's thyroiditis

E. Emphysema

Skin

149. A 63-year-old male was found dead in bed by his wife. He had come into the house after shoveling snow, complaining of being fatigued and gone to sleep. An autopsy was performed and identified the pathologic lesion illustrated in the figure. No mass was identified. Of the following, what pre-existing medical condition was the most significant contributor to his final cause of death?

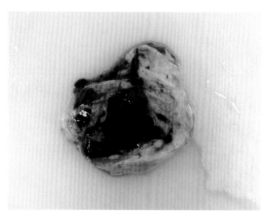

A. Cirrhosis of the liver

B. Polyarteritis nodosa

C. Hypertension

D. Multiple sclerosis

E. Amyotrophic lateral sclerosis

Brain

150. A 61-year-old male with a long history of smoking presents to an acute care clinic with complaints of shortness of breath and coughing, with occasional blood being coughed up. A chest X-ray reveals a mass in the left lung. A biopsy of the mass reveals changes illustrated in the figure. Of the following, which feature best identifies that the mass is malignant and is present in the image?

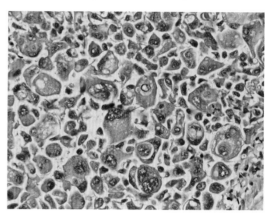

A. High mitotic rate

B. Nuclear pleomorphism

C. Nucleoli

D. Vacuoles in the neoplastic cells

E. Abnormal mitotic figures

Lung

151. A 63-year-old has a persistent headache. Her family physician orders a CT scan, which identifies a mass. A neurosurgeon removes the mass, and it is examined by a pathologist. The histologic appearance is illustrated in the figure. Of the following, what is the diagnosis?

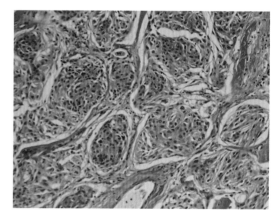

A. A low-grade astrocytoma

B. An oligodendroglioma

C. An ependymoma

D. A meningioma

E. A pilocytic astrocytoma

Brain

152. A 36-year-old male is found unresponsive by his friends when they go to visit him. An ambulance is called and he is taken to the hospital, unconscious, but breathing. Laboratory testing reveals a BUN of 42 mg/dL and a creatinine of 4.3 mg/dL. The patient has no significant past medical history. The pathologic process is illustrated in the figure. Of the following, what is the most likely diagnosis?

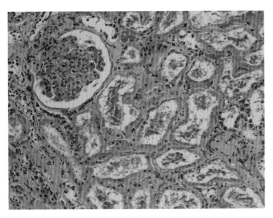

A. Warm autoimmune hemolytic anemia

B. Membranous glomerulonephropathy

C. Ethylene glycol poisoning

D. Acute pyelonephritis

E. Urinary tract obstruction

Kidney

153. A 37-year-old male is brought to the emergency room by friends because he has been acting confused. They also report that earlier he complained of a headache. He has no significant past medical history other than a heart murmur he has had since birth, which he told his friends about and said it had never caused him any problems. Of the following, what is the most likely cause of the pathologic lesion illustrated in the figure?

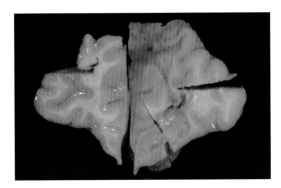

A. A neoplasm

B. A recent fall on the back of his head

C. Alcohol consumption

D. Endocarditis

E. Cirrhosis of the liver

Brain

154. A pathologist is performing an autopsy on a 43-year-old male. Removal of the brain reveals the pathologic lesions illustrated in the figure. Of the following, what was the most likely cause?

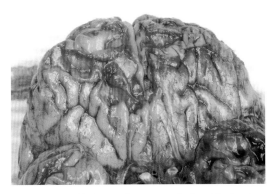

A. A blow to his face a day or two before his death

B. A fall on the back of his head weeks to months earlier

C. HSV encephalitis

D. Fat emboli

E. Metastatic tumor

Brain

155. A 41-year-old woman identifies a possible nodule during a breast self-examination. After meeting with her gynecologist, a breast biopsy is performed. The results are illustrated in the figure. Of the following, what is the diagnosis?

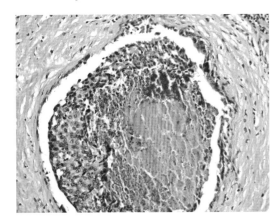

A. Lobular carcinoma in situ

B. Invasive lobular carcinoma

C. Low-grade ductal carcinoma in situ

D. High-grade ductal carcinoma in situ

E. Invasive ductal carcinoma

Breast

337

156. A 63-year-old male is brought to the emergency room by his family because of a change in sensation and muscle weakness that developed very suddenly. He is admitted to the hospital, and, despite treatment, including reperfusion therapy, dies three days later. An autopsy is performed, and the pathologist identifies the pathologic lesion illustrated in the figure. Of the following, what is the most likely diagnosis?

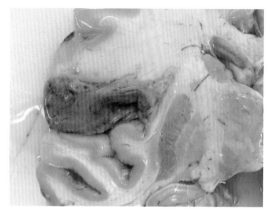

Consider this figure for questions 156, 157, and 158

A. Acute cerebral infarct

B. Remote cerebral infarct

C. Intracerebral hemorrhage

D. Encephalitis

E. Fatty emboli syndrome

Brain

157. Of the following, which artery has the defect that caused his symptoms?

A. Left anterior cerebral artery

B. Anterior communicating artery

C. Branch of left middle cerebral artery

D. Branch of the left posterior cerebral artery

E. Branch of the left vertebral artery

Brain

158. Of the following, what form of muscle weakness and loss of sensation did the patient most likely experience?

A. Loss of vision and weakness of extraocular muscles

B. Loss of hearing and weakness of muscles in the legs

C. Loss of fine touch sensation in the toes and weakness of muscles in the legs

D. Loss of fine touch sensation and weakness in the hands

E. Loss of fine touch sensation and weakness in the abdomen

Brain

159. A 71-year-old male died from injuries sustained in a car accident. At autopsy, the pathologist identified the lesion illustrated in the figure. The man had a past medical history of hypertension and diabetes mellitus type 2. Of the following, what was the most likely cause of the abnormality in the image?

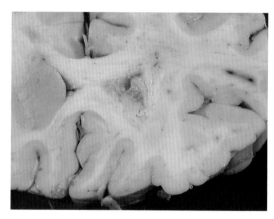

A. Encephalitis

B. A neoplasm

C. Atherosclerosis of the carotid arteries

D. Endocarditis on a calcified tricuspid aortic valve

E. Trauma

Brain

160. A 64-year-old male presents to his family physician because of complaints of fatigue. Laboratory evaluation reveals a hemoglobin of 11.3 g/dL. His stool is positive for occult blood. A GI procedure identifies an ulcerated mass in his gastrointestinal tract. The mass is resected, and a representative section of the mass is illustrated in the figure. Of the following, what characteristic is this mass most likely to have?

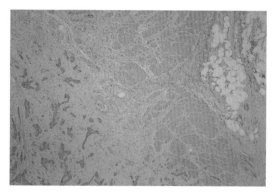

A. It was in the small intestine.

B. It was unlikely to be a cause of his anemia.

C. It has a good prognosis.

D. It is most likely to metastasize to the liver.

E. The presence of lymph node metastases predicts a worse prognosis than the features in the image.

Liver

161. A 35-year-old male presents to an acute care clinic with a history of a cough, which produces sputum, and difficulty breathing. In the past, he has had several cases of pneumonia, including once with *Aspergillus*, which almost caused his death. His vital signs include a temperature of 101°F. A chest radiograph reveals bilateral diffuse pulmonary infiltrates that are symmetric in nature, with the exception of an area of more prominent consolidation in the lower lobe of the right lung. He is diagnosed with pneumonia, but a subsequent lung biopsy reveals the histologic findings in the figure. He has no history of hypertension, high cholesterol, or valvular abnormalities. Of the following, what is his most likely underlying diagnosis?

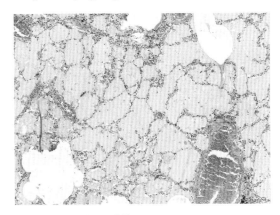

A. Congestive heart failure

B. Usual interstitial pneumonia

C. *Mycoplasma pneumoniae*

D. Alveolar proteinosis

E. Goodpasture's syndrome

Lung

162. A 64-year-old male is being followed by a physician because of some dyspnea with exertion, which does not significantly impair his ability to work or otherwise function at various tasks. A biopsy of his lung would reveal the pathologic lesions illustrated in the figure. The findings in the image are representative of his disease process. Of the following, what is the most likely diagnosis?

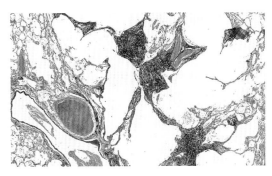

A. Metastatic melanoma

B. Congestive heart failure

C. Simple coal worker's pneumoconiosis

D. Progressive massive fibrosis

E. Emphysema

Lung

163. A 60-year-old male presents to his family physician with complaints of a lingering cough. With the cough, he does not usually produce sputum. A chest X-ray reveals a patchy infiltrate in the lower lobe of the right lung. He is treated for a pneumonia; however, the symptoms persist. A lung biopsy is performed, revealing the pathologic changes in illustrated in the figure. Of the following, what is the most likely diagnosis?

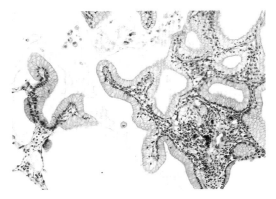

A. *Legionella* pneumonia

B. Type II pneumocyte hyperplasia secondary to bacterial pneumonia

C. Adenocarcinoma in situ

D. Minimally invasive adenocarcinoma

E. Caseous necrosis associated with tuberculosis infection

Lung

164. A 53-year-old homeless chronic alcoholic is found deceased at his campsite in a remote section of a minimally used public park. At autopsy, the pathologist notes numerous white-yellow nodules in the lung that are approximately 1 mm in size. The nodules are illustrated in the figure. Of the following, what was the mechanism for this production?

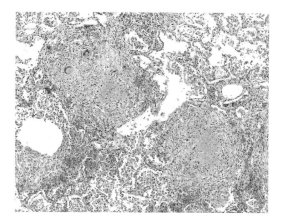

A. Blood vessel invasion

B. Lymphatic invasion

C. Release of vasoactive mediators

D. Aspiration of stomach contents

E. Parasite migration

Lung

165. A 23-year-old female who is pregnant and at 18 weeks gestation presents to her obstetrician because she is having some uterine bleeding, and has passed a few fragments of tissue. She undergoes a dilation and curettage that reveals the pathologic findings illustrated in the figure. The changes were consistent throughout the specimen. Of the following, what is the most likely diagnosis?

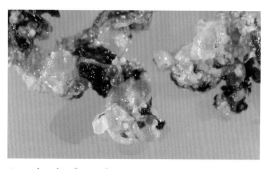

Consider this figure for questions 165 and 166

A. Sarcoma botroides

B. Partial hydatidiform mole

C. Complete hydatidiform mole

D. Choriocarcinoma

E. Ectopic pregnancy

166. Of the following, which is most characteristic of the preceding pathologic condition?

A. There is no risk for the development of choriocarcinoma.

B. An embryo is often present.

C. The karyotype is 46,XX.

D. The risk of persistence after initial treatment is only about 5%.

E. Patients often have a concomitant granulosa cell tumor of the ovary.

Uterus

167. At autopsy, a pathologist identifies the lesions illustrated in the figure in a 43-year-old female. Of the following, what is most characteristic of her disease process?

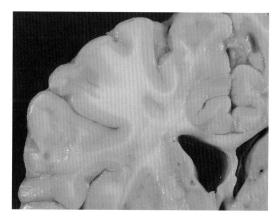

A. The condition is caused by abnormal prion proteins.

B. Damaged ependymal cells produce the lesions.

C. Microscopic examination will reveal microglial nodules and perivascular cuffing with lymphocytes.

D. All lesions identified in the CNS developed at the same time.

E. Involvement of the optic nerves is common.

Brain

168. A neuropathologist is examining the brain of a 29-year-old male that was submitted for examination. On gross examination, she identifies punctate hemorrhages in the corpus callosum and brainstem. Microscopic examination reveals the pathologic findings illustrated in the figure. Of the following, which is most characteristic of this lesion?

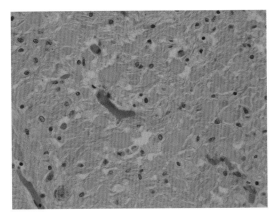

A. It indicates a viral infection.

B. It indicates a fungal infection.

C. The lesions in the slide will stain with Congo red.

D. The person most likely sustained a long bone fractures.

E. The lesions in the slide will stain with β-amyloid precursor protein.

Brain

169. A 41-year-old male with a history of two back injuries, both requiring surgeries, and resultant chronic pain, who refuses to use opioid medications presents to an acute care clinic because of blood in his urine. Physical examination reveals a temperature of 98.7°F, blood pressure of 147/91 mm Hg, and pulse of 86 bpm. A physical examination reveals no costovertebral angle tenderness or suprapubic discomfort. Laboratory testing reveals a hemoglobin of 12.1 g/dL. Of the following, what is the most likely diagnosis?

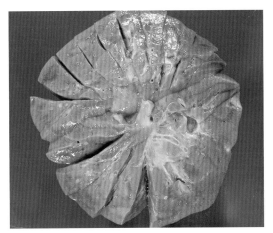

A. Nephrolithiasis

B. Multicentric renal cell carcinoma

C. Papillary necrosis

D. Xanthogranulomatous pyelonephritis

E. Multiple myeloma

Kidney

170. A 28-year-old male is having a yearly physical examination when he is found to have a blood pressure of 146/93 mm Hg. He is treated with an ACE inhibitor. Four years later, he develops hematuria. A urinalysis reveals 2+ red blood cells and 1+ protein. The pathologic condition causing his symptoms is illustrated in the figure. Of the following, what is most characteristic of the disease process?

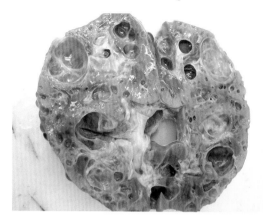

A. The disorder has an autosomal recessive inheritance.

B. Genetic analysis would reveal a mutation in the *WT1* gene.

C. Patients rarely (< 1% of patients) die of an intracranial hemorrhage.

D. Cysts of the liver are common (about 25% of patients).

E. Most of the nephrons in the kidney develop cysts.

Kidney

171. A 36-year-old female presents to the emergency room. Over the past two days, she has developed chills and pain in her lower back. She has also felt febrile, but has not taken her temperature. Her vital signs include a temperature of 101°F. Physical examination reveals costovertebral angle tenderness. Urinalysis reveals white blood cell casts. She has no significant past medical history. Of the following, based on the pathology illustrated in the figure, what is the diagnosis?

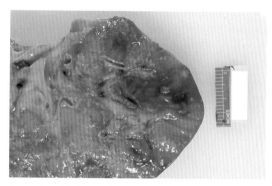

Consider this figure for questions 171 and 172

A. Miliary tuberculosis

B. Acute pyelonephritis

C. Multifocal renal cell carcinoma

D. Papillary necrosis

E. Renomedullary interstitial cell tumors

Kidney

172. Of the following, what is most characteristic of the preceding condition?

A. *Staphylococcus aureus* is the most common cause.

B. Bilateral infection of the kidneys essentially always occurs.

C. The patient may have endocarditis.

D. A complete blood count will likely be normal.

E. Males more commonly develop the condition than females.

Kidney

173. A 56-year-old female presents to her family physician with complaints of blood in her urine. A urinalysis reveals 4+ red blood cells, but no red blood cell casts. A CT scan of the abdomen reveals a mass in the left kidney. The histologic features of the mass are illustrated in the figure. Of the following, what is the most likely diagnosis?

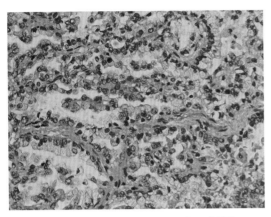

Consider this figure for questions 173 and 174

A. Renal cell carcinoma, clear cell type

B. Renal cell carcinoma, papillary type

C. Angiomyolipoma

D. Wilms' tumor

E. Metastatic colonic adenocarcinoma

Kidney

174. Of the following, what is most characteristic of this tumor?

A. Mutations of the *VHL* gene are rare.

B. Tobacco use is only associated with about 1 to 2% of tumors.

C. Some can produce a PTH-like hormone.

D. It is commonly associated with sickle cell disease.

E. The grade of the tumor is the most significant prognostic indicator.

Kidney

175. A 54-year-old male presents to his family physician because of blood in his urine. A urinalysis reveals 3+ red blood cells, but no red blood cell casts. A CT scan reveals a mass in the right kidney. Of the following, what is the most likely diagnosis?

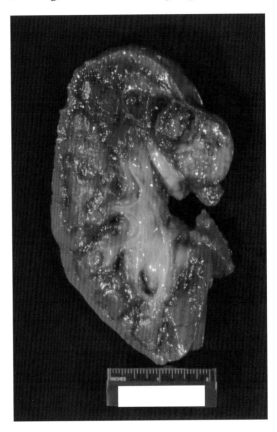

A. Clear cell renal cell carcinoma

B. Metastatic colonic adenocarcinoma

C. Transitional cell carcinoma

D. Angiomyolipoma

E. Pheochromocytoma

Kidney

176. A 37-year-old male presents to the emergency room because of excruciating back pain. The pathologic lesion causing the pain is illustrated in the figure. The two lesions were both radiolucent. Of the following, what is the most likely diagnosis?

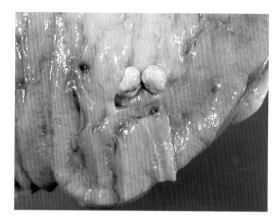

A. Calcium calculi

B. Staghorn calculi

C. Uric acid calculi

D. Cystine calculi

E. Calcified urothelial polyps

Kidney

177. A 29-year-old male with a history of ascites and cirrhosis of the liver is brought to the emergency room by friends because he vomited blood. His diagnosis of cirrhosis of the liver was made by doing liver biopsy, which is illustrated in the figure. The stain used in the image is a periodic acid–Schiff with diastase digestion. Of the following conditions, which is the patient at the greatest risk for developing?

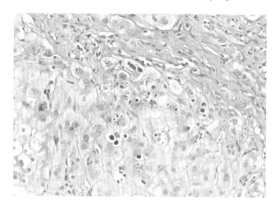

A. Kayser-Fleischer rings

B. Primary sclerosing cholangitis

C. Chronic pancreatitis

D. Emphysema

E. Cerebellar vermal atrophy

Liver

178. A 44-year-old female has been having recurrent pelvic pain for 6 months, which has been associated with pain on sexual intercourse. In consultation with her gynecologist, she elects to have a hysterectomy, as she is a mother of four children and desires no more. The figure illustrates the pathologic process identified in her uterus. Of the following, what is the most likely diagnosis?

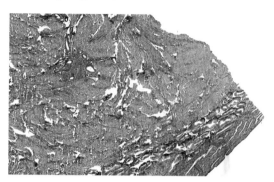

A. Invasive molar pregnancy

B. Invasive endometrial adenocarcinoma

C. Leiomyoma

D. Adenomyosis

E. Endometrial stromal sarcoma

Uterus

179. A pathologist is examining a microscopic section from a kidney lesion, which is illustrated in the figure. Of the following, what is most characteristic of this disease process?

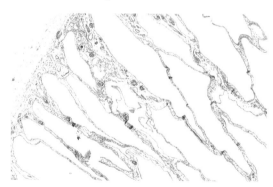

A. Metastases to the brain are common.

B. The renal papillae are most frequently involved and patients are usually asymptomatic.

C. It is associated with a mutation of the gene for fibrillin.

D. Death in the neonatal period due to pulmonary hypoplasia is common.

E. Patients often develop berry aneurysms.

Kidney

180. A 37-year-old male is brought to the emergency room by his wife, because, while they were working in the backyard, he suddenly fell over, and told her that his left leg had become very weak. He is admitted to the hospital with the diagnosis of a stroke. He has no history of hypertension, diabetes mellitus, or hypercholesterolemia. During the following evaluation, an echocardiogram of the heart reveals a mass, which is illustrated in the figure. His foramen ovale is noted to be closed. Of the following, where did this mass most likely originate?

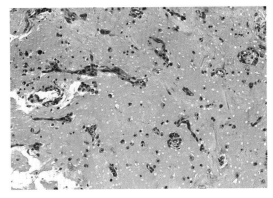

A. Wall of left atrium

B. Mitral valve

C. Ventricular septum

D. Tricuspid valve

E. Wall of right atrium

Heart

181. A 43-year-old male has a 10-year history of intermittent heartburn that he has treated with over-the-counter medications. He presents to his family physician because of pain with swallowing. After hearing his history, the physician schedules a consult with a gastroenterologist, who recommends and later performs an EGD. Biopsies of the gastroesophageal junction are taken and illustrated in the figure. Of the following, which is most characteristic of the lesion?

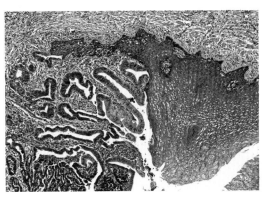

A. His history of heartburn is unrelated.

B. Immunohistochemical staining would be positive for herpes simplex virus.

C. At the least frequent repeat biopsies would be recommended.

D. The disease is due to damage to the myenteric plexus.

E. It is due to prolonged vomiting.

Esophagus

182. A 67-year-old male presents to his family physician because of a growth on his nose. His family physician notes that it looks like a pearly papule, and does a shave biopsy. The histologic features of the lesion are illustrated in the figure. Of the following, what is the most likely diagnosis?

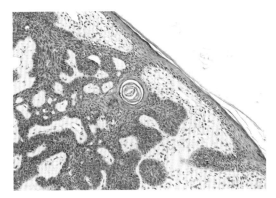

A. Basal cell carcinoma

B. Squamous cell carcinoma

C. Malignant melanoma

D. Actinic keratosis

E. Seborrheic keratosis

Skin

345

183. A 29-year-old female, who has not seen a gynecologist in three years, has an abnormal Pap smear and subsequently undergoes a cervical biopsy. The results of the biopsy are illustrated in the figure. Of the following, which is most likely regarding the lesion?

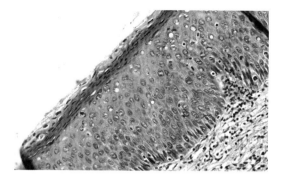

A. The cause was infection with HPV type 6 or 11.

B. The Pap smear most likely was interpreted at LSIL.

C. The mechanism of histologic change is accumulation of virus particles.

D. Without treatment she will progress to invasive squamous cell carcinoma.

E. A similar disease can affect the vagina in older women.

Cervix

184. A 31-year-old female has a Pap smear performed as part of her annual examination. Because of the results of the Pap smear, a biopsy of the cervix is performed. The figure illustrates the results of this biopsy. Of the following, what is the most likely diagnosis?

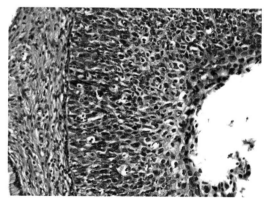

A. Normal cervix

B. CIN I

C. CIN III

D. Invasive squamous cell carcinoma

E. Small-cell carcinoma of the cervix

Cervix

185. A 37-year-old male presents to the emergency room with complaints of a fever and shortness of breath. A chest X-ray reveals some diffuse subtle infiltrates. The pathologic condition causing his symptoms is illustrated in the figure. Of the following, what is the most likely diagnosis?

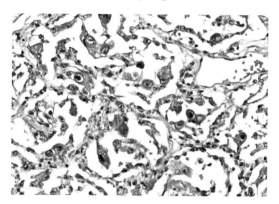

A. Adenocarcinoma in situ

B. Diffuse alveolar damage

C. Cytomegalovirus pneumonia

D. Influenza pneumonia

E. Usual interstitial pneumonia

Lung

186. A 53-year-old female has her annual mammogram, which detects micro calcifications in her left breast. She subsequently undergoes a biopsy. The results of the biopsy are illustrated in the figure. Of the following, what is the most likely diagnosis?

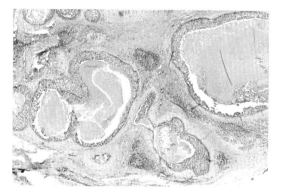

A. Fibrocystic disease of the breast

B. Low-grade ductal carcinoma in situ

C. High-grade ductal carcinoma in situ

D. Invasive ductal carcinoma

E. Small-cell carcinoma of the breast

Breast

187. A 34-year-old male's wife notices a dark brown-black macule on his back one day while they are at the beach. Knowing about melanoma, she asks him to see a dermatologist to get it removed. The histologic features of the macule are illustrated in the figure. Of the following, what is the most likely diagnosis?

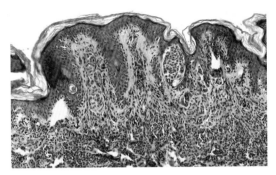

A. Intradermal nevus

B. Junctional nevus

C. Compound nevus

D. Dysplastic nevus

E. Malignant melanoma

Skin

188. A 54-year-old female has her yearly mammogram, in which the radiologist identifies a change from the previous year in her right breast. To investigate this change, she undergoes a breast biopsy. The results of the biopsy are illustrated in the figure. Of the following, what is most characteristic regarding the lesion in the image?

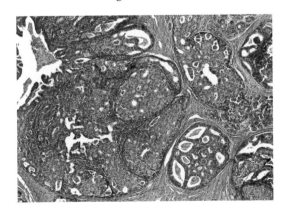

A. The cells will be negative for E-cadherin.

B. If invasive carcinoma develops, this lesion indicates that such a tumor might involve the left breast.

C. Physical examination could reveal erythema of the breast associated with this lesion.

D. Surgical excision is not curative, and adjuvant radiation or chemotherapy is needed.

E. Bloody nipple discharge is common.

Breast

189. A 51-year-old has her first annual colonoscopy, and the gastroenterologist performing the procedure identifies a small mass in the descending colon, measuring about 1.0 cm. The mass is resected. The histologic features of the mass are illustrated in the image. Of the following, what is the most likely diagnosis?

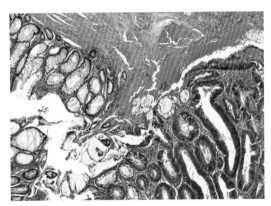

Consider this figure for questions 189 and 190

A. Hyperplastic polyp

B. Tubular adenoma

C. Invasive colonic adenocarcinoma

D. Juvenile polyp

E. Lymphoid polyp

Colon

190. Of the following, what is most characteristic regarding the preceding lesion?

A. The presence of hundreds is associated with a mutation of *hMSH2* or *hMLH1*.

B. They are common in children.

C. Cigarette use is a risk factor.

D. If more sections of the mass were reviewed, invasive carcinoma would most likely be found.

E. They commonly occur in the small intestine.

Colon

347

191. A 52-year-old female palpates a mass in her left breast. She discusses her finding with her gynecologist at her next visit. He assures her that the mass is benign; however, she is concerned and requests a biopsy for confirmation. A biopsy is performed, and the figure illustrates the pathologic lesion. Of the following, what is the most likely diagnosis?

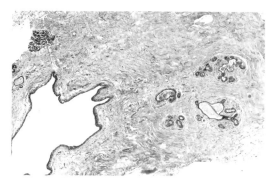

A. Fibrocystic disease

B. Sclerosing adenosis

C. Ductal carcinoma in situ

D. Invasive ductal carcinoma

E. Fat necrosis

Breast

192. A 47-year-old male has had intermittent pain in his left big toe for about 5 years. His friends tell him that he has gout and that he should seek treatment; however, he refuses because he lacks medical insurance. Ultimately, he develops a mass in his left big toe, and goes to an acute care clinic. The histologic appearance of the mass is illustrated in the figure. Of the following, what is the most likely diagnosis?

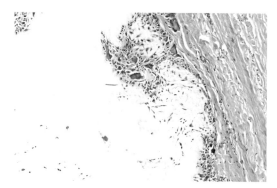

Consider this figure for questions 192 and 193

A. Chondrosarcoma

B. Giant cell tumor

C. Osteosarcoma

D. Tophus

E. Charcot joint

Joint

193. Of the following, which is most characteristic of the preceding disease process?

A. The source of the deposits in the joints is pyrimidines.

B. The material in the deposits is normally excreted from the body in both the urine and the feces.

C. The condition occurs in individuals with Neiman-Pick disease.

D. Certain leukemias are a risk factor.

E. The patient's presentation is unusual.

Joint

194. A 37-year-old male presents to his family physician. He says that over the last 6 months he has noticed that he has become much more anxious and nervous. In addition, he has lost 35 lbs. During his review of systems, he reports some intolerance to heat, excessive sweating, and occasional palpitations. The figure illustrates the pathologic process causing his symptoms. Of the following, what is the most likely diagnosis?

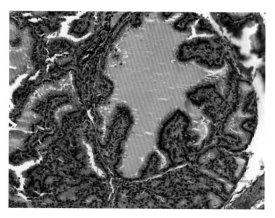

A. TSH-producing pituitary adenoma

B. Graves' disease

C. Hashimoto's thyroiditis

D. Pheochromocytoma

E. Papillary thyroid carcinoma

Thyroid gland

195. A 59-year-old female is performing her monthly breast self-examination when she notices a lump. She refers her finding to her gynecologist, who recommends a biopsy. The figure illustrates the histologic features of the biopsy. Of the following, what is the most likely diagnosis?

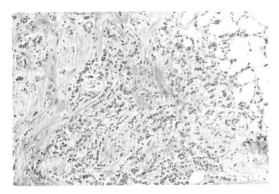

A. Sclerosing adenosis

B. Ductal carcinoma in situ

C. Invasive ductal carcinoma

D. Invasive lobular carcinoma

E. Tubular carcinoma

Breast

196. A 28-year-old male twice has an unexplained elevation in his alkaline phosphatase. The first elevation was unexpected, and the second elevation confirmed it was not spurious. To assist in the determination of the cause, he undergoes a liver biopsy. The results of the biopsy are illustrated in the figure. Of the following, what other medical condition is he most likely to have?

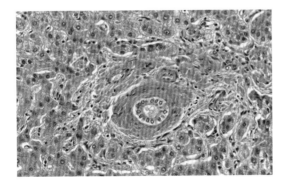

A. Cholelithiasis

B. A marginal zone lymphoma

C. Renal calculi

D. Ulcerative colitis

E. Restrictive cardiomyopathy

Liver

197. A 35-year-old male presents to his family physician after having palpated a nodule in his left testis during a self-examination. He is referred to a urologist, who performs an ultrasound, confirms the solid nature of the mass, and proceeds with an orchiectomy. The figure illustrates the histologic features of the tumor. The cells are CD117 positive. Of the following, what is the most likely diagnosis?

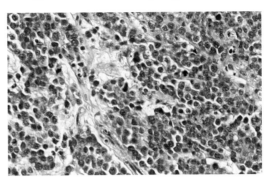

A. Seminoma

B. Spermatocytic seminoma

C. Yolk sac tumor

D. Malignant lymphoma

E. Choriocarcinoma

Testis

198. A 56-year-old female is being seen for the third time in two months by her family physician because of complaints of diarrhea. She says that the diarrhea is watery and has no blood in it. She has been drinking a lot of water to stay hydrated. During her physical examination, her physician palpates a nodule in the right lobe of the thyroid gland. It is subsequently resected, and the histologic appearance is illustrated in the figure. Of the following, what is the most likely diagnosis?

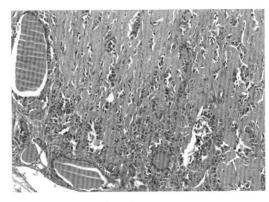

A. Papillary thyroid carcinoma

B. Follicular carcinoma

C. Medullary thyroid carcinoma

D. Anaplastic carcinoma

E. Metastatic osteosarcoma

Thyroid gland

199. A 61-year-old male is having a surveillance colonoscopy, when the gastroenterologist identifies two polyps, both 1.0 cm in size. The first polyp is diagnosed as a tubular adenoma. The histologic features of the second polyp are illustrated in the figure. Of the following, which is true?

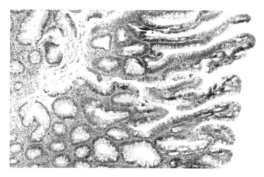

A. The second polyp has no risk of harboring a neoplasm.

B. The second polyp has a lesser risk of harboring a neoplasm than the first polyp.

C. The second polyp has an equal risk of harboring a neoplasm as the first polyp.

D. The second polyp has a greater risk of harboring a neoplasm than the first polyp.

E. The second polyp is an invasive adenocarcinoma.

Colon

200. A 3-year-old male is brought to the emergency room by his parents because they have noted blood in his urine. Physical examination reveals a right-sided abdominal mass. Surgery is performed, and the mass is resected. Of the following, what statement is most characteristic about this mass?

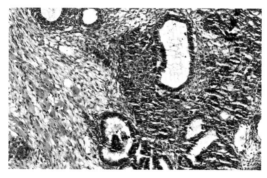

A. Most cases occur in adults.

B. Patients often have a loss of imprinting defect on chromosome 12.

C. The survival rate is very low.

D. Anaplasia is a good prognostic sign.

E. The tumor occurs as a part of Beckwith-Wiedemann syndrome.

Kidney

201. During histologic examination of a section of skeletal muscle removed at autopsy, the lesion illustrated in the figure is identified. Of the following, how was this condition most likely acquired?

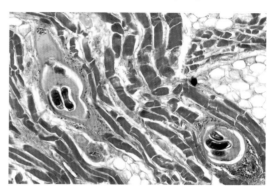

A. Hiking in the San Joaquin valley

B. Eating poorly cooked pork

C. Tick bite

D. Bite of reduviid bug

E. Drinking unfiltered stream water

Diaphragm

202. A 67-year-old woman presents to the emergency room with her husband. She has had an intermittent headache for a while, but, this evening, she developed blindness in her right eye. After evaluation, she is referred to a rheumatologist, who orders a temporal artery biopsy. The results of the biopsy are illustrated in the figure. Of the following, what is the most likely diagnosis?

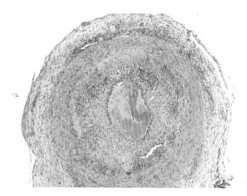

A. Polyarteritis nodosa

B. Microscopic polyangiitis

C. Takayasu's arteritis

D. Temporal arteritis

E. Granulomatosis with polyangiitis

Cardiovascular

203. A 43-year-old male presents to his family physician because of complaints of blood in his urine. He has a 50-pack-per-year smoking history and hypertension treated with an ACE inhibitor, but otherwise he has no known medical conditions. His physical examination is unrevealing. He is referred to a urologist, who performs a cystoscopy, and biopsies the lesion illustrated in the figure, which he described as papillary in architecture. Of the following, what is the most likely diagnosis?

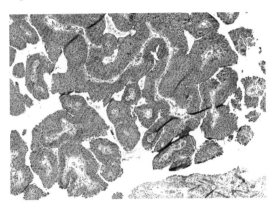

A. Inverted papilloma

B. Urothelial papilloma

C. Low-grade papillary urothelial carcinoma

D. Invasive urothelial carcinoma

E. Squamous cell carcinoma

Bladder

204. A 34-year-old male is brought to the emergency room by his family. They say he rapidly has gone from having no medical conditions to being very upset and not being able to remember his name or where he is. While in the emergency room, the patient has a seizure. Over the next two days, despite medical care, he develops spasms in his throat, has difficulty swallowing, and ultimately dies. An autopsy is performed, and the findings are illustrated in the figure. Of the following, what does the image show?

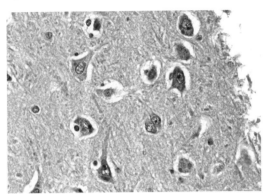

A. Normal neurons

B. HSV inclusions

C. Negri bodies

D. Prion infection

E. *Naegleria fowleri*

Brain

205. A 7-year-old child is in the intensive care unit at a children's hospital. A liver biopsy reveals the cause of his admission. Of the following, what is the most likely scenario that best describes his need for hospital admission?

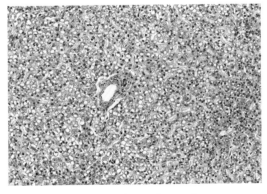

A. Infection with hepatitis A virus at day care

B. Aspirin use during a recent chickenpox infection

C. Recent blood transfusion

D. Thrombus of the hepatic vein

E. Accidental ingestion of alcohol

Liver

351

206. A 21-year-old female presents to her obstetrician for an examination. She is estimated to be at 12 weeks gestational age. On physical examination, her physician identifies that her uterus is large for her gestational age. A dilation and curettage is performed, and histologic examination of the tissue obtained is illustrated in the figure. Of the following, what is the most likely diagnosis?

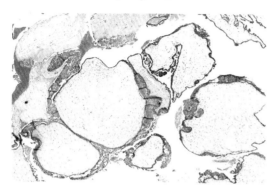

A. Choriocarcinoma
B. Partial hydatidiform mole
C. Complete hydatidiform mole
D. Placental site trophoblastic tumor
E. HELLP syndrome

Uterus

207. A 27-year-old male presents to his family physician. He has noticed recent growths on the skin adjacent to his penis. He is concerned about having acquired a sexually transmitted disease through one of several recent sexual encounters. The physician notes that the lesions are smooth dome-shaped papules with a central depression. The figure illustrates the histologic appearance of these lesions. Of the following, what is the most likely diagnosis?

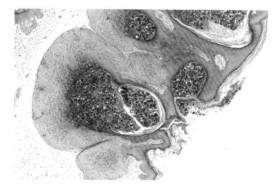

A. Syphilis
B. Lymphogranuloma venerum
C. Molluscum contagiosum
D. Human papillomavirus
E. Scabies

Skin

208. A 47-year-old female presents to her family physician. She says that for the past several months she has noticed an enlargement in her neck. As the enlargement was not painful, and as she had no other symptoms, she did not think it was necessary to seek immediate care. On physical examination, her physician identifies an enlarged and firm thyroid gland. The disease process is illustrated in the figure. Of the following, what is the most likely diagnosis?

A. Papillary thyroid carcinoma
B. Graves' disease
C. Hashimoto's thyroiditis
D. Riedel's thyroiditis
E. de Quervain's thyroiditis

Thyroid gland

209. A 29-year-old male is brought to the emergency room by his wife. Over the past several days, he has begun to act more confused, sometimes forgetting the day or where he was at. She has not noticed any focal weakness, and he has not complained of any focal areas of loss of sensation. The figure illustrates the pathologic process causing his symptoms. Of the following, what is the diagnosis?

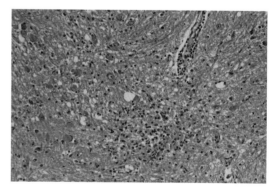

A. Acute cerebral infarct
B. Multiple sclerosis
C. Encephalitis
D. Low-grade astrocytoma
E. Marchifava-Bignami disease

Brain

210. A 37-year-old female is having her annual examination when her gynecologist palpates a mass in her left ovary. Surgery is subsequently scheduled, and the mass is removed. The figure illustrates the histologic features of the mass. Of the following, what is the diagnosis?

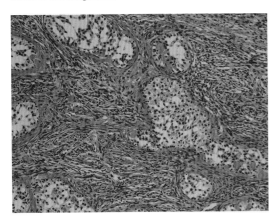

A. Dysgerminoma

B. Brenner's tumor

C. Granulosa cell tumor

D. Serous cystadenocarcinoma

E. Endometriosis

Ovary

211. A 47-year-old female has a breast biopsy to further investigate an irregular area appearing on her mammogram. One of the histologic findings identified in the biopsy is illustrated in the figure. Of the following, what is the diagnosis?

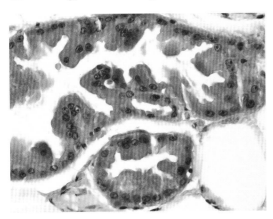

A. Lobular carcinoma in situ

B. Ductal carcinoma in situ

C. Sclerosing adenosis

D. Apocrine metaplasia

E. Normal glandular elements

Breast

212. A 71-year-old male presents to his family physician, complaining of shortness of breath and coughing up occasional blood. A CT scan of the chest reveals numerous masses, measuring up to 2.5 cm, in both lobes of the lung. A biopsy reveals the histologic appearance illustrated in the figure. Of the following, what was the tissue of origin for the metastatic neoplasm?

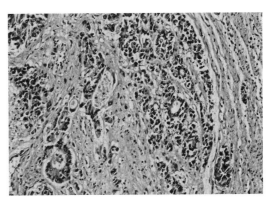

A. Stratified squamous epithelium

B. Transitional epithelium

C. Glandular epithelium

D. Adipose tissue

E. Smooth muscle

Lung

213. A 43-year-old male presents to an acute care clinic because of recurrent episodes of diarrhea associated with weight loss. He has, in the past, had several episodes of severe abdominal pain, several of which required treatment of the underlying disorder. The pathologic process producing his symptoms is illustrated in the figure. Of the following, what is the most likely diagnosis?

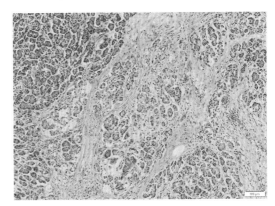

Consider this figure for questions 213 and 214

A. Acute pancreatitis

B. Chronic pancreatitis

C. Pancreatic adenocarcinoma

D. Metastatic colonic adenocarcinoma

E. Nesidioblastosis

Pancreas

353

214. Of the following, what was the most likely cause of the preceding condition?

A. Congenital malformation

B. Fungal infection

C. Gallstones

D. Invasive neoplasm

E. Hypertriglyceridemia

Pancreas

215. A 72-year-old male has a diagnosis of dementia. Following his death, his family requests an autopsy to determine the cause of his dementia. The figure illustrates histologic features of his dementia. Of the following, what is the most likely diagnosis?

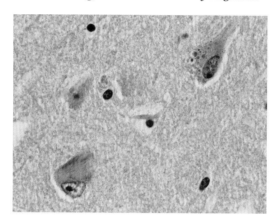

A. Alzheimer's disease

B. Pick's disease

C. Parkinson's disease

D. Acute hemorrhagic encephalitis

E. Diffuse Lewy body disease

Brain

216. A 43-year-old alcoholic has a chronic cough. He presents to the emergency room, and a chest X-ray reveals a mass in the upper lobe of the right lung. Of the following, an inflammatory process composed of what type of cell would most likely accompany the findings illustrated in the figure?

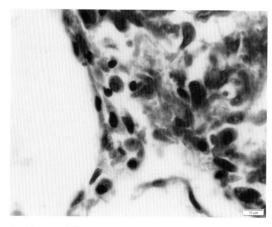

A. Neutrophils

B. Eosinophils

C. Lymphocytes

D. Macrophages

E. Basophils

Lung

217. A 19-year-old female is brought to the emergency room because of blood in her urine. A CT scan is performed, which reveals a mass. The mass is excised, and the figure illustrates the histologic features of the mass. Of the following, what syndrome does this patient most likely have?

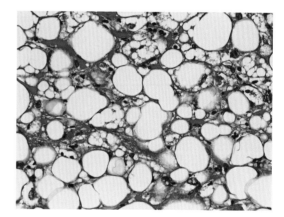

A. von Hippel–Lindau

B. Cystic fibrosis

C. Tuberous sclerosis

D. Hereditary hemochromatosis

E. Ollier's syndrome

Kidney

218. A 53-year-old male at autopsy was found to have the condition illustrated in the figure. Of the following, what other condition, related to the disease process in the image, would be most likely to be identified?

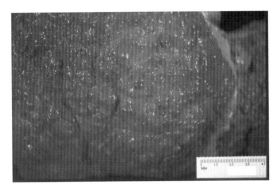

A. Intracerebral hemorrhage

B. Papillary thyroid carcinoma

C. Pulmonary emphysema

D. Spider angiomas

E. Budd-Chiari syndrome

Liver

219. A 36-year-old female is having her annual physical examination when her gynecologist palpates a mass in her right ovary. A CT scan confirms the mass, and surgery to remove it is subsequently performed. The figure illustrates the histologic appearance of the mass. Of the following, what is the diagnosis?

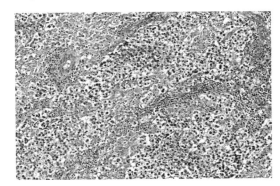

A. Choriocarcinoma

B. Sertoli-Leydig cell tumor

C. Mucinous cystadenoma

D. Dysgerminoma

E. Seminoma

Uterus

220. A 41-year-old male was found in his apartment with a gunshot wound of the head, having committed suicide. A physical examination of his body at autopsy reveals the features illustrated in the figure. Of the following, which is also commonly found in this disease process?

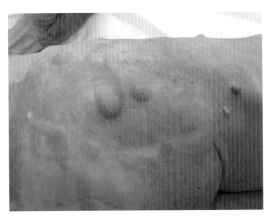

Consider this figure for questions 220 and 221

A. Kayser-Fleischer ring

B. Koplik spots

C. Lisch nodules

D. Subependymal nodules

Skin

221. Of the following, which neoplastic condition was the preceding man at most risk for having?

A. Malignant melanoma

B. Basal cell carcinoma

C. Malignant peripheral nerve sheath tumor

D. Hepatocellular carcinoma

E. Colonic adenocarcinoma

Skin, peripheral nerve

355

222. A 37-year-old female presents to her family physician complaining of an increased need to urinate, often at night. She has been drinking an increased amount of water to prevent dehydration. Her past medical history includes at least four documented urinary tract infections. Laboratory testing reveals a glucose of 81 mg/dL, BUN of 26 mg/dL, and creatinine of 2.7 mg/dL. The figure illustrates the pathologic process causing her symptoms and laboratory abnormalities. Of the following, what is the most likely diagnosis?

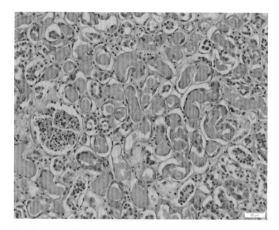

A. Acute pyelonephritis
B. Chronic pyelonephritis
C. Renal cell carcinoma
D. Acute tubular necrosis
E. Interstitial nephritis

Kidney

223. A 34-year-old male presents to his family physician with complaints of a mass at his left knee. He says that the mass has been present for 1 year; however, he thought it was a healing injury and did not seek care earlier. A CT scan of the knee is performed, revealing a solid mass. He undergoes surgery, and the histologic appearance of the mass is illustrated in the figure. Of the following, what is the most likely diagnosis?

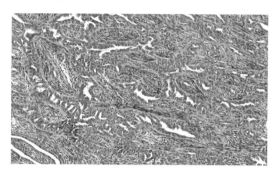

A. Baker's cyst
B. Extra-articular rheumatoid arthritis
C. Nodular fasciitis
D. Synovial sarcoma
E. Osteosarcoma

Musculoskeletal

224. A 61-year-old male presents to his family physician with complaints of fatigue. He also complains of recent development of intermittent pain in his left big toe. His vital signs are a temperature of 99.1°F, pulse of 108 bpm, and blood pressure of 124/81 mm Hg. Physical examination reveals an enlarged spleen. Laboratory evaluation reveals a hemoglobin of 10.1 g/dL, white blood cell count of 12,100 cells/μL, and platelet count of 112,000 cells/μL. The blood smear reveals the red blood cell morphology illustrated in the figure. Of the following, what is the most likely diagnosis?

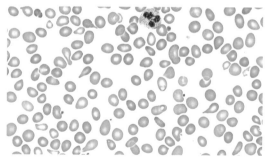

A. Megaloblastic anemia
B. Acute lymphoblastic leukemia
C. Hairy cell leukemia
D. Infectious mononucleosis
E. Myelofibrosis

Heme

225. A 64-year-old male with a past history of hypertension, gout, and a 70-pack-per-year smoking history presents to an acute care clinic with complaints of increasing shortness of breath and a cough, which occasionally has blood-tinged sputum. A CT scan of the chest reveals a 3.0 cm mass in the hilum of the left lung. The figure illustrates the histology of this mass. Of the following, what form of molecular abnormality is most likely to be identified in this tumor?

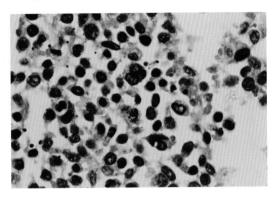

A. t(15;17)

B. *ALK* rearrangment

C. *EGFR* mutation

D. *KRAS* mutation

E. 3p deletion

Lung

226. A 31-year-old male who lives in and is from North Dakota is found unresponsive by his wife. He has been complaining of a cough and congestion for a few days prior. An autopsy is performed. Histologic examination of the heart reveals the findings illustrated in the figure. Of the following, what organism is most likely responsible for these changes?

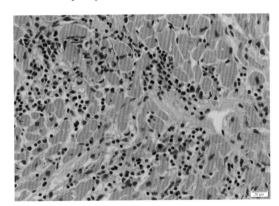

A. *Mycobacterium tuberculosis*

B. *Aspergillus niger*

C. *Trypanosoma cruzi*

D. Coxsackievirus B

E. *Staphylococcus aureus*

Heart

227. A 62-year-old male has a diagnosis of dementia, in addition to other medical conditions. The figure illustrates histologic features of the neurologic condition causing his dementia. Of the following, what is his most likely diagnosis?

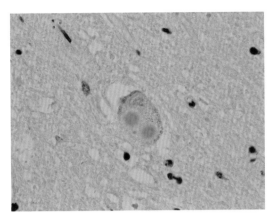

A. Alzheimer's disease

B. Multi-infarct dementia

C. Parkinson's disease

D. Amyotrophic lateral sclerosis

E. Rabies encephalitis

Brain

228. A 41-year-old male who sustained a fracture of his right ankle two weeks ago presented to an acute care clinic with complaints of sudden onset of difficulty breathing associated with sharp chest pain. He was diagnosed with costochondritis and sent home. Three days following this visit to an acute care clinic, he was found unresponsive on the floor of the living room by his wife. He has no history of hypertension, high cholesterol, or sudden deaths in his family. The figure illustrates a pathologic finding at the time of autopsy. Of the following, what was the most likely cause of his death?

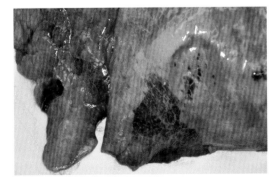

A. Fat embolism

B. Acute bronchopneumonia

C. Pulmonary thromboembolus

D. Acute myocardial infarct

E. Ruptured peptic ulcer

Lung

357

229. During her annual physical examination, a 31-year-old female is identified to have a small mass in her left breast. A biopsy is performed and reveals the histologic features illustrated in the figure. Of the following, what is the most likely mechanism for formation of her mass?

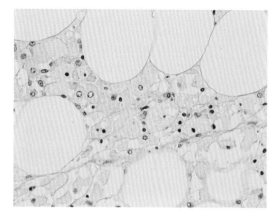

A. Inheritance of *BRCA1*

B. Trauma

C. Amoebic infection

D. *Mycobacterium tuberculosis* infection

E. Bacterial infection

Breast

230. A 49-year-old female presents to her family physician with complaints of unsightly worm-like structures on her legs, which have developed over several years. She has a history of Hashimoto's thyroiditis, but no other medical conditions. The figure illustrates her pathologic process. Of the following, what is the most likely mechanism for the formation of the lesions?

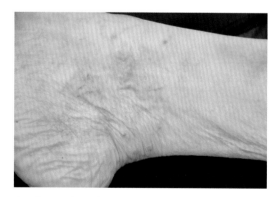

A. Obstruction of venous blood flow

B. Incompetence of venous valves

C. Neoplastic infiltration of lymphatic vessels

D. Heart failure

E. Autoantibodies

Cardiovascular

231. A 71-year-old with a history of a stroke that has left her unable to ambulate well is a resident of a nursing home. When moving her to change her bedsheets, a nursing assistant notices the lesion pictured in the figure on the posterior surface of her right thigh. Of the following, what is the most likely diagnosis?

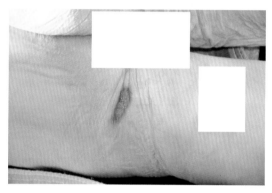

A. Squamous cell carcinoma

B. Basal cell carcinoma

C. Decubitus ulcer

D. Traumatic abrasion

E. Bullous pemphigoid

Skin

232. A 32-year-old male has had an upper respiratory infection for about 5 days. He is playing basketball with friends when he collapses and becomes unresponsive. Despite resuscitation attempts, he dies. An autopsy reveals the lesion illustrated in the figure. Of the following, what is the most likely etiology?

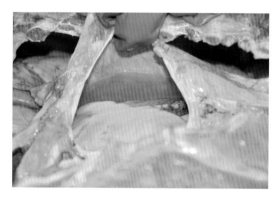

A. Metastatic papillary thyroid carcinoma

B. *Staphylococcus aureus* infection

C. Recent acute myocardial infarction

D. Coxsackievirus B infection

E. Chest trauma

Cardiovascular

233. A 56-year-old male presents to his family physician because of pain in his extremities and a recurring headache. X-rays of his body reveal numerous lytic bone lesions. A subsequent bone marrow biopsy reveals a plasma cell count of 35%, some of which are atypical. Also within the bone marrow is the histologic finding illustrated in the figure. Of the following, what is the name for this lesion?

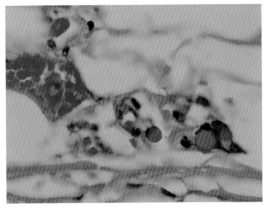

A. Intranuclear inclusions

B. Reed-Sternberg cell

C. Russell bodies

D. Negri bodies

E. Psammoma bodies

Heme

234. A 52-year-old male is having a routine colonoscopy, when the gastroenterologist identifies a small 0.3-cm polyp in the descending colon, which he biopsies. The biopsy is examined by a pathologist, who sees the features illustrated in the figure. Of the following, what is the diagnosis?

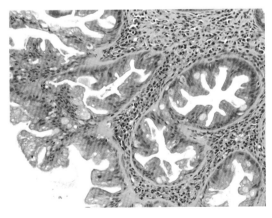

A. Hyperplastic polyp

B. Tubular adenoma

C. Villous adenoma

D. Invasive adenocarcinoma

E. Barrett's metaplasia

Gastrointestinal

235. A pathologist performs an autopsy on a 51-year-old male who died as the result of blunt force injuries sustained in a motor vehicle accident. Histologic examination of the kidneys reveals the vascular abnormality illustrated in the figure. Of the following, what diagnosis, which would cause the vascular change, did the decedent most likely have?

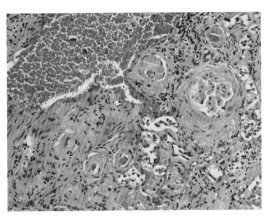

A. Hypercholesterolemia

B. Excessive tobacco use

C. Hypertension

D. Polyarteritis nodosa

E. Syphilis

Cardiovascular

236. A 17-year-old male is brought to an acute care clinic by his parents because of a one-week history of a sore throat, swollen nodules in his neck, and a fever up to 101°F. A physical examination reveals an enlarged spleen. A blood smear reveals the cell type illustrated in the figure. Of the following, what test would most likely be positive?

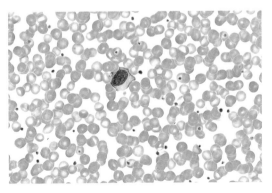

A. ANA

B. Anti-hepatitis C antibody

C. Monospot test

D. Analysis for t(9;22)

E. Anti-streptolysin O

Heme

359

237. A 53-year-old chronic alcoholic is brought to the emergency room by his friends. For two days, he has been complaining of a headache, and he has felt warm to the touch. The figure illustrates the pathologic process causing his symptoms. Of the following, what is the most likely etiologic agent?

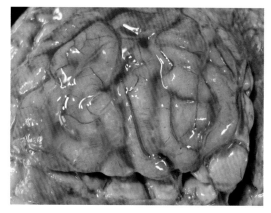

A. *Neisseria meningitidis*

B. *Streptococcus pneumoniae*

C. *Pseudomonas aeruginosa*

D. *Mycobacterium tuberculosis*

E. *Aspergillus niger*

Brain

238. A 31-year-old female is found at autopsy to have the lesion illustrated in the figure. Of the following, what would have been her most likely presenting symptom?

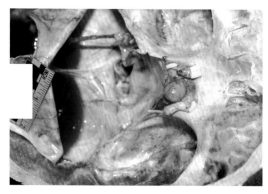

A. Galactorrhea

B. Palpitations

C. Oral hyperpigmentation

D. Axillary and femoral hyperpigmentation

E. Seizures

Pituitary gland

239. A 71-year-old male presents to his family physician for a nonhealing skin lesion on his forearm. He is a retired farmer. His physician is concerned for a malignancy and excises the lesion. The figure illustrates the histologic appearance of the lesion. Of the following, what is the diagnosis?

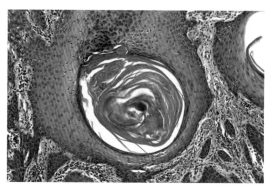

A. Seborrheic keratosis

B. Lipoma

C. Basal cell carcinoma

D. Squamous cell carcinoma

E. Malignant melanoma

Skin

240. A 3-year-old child sustains lethal injuries during a car accident and dies. An autopsy is performed. Histologic examination of the organs reveals the findings illustrated in the figure. Which type of tumor would this child have been at risk for developing?

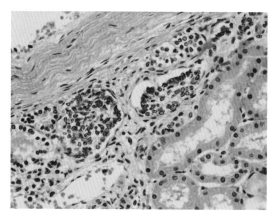

A. Retinoblastoma

B. Neuroblastoma

C. Wilms' tumor

D. Pancreatic adenocarcinoma

E. Pilocytic astrocytoma

Kidney

241. A 63-year-old female presents to her family physician. She says that for the past 6 months she has been having intermittent vaginal bleeding. An endometrial biopsy is performed followed by a hysterectomy and bilateral salpingo-oophorectomy. The resected uterus is exhibited in the figure. Of the following, which tumor type may also be present and have contributed to the development of the uterine lesion?

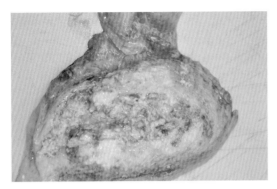

A. Invasive ductal carcinoma of the breast

B. Hepatocellular carcinoma

C. Colonic adenocarcinoma

D. Dysgerminoma

E. Granulosa cell tumor

Uterus

242. A 63-year-old female with a history of hypertension and diabetes mellitus type 2 is found dead on the floor of the kitchen by her husband when he comes home from work. An autopsy reveals a thrombus in the left anterior descending coronary artery and the lesion illustrated in the figure. She has no other medical conditions. Of the following, what other condition is most likely to be identified at autopsy?

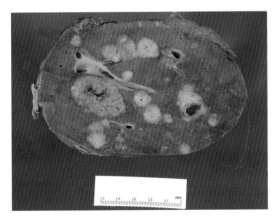

A. Crohn's disease

B. Colonic adenocarcinoma

C. Glioblastoma multiforme

D. Nephrolithiasis

E. Granulomatosis with polyangiitis

System

243. At the autopsy of a 54-year-old male, the condition illustrated in the figure was identified. Of the following, what is the most accurate statement regarding the etiology/clinical presentation of this lesion in this man?

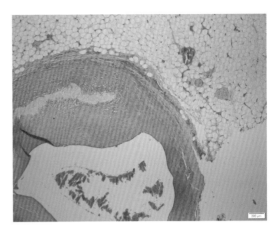

A. He was having consistent, unchanging chest pain with exertion.

B. He was having increasing amounts of chest pain with the same level of exertion.

C. The lesion was his cause of death.

D. His hyperhomocysteinemia is a risk factor.

E. The lesion does not contain cholesterol.

Heart

244. A 63-year-old male commits suicide by a gunshot wound of the head. His past medical history includes depression and recent diagnosis of colonic adenocarcinoma. Based on the appearance of his heart as illustrated in the figure, of the following, what other medical condition did he most likely have?

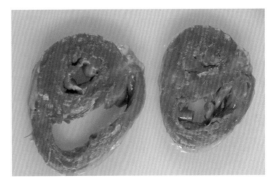

A. Systemic hypertension

B. Amyloidosis

C. Hypertrophic cardiomyopathy

D. Chronic obstructive pulmonary disease

E. Cirrhosis of the liver

Heart

245. The pathologic lesion illustrated in the figure was identified in the left anterior descending coronary artery of a 56-year-old male, who presented to the hospital with chest pain and was subsequently found to have a troponin I of 9.6 ng/mL. The chest pain has been occurring for 2 days. He died suddenly during evaluation in the emergency room, without receiving treatment. Based on the appearance of the lesion and the laboratory testing, what would gross examination of the heart reveal?

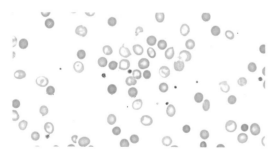

A. Circumferential subendocardial pallor

B. Subendocardial pallor and yellow discoloration in the anterior wall of the left ventricle

C. Transmural pallor and yellow discoloration in the anterior wall of the left ventricle

D. Subendocardial pallor and yellow discoloration in the inferior wall of the left ventricle

E. Transmural pallor and yellow discoloration in the inferior wall of the left ventricle

Heart

246. A 31-year-old male presents to his family physician complaining of fatigue. A physical examination reveals an enlarged spleen. A complete blood cell count reveals a hemoglobin of 9.1 g/dL. Both his mother and his maternal grandmother have a history of anemia. His blood smear is illustrated in the figure. Of the following, what is the most likely diagnosis?

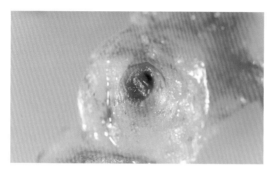

Consider this figure for questions 246 and 247

A. Sickle cell anemia

B. Glucose-6-phosphate dehydrogenase deficiency

C. Hereditary spherocytosis

D. Malaria

E. Iron deficiency anemia

Heme

247. Of the following, which infectious agent was the most likely the cause of the preceding patient's acute presentation?

A. Cytomegalovirus

B. Hepatitis A

C. Parvovirus B19

D. Coxsackievirus A

E. Malaria

Heme

248. A 48-year-old male presents to his family physician. Over the past 2 months, he has been fatigued with exertion and has noticed some bleeding when he brushes his teeth, both of which are new for him. His complete blood cell count includes a white blood cell count of 110,000 white blood cells/µL. A blood smear is illustrated in the figure. The cells of interest are CD33 positive. Of the following, what is the most likely diagnosis?

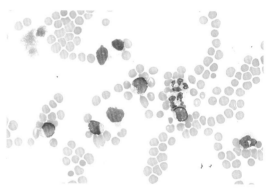

A. ALL

B. CLL

C. AML

D. CML

E. Leukemoid reaction

Heme

249. A 61-year-old female is having a physical examination by her family physician who notes some cervical lymphadenopathy. She had told him about some increasing shortness of breath with exertion and fatigue over the past year. A blood smear is illustrated in the figure. Of the following, what is the most likely diagnosis?

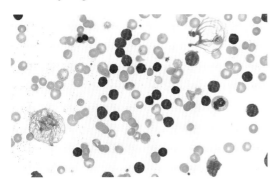

A. ALL

B. CLL

C. AML

D. CML

E. Hairy cell leukemia

Heme

250. A 41-year-old male presents to his family physician stating that he has just not felt good for about 6 months. He has been weak and unable to enjoy his favorite hobby, golfing. Also, he has lost 25 lbs. A physical examination reveals an enlarged spleen. As part of his evaluation, a blood smear is performed, which is illustrated in the figure. Of the following, what is the most likely diagnosis?

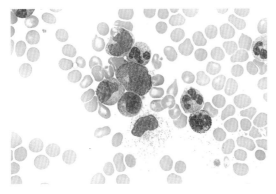

A. ALL

B. CLL

C. AML

D. CML

E. Hairy cell leukemia

Heme

251. A 61-year-old male presents to his family physician with complaints of fatigue and, occasionally, shortness of breath with exertion. These symptoms have developed over the past several months. A blood smear reveals the pathologic changes illustrated in the figure. Of the following, what is the most likely diagnosis?

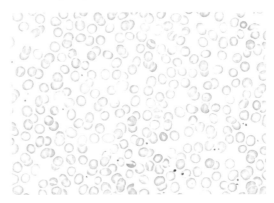

A. ALL

B. Hereditary spherocytosis

C. Iron deficiency anemia

D. Megaloblastic anemia

E. Hairy cell leukemia

Heme

252. A 53-year-old male presents to the emergency room, having had an episode of right-sided sharp chest pain followed by difficulty breathing, which has been increasing. A needle catheter is inserted into his right chest, which causes a release of air. The underlying cause of his symptoms is illustrated in the figure. Of the following, what is the most likely diagnosis?

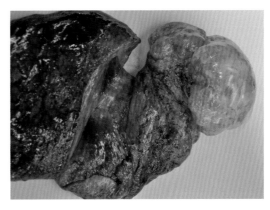

A. Adenocarcinoma

B. Asthma

C. Bronchiectasis

D. Bullous emphysema

E. *Echinococcus* infection

Lung

363

253. A 52-year-old male with a 75-pack-per-year smoking history presents to his family physician with complaints of increasing shortness of breath during periods of exertion, which has developed and increased over the last year or more. The pathologic lesion causing his symptoms is illustrated in the figure. Assuming the changes are diffuse throughout the lung biopsy, which of the following is his most likely diagnosis?

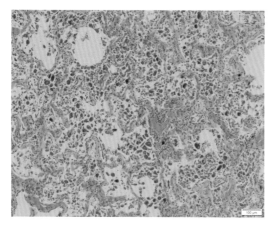

A. Usual interstitial pneumonitis

B. Nonspecific interstitial pneumonitis

C. Desquamative interstitial pneumonitis

D. Acute bronchopneumonia

E. Emphysema

Lung

254. A 33-year-old female presents to her family physician because she is febrile and has had blood in her urine. For the past week, she says that she has had pain with urination, and she says that her urine has smelled bad. Her vital signs include a temperature of 101°F, and on physical examination, she has pain to palpation of the lower back. Her disease process is illustrated in the figure. Of the following, what is the most likely diagnosis?

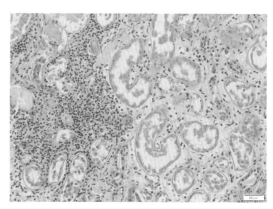

A. Drug-induced interstitial nephritis

B. Renal cell carcinoma

C. Malignant hypertension

D. Acute pyelonephritis

E. Hemolytic uremic syndrome

Kidney

255. A 67-year-old male presents to his family physician because over the past week he has had blood in his urine three times. As a part of his workup, a CT scan of his abdomen is performed, revealing a mass in the left kidney. No stones are identified. The histologic features of the mass are exhibited in the figure. Of the following, what is the most likely diagnosis?

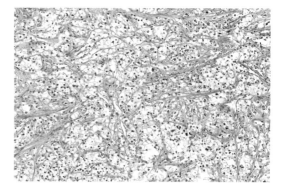

A. Clear cell sarcoma

B. Papillary renal cell carcinoma

C. Metastatic colonic adenocarcinoma

D. Clear cell renal cell carcinoma

E. Xanthogranulomatous pyelonephritis

Kidney

256. A 35-year-old female presents to her family physician with complaints of blood in her urine and a fever. She is concerned about a urinary tract infection, as she has had one before. Further interviewing reveals that she received rifampin about 3 weeks ago, after a possible meningitis scare at the daycare center where she works. The figure illustrates the pathologic process causing her symptoms. Of the following, what is the most likely diagnosis?

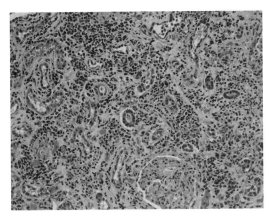

A. Acute pyelonephritis

B. Follicular lymphoma

C. Drug-induced interstitial nephritis

D. Papillary renal cell carcinoma

E. Cytomegalovirus infection

Kidney

257. An autopsy was performed on a 23-year-old male with a history of depression who committed suicide by ingesting antifreeze. Histologic examination of the kidney reveals the findings illustrated in the image. Of the following, which enzyme is responsible for these changes?

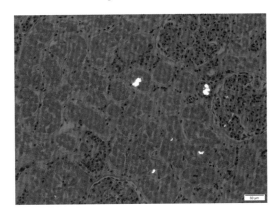

A. Alcohol dehydrogenase

B. Aldehyde dehydrogenase

C. Superoxide dismutase

D. Glutathione transferase

E. UDP-glucuronyl transferase

Kidney

258. A 52-year-old male who complained of a severe headache to his wife suddenly became unresponsive and, despite treatment, died shortly thereafter. An autopsy reveals his cause of death to be an intracerebral hemorrhage. Histologic examination of the kidney reveals the pathologic lesion illustrated in the figure. Of the following, what is most characteristic of this disease process?

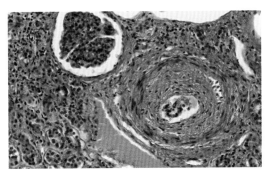

A. Testing for p-ANCA is often positive.

B. The inheritance pattern is autosomal dominant in almost all cases.

C. Infection with schistosomiasis is a risk factor.

D. Retinal hemorrhage often occurs.

E. The intracerebral hemorrhage is unrelated.

Kidney

259. At autopsy, the pathologic lesion illustrated in the figure was identified in the heart of a 47-year-old male who died as the result of a methadone overdose. Of the following, which is most characteristic of the lesion?

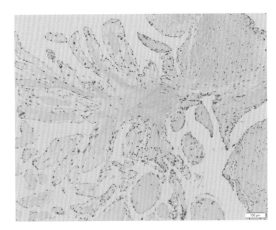

A. It most commonly occurs on the atrial septum.

B. Malignant transformation is common.

C. It is a result of acute rheumatic fever.

D. Patients can develop an acute cerebral infarct.

E. Culture of the lesion would most likely grow viridans streptococci.

Heart

260. A 58-year-old male presents to his family physician complaining of a slow-growing mass just anterior to his ear. After his evaluation, the physician schedules surgery. The histologic appearance of the mass is illustrated in the figure. Of the following, what is the most likely diagnosis?

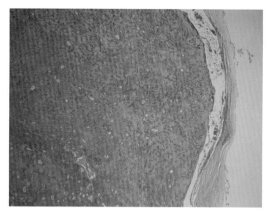

A. Meningioma

B. Chondrosarcoma

C. Pleomorphic adenoma

D. Mucoepidermoid carcinoma

E. Warthin's tumor

Parotid gland

261. A 32-year-old male presents to his family physician with complaints of recurrent heartburn, which has been going on for about 2 years now. An appointment with a gastroenterologist is scheduled, and the man undergoes an EGD. Biopsies of the stomach reveal the pathologic lesion illustrated in the figure. Of the following, what is the most likely diagnosis?

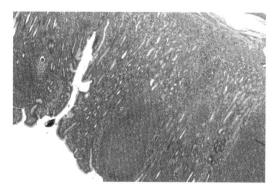

A. Acute gastritis

B. Stress ulcers

C. Chronic gastritis

D. Malignant lymphoma

E. Gastric adenocarcinoma

Stomach

262. A 53-year-old male dies as the result of a self-inflicted gunshot wound. Other than depression and a recent divorce, he had no other medical conditions or significant psychosocial factors. At autopsy, the condition illustrated in the figure is diagnosed. Of the following, what is the most likely diagnosis?

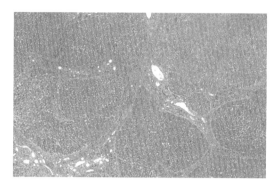

A. Cavernous hemangioma

B. Hepatocellular carcinoma

C. Cirrhosis

D. Metastatic colonic adenocarcinoma

E. Hepatitis A

Liver

263. A 52-year-old male was involved in a motor vehicle accident. He was the driver of a car that struck another car. He was pronounced dead at the scene, and an autopsy was ordered by the coroner. At the time of autopsy, the condition illustrated in the figure was identified. Of the following, what etiologic agent was most likely the cause of the condition?

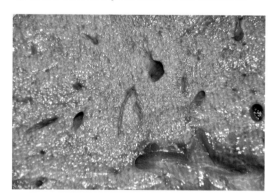

A. Iron

B. Amyloid

C. Alcohol

D. Hepatitis A

E. *Clonorchis sinensis*

Liver

264. A pathology resident is performing an autopsy on a 57-year-old male who died in the hospital. He tells his attending physician that he has found an infarct in the liver. His attending physician explains that infarcts in the liver are very rare and that most likely it is something else. The figure illustrates the pathologic lesion in the liver. Of the following, what is the diagnosis?

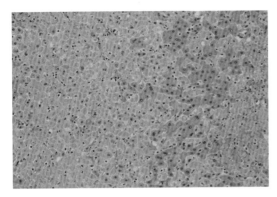

A. Caseous necrosis

B. Liquefactive necrosis

C. Coagulative necrosis

D. *Entamoeba histolytica* infection

E. Acute myeloid leukemia

Liver

265. A 40-year-old male is found unresponsive in his apartment by friends who came to check on him. In the toilet bowl and on the bathroom floor is a large amount of blood. At autopsy, the forensic pathologist identifies a tear at the gastroesophageal junction. Histologic examination of his liver reveals the findings illustrated in the figure. Of the following, which is present in the image?

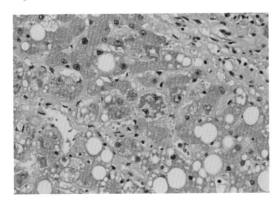

A. Amyloid

B. Intrahepatic fibrosis

C. Mallory's hyaline

D. Schistosomiasis

E. Russell bodies

Liver

266. A 37-year-old male undergoes a liver biopsy after his family physician identifies persistently elevated AST and ALT. The figure illustrates the results of the biopsy. The pathologist reading the biopsy does note that there are no ground-glass hepatocytes identified, and that in some areas of the biopsy, lymphoid aggregates and some proliferation of bile duct epithelium are noted. Of the following, what is the most likely diagnosis?

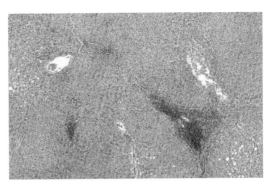

A. Chronic hepatitis A infection

B. Chronic hepatitis B infection

C. Chronic hepatitis C infection

D. Primary sclerosing cholangitis

E. Hepatocellular carcinoma

Liver

267. An autopsy is being performed on a 27-year-old female who died as the result of injuries sustained in a motor vehicle accident. The pathologist performing the autopsy identifies three lesions, all appearing as illustrated in the figure. Of the following, what is the most likely etiology of the lesion?

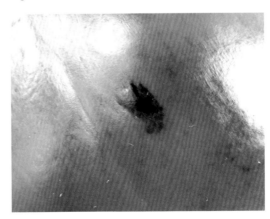

A. Trauma

B. Infection

C. Tumor metastases

D. Benign proliferation of cells

E. Drug-induced

Liver

367

268. A 48-year-old male is being followed by a hepatologist for cirrhosis of the liver. He has also, in the past year, developed insulin-dependent diabetes mellitus, and he has increased pigmentation of his face and forearms. The figure illustrates the pathologic changes in his liver. Of the following, which stain would highlight the dark brown material?

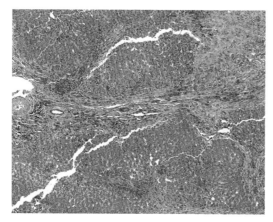

Consider this figure for questions 268 and 269

A. Warthin-Starry

B. Congo red

C. Oil-Red O

D. Prussian blue

E. Trichrome

Liver

269. Of the following, which statement is most characteristic of the preceding disease process?

A. It develops due to impaired urinary excretion of iron.

B. There is complete penetrance.

C. While cirrhosis can develop, the risk for hepatocellular carcinoma is very low.

D. The disease causes some patients to develop arthritis.

E. The disease causes some patients to develop dementia.

Liver

270. A 39-year-old obese female has had intermittent right upper quadrant pain for over a year. She is referred to a surgeon, who proceeds with a cholecystectomy. Her resected gallbladder is illustrated in the figure. Of the following, what is the most likely diagnosis?

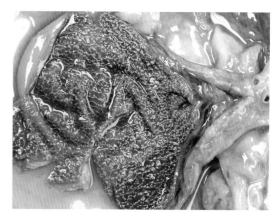

A. Normal gallbladder

B. Cholesterolosis

C. Acute cholecystitis

D. Cholelithiasis

E. Adenocarcinoma of the gallbladder

Gallbladder

271. A 41-year-old obese female with three children has been having intermittent right upper quadrant pain for the past two years. She presents to an acute care clinic with a two-day history of abdominal pain and chills. She has no history of foreign travel. Her vital signs include a temperature of 101°F, and she has scleral icterus. The pathologic process causing her symptoms is illustrated in the figure. Of the following, what is the most likely diagnosis?

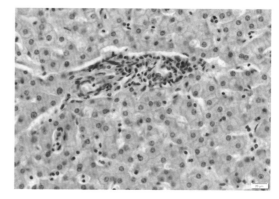

A. Primary biliary sclerosis

B. Acute hepatitis B infection

C. Acute cholangitis

D. *Clonorchis sinensis* infection

E. Alcoholic hepatitis

Gallbladder

272. A 41-year-old male has been seeing his family physician for 1 year because of complaints of heartburn. An EGD is scheduled with a gastroenterologist, who obtains a biopsy that reveals the finding illustrated in the figure. Of the following, what is the most likely diagnosis?

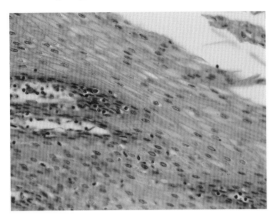

A. Crohn's disease

B. Esophageal parasite

C. Reflux esophagitis

D. Eosinophilic esophagitis

E. Barrett's esophagus

Gallbladder

273. A 47-year-old chronic alcoholic who is homeless and has received no medical care in 15 years was found dead by a fellow homeless person. An autopsy is performed, which reveals the finding illustrated in the figure. Of the following, what is the most likely diagnosis?

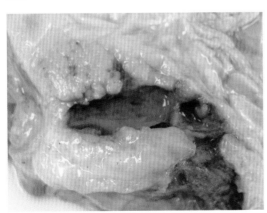

A. Congenital pancreatic cyst

B. Acquired pancreatic cyst

C. Pancreatic pseudocyst

D. Serous cystadenoma

E. Mucinous cystadenoma

Esophagus

274. A 38-year-old male presents to an acute care clinic because of severe abdominal pain. Laboratory testing reveals an amylase of 720 U/L and a lipase of 320 U/L. The pathologic process causing his symptoms is illustrated in the figure. Of the following, what is the most likely diagnosis?

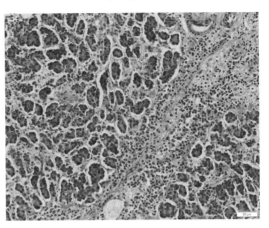

A. Acute pancreatitis

B. Chronic pancreatitis

C. Pancreatic adenocarcinoma

D. Type III hypersensitivity reaction

E. Malignant lymphoma

Pancreas

275. During his annual physical examination, a 67-year-old male has a palpable nodule detected by his family physician during his rectal examination. His PSA is 9 ng/mL. He undergoes a biopsy of his prostate gland, the results of which are illustrated in the figure. Of the following, what is the diagnosis?

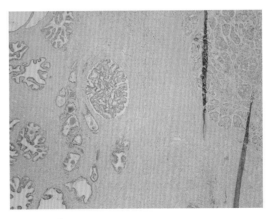

A. Normal prostate

B. Acute prostatitis

C. Benign prostatic hyperplasia

D. Prostatic adenocarcinoma

E. Invasive colonic adenocarcinoma

Prostate

276. A 43-year-old female presents to her gynecologist with complaints that her periods have been heavier than usual. The figure illustrates the pathologic process causing her symptoms. Of the following, what is the most likely diagnosis?

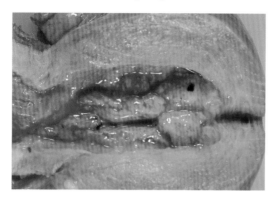

A. Dysfunctional uterine bleeding due to transition into menopause

B. Endometrial polyps

C. Intramural leiomyoma

D. Endometrial carcinoma

E. Pelvic inflammatory disease

Uterus

277. A 51-year-old female palpates a mass in her left breast during her monthly self-examination. She visits her gynecologist, who confirms the mass and refers her to a general surgeon, who excises the mass. The figure illustrates the histologic appearance of the mass. Of the following, what is the most likely diagnosis?

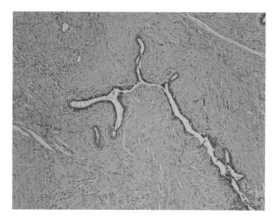

A. Fibroadenoma

B. Phylloides tumor

C. Invasive ductal carcinoma

D. Myxoid stromal sarcoma

E. Dysgerminoma

Breast

22.2 Images—Answers and Explanations

Easy	Medium	Hard

1. Correct: Asthma (D)

The image illustrates an airway (bottom of the figure). The airway has collagen deposition under the basement membrane, giving it a thickened appearance; smooth muscle hypertrophy; and a prominent infiltrate of eosinophils, which are the characteristic microscopic features of asthma (**D**). Two other findings which can be present in asthma are Charcot-Leyden crystals and Curschmann spirals. The Charcot-Leyden crystals are accumulations of major basic protein, and Curschmann spirals are casts of sloughed epithelial cells. The histologic features are not characteristic of the other conditions that are listed (**A-C, E**).

2. Correct: Fibrinous pericarditis (E)

The epicardial surface of the heart has the classic "bread and butter" appearance, which is associated with fibrinous pericarditis (**B**). Microscopic examination of the epicardium would reveal proteinaceous material (i.e., the fibrin). Grossly, the adhesions are easily lysed. Serous pericarditis would be a watery fluid filling the pericardial sac (**A**). Fibrous pericarditis would be fibrous scarring of the pericardial sac, and it could not be removed leaving the pericardial surface intact (**E**). Fibrous adhesions must be cut, and cannot be lysed with palpation. The image shows neither hemorrhage nor purulence (**C, D**).

3. Correct: Uremia (D)

The heart has a fibrinous pericarditis. Fibrinous pericarditis, a "bread and butter" pericarditis, is most commonly associated with uremia (**D**); however, it can also occur following a myocardial infarct, or in association with a collagen vascular disease. Coxsackievirus A infection would cause a serous pericarditis, and watery fluid would be in the pericardial sac (**A**). Metastatic tumor most commonly is associated with a hemorrhagic pericarditis (**B**), and a bacterial infection with a purulent pericarditis (**C**). Tuberculosis is also frequently associated with a hemorrhagic pericarditis (**E**).

4. Correct: Sarcoidosis (D)

The image illustrates a noncaseating granuloma, which is characteristic of sarcoidosis (**D**). Characteristically, tuberculosis produces caseating granulomas (**C**); however, the negative acid-fast bacillus stain also confirms the diagnosis is not tuberculosis. There is no histologic evidence of carcinoma (**A, B**), and *Streptococcus pneumoniae* does not normally produce granulomas (**E**).

5. Correct: Asteroid bodies (A)

The image illustrates a noncaseating granuloma. In a pulmonary lymph node (as well as at other locations, as the disease process can affect virtually any organ), a noncaseating granuloma is consistent with sarcoidosis. Two histologic findings associated with granulomas in sarcoidosis are asteroid bodies and Schaumann bodies (**A**). Ferruginous bodies are associated with asbestosis (**B**). Keratin pearls are associated with squamous cell carcinoma (**C**). Fibroblastic foci are associated with usual interstitial pneumonia (**D**). and Charcot-Leyden crystals are associated with asthma (**E**).

6. Correct: Cardiac tamponade (C)

The image illustrates a cardiac rupture due to an underlying myocardial infarct. The yellow discoloration surrounding the tear in the myocardium indicates the myocardial infarct is around 1 to 4 days in age. A tear in the free wall of the left ventricle leads to blood entering the pericardial sac, which causes a cardiac tamponade (**C**). Acute myocardial infarcts can also cause death due to a dysrhythmia or acute mitral insufficiency (**B, D**). Mural thrombi can form as a result of a myocardial infarct and can subsequently embolize, potentially to the brain, causing an infarct (**E**). Any time a patient is less mobile, the patient is at risk for the formation of deep venous thrombi and subsequent pulmonary thromboembolus (**A**).

7. Correct: 4 days (C)

The image illustrates an acute myocardial infarct, with extensive and well-developed coagulative necrosis combined with a prominent neutrophilic infiltrate. At 1 minute, no histologic change in the heart would be present (**A**). At 1 day, coagulative necrosis and a neutrophilic infiltrate can be present, but would not be well-developed (**B**). At around 4 to 5 days, macrophages begin to appear and break down the dead tissue and inflammatory cells (**C**), following which granulation tissue develops beginning around 7 to 10 days (**D**), and progresses to a dense fibrous scar by 2 months (**E**).

8. Correct: Ruptured abdominal aortic aneurysm (D)

The image illustrates a ruptured abdominal aortic aneurysm, which has been further opened to reveal a lumen filled with thrombus. The forceps at the top of the image are reflecting the wall of the aneurysm, and the aneurysmal cavity is at the top of the image. On the left side of the image are the two iliac arteries, which assist in determining the location of the aneurysm. Syphilitic aneurysms and aneurysms due to giant cell arteritis normally occur in the thoracic aorta (**A, B**). An aortic dissection would have hemorrhage in the wall of the aorta, and it does not form an aneurysm (**C**). The lesion is not a vascular angiosarcoma, which would present as a mass (**E**).

9. Correct: Apoptosis (C)

On the left side of the image, there is a single eosinophilic cell, with no surrounding inflammation. This is a Councilman body, which can be seen in hepatitis, and represents apoptosis of a hepatocyte. Apoptosis causes breakdown of a cell without generating an inflammatory response (**C**); whereas, with coagulative necrosis, although the cell may appear similar, the process generates an inflammatory response (**A**). Liquefactive necrosis would involve dissolution of cellular architecture (**B**). The cell represents neither metaplasia nor dysplasia (**D, E**).

10. Correct: No abnormality (E)

The image illustrates an adrenal adenoma. Most adrenal adenomas are nonfunctional and represent an incidental finding, and therefore, in most patients, such a finding would not result in any laboratory abnormalities (**E**). In addition, if the adrenal adenoma were secreting cortisol and causing Cushing's syndrome, the ACTH concentration would be decreased (**A, B**), and, because of decreased stimulus, the surrounding non-neoplastic adrenal gland would be atrophic, which is not evident in the image. Urinary metanephrines are found in individuals with a pheochromocytoma (**C**), which would be centered on the adrenal medulla. Low plasma renin activity would indicate an aldosterone-secreting tumor (**D**).

11. Correct: Decreased serum ACTH (B)

The patient has adrenal gland hyperplasia, which can be the primary source of Cushing's syndrome. As the adrenal gland is producing cortisol, it will feed back into the pituitary gland and suppress secretion of ACTH (**A, B**). Neither a low-dose nor a high-dose dexamethasone will suppress secretion of cortisol, when the source is adrenal gland hyperplasia or an adrenal gland adenoma (**C, D**). A high-dose dexamethasone suppression test would only cause a lowered cortisol concentration if the source of the ACTH is a pituitary adenoma. Obesity, hypertension, and osteoporosis are features of Cushing's disease and Cushing's syndrome. The hypertension does not indicate a pheochromocytoma (**E**), and the image is of a nodular adrenal cortex and not a single mass in the adrenal medulla.

12. Correct: t(15;17) (C)

The image illustrates myeloblasts, and, in the center, is a myeloblast with numerous Auer rods. Auer rods are found in acute myeloblastic leukemia, and, while in most cases there is only one Auer rod per cell, in AML with t(15;17), myeloblasts can contain numerous Auer rods (C). A t(8;21) and an inv(16) are causes of acute myeloblastic leukemia; however, in these types, multiple Auer rods in a given cell would most likely not occur (A, B). A t(1;14) translocation is found in marginal zone lymphoma (also called

MALTomas) (D), and a t(11;14) translocation is found in mantle cell lymphomas (E), neither of which have Auer rods. Patients with AML with the t(15;17) can present with disseminated intravascular coagulation and can develop hemorrhages, including intracerebral hemorrhage.

13.   Correct: Emphysema (B)

The image depicts lungs with anthracotic pigment, the black material on the surface and within the pleural lymphatics. The accumulation of anthracotic pigment occurs in individuals who use tobacco or who live in polluted environments. As anthracosis indicates the exposure to cigarette smoke (or similar exposure), of the disease processes listed, he is most likely to develop emphysema (B). With the exception of a few people, the vast majority of people with emphysema develop the condition due to tobacco use. Anthracotic pigment accumulation is not directly associated with the other disease processes listed. (A, C-E).

14.   Correct: Bicuspid aortic valve (D)

Three pathologic processes are evident—the left ventricle is dilated, there is a bicuspid aortic valve, and there is an aortic dissection (B). The dissection is near the cut edge of the aorta, and only a small residual tag of tissue holds the aorta together. The portion of the aortic valve present is two cusps, yet they are fused, having a midline raphe, which indicates an aortic valve. The dilated left ventricle is not a dilated cardiomyopathy, and instead resulted from regurgitation through an insufficient aortic valve (A). The bicuspid valve best explains all pathologic findings—it explains the valve abnormality, the dilated left ventricle, and aortic dissection is associated with bicuspid aortic valves (D). Neither an aortic aneurysm or myocarditis would explain the pathologic findings in the image (C, E).

15.   Correct: Aortic dissection (B)

The image illustrates an unopened pericardial sac containing blood, a hemopericardium. The two more common causes of a hemopericardium, other than trauma, include a ruptured myocardial infarct and aortic dissection (B). However, if the interventricular septum ruptures, a left-to-right shunt between the left ventricle and the right ventricle forms, not a hemopericardium (C). Rupture of a coronary artery aneurysm could cause a hemopericardium; however, coronary artery aneurysms essentially always occur as a complication of Kawasaki's disease, and compared to the incidence of aortic dissection, are much less common (D). A ruptured abdominal aortic aneurysm or a pulmonary thromboembolus would not result in bleeding into the pericardial sac (A, E).

16.   Correct: Diastolic dysfunction (C)

The patient has a hemopericardium. The blood filling the pericardial sac will put pressure on the wall of the heart from the outside and impair dilation of the ventricles during diastole, which impairs filling (C). Contractility of the heart is not impaired; however, the chambers do not adequately fill with blood (A, B). While an aortic dissection can lead to aortic insufficiency if it involves the valve root, the main effect of a hemopericardium itself is not aortic insufficiency (D). The blood in the pericardial sac is outside the normal flow of blood, so while with survival thrombi can form in the pericardial sac, they would not embolize (E).

17.   Correct: Cystic medial degeneration (C)

The lesion illustrated in the image is the proximal aorta and aortic valve. Above the coronary artery ostium near the center of the image is a tear in the intima, which is consistent with an aortic dissection. The underlying histologic change associated with aortic dissections is often cystic medial degeneration (C). If the patient survived the acute event, hemosiderin would be deposited, because of hemorrhage within the wall of the aorta, but it would not be present acutely, as it takes around 2 to 5 days to start to appear after a hemorrhage (B). Granulomatous inflammation of the aorta is associated with giant cell arteritis and Takayasu's arteritis, which are both associated with thoracic aortic aneurysms but not commonly with aortic dissections (A). The pathologic process pictured in the image is neither bacterial nor neoplastic in origin (D, E).

18.   Correct: Acute appendicitis (D)

The image is that of a tubular structure, with attached adipose tissue. Some of the adipose tissue is more red because it is inflamed. The white material on the tip is purulence. Although diverticulitis and ulcerative colitis appear in a tubular structure (i.e., the colon), the image does not show tenia coli (A, C). Also, ulcerative colitis is a mucosal and submucosal process and not transmural. The structure present is not the stomach, and the duodenum, being mostly retroperitoneal, should have attached tissue to the serosal surface (E). When considering the choices given, acute appendicitis is most consistent with the clinical scenario (D). In the image, there is no evidence of a fetus (B).

19.   Correct: Mesothelioma (C)

The image illustrates a ferruginous body, which is most commonly associated with asbestos exposure. The ferruginous body results from a macrophage engulfing an asbestos fiber and then coating it with iron. Other features of asbestos exposure include mesothelioma, pleural plaques, and asbestosis (an interstitial lung disease) (**C**). In addition to mesothelioma, asbestos exposure also increases the likelihood of the development of bronchogenic carcinoma. Progressive massive fibrosis is associated with coal and silica exposure (**A**), Schaumann bodies are associated with sarcoidosis (**B**), and both bilateral apical scars and caseating granulomas are associated with tuberculosis (**D**, **E**). Tuberculosis, especially reactivation, can involve the apices of the lungs, as that is the best oxygen content for the organism, and scarring can result.

20. Correct: Acute rheumatic fever (B)

The pathologic finding illustrated in the image is an Aschoff nodule, which is the characteristic pathologic lesion found in acute rheumatic fever (**B**). The finding of a rash, arthralgia, and dyspnea (due to cardiac involvement) is consistent with acute rheumatic fever, which is the result of cross-reactivity of antibodies directed at *Streptococcus pneumoniae* antigens, which cross-react with cardiac antigens. Giant cell myocarditis is essentially just giant cells (**D**), and lymphocytic myocarditis, commonly due to enteroviruses such as coxsackie virus A and B, with lymphocytes and myocyte necrosis (**A**). The image is consistent with neither of these conditions, and there are no noncaseating granulomas in the image, ruling out sarcoidosis (**C**). The lesion is not a neoplastic proliferation of muscle cells, and the clinical presentation is not consistent with a rhabdomyoma (**E**).

21. Correct: Cardiac dysrhythmia (C)

In the center of the image is an asteroid body, and near the center of the bottom of the image is a giant cell. These features are consistent with sarcoidosis. Sarcoidosis can involve many organ systems and produce a variety of extrapulmonary disease, including uveitis, iritis, and erythema nodosum. In addition, granulomas can develop in a wide range of organs, including the liver, spleen, and kidney. Involvement of the heart can lead to the possibility of a cardiac dysrhythmia (**C**). None of the other conditions listed are commonly associated with sarcoidosis (**A-B, D-E**).

22. Correct: Deep venous thrombus embolizing to the brain (B)

The image illustrates an atrial septal defect. While atrial septal defects would allow for a left-to-right shunt, the shunt would be atrial and not ventricular (**A**). Also, with the development of right ventricular dilation and hypertrophy, the shunt can become right-to-left. An atrial septal defect can allow a venous thrombus to enter the systemic circulation, which is termed a paradoxical embolus (**B**). An atrial septal defect is not a risk factor for an atrial myxoma,

myocarditis, or Kawasaki's syndrome (**C-E**). The most common location for an atrial myxoma, however, is in the left atrium adjacent to the fossa ovalis.

23. Correct: Stable angina (A)

The image illustrates atherosclerosis of a coronary artery. The plaque is stable and does not have any acute changes. The purple-blue material in the wall is calcification. The plaque does obstruct more than 75% of the lumen, however, and thus, the patient could develop stable angina (**A**). Unstable angina, ST-elevation myocardial infarct, and non-ST-elevation myocardial infarct are all due to an acute plaque change, including hemorrhage and thrombosis due to plaque ulceration or rupture, none of which is present (**B-D**). Coronary artery dissection is a rare condition, most commonly occurring in pregnant females. Atherosclerosis is not by itself a risk factor; however, if patients undergo coronary artery angiography, the procedure can induce a dissection on rare occasions (**E**).

24. Correct: Collateral circulation (C)

The image shows complete obstruction of the coronary artery, which will completely block the flow of blood and nutrients to the myocytes; however, if this lesion develops over time, collateral vessels in the form of capillaries and other small vessels, not full-sized coronary arteries, can develop and allow blood to bypass the obstruction, and therefore, although the vessel is completely obstructed, no infarct is present corresponding to the distribution of blood flow (**C**). An acute myocardial infarct will never completely resolve; once it occurs, a scar will be formed (**A**). Diabetes mellitus contributes to the development of atherosclerosis (**B**). A paired left anterior descending coronary artery would be an exceptionally rare anomaly (**D**). Oxygen from the ventricular blood can reach the first layers of cardiac myocytes underneath the endocardium, but could never sustain the entire wall of the left ventricle (**E**).

25. Correct: Sex of the patient (D)

The lesion in the aorta is atherosclerosis. Atherosclerosis has risk factors that can be modified with lifestyle changes, namely hypertension, smoking, high cholesterol, and diabetes mellitus (**A, B, E**), and risk factors that cannot be modified, namely sex of the patient (with increased risk in males) and age of the patient (**D**). Gout is not commonly associated with a significantly increased risk for the development of atherosclerosis (**C**).

26. Correct: Adenocarcinoma in situ (C)

The image illustrates lepidic growth, which is characteristic of adenocarcinoma in situ, and adenocarcinoma in situ can present as an apparent bronchopneumonia that then fails to respond to the normal treatment (**C**). Type II pneumocytes are similar to the cells in the image, as they are tall cells; however, type II pneumocyte hyperplasia is induced by damage to the underlying alveolar septum, most commonly fibrosis, and, in the image, the alveolar septa, other than the neoplastic cells, appear normal (**D**). There are no granulomas, fibroblastic foci and honeycomb change, or neutrophilic infiltrates, ruling out the other three diagnoses (**A, B, E**).

27. Correct: Barrett's esophagus (D)

The image illustrates the esophagus (i.e., the tubular structure in the center of the image), the gastroesophageal junction, and a portion of the stomach. The gastroesophageal junction is approximately at the level of the bend of the tubular structure; however, note that mucosa similar to that lining the stomach is present to the cut edge of the esophagus (to the right side of the tubular structure) (**D**). The esophagus itself is not dilated, there is no mass, there are no varices, and the mucosa is not eroded (**A-C, E**). In the case of erosive esophagitis, the mucosa would be more blackened and sloughed.

28. Correct: Normal squamous epithelium (A)

In Barrett's esophagus, the esophageal mucosa is exposed to gastric contents, which causes it to change in structure from squamous epithelium to glandular epithelium. Squamous epithelium is thicker, and hence, the white appearance (**A**), while the glandular epithelium appears more like the lining of the stomach (**B**). Within the metaplastic glandular epithelium, areas of dysplasia and ultimately neoplasia can occur, and thus, patients with Barrett's esophagus often need to make screening biopsies. The white areas are not metaplasia or dysplasia (**C-E**).

29. Correct: Congenital (B)

The image is that of a bicuspid aortic valve. Note the midline raphe at 12 o'clock and that of the other two commissures are unfused (**B**). Wear and tear would produce nodules of calcium on the sinus side of the cusp and would not normally be present in a 42-year-old (**A**). Rheumatic fever, when it involves the aortic valve, causes fusion of all three commissures (**C**). Myxomatous degeneration of the aortic valve is rare and would not produce a bicuspid aortic valve, and neither is a neoplastic process likely to (**D, E**).

30. Correct: Bronchiolitis obliterans–organizing pneumonia (B)

The image is that of a fibroblastic plug, which is filling the airway in which it is found and is branching into other airways. These are characteristic of both BOOP and COP; however, given that there is an etiology for the lung condition (i.e., the near fatal drug overdose), the correct diagnosis is BOOP, as the etiology is not

unknown (**B, C**). Usual interstitial pneumonia has fibroblastic foci, which appear very similar; however, in UIP, instead of being in the airways, the fibroblastic foci are within the alveolar septa (**D**). Diffuse alveolar damage (i.e., acute respiratory distress syndrome) has hyaline membranes (**A**), and desquamative interstitial pneumonitis has alveolar airspaces filled with finely pigmented macrophages (**E**).

31. Correct: Axonal spheroids (C)

In the center of the image is a cluster of multiple acellular globular eosinophilic masses. These are axonal spheroids, which are seen in diffuse axonal injury, which can occur as a result of head trauma (**C**). Lewy bodies are found within neurons in the substantia nigra most commonly and are associated with Parkinson's disease (**A**). They can also be found in the cerebral cortex in diffuse Lewy body disease, a form of dementia. Negri bodies are inclusions associated with rabies (**B**). Red neurons are eosinophilic neurons that are a result of hypoxic or ischemic injury (**D**). Rosenthal fibers are found associated with some forms of brain tumors, often the slower-growing ones, such as pilocytic astrocytomas in children (**E**).

32. Correct: *Staphylococcus aureus* (D)

The left corner has an inflammatory infiltrate (neutrophils) filling the alveolar airspaces; however, in the upper right corner, there is only edema and no inflammatory infiltrate. As the lung is involved in a patchy distribution, the diagnosis is a bronchopneumonia. Of the etiologic agents listed, *Staphylococcus aureus* would cause a bronchopneumonia (**D**). Both *Mycobacterium tuberculosis* and *Coccidioides immitis* would cause a granulomatous inflammation (**B, C**). Influenza A would cause an interstitial infiltrate, and the airspaces would be open (**A**). *Pneumocystis jiroveci* causes a more fluffy eosinophilic exudate in the alveolar airspaces (**E**), vaguely similar to edema or alveolar proteinosis in appearance.

33. Correct: t(8;14) (E)

A t(8;14) is associated with Burkitt's lymphoma and results from the combining of MYC on chromosome 8 and the Ig heavy chain gene. The image shows a starry sky pattern, which is characteristic of Burkitt's lymphoma (**E**). A t(14;18) is associated with follicular lymphoma and diffuse large B-cell lymphoma and moves the *BCL2* gene adjacent to the Ig heavy chain gene (**A**). A t(11;14) is associated with mantle cell lymphoma and moves cyclin D1 adjacent to the Ig heavy chain gene (**B**). A t(9;22) is associated with chronic myelogenous leukemia and certain forms of acute lymphoblastic leukemia, and is the result of the combination of *ABL* and *BCR* (**C**). A t(15;17) is associated with acute myelogenous leukemia and results from the combination of *PML* and *RARA* (**D**).

34. Correct: A common location is near the ileocecal valve. (C)

The histologic image is that of a starry sky appearance, which is characteristic of Burkitt's lymphoma. Burkitt's lymphoma is associated with EBV virus infection (many cases of Burkitt's lymphoma in the United States and essentially all cases in Africa) (**A, E**) and is a B-cell neoplasm and therefore, CD10, CD19, and CD20 positive, but not CD5 in most cases (**D**). Tumor lysis syndrome is common because the neoplasm is rapidly growing and thus has a high turnover rate (**B**). Tumor lysis syndrome can lead to metabolic acidosis, hyperuricemia, and acute renal failure. Burkitt's lymphoma commonly is located near the ileocecal valve but also in the retroperitoneum or the ovaries (**C**).

35. Correct: Adenocarcinoma (B)

On the lower left side is a mass. Most frequently, adenocarcinoma is peripheral, such as this tumor, while squamous cell carcinoma is centrally located and often has central cavitation (**A, B**). A pulmonary hamartoma is a nodule of cartilage (**C**). Adenocarcinoma in situ does not normally form a well-defined mass (**D**). A pulmonary abscess would be caveated and contain pus (**E**).

36. Correct: Pulmonary tuberculosis (E)

The image is that of caseating granulomas, characterized by central necrosis of the granulomas, which is consistent with a diagnosis of pulmonary tuberculosis (**E**). Sarcoidosis and chronic hypersensitivity pneumonitis both have granulomas as a characteristic histologic feature; however, the granulomas are most frequently noncaseating and, in chronic hypersensitivity pneumonitis, are within the alveolar septa (**A, B**). The image does not represent a neoplasm (**C, D**).

37. Correct: Contraction band necrosis (C)

To the right of center, and toward the top of the image, the cardiac myocytes are traversed by dark eosinophilic bands, which represent contraction band necrosis (**C**). An intercalated disk would appear similar; however, the normal concentration of intercalated disks would never match that of the image (**D**). Cystic medial degeneration occurs in the aorta associated with hypertension, and the histologic lesion has no characteristics of liquefactive necrosis or myocarditis (**A, B, E**).

38. Correct: Brainstem hemorrhage (D)

The pathologic condition illustrated in the image is cerebral edema. Notice that instead of being convoluted, the gyri are flattened, and the sulci, instead of being open, are closed and essentially obliterated. Complications of cerebral edema include cingulate, uncal, cerebellar tonsillar, and brainstem herniation. Brainstem herniation leads to midline hemorrhages in the brainstem, called Duret's hemorrhages (**D**). Cerebral edema is not a risk factor for subarachnoid hemorrhage, meningitis, or astrocytoma, and, as the condition is diffuse and not focal, it would not cause focal neurological deficits such as loss of motor function and sensation in the left lower extremity (**A-C, E**).

39. Correct: Supersaturation of bile with cholesterol (C)

Given the multitude of stones in the image, cholelithiasis and not nephrolithiasis is the most likely diagnosis. Increased uric acid and cystine concentrations are not associated with cholelithiasis (**A, E**). The two types of gallstones are cholesterol and pigment. Pigment stones are darker in coloration, while cholesterol stones are yellow or yellow-green. The mechanism of formation of cholesterol stones in the gallbladder begins with supersaturation of bile with cholesterol (**C**). Neither hemolysis nor conversion of ethylene glycol to oxalic acid affect the production of cholesterol stones; however, the mechanism for formation of pigment stones is hemolysis (**B, D**).

40. Correct: In some patients, the stone can cause obstruction of the small intestine. (D)

The patient has cholelithiasis. Most patients with cholelithiasis are asymptomatic (**A**). The stones in the image are consistent with cholesterol stones, which, in most cases, are radiolucent and would not be identified by X-ray (**B**). Cholesterol stones are due to supersaturation of bile with cholesterol, causing crystallization of the cholesterol and the production of stones. Pigment stones are due to increased amounts of unconjugated bilirubin, such as would occur with increased red blood cell breakdown (**C**). Women are more likely than men to have gallstones, and the incidence increases as the age of the patient increases (**E**). In some cases, a fistula forms between the gallbladder and the small intestine, allowing for a calculus of some size to enter the small intestine, which can lead to obstruction (**D**).

41. Correct: Alcohol use (C)

The organ is the pancreas, and the sections at the bottom illustrate chronic pancreatitis, with calcification and pseudocyst formation. The two main causes of pancreatitis are alcohol use and gallstones (**C**). None of the other conditions listed is a common cause of pancreatitis, although each could potentially contribute to its development (**A-B, D-E**).

42. Correct: Congestive heart failure (D)

The clinical scenario is consistent with congestive heart failure, as patients with left-sided heart failure will develop pleural effusions due to increased hydrostatic pressure in the pulmonary vasculature, then leakage of fluid into the alveolar airspaces and the pleural cavities. Over time, this leads to fibrosis of the alveolar septa and accumulation of hemosiderin-laden macrophages. The pathologic condition is termed chronic passive congestion of the lungs (**D**). The histologic changes are not, given the scenario, consistent with the remainder of the diagnoses (**A-C, E**).

43. Correct: Autoantibodies directed at cardiac antigens (D)

The image illustrates fusion and thickening of the chordae tendineae and thickening of the mitral valve leaflets, which is consistent with chronic rheumatic mitral valvulitis. Acute rheumatic fever is due to antibodies formed against bacterial antigen that cross-react with normal cardiac antigens (**D**). Although endocarditis can involve the valves, it would be very unusual for it to completely mimic chronic rheumatic mitral valvulitis (**A**). Carcinoid tumor typically produces changes in the tricuspid valve, with thickening of the leaflets (**C**). Eosinophilic infiltrates are most often associated with endocardial thickening (**E**). Amyloid could deposit in the cardiac valves, but would be rare for it to produce the same gross appearance as chronic rheumatic mitral valvulitis (**B**).

44. Correct: Hemorrhoids (D)

The condition illustrated in the image is cirrhosis of the liver. Cirrhosis of the liver is due to alcohol use, hepatitis B and C, hemochromatosis, and other conditions. It is not a risk factor for primary sclerosing cholangitis or hiatal hernias (**A, E**). Cirrhosis of the liver is a risk factor for hepatocellular carcinoma, but not hepatic hemangiomas (**C**). Alcohol is a risk factor for both cirrhosis and acute pancreatitis, but cirrhosis is not independently a risk factor for acute pancreatitis (**B**). Hemorrhoids develop due to portal hypertension. As the pressure in the liver increases, blood will follow alternate, lower-pressure routes back to the heart, leading to the formation of esophageal varices, caput medusae, and hemorrhoids (**D**).

45. Correct: Micronodular cirrhosis of the liver (C)

The cut surface of the liver exhibits a very fine nodularity, with the nodules being less than 3 mm in size, which is micronodular cirrhosis of the liver (**C**). Although the entire liver is yellow, a diffuse fatty liver by itself has no nodularity (**D**). The hepatocytes in cirrhosis of the liver can exhibit the various histologic changes of normal hepatocytes, including fatty accumulation, bile production, and Mallory's hyaline. Metastatic adenocarcinoma would be more discrete nodules, the nodules would likely be white or tan-white, and there would produce more variation in size, with many much larger (**E**). Miliary tuberculosis would also present as more discrete nodules, which would likely be more white in coloration (**A**). The changes are not consistent with a lymphoma (**B**).

46. Correct: Chronic lymphocytic leukemia (D)

The white blood cells illustrated in the image have a lymphocytic appearance with a large nuclear-to-cytoplasmic ratio. The nuclei do not appear as blasts, in that the chromatin is not smooth and nucleoli are not present; instead, the chromatin is more heterogeneous, described as a cracked earth or gingersnap appearance. These features are consistent with CLL (**D**). As the cells do not appear as blasts, (**A, B**) are incorrect, and as the cells appear lymphoid instead of myeloid, (**C**) is incorrect. The cells are not morphologically consistent with a hairy cell leukemia (**E**).

47. Correct: Patients can have a hypogammaglobulinemia (D)

CLL is a leukemia that is derived from B cells (**E**); however, the cells do express CD5, which is normally a T cell marker (**A**). Patients with CLL will often survive ten years or more after the time of their diagnosis (**B**). CLL is most common in adults (**C**). Despite the fact that the neoplasm is derived from B cells, patients can have a hypogammaglobulinemia, and they can also produce abnormal antibodies, resulting in either hemolytic anemia or thrombocytopenia.

48. Correct: Chronic myelogenous leukemia (C)

The cells have a myeloid appearance, with a small nuclear-to-cytoplasmic ratio, and there are myeloid cells of various maturational stages, including band neutrophils. No myeloblasts are present (**A, B**). These changes are consistent with chronic myelogenous leukemia (**C**). The cells are not lymphoid in appearance (**B**), and the morphology is not consistent with hairy cell leukemia (**E**).

49. Correct: The early satiety is most likely caused by splenomegaly. (D)

The image illustrates chronic myelogenous leukemia. CML most commonly occurs in adults (although a juvenile form of CML does exist, it is not as prevalent) (**A**). CML is a fairly common form of leukemia, representing around 1/5 of cases of all leukemias (**C**). If patients enter a blast crisis, they have a poor prognosis (**B**), and the blast crisis can be either AML or ALL. The translocation is t(9;22); however, the two genes involved are *BCR* and *ABL* (**E**). CML is associated with splenomegaly, and an enlarged spleen can put pressure on the stomach and cause early satiety (**D**).

50. Correct: Cytomegalovirus infection (C)

In the center of the image is an enlarged cell with a prominent intranuclear inclusion, whose appearance is consistent with cytomegalovirus (**C**). While the cell in the center does not appear similar to the classic Reed-Sternberg cell in Hodgkin's lymphoma, as it does not have an owl's-eye appearance, variant Reed-Sternberg cells could appear similar; however, Hodgkin's lymphoma involving the stomach would be exceptionally rare (**D**). The image contains numerous neutrophils, consistent with the acute inflammation, and not eosinophils (**E**). No neoplastic cells, including signet ring cells, are present (**A**). While the infection with the CMV could lead to an ulcer, it would not be the characteristic peptic ulcer, and the definitive diagnosis of a peptic ulcer from the image provided would not be possible (**B**).

51. Correct: Coronary artery atherosclerosis (C)

The image illustrates coagulative necrosis associated with a prominent neutrophilic infiltrate. Many of the neutrophils are degenerating, producing stippled debris in the interstitium. The image illustrates an acute myocardial infarct. Both coronary artery atherosclerosis and a coronary artery dissection can cause an acute myocardial infarct, but by far the more common of the two is coronary artery atherosclerosis; with coronary artery dissection is relatively rare and most commonly associated with pregnant females (**C, D**). There are no lymphocytes or granulomas, and septic emboli would have a large collection of bacterial cocci or bacterial rods associated with the inflammation (**A, B, E**).

52. Correct: Unprotected anal intercourse (C)

The image illustrates an anal condyloma, which can appear as a nodule with a polypoid-like surface architecture. The main risk factor for condylomas is exposure to human papillomavirus, which, in males, would be acquired through unprotected anal intercourse (**C**). The mass is not an adenocarcinoma, and thus chemical carcinogens in the diet and ulcerative colitis are not risk factors (**A, B**). Cirrhosis of the liver increases the risk for development of hemorrhoids, but a hemorrhoid is a dilated vein and would not appear as the mass in the image (**E**). Quadriplegia is not a risk factor for condylomas (**D**).

53. Correct: Brain (A)

The image illustrates a *Cryptococcus neoformans* infection of the lung; however, in patients with AIDS, the disease is most commonly associated with the brain, causing a meningitis (**A**). The other answers are incorrect (**B-E**).

54. Correct: Aortic dissection (C)

The image illustrates cystic medial degeneration. There are amorphous collections of acellular pale blue material between elastic fibers in the wall of the aorta. Cystic medial degeneration is associated with hypertension and Marfan's syndrome. Of the conditions listed, the underlying cause of an aortic dissection is most frequently hypertension (**C**), although they can also occur in people with Marfan's syndrome and Ehlers-Danlos. The other conditions listed are not associated with aortic dissection or hypertension (**A-B, D-E**).

55. Correct: Acute respiratory distress syndrome (C)

The image illustrates hyaline membranes, which are the characteristic histologic feature of acute respiratory distress syndrome (ARDS) (**C**). The pathologic term used is diffuse alveolar damage. The appearance of the hyaline membranes in adults is essentially the same as their appearance in hyaline membrane disease in infants; however, the etiology is different. Hyaline membranes in infants are due to prematurity and lack of surfactant, whereas hyaline membranes in adults are due to a wide variety of insults that damage either the epithelium or the endothelium in the alveolar septum and allow leakage of protein. A common cause is sepsis. The image has no features of pulmonary edema, UIP, bacterial pneumonia, or influenza (**A-B, D-E**).

56. Correct: Dilated cardiomyopathy (D)

The image illustrates a globular heart (i.e., one with a rounded outline, instead of coming to a relative point at the apex). This gross appearance is most consistent with a dilated cardiomyopathy (**D**). Examination of the heart based on the image provided would not allow for the diagnosis of any of the other conditions listed (**A-C, E**).

57. Correct: Exposure to alcohol (D)

The image illustrates diffuse fatty change, with essentially every hepatocyte containing one large vacuole, which is macrovesicular steatosis. Fatty change in the liver can occur due to a variety of insults, including alcohol use, obesity, and diabetes mellitus (with obesity and diabetes mellitus responsible for many cases of nonalcoholic steatohepatitis) (**D**). Hepatitis B infection, accumulation of α-1-antitrypsin, iron deposition, and bile duct obstruction are associated with liver damage and can lead to cirrhosis; however, they are not associated with such extensive fatty change (**A-C, E**). Hepatitis C can be associated with some fatty change.

58. Correct: Diverticulosis (C)

The image illustrates multiple colonic diverticula (**C**). The diverticula are false diverticula caused by outward expansion of mucosa and submucosa through weak spots in the muscularis. Meckel's diverticulum occurs in the terminal ileum, is a true diverticulum, and is single (**E**). The appearance is not consistent with ulcerative colitis, rectal adenocarcinoma, or familial polyposis, as these conditions affect the mucosa (**A, B, D**). Extension through the wall by a rectal adenocarcinoma could occur, but the serosa would not appear normal.

59. Correct: Diffuse large B-cell lymphoma (C)

As the name indicates, the tumor is a homogenous proliferation of essentially one cell type. The image does not show the follicular pattern seen in follicular lymphoma, the starry sky pattern seen with Burkitt's lymphoma, or Reed-Sternberg cells in the background of a heterogenous cell population (**A, B, E**). The tumor cells do not appear like plasma cells (**D**). The fact that the neoplasm is CD20+ could help in a differential diagnosis of primary brain tumors or metastatic disease versus a lymphoma.

60. Correct: Ectopic pregnancy (C)

The image illustrates Fitz-Hugh–Curtis syndrome, in which individuals develop adhesions between the diaphragm and liver. It is associated with pelvic inflammatory disease, which can occur as the result of an infection with *Neisseria gonorrhoeae* or *Chlamydia trachomatis*. Pelvic inflammatory disease, because of causing adhesions affecting the uterus, ovaries, and even small intestine, can lead to infertility, ectopic pregnancy, and bowel obstruction (**C**). Pelvic inflammatory disease and Fitz-Hugh–Curtis syndrome are not risk factors for the other listed conditions. (**A-B, D-E**). Fitz-Hugh–Curtis syndrome can cause right upper quadrant pain and mimic cholecystitis.

61. Correct: Congestive heart failure (C)

The image illustrates a pleural effusion. The pleural effusion is watery and straw-colored, which is consistent with a transudate due to congestive heart failure (**C**). An empyema would be more cloudy and yellow-green or yellow-white, and a chylothorax would appear more milky (**A, B**). Pleural effusions due to an empyema or chylothorax would be rare compared to pleural effusions due to congestive heart failure. A pleural effusion due to pulmonary neoplasm would be more cloudy as well (**D**). An autoimmune disorder can cause a serositis and pleural effusion, but his past history does not indicate such a condition (**E**). The clinical scenario (i.e., repeat admissions for pleural effusions) is also consistent with congestive heart failure.

62. Correct: The lesion is most common in the apices of the lungs. (D)

The image illustrates pulmonary emphysema. Patients with pulmonary emphysema have a decreased FEV1/FVC ratio (**A**), are normally older individuals (**B**), and the main cause of the condition is tobacco/cigarette use (**C**). Microscopic examination would reveal loss of pulmonary parenchyma, but essentially no fibrosis (**E**). Cigarette smoke tends to rise, and therefore, the apices of the lung are the most commonly involved (**D**). In α-1-antitrypsin deficiency, patients can develop both emphysema and cirrhosis. Unlike the emphysema due to cigarette smoke, the emphysema in α-1-antitrypsin deficiency diffusely involves the lungs (i.e., is present in each lobe equally); however, the majority of cases of emphysema are associated with cigarette use and not α-1-antitrypsin deficiency.

63. Correct: Raised tender lesions on the fingers can occur. (E)

The image illustrates a vegetation in an individual with endocarditis. Bacterial endocarditis commonly involves the aortic and mitral valves, as well as the tricuspid valve in intravenous drug users, but the pulmonary valve would be the least likely to be involved (**B**). Common bacteria causing bacterial endocarditis are viridans streptococci and *Staphylococcus aureus*. *Pseudomonas aeruginosa* could cause endocarditis, but the incidence would be low (**C**). The lesion is not an atrial myxoma, which occurs most commonly in the left atrium adjacent to the fossa ovalis, and it is not a precursor to a papillary fibroelastoma (**A, D**). Complications and manifestations of bacterial endocarditis include raised tender lesions on the fingers (Osler nodes), erythematous lesions on the palm or sole (Janeway lesion), splinter hemorrhages, septic emboli, valvular regurgitation, and glomerulonephritis, due to immune complex deposition (**E**).

64. Correct: Cirrhosis of the liver (C)

The image illustrates the esophagus (tubular structure), the gastroesophageal junction, and an opened portion of the stomach. The esophagus has been turned inside-out to reveal the mucosal surface. The mucosal surface of the esophagus normally does not have visible blood vessels. In this case, the visible blood vessels represent esophageal varices. The most common cause of esophageal varices, and essentially the only cause, is cirrhosis of the liver (C). Gastroesophageal reflex would lead to glandular metaplasia (**B**), prolonged vomiting can lead to a mucosal tear (i.e., a Mallory-Weiss laceration) (**D**), and ingestion of lye would damage the mucosa, as would a viral infection (**A, E**).

65. Correct: Long bone fracture (D)

The clinical scenario is consistent with fatty emboli syndrome. The image illustrates a small vessel in the lung filled with several clear spaces, which are fat. To retain the fat in the lung, special procedures must be followed, or fresh lung can be cut from a frozen section and stained with an Oil-Red-O stain. Fatty emboli syndrome most commonly is associated with long bone fractures (**D**), occurring several days after the fracture, but has also been associated with acute pancreatitis and fatty trauma. None of the other conditions listed are a risk factor for fatty emboli (**A-C, E**).

66. Correct: Males with the condition can have gynecomastia and testicular atrophy. (D)

The image illustrates cirrhosis of the liver. While hepatitis B and C (and D, if B already infects the patient) can lead to cirrhosis, hepatitis A causes an acute disease, but not a chronic form (**A**). While cirrhosis can affect children (e.g., those with galactosemia), it most commonly affects adults (**B**). It is not a risk factor for an acute myocardial infarct, and microscopic examination will reveal a hepatic parenchyma divided into nodules by fibrous septa (**C, E**). Granulomas are not a component of cirrhosis (**E**). Due to changes in hormones induced by the condition, males can develop gynecomastia and testicular atrophy (**D**).

67. Correct: Fatty streaks (D)

The image illustrates fatty streaks in the aorta (**D**). The openings in the wall of the aorta are for the intercostal arteries. Syphilic aortitis is a late-term complication of the disease and would be unlikely in a young adult, and the intima more characteristically has a tree-bark appearance (**A**). Polyarteritis nodosa does not affect the aorta (**B**), and Takayasu's arteritis usually affects the thoracic aorta or its major branches, such as the subclavian artery (**E**). The lesions are not tears (**C**).

68. Correct: The neoplastic cells frequently stain with CD20. (D)

The image illustrates a follicular lymphoma, with back-to-back follicles present. Follicular lymphoma most commonly occurs in adults (**A**), and patients usually live around 5 to 10 years after initial diagnosis (**B**), even though most patients are initially diagnosed at a high stage. The tumor is most frequently associated with a t(14;18); however, the two genes involved are the *BCL2* gene, and the Ig heavy chain gene (**C**). Follicular hyperplasia, which occurs due to an infectious process, has a similar appearance to follicular lymphoma, and without due care, a follicular lymphoma can be misdiagnosed as a benign process, or a benign process can be misdiagnosed as a malignant neoplasm (**E**). As the cells of origin in follicular lymphoma are B cells, the neoplastic cells stain with CD20 (**D**).

69. Correct: A nutrient deficiency (C)

The image illustrates a nodular goiter, with its colloid appearance visible in the cut sections. Goiter most commonly develops due to a deficiency of iodine (**C**). Although the thyroid gland is greatly enlarged, patients are usually euthyroid, with the increased size of the thyroid representing the body's adaptation to the low iodine levels, creating a condition that will recycle as much iodine as possible. The other conditions listed will not produce a nodular goiter (**A-B, D-E**).

70. Correct: Noncaseating granuloma (C)

The image illustrates a noncaseating granuloma (**C**). A granuloma is composed of epithelioid histiocytes, which can have giant cells (note: the giant cells are not necessary components of a granuloma but help in their identification). In a caseating granuloma, there is central necrosis, which is not present in the image (**B**). There is no significant number of neutrophils in the image, no amyloid, and no neoplastic cells (**A, D, E**).

71. Correct: Increased TSH (A)

The image illustrates Hashimoto's thyroiditis. Residual thyroid follicles are present as well as lymphocytic clusters with germinal centers and oncocytic change. Patients with Hashimoto's thyroiditis would have elevated TSH (**A**), because the decreased function of the thyroid gland stimulates the pituitary gland, which releases TSH. The other choices are incorrect (**B-F**).

72. Correct: Antithyroglobulin antibodies (B)

The image illustrates Hashimoto's thyroiditis. Patients with Hashimoto's thyroiditis can have antithyroglobulin or antithyroid peroxidase antibodies (**B**). Anti-TSH receptor antibodies are found in Graves' disease (**A**). Anti-21-hydroxylase antibodies are found in Addison's disease (**C**). Antimitochondrial antibodies are found in primary biliary cirrhosis (**D**). Anti–smooth muscle antibodies are found in autoimmune hepatitis (**E**).

73. Correct: Hepatocellular carcinoma (E)

Hepatocellular carcinomas can exhibit features that are normally found associated with non-neoplastic hepatocytes, including fat accumulation, Mallory's hyaline, and bile production. The nuclei in this histologic section are pleomorphic, consistent with a neoplasm, since hepatocyte nuclei are usually round and regular. The cells contain fat, and abundant Mallory's hyaline is present (**E**). The histologic features are not consistent with the remainder of the choices (**A-D**).

74. Correct: Positive test for tartrate-resistant acid phosphatase (C)

The clinical scenario (an older male with pancytopenia and splenomegaly) is consistent with hairy cell leukemia, and the cell illustrated in the blood smear in the image is hairy cell leukemia. The characteristic laboratory abnormality in hairy cell leukemia is a positive test for tartrate-resistant acid phosphatase (**C**). A t(9;22) translocation is found in CML and some forms of ALL (**A**). A t(11;14) is found in mantle cell lymphoma (**B**). A positive mono spot test would indicate an EBV infection (**E**), which can result in atypical lymphocytes, but these have a more abundant cytoplasm and abut adjacent red blood cells. Antibodies directed against the A blood group antigen are not characteristic of hairy cell leukemia (**D**).

75. Correct: Hypertrophic cardiomyopathy (C)

The image illustrates myocardial disarray, which is also referred to as whorled or pin-wheeled, and fibrosis, which are the characteristic microscopic features of hypertrophic cardiomyopathy (**C**). The clinical scenario is also consistent with this diagnosis—the sudden death of a young individual while engaged in physical activity. The histologic features are not consistent with the remainder of the choices (**A-B, D-E**).

76. Correct: Endocardial fibrosis of the left ventricular outflow tract (C)

The histologic features are consistent with hypertrophic cardiomyopathy. The characteristic gross features of hypertrophic cardiomyopathy are asymmetrical thickening of the interventricular septum and endocardial fibrosis of the left ventricular outflow tract (C). The fibrosis of the left ventricular outflow tract corresponds to the location of the anterior leaflet of the mitral valve, where it would contact the thickened interventricular septum. The other changes listed are not characteristic of hypertrophic cardiomyopathy (A-B, D-E).

77. Correct: The lesion can cause death. (D)

The image illustrates a cavernous hemangioma. Cavernous hemangiomas are relatively common incidental findings in the liver. They usually occur in visceral organs, and not usually in the skin (A). Capillary hemangiomas most often are found in the skin. While capillary hemangiomas are likely to regress, cavernous hemangiomas do not (B). Malignant transformation of a cavernous hemangioma to an angiosarcoma would be extremely rare (C), and the lesion is not usually associated with neurofibromatosis (E). Patients with a hepatic hemangioma can die if the mass ruptures, causing an intraperitoneal hemorrhage (D).

78. Correct: Hemochromatosis (C)

The clinical history is consistent with hemochromatosis (C), with organ involvement of the pancreas causing diabetes mellitus, and the liver, causing cirrhosis. Bronze discoloration of the skin is also characteristic of the disease; hence the name "bronze diabetes." The image illustrates a Prussian blue stain of the liver showing extensive iron deposition. The histologic features are not consistent with the other choices (A-B, D-E).

79. Correct: Trauma (C)

The image illustrates extensive hemosiderin deposition. Hemosiderin accumulates after the breakdown of red blood cells. Although hemorrhage can occur as a result of infection and neoplasms, it is not usually the major component of the process, and, given that the hemorrhage is in the soft tissue of an extremity, the most likely underlying cause is trauma (C). The other choices are not the best option (A-B, D-E).

80. Correct: Hodgkin's lymphoma (C)

The histologic features are consistent with Hodgkin's lymphoma (C). Reed-Sternberg cells are present, and the background inflammation includes lymphocytes and eosinophils. Follicular lymphoma would have back-to-back follicles (A). Diffuse large B-cell lymphoma would have a proliferation of homogeneous-appearing cells (B). Small-cell carcinoma has small cells with a high nuclear-to-cytoplasmic ratio and exhibits nuclear molding (D). Squamous cell carcinoma would have malignant squamous cells with intercellular bridges and keratin pearls (E).

81. Correct: Systemic hypertension (A)

The histologic change illustrated in the image is hyaline arteriolosclerosis. Hyaline arteriolosclerosis can occur in either systemic hypertension or diabetes mellitus (A). The mechanism is different, but the histologic appearance is the same. The hypertension damage to the endothelium allows serum proteins to leak into and accumulate within the wall of the blood vessel, while in diabetes mellitus, the histologic appearance is due to accumulation of advanced glycosylation end products. The other conditions have a different histologic appearance (B-E).

82. Correct: Hypertension (D)

The image illustrates cardiac hypertrophy. Although it is difficult to identify enlarged cardiac myocytes, the nuclei can be used to identify hypertrophy. A hypertrophied cardiac myocyte has an enlarged, rectangular nucleus, referred to as a boxcar nucleus. More irregularity in shape and even multinucleation is also possible. One of the main causes of cardiac hypertrophy is hypertension (D). The image has no histologic features consistent with any of the other answers (A-C, E).

83. Correct: Acute myocardial infarct (C)

In the inferoseptal region of the heart is a pale region that corresponds to an acute myocardial infarct (C). The interventricular septum is not thickened, as would be expected in hypertrophic cardiomyopathy (A). Myocarditis would have a patchy pallor throughout the entire left ventricle (B). Cardiac amyloidosis would also most likely be patchy and involve the entire left ventricle (D). The left ventricle and right ventricle are not dilated (E).

84. Correct: 1 day (C)

For an acute myocardial infarct to be identified in the myocardium grossly, about 1 day must have passed since the infarct occurred (A-C). Treatment with chemicals can allow for identification of earlier infarcts (i.e., those less than 1 day of age), but these chemicals are not commonly used because of their carcinogenic nature. At 2 to 3 days, the infarct will be well established and usually yellow in color. At 3 to 5 days, macrophages begin to infiltrate the infarct, engulfing necrotic debris, causing the infarct to be somewhat retracted from the cut surface (D). At 10 days, granulation tissue should be developing (E). Of importance, from 2 months on, there is a dense fibrous scar; however, sometimes a scar (indicative of greater than 2 months from the time of the infarct to the time of examination of the heart) can mimic an acute infarct, appearing as a pale region. Histologic confirmation is necessary.

85. Correct: Right (E)

In the infero-septal region of the left ventricle is a pale discoloration of the myocardium. The right coronary artery, in a right-dominant individual, is the vessel that supplies this region of the heart (**E**). To identify the position in the left ventricle, remember that the mitral valve has an anterolateral and posteromedial papillary muscle, which are both visible in this section, and that the inferior wall of the right ventricle is thicker than the anterior wall. The other choices are not correct (**A-D**).

86. Correct: Squamous cell carcinoma (A)

The image illustrates a keratin pearl, which is found in squamous cell carcinomas that are well or moderately differentiated (**A**). A poorly differentiated tumor may not have any of the characteristic histologic features from its cell of origin. The histologic features are not consistent with the other tumors listed, although it is possible for a mature teratoma to develop a squamous cell carcinoma (**B-E**).

87. Correct: Hypoxia-ischemia (D)

The image illustrates red neurons. Red neurons occur due to hypoxic or ischemic injury (**D**). Although the other four conditions can contribute to hypoxic-ischemic injury, the only histologic finding is the red neurons, and there is nothing else to suggest an etiology for the hypoxic-ischemic event (**A-C, E**).

88. Correct: Diabetes mellitus (B)

Diabetes mellitus is a significant risk factor for non-healing ulcers of the feet (**B**). People with diabetes mellitus have damage to both arteries and nerves. Nerve damage leads to an inability to feel minor trauma to the feet, allowing injuries to occur and go unnoticed, and, because of damage to the arteries, the feet have poor vascular supply, and injuries do not heal well. Amyloidosis affects vessels, but would be a rare cause of a nonhealing ulcer (**D**). Thromboangiitis obliterans can cause ulceration of the extremities, but is rare compared to diabetes mellitus (**C**). Congestive heart failure can cause chronic venous stasis and ulceration of the skin; however, amputation would rarely be required (**A**). Poorly healed trauma could lead to ulceration, but, compared to diabetes mellitus, would be rare. As long as an individual seeks treatment for the trauma, and is careful, the injuries should heal completely, albeit with variable loss of function depending on the extent of the injury (**E**).

89. Correct: Diabetic nephropathy (C)

The image illustrates a classic Kimmelstiel-Wilson lesion, which is the characteristic histologic features of diabetic nephropathy (**C**). The other choices are incorrect (**A-B, D-E**).

90. Correct: Acute pancreatitis (B)

The image illustrates three cross-sections of the pancreas, each suffused with blood. The image is that of acute hemorrhagic pancreatitis (**B**). Acute pancreatitis is a serious condition and can have a fairly high mortality rate, as it leads to diffuse alveolar damage and disseminated intravascular coagulation. There is no evidence of a mass or of chronic pancreatitis, which would show fibrosis, calcification, and possible pseudocyst formation (**A, C**). Given the protected location of the pancreas, abdominal trauma is less likely, and diffuse infiltration of the pancreas with blood would not be usual (**D**). Waterhouse-Friderichsen syndrome is a diffuse infiltration of the adrenal glands with blood and is associated with *Neisseria meningitidis* (**E**), which is not consistent with the clinical history.

91. Correct: Coxsackievirus A infection (C)

The image illustrates lymphocytic myocarditis, which is characterized by a lymphocytic infiltrate and cardiac myocyte damage. One of the most common causes of lymphocytic myocarditis is coxsackievirus A or B infection (**C**). Coronary artery atherosclerosis does not cause the histologic changes shown (**A**). A recent medication change would be associated with a hypersensitivity myocarditis, which is characterized by perivascular infiltrates of eosinophils (**B**). Hypertrophic cardiomyopathy has myocyte disarray (**D**), and sarcoidosis has granulomas (**E**), neither of which are present in the image.

92. Correct: Steatohepatitis (B)

In the center of the image is a fat vacuole rimmed with neutrophils, which is the characteristic histologic appearance of steatohepatitis (**B**). Steatohepatitis can occur in alcoholics, and it can also occur in nonalcoholics (nonalcoholic steatohepatitis, NASH). NASH is more common in people who are obese and those who have diabetes mellitus. This condition, if persistent and severe, can lead to cirrhosis of the liver. The image does not have histologic features consistent with the other choices (**A, C-E**).

93. Correct: Pulmonary thromboembolus (D)

The image illustrates a vessel with a thrombus. Within that thrombus are lines of Zahn, which indicate that the thrombus formed in a vessel, which results in the intermittent layering of red blood cells and white blood cells. This thrombus then embolizes, which would create a pulmonary thromboembolus (**D**). The features in the blood vessel are not consistent with the other listed diagnoses (**A-C, E**).

94. Correct: Recent use of antibiotics (D)

The image illustrates pseudomembranous colitis. Pseudomembranous colitis can arise after antibiotic use, with the antibiotics killing the normal gut flora and allowing the overgrowth of *Clostridium difficile* (**D**). Pseudomembranes can also occur in some bacterial infections (e.g., *Shigella*, certain *Staphylococcus* infections) and in ischemia. Drinking water from a stream is a risk for *Giardia lamblia* (**A**), sensitivity to gluten can lead to celiac disease (**B**), the *NOD2* gene most likely plays a role in inflammatory bowel disease (**C**), and weakness of the colonic wall can contribute to diverticula (**E**). None of these choices are associated with pseudomembranes.

95.   Correct: Age-related changes (B)

The image illustrates a heart with lipofuscin pigment surrounding each nucleus in the cardiac myocytes. Lipofuscin deposition is normally perinuclear. Lipofuscin is a wear-and-tear pigment, with increasing amounts accumulating as a person ages (**B**). The histologic section has no evidence of any of the other choices (**A, C-E**).

96.   Correct: Congestive heart failure (D)

The image illustrates pitting edema, which is a characteristic physical finding in congestive heart failure (**D**). Metastatic carcinoma and cirrhosis of the liver would not normally produce edema in the lower extremities, and peripheral vascular disease would not normally cause shortness of breath (**B-C, E**). Both a pulmonary thromboembolus and congestive heart failure can cause edema of the lower extremities and shortness of breath; however, pitting edema is characteristic for congestive heart failure, and deep venous thrombi do not normally cause pitting edema (**A**).

97.   Correct: Interstitial lung disease (D)

The pathologic lesion is a pleural plaque. Although not diagnostic, pleural plaques are very suggestive of prior asbestos exposure. In addition to pleural plaques, asbestos exposure can also lead to a pleural mesothelioma and asbestosis, an interstitial lung disease (**D**). The characteristic microscopic finding in asbestos exposure is a ferruginous body; however, none are normally found in the pleural plaques, which are usually located only in the pulmonary parenchyma. The other conditions listed are not normally associated with pleural plaques (**A-C, E**).

98.   Correct: Small spleen (D)

The sinusoids in the liver contain sickled red blood cells. The multiple admissions to the hospital were most likely for painful crises, due to necrosis of bone marrow secondary to ischemia caused by sickled red blood cells obstructing the vasculature. This same process can lead to autoinfarction of the spleen (**D**), with the patient then being at greater risk for infection with encapsulated organisms. The other features listed are not characteristic of sickle cell anemia (**A-C, E**).

99.   Correct: Hepatitis A infection (B)

The patient has jaundice. Although excessive amounts of carotene and betadine staining of the skin could mimic jaundice, the elevated AST is not consistent with these mechanisms (**D, E**). The other three conditions could each contribute to increased bilirubin; however, the normal haptoglobin concentration rules out hemolysis, excluding TTP (**A**), and the fact that the AST is markedly elevated, but the alkaline phosphatase is normal, favors a hepatic process over the cholestatic process, excluding ascending cholangitis (**C**). Of the choices, the clinical scenario is most consistent with hepatitis A infection (**B**).

100.   Correct: A positive Homans' sign (A)

The image illustrates a pulmonary thromboembolus. The underlying cause of a pulmonary thromboembolus is immobility, endothelial damage, and hypercoagulability (Virchow triad). These factors contribute to the development of deep venous thrombi, which can then break free and embolize to the lung, causing sudden death or pulmonary infarcts. The presence of a deep venous thrombi can lead to a positive Homans' sign (**A**), pain on palpation of the calf when the foot is dorsiflexed. A positive Babinski's sign is an upgoing toe when the foot is stroked, and indicates an upper motor neuron defect (**B**). A positive Auspitz's sign is seen in psoriasis (**C**), a positive Nikolsky's sign in pemphigus vulgaris (**D**), and a positive Kernig's sign in meningitis (**E**).

101.   Correct: Patients can develop a restrictive cardiomyopathy. (E)

The bone marrow contains a prominent number of plasma cells. Given the lytic bone lesions in the skull, the patient most likely has multiple myeloma. The majority of patients (about 80%) with multiple myeloma will have an M spike (**A**). The most common immunoglobin is IgG (about 60%), with IgA less frequent, and, in some cases, the patient will produce only light chains (**B**). Because of the abnormal production of immunoglobulins, the risk of infection is quite high (**C**), and often, the cause of death for patients with myeloma is an infection. The normal age range in which multiple myeloma occurs is around 50 to 60 years of age (**D**). Patients with myeloma can develop amyloidosis, due to deposition of the immunoglobulin chains being produced, and amyloidosis can present as a restrictive cardiomyopathy (**E**).

102.   Correct: Papillary carcinoma (A)

The image illustrates a papillary architecture, with the neoplastic cells having cleared-out nuclei, which, of the choices, is most consistent with papillary thyroid carcinoma. At the bottom of the image is a psammoma body, which is also characteristic for papillary thyroid carcinoma (**A**). Microscopic examination of the tumor reveals no follicles, amyloid deposition, anaplastic features, or lymphoid cells (**B-E**).

103. Correct: Congestive heart failure (C)

The image illustrates a nutmeg liver, which is caused by centrilobular congestion, leading to ischemic injury, which can cause atrophy or necrosis and possible scarring. Individuals with long-term centrilobular congestion, such as from congestive heart failure, and the other mentioned changes can develop cirrhosis of the liver, so-called cardiac cirrhosis (**C**). The appearance of the liver very much resembles the cut surface of a nutmeg. The liver is not cirrhotic, and the evenly distributed areas of hemorrhagic discoloration are the congestion of the centrilobular sinusoids and not a bleeding, neoplastic, or metastatic process (**A-B, D-E**).

104. Correct: Pulmonary anthracosis (C)

The image illustrates squamous metaplasia of an airway. Squamous metaplasia is due to irritants to the bronchial epithelium, necessitating a switch to a more protective epithelial type (i.e., from respiratory-type epithelium to squamous-type epithelium). If the irritants continue, squamous metaplasia can lead to dysplasia and ultimately neoplasia, explaining why cigarette smokers can develop squamous cell carcinoma of the lung. The only other condition listed that is commonly associated with cigarette use is pulmonary anthracosis (**C**), which is the black pigmentation of the pleural surface of the lungs due to accumulation of carbonaceous pigment in macrophages and within lymphatics. The other conditions listed are not usually associated with tobacco use (**A-B, D-E**).

105. Correct: Anti-SSA or anti-SSB (D)

The image illustrates a salivary gland, with normal glandular elements being found in the upper left corner. Also throughout the specimen is a lymphocytic infiltrate. This individual has Sjögren's syndrome, which is marked by a dry mouth and dry eyes and is an autoimmune disorder most often associated with rheumatoid arthritis. Although testing for ANAs can be positive (**A**), anti-SSA or anti-SSB are more specific for Sjögren's syndrome (**D**). Anti-dsDNA and anti-Smith antibodies are associated with SLE (**B, C**), and anti-U1 RNP antibodies are associated with mixed connective tissue disorder (**E**).

106. Correct: Acute alcohol intoxication (C)

The image illustrates aspiration pneumonia. In the airway in the center of the image, which is filled with neutrophils, is foreign material, possibly degenerated vegetable matter. Aspiration pneumonia occurs in those individuals who have neuromuscular impairment, such as would occur with acute alcohol intoxication (C). There are no histologic features consistent with or specific to the other diagnoses (**A-B, D-E**).

107. Correct: Pheochromocytoma (B)

The image illustrates a pheochromocytoma (**B**). A strip of normal adrenal gland is present along the inferior aspect of the pathologic specimen. After fixation, the tumor develops a more brown-red coloration. A pheochromocytoma is a cause of secondary hypertension, with patients often having episodic hypertension corresponding to intermittent release of catecholamines. Testing for metanephrines in the urine can assist in the diagnosis. Although the other conditions listed could appear similar to a pheochromocytoma (with the exception of sarcoidosis, which would be more likely to be a white, or tan-white color), none are a common cause of secondary hypertension when manifested in the adrenal gland (**A, C-E**).

108. Correct: Hypotension (C)

The bowel is dilated, and one segment has a darker red discoloration of the serosal surface. The gross changes are consistent with ischemic bowel. Ischemic bowel due to hypotension most often develops at the watershed areas, including the splenic flexure (**C**). The changes illustrated in the image are not characteristic of any of the other conditions that are listed (**A-B, D-E**).

109. Correct: Meckel's diverticulum (E)

The pathologic condition illustrated involves the intestine, so it is not an aneurysm (**A**). The involved organs are loops, and the serosa has no attached soft tissue, so it is not Zenker's diverticulum, which occurs in the esophagus (**C**). The lesion is not at the gastroesophageal junction and instead occurs within a tubular structure; therefore it is not a hiatal hernia (**D**). The intestine in the image is small and not the large intestine, as there are no taeniae coli; therefore, of the choices, the best is Meckel's diverticulum (**B, E**). A Meckel's diverticulum is a remnant of the vitelline duct and commonly occurs in the small intestine near the ileocecal valve. In addition to small intestine mucosa, they can also contain gastric or pancreatic tissue.

110. Correct: Hyaline membranes (C)

The image illustrates hyaline membranes (**C**). Hyaline membranes, in adults are termed diffuse alveolar damage, which corresponds to the clinical diagnosis of acute respiratory distress syndrome, which can occur due to a variety of conditions, including, commonly, sepsis. Hyaline membrane disease occurs in premature infants due to a lack of surfactant and has a similar histologic appearance. The histologic changes are not specific for any of the other conditions listed (**A-B, D-E**).

111. Correct: Thrombotic thrombocytopenic purpura (C)

The image illustrates schistocytes. The findings of microangiopathic hemolytic anemia, thrombocytopenia, fever, mental status changes, and acute renal failure are characteristic for thrombotic thrombocytopenic purpura (**C**). Although disseminated intravascular coagulation (DIC) can also cause schistocytes, in DIC the PT and PTT would be elevated, whereas they are normal in TTP (**A**). ITP would affect the platelets but would not cause the other changes (**B**). von Willebrand's disease would present with bleeding (**D**), and in essential thrombocythemia, a chronic myeloproliferative disorder, the platelet count should be elevated (**E**).

---

112. Correct: ADAMTS-13 (B)

The clinical scenario is consistent with thrombotic thrombocytopenic purpura (TTP). TTP is due to a deficiency of ADAMTS-13, which is an enzyme that breaks down very high-weight multimers of von Willebrand's factor (**B**). A G6PD deficiency is associated with the finding of Heinz bodies, which are denatured hemoglobin, and bite cells, a result of phagocytes removing the Heinz bodies from the red blood cell (**A**). Individuals with G6PD deficiency are often asymptomatic until they encounter some form of oxidative stress. Deficiencies of hexokinase, glucose phosphate isomerase, and enolase could present with a hemolytic anemia, but not the other clinical symptoms (**C-E**). Hexokinase deficiency and enolase deficiency are very rare.

---

113. Correct: Psammoma body (C)

The clinical scenario indicates a thyroid neoplasm. The histologic features of the tumor illustrated are consistent with papillary thyroid carcinoma. One feature of papillary thyroid carcinoma is a psammoma body (**C**). Psammoma bodies are also found in meningiomas. Asteroid bodies and Schaumann bodies are associated with sarcoidosis (**A, B**). Schiller-Duval bodies are associated with yolk sac tumors (**D**). Michaelis-Gutmann bodies are associated with malakoplakia (**E**).

---

114. Correct: Coronary artery plaque hemorrhage (D)

The image illustrates hemorrhage into a coronary artery atherosclerotic plaque, with associated thrombus of the lumen. The man is having unstable angina, which could continue to the development of an acute myocardial infarction if he is not treated quickly. Unstable angina is due to an acute change in a plaque, as is present in this case, whereas stable angina results from a plaque that has increased in size enough to produce significant obstruction to the flow of blood but without an acute change (**A, D**). Kawasaki's disease causing an arteritis would present at a much younger age and, in an older person, would present as a coronary artery aneurysm (**E**). A dissection would be in the media, and not the intima, and there is no mass lesion, such as would occur with a hemangioma (**B, C**).

---

115. Correct: Myxomatous mitral valve (D)

The image illustrates a mitral valve. Note the thick myocardium, representing the left ventricle, and not the right ventricle, and the chordae tendineae, which are not a feature of the aortic valve (**A**). The leaflets also are not similar to those of the aortic valve. The

leaflets are thickened and ballooned upward (also described as redundant), which is characteristic of a myxomatous mitral valve, or floppy mitral valve, which is responsible for the clinical entity of mitral valve prolapse (**D**). Carcinoid syndrome is much less common than a myxomatous mitral valve and normally affects the tricuspid valve (**C**). There is no evidence of endocarditis or mitral annular calcification (**B, E**). A myxomatous mitral valve can lead to regurgitation, which can cause dyspnea and fatigue.

---

116. Correct: Sudden death can result. (C)

The image illustrates a myxomatous mitral valve. Although a myxomatous mitral valve is commonly asymptomatic, the condition can result in mitral regurgitation and, occasionally, sudden death (**C**). The condition is common, occurring in a small percent of the population (**A**), and it affects both women and men (**D**). As the valve is abnormal, it presents a risk factor for the development of endocarditis (**B**). The change in the leaflet is from myxoid deposition thickening the leaflet and not adipose tissue infiltration (**E**).

---

117. Correct: He may develop neuromuscular complaints related to the tumor. (E)

The image illustrates small-cell carcinoma. Small-cell carcinoma has small cells with a very high nuclear-to-cytoplasm ratio (i.e., the cell is mostly nucleus, with only a tiny amount of cytoplasm), and there is nuclear molding, in which one cell adjacent to another will indent the nucleus. Most small-cell carcinomas are centrally located (**A**), associated with cigarette use, and have a poor prognosis (**D**), as they are considered to have metastasized at the time they are diagnosed. Paraneoplastic syndromes related to small-cell carcinoma are production of ACTH and ADH, as well as Lambert-Eaton syndrome, which produces proximal muscle weakness (**E**). Squamous cell carcinoma is most characteristic for producing parathyroid-like hormone (**C**). Asbestos exposure is a risk factor for mesotheliomas and bronchogenic carcinomas, but is not necessarily a major risk factor for small-cell carcinoma (**B**).

---

118. Correct: Peptic ulcer (D)

The image illustrates gastric mucosa with *Helicobacter pylori* on the mucosal surface. *H. pylori* infection is a very common cause of gastric peptic ulcers (with NSAID use also well associated with gastric peptic ulcers), and it is almost always the underlying cause for duodenal peptic ulcers (**D**). *H. pylori* infection is not associated with the remainder of the conditions that are listed (**A-C, E**).

---

119. Correct: Kawasaki's disease (C)

The image illustrates an intramyocardial artery with extensive thickening of the intima. The symptoms described (fever, cervical lymphadenopathy, oral erythema, and rash of the palms and soles) occurring in a young child are consistent with Kawasaki's disease. Kawasaki's disease affects the coronary arteries, causing coronary artery aneurysms, but it can also cause intimal thickening (**C**). The changes are not consistent with hyaline or hyperplastic arteriolosclerosis, such as could occur in patients with hypertension (**A**). Chronic rheumatic fever affects the cardiac valves and is not associated with coronary artery changes (**B**). The intimal thickening is cellular, but not in concentric layers, such as would be seen in hyperplastic arteriolosclerosis. Thromboangiitis obliterans essentially affects only smokers, and it affects arteries of the distal portion of the extremities (**E**). Polyarteritis nodosa would have either a transmural necrotizing inflammation or resultant scarring (**D**).

120. Correct: Subacute combined degeneration of the spinal cord. (C)

The image illustrates a hyper-segmented neutrophil, which is characteristic of megaloblastic anemia; other findings on a blood smear can include oval macrocytes. Megaloblastic anemia is due to either folate or B12 deficiency. As the patient had a gastrectomy, with subsequent decreased ability to absorb B12 because of the loss of intrinsic factor production by parietal cells of the stomach, a B12 deficiency is most likely. A B12 deficiency, but not a folate deficiency, is a cause of peripheral neuropathy and subacute combined degeneration of the spinal cord, which involves the posterior and lateral columns (**C**). Central pontine myelinolysis is associated with rapid correction of hyponatremia and with alcoholism (**A**). Descending Wallerian degeneration is due to damage to an axon, with subsequent breakdown of the segment distal to the injury (**B**). A B12 deficiency is not a risk factor for multiple sclerosis or a brainstem astrocytoma (**D, E**).

121. Correct: Hypoxic injury (A)

The image illustrates red neurons, which are the histologic change occurring following hypoxic or ischemic injury. The change essentially represents coagulative necrosis of the neuron (**A**). There is no evidence of microglial nodules or perivascular cuffing of vessels with lymphocytes, foamy macrophages, a neoplastic process, or injuries, such as contusions (**B-E**).

122. Correct: Alzheimer's disease (D)

The image illustrates neurofibrillary tangles, which, along with senile plaques, are the characteristic histologic finding in Alzheimer's disease (**D**). These changes also occur with aging, and thus, the diagnosis of Alzheimer's disease requires a clinical-pathologic correlation. There are no Pick bodies or Lewy bodies (**A, C**). The diagnosis of multi-infarct dementia and chronic subdural hemorrhage would require examination of the brain grossly; however, their incidence is lower (**C, E**).

123. Correct: Basal cell carcinoma (C)

In the dermis is a neoplasm composed of nests of relatively bland cells with peripheral palisading. This appearance is consistent with a basal cell carcinoma, and these neoplasms usually occur on sun-exposed skin (**C**). Notice that the neoplasm has an epithelial appearance, as opposed to nevi that are more neural-appearing (**A, B**). The lesion does not appear like a squamous cell carcinoma nor like a melanoma (**D, E**).

124. Correct: Subarachnoid hemorrhage (D)

Just anterior to the optic chiasm, between the olfactory tracts, and in the midline of the brain, is a calcified berry aneurysm. The aneurysm is in a common location, being in the anterior circulation near the junction of the anterior cerebral and anterior communicating cerebral arteries. Berry aneurysms have a risk for rupture, following which the patient will develop a subarachnoid hemorrhage, and sudden death can occur, with a ruptured berry aneurysm having about a 50% mortality rate (**D**). A berry aneurysm is not a risk factor for the other listed conditions (**A-C, E**).

125. Correct: Benign prostatic hyperplasia (B)

The diagnosis is benign prostatic hyperplasia (**B**). To the left and right of the urethra are multiple nodules that bulge from the cut surface. Their location leads to blockage of urine flow, and the reported symptoms. Prostatic adenocarcinoma is usually located posterior, and can be felt with a rectal examination (i.e., the finger would be palpating the portion of the prostate at the inferior part of the image) (**C**). Although a leiomyoma would have a similar appearance (i.e., being a well-circumscribed mass that bulges from the cut surface), it would be a rare tumor of the prostate (**D**). Acute prostatitis will often have abscess formation, which is not present; would not be as common; and would most likely develop much more quickly (**A**). There is no mass in the urethra to suggest a transitional cell carcinoma (**E**).

126. Correct: Thrombocytopenia can occur. (E)

The pathologic lesion is a capillary hemangioma. Capillary hemangiomas occur commonly in the skin, and although surgical resection is curative (**D**), it is not usually warranted, as the lesion is likely to regress (**B**); therefore, forgoing surgical removal can prevent a scar or other dysfunction. Capillary hemangiomas cause a functional decrease in the number of platelets by accumulating them within the substance of the tumor, leading to thrombocytopenia (e.g., Kasabach-Merritt syndrome) (**E**). Often capillary hemangiomas are sporadic, and the presence of an internal malignancy is unlikely (**C**). Kaposi sarcoma is associated with HHV8 (**A**).

127. Correct: Bladder (E)

The image illustrates a keratin pearl, which is a histologic feature of squamous cell carcinoma. Excluding metastases, squamous cell carcinomas essentially do not occur in the brain, thyroid gland, liver, or adrenal gland (**A-D**); however, they can develop in the bladder (**E**). In the bladder, squamous cell carcinoma is associated with schistosomiasis and with chronic inflammation, such as from an indwelling catheter.

128. Correct: Dysplasia (C)

The glands at the top of the image have a similar architecture to the glands at the bottom of the image; however, the nuclei are larger and more hyperchromatic. This change represents dysplasia (**C**), which is a component of tubular adenomas, tubulovillous adenomas, and villous adenomas. Dysplasia can progress to neoplasia; however, neoplasia is not present (**D**) and neither are hyperplasia, metaplasia, or atrophy (**A, B, E**).

129. Correct: Glioblastoma multiforme (D)

The histologic section reveals a neural-appearing neoplasm, ruling out melanoma (**E**), with marked cellularity, necrosis, palisading around the areas of necrosis, and microvascular proliferation. Closer examination would reveal numerous mitotic figures. The presence of pleomorphism, necrosis, mitotic figures, and microvascular proliferation is characteristic of a high-grade astrocytoma, a glioblastoma multiforme (**D**). The characteristic microscopic feature of these tumors is nuclear palisading around the areas of necrosis. The histologic features are not consistent with the remainder of the conditions listed (**A-C**).

130. Correct: The condition is estrogen sensitive. (D)

The mass in the myometrium is a leiomyoma, which is also commonly called a fibroid. Leiomyomas are benign tumors composed of interlocking fascicles of smooth muscle (**C**) that very rarely undergo malignant degeneration (**A**), with pelvic radiation being a risk factor for malignant degeneration. Leiomyomas are a significant cause of infertility (**B**), premature labor, and spontaneous abortions, and they are estrogen sensitive (**D**), increasing in size during pregnancy and decreasing in size during menopause. The tumors occur in women of all ancestries and not just almost exclusively in white females (**E**).

131. Correct: They commonly have progesterone receptors. (E)

The image illustrates a meningioma. Meningiomas are most often benign (**B**) and do not invade or metastasize; however, some cases are aggressive. Meningiomas most commonly occur at the cranial vault (**C**). Microscopic examination will reveal whorls of meningothelial cells, and often psammoma bodies., not Schaumann bodies (**D**). Meningiomas are associated with neurofibromatosis 2 (**A**), and they are more frequent in women and often have progesterone receptors (**E**).

132. Correct: Phimosis (D)

The foreskin is contracted tightly, and will not retract, which is phimosis (**D**). Epispadias and hypospadias consist of the urethral orifice being on the dorsal or ventral (respectively) surface of the shaft of the penis (**A, B**). Condyloma would have a papillated or pedunculated mass (**E**). Penile carcinoma would be a mass (**C**).

133. Correct: Prostatic adenocarcinoma (D)

The diagnosis of prostatic adenocarcinoma is essentially a low-power diagnosis. Prostatic adenocarcinoma appears as small glands that are back to back, compared to the normal prostatic glands, which are larger and more widely spaced (**D**). No neutrophil clusters or abscesses are present (**B**). Prostatic infarcts would most commonly have an area of coagulative necrosis surrounded by squamous metaplasia (**C**). Pelvic intraepithelial neoplasia is a precursor of prostatic adenocarcinoma and appears as papillary-type epithelium within otherwise fairly normal-sized prostatic ducts (**E**). As the lesion is a neoplasm, it is not a hyperplastic process (**A**).

134. Correct: Mutation of the glutathione S-transferase gene promoter is often present (B)

Prostatic adenocarcinoma is most known for producing osteoblastic metastases (**A**), which can cause an elevated concentration of alkaline phosphatase (**D**), and which commonly involve the spine. Although the diagnosis can essentially be made on lower-power examination, high-power examination reveals the neoplastic glands to have one cell layer (**C**), and often blue mucin or crystals are present. Nucleoli are prominent. Prostatic adenocarcinoma is a common cause of death (**E**). Mutation of the glutathione S-transferase gene promoter is often present (**B**).

135. Correct: Hyperplastic arteriolosclerosis (C)

The vessel in the image has concentric cellular rings, which is characteristic of hyperplastic arteriolosclerosis (**C**). In hyaline arteriolosclerosis, the vessel wall is thick, eosinophilic, and acellular (**B**). Hyperplastic arteriolosclerosis is associated with malignant hypertension, and the precursor lesion is fibrinoid necrosis. The glomerulus in the image is essentially normal (**A**). Both polyarteritis nodosa and microscopic polyarteritis, in a single section with only one vessel, would appear as either transmural inflammation or scarring of the vessel wall (**D, E**).

136. Correct: HPV33 (B)

The image illustrates cervical intraepithelial neoplasia III (CINIII)/carcinoma in situ (CIS). There is full-thickness dysplasia, with atypical cells present all the way to the surface of the mucosa. CIN is essentially a sexually transmitted disease, being caused by infection with human papilloma virus (HPV). There are many different types of HPV. HPV11 is associated with a more low-grade dysplasia, such as CINI (**A**), while HPV33 is associated with a higher-grade dysplasia, like CINIII, which is more likely to progress to invasive squamous cell carcinoma of the cervix (**B**). The other conditions listed are not associated with an increased risk of CIN or invasive squamous cell carcinoma (**C-E**).

137. Correct: *Neisseria gonorrheae* (E)

The condition is Fitz-Hugh–Curtis syndrome, and results from *Neisseria gonorrheae* infection (**E**). The condition has also been associated with *Chlamydia trachomatis* infection but is not associated with the other conditions that are listed (**A-D**).

138. Correct: Mucinous cystadenoma (B)

The mass is multiloculated. Mucinous tumors tend to be multiloculated, while serous tumors tend to be uniloculated (**A, B**). Also, mucinous tumors are more likely to be benign than serous tumors; however, the majority of both mucinous and serous tumors are benign. The benign version of the tumor is termed a cystadenoma, and the malignant version is termed a cystadenocarcinoma. Between benign and malignant is a borderline category. Neoplastic tumors tend to be more complex, with papillary projections from the walls of the cysts and more solid areas throughout (**C, D**). A mature cystic teratoma would have hair, sebaceous material, and even teeth (**E**). In the image, the production of mucus can be seen (**B**).

139. Correct: *Streptococcus pneumoniae* (B)

The image illustrates meningitis. The meninges have a thick yellow-green exudate. In *Neisseria meningitidis* infection, no gross changes are usually appreciated, because the organism can cause death so quickly, before a good inflammatory infiltrate can develop (**A**). *Aspergillus flavus* and *Naegleria fowleri* can both cause meningitis but are very rare (**D, E**). *Cryptococcus neoformans* would produce more of a cystic and mucoid-type appearance (**C**). *Streptococcus pneumoniae* is the most common cause of meningitis in this type of patient (**B**).

140. Correct: It can lead to high-pitched bowel sounds and tympany to percussion. (E)

The image illustrates pelvic inflammatory disease, with the ovary and fallopian tube adherent to each other. Pelvic inflammatory disease is caused by *Neisseria gonorrheae* or *Chlamydia trachomatis* infection (**D**). It is not a risk factor for ovarian carcinoma (**A**); however, it is a risk factor for infertility and bowel obstruction (**C**). A bowel obstruction can produce high-pitched bowel sounds and tympany to percussion (**E**). Glands, stroma, and hemosiderin are indicative of endometriosis; however, no nodularity or mass lesion is present in this case. Only two of the three findings (glands, stroma, or hemosiderin) are required for the diagnosis of endometriosis (**B**).

141. Correct: Parkinson's disease (C)

The image illustrates Lewy bodies in neurons in the substantia nigra. The black pigment helps identify the location, although the locus ceruleus also has pigmented neurons. The Lewy bodies are the round eosinophilic inclusions with the surrounding clearings. Of the diseases listed, only Parkinson disease has Lewy bodies (**A-E**).

142. Correct: Cogwheel rigidity and flat affect (C)

The pathologic feature is Lewy bodies, which, based on the presence in pigmented neurons, is most likely in the substantia nigra, and represents Parkinson's disease. Parkinson's disease patients have cogwheel rigidity, flat affect, a pill-rolling tremor, a shuffling gait, and bradykinesia (**C**). Chorea is associated with Huntington's disease (**A**), and memory loss and diminished cognitive function are associated with dementia (**B**). About 20% of Parkinson's disease patients can also manifest dementia. Aphasia and cranial nerve palsies are not normally associated with Parkinson's disease (**D, E**).

143. Correct: Ruptured berry aneurysm (D)

The patient has a subarachnoid hemorrhage. Without a history of trauma, the most common cause of a subarachhnoid hemorrhage is a ruptured berry aneurysm (**D**). An intracerebral hemorrhage, which would be unlikely in this young patient without another underlying disease process, can rarely rupture through the cortical surface but would not cause a bilateral subarachnoid hemorrhage, and, under such circumstances, it usually produces a subdural hemorrhage as well (**B**). Meningitis is rarely hemorrhagic (**C**), and it would likely be in association with a fungal meningitis, which is rare in otherwise healthy individuals. A ruptured brain tumor would not likely cause a bilateral subarachnoid hemorrhage (**E**), and would be rare to rupture. AML would also be a rare cause (**A**).

144. Correct: Rapidly progressive glomerulonephritis (D)

The image illustrates rapidly progressive glomerulonephritis (**D**). The glomerulus has a crescent, which is characteristic of this disease process. The presenting symptoms are consistent with nephritic syndrome. FSGS and membranous glomerulonephropathy cause nephrotic syndrome (**A, B**), and postinfectious glomerulonephritis and rapidly progressive glomerulonephritis cause nephritic syndrome, but postinfectious glomerulonephritis does not have crescents (**C**), and membranoproliferative glomerulonephritis can present with either nephrotic or nephritic syndrome (**E**).

145. Correct: Cerebral edema (C)

The gyri are flattened and the sulci are closed, giving the surface of the brain a smooth texture, which is consistent with cerebral edema (**C**). An overdose on an opioid-type medication can lead to cerebral edema. The gyri are otherwise normal, and thus neither polymicrogyria or pachencephaly is present (**A, B**). There is no evidence of hemorrhage or purulence (**D, E**).

146. Correct: Seborrheic keratosis (E)

Seborrheic keratoses are common skin lesions in older patients. They appear dark brown and have a stuck-on appearance (**E**). A nevus would not be normally raised, or only raised slightly, from the surface of the skin (**A, B**). Nodular malignant melanoma would not be so well demarcated at its edges, and would not occur at multiple points (**C**) around the body. An actinic keratosis occurs in sun-exposed skin as a roughened area and is a precursor to squamous cell carcinoma (**D**).

147. Correct: Subdural hemorrhage (B)

On the floor of the left middle cranial fossa and extending into the posterior fossa is a subdural hemorrhage (note that the dura mater is still in place in the figure) (**B**). Although the amount of hemorrhage in the image is insufficient to cause death, it is representative of the process that was identified prior to removal of the brain. The fall caused a subdural hemorrhage, which increased in size slowly, allowing the man to return home, and, once it reached a critical size, caused his death. The other choices are incorrect (**A, C-E**).

148. Correct: Hashimoto's thyroiditis (D)

The man has vitiligo of the hand. Vitiligo may be of autoimmune origin in some cases, and is sometimes associated with an underlying autoimmune disorder. Hashimoto's thyroiditis could cause weight gain and fatigue and, of the choices, is the only primary autoimmune disorder (**D**). The other choices (**A-C, E**) are not commonly associated with vitiligo.

149. Correct: Hypertension (C)

The image illustrates a hemorrhage in the brainstem. The main cause of an intracerebral hemorrhage, not associated with trauma or cerebral edema, is hypertension (**C**). The most common sites for a hypertensive intracerebral hemorrhage are the basal ganglia, the cerebellum, and the brainstem. In the elderly, cerebral amyloid angiopathy is also a significant cause. The

other conditions listed are not routinely associated with an intracerebral hemorrhage (**A-B, D-E**).

150. Correct: Abnormal mitotic figures (E)

Although histologic features used to determine whether a mass is benign or malignant include pleomorphism and a high mitotic rate (**A, B**), there are benign neoplasms, and benign nonneoplastic processes that have such features; however, abnormal mitotic figures are consistent with a malignant process, and on the right side of the image is a tripolar mitosis (**E**). The presence of nucleoli and vacuoles is in general not useful for distinguishing between benign and malignant (**C, D**).

151. Correct: A meningioma (D)

The histologic appearance is that of clusters of cells with a whorled appearance, which is characteristic of a meningioma (**D**). No psammoma bodies, another histologic feature of meningiomas, are present in the section. The histologic features are not consistent with the other listed conditions (**A-C, E**).

152. Correct: Ethylene glycol poisoning (C)

The image illustrates acute tubular necrosis. The tubule epithelial cells are flattened, the lumens of the tubules are dilated, and there is coagulative necrosis of the tubular epithelial cells. When ethylene glycol is metabolized by the body, oxalic acid is formed, which deposits in the kidney (**C**). A warm autoimmune hemolytic anemia would cause prerenal failure with a BUN/Cr ratio of > 20 (**A**). There is no evidence of an infectious process, as pyelonephritis would have infiltrates of neutrophils in the interstitium and filling tubules (**D**). Membranous glomerulonephropathy would not likely present so acutely (**B**), and the one glomerulus pictured is not consistent with the disease process. There is no evidence of a urinary tract obstruction (**E**).

153. Correct: Endocarditis (D)

The image illustrates a cerebral abscess, which is in the inferior portion of the right frontal lobe. Of the choices, the most likely underlying cause is endocarditis, with the abscess the result of a septic embolus (**D**). The heart murmur may represent a congenital bicuspid aortic valve, which is a risk factor for endocarditis. The lesion present is not a contusion, such as would occur in the frontal lobes after a fall on the back of the head (a contre-coup contusion) (**B**). No features indicative of a neoplasm, alcohol consumption, or cirrhosis of the liver are present (**A, C, E**).

154. Correct: A fall on the back of his head weeks to months earlier (B)

The image illustrates contusions on the undersurface of the frontal lobes of the brain. These contusions have a yellow-brown discoloration, which indicates the deposition of hemosiderin and that the injuries are not recent. Contusions on the undersurface of the frontal lobe essentially always indicate contre-coup contusions, which are due to a fall on the back of the head and not a blow to the face (**A, B**). HSV encephalitis affects the temporal lobes most prominently (**C**). The lesions are not petechiae, such as would be seen in fatty emboli (**D**), and there is no evidence of a metastatic tumor, as no masses are present (**E**).

155. Correct: High-grade ductal carcinoma in situ (D)

The duct is filled with a proliferation of cells; however, there is no invasion of the surrounding tissue (**B, E**). The proliferation of cells is within a duct, not a lobule. Lobular carcinoma in situ would have a generalized proliferation of cells with an overall architecture of a lobule (**A**). Ductal carcinoma can be low-grade or high-grade, and comedonecrosis, which is necrosis of the center of the proliferating cells, is considered high-grade (**C, D**).

156. Correct: Acute cerebral infarct (A)

The image illustrates a hemorrhagic lesion in the lateral portion of the left frontal lobe. The changes are consistent with a reperfused cerebral infarct, with blood leaking from damaged blood vessels (**A**). A remote cerebral infarct would appear as a cystic space (**B**), and intracerebral hemorrhage causes splitting of the cerebral parenchyma by the hemorrhage, and not suffusion of the tissue (**C**). Both encephalitis and fatty emboli syndrome would usually be a more widespread process and may not have any gross abnormalities, although fatty emboli syndrome will usually have petechial hemorrhages (**D, E**).

157. Correct: Branch of left middle cerebral artery (C)

The area of the brain affected is the lateral portion of the left frontal lobe, which is supplied by the left middle cerebral artery (**C**). If the entire artery had been obstructed, the size of the infarct would have been greater; therefore, only a branch vessel was affected. The left anterior cerebral artery supplies about the anterior three-fourths of the medial portion of the left cerebral hemisphere (**A, B**). The posterior cerebral artery supplies the occipital lobes and posterior portion of the parietal lobes (**D**). The left vertebral artery combines with the right vertebral artery to form the basilar artery (**E**).

158. Correct: Loss of fine touch sensation and weakness in the hands (D)

The area of the body with sensation and muscle control affected by the region of the brain with the pathologic change includes the upper extremities (**D**). A lesion at this site would not produce the other neurologic changes in the other choices (**A-C, E**).

159. Correct: Atherosclerosis of the carotid arteries (C)

The image illustrates an organizing infarct centered on the anterior portion of the right caudate nucleus. Cerebral infarcts are most commonly due to an atherosclerotic plaque that embolizes from the carotid artery and obstructs a vessel (**C**). The pathology is not consistent with encephalitis, a neoplasm, a septic embolus from a calcified aortic valve, or trauma. Encephalitis is a more diffuse process and often has no gross changes (**A**). A neoplasm can be cystic, but the incidence of cerebral neoplasms compared to cerebral infarction is much less (**B**). The lesion would be very unusual for trauma, as there is no hemorrhage or evidence of past hemorrhage (**E**). Embolization from endocarditis would be uncommon compared to infarction, and the appearance of the lesion would be more like an abscess, a collection of pus (**D**).

160. Correct: It is most likely to metastasize to the liver. (D)

The image illustrates an invasive adenocarcinoma. Given the clinical scenario, it is most likely a colonic adenocarcinoma, as tumors of the small intestine are rare compared to tumors of the colon (**A**). Given that the tumor was ulcerated, it was likely bleeding and served as the source of the positive fecal occult blood test and the anemia (**B**). In the image, the tumor can be seen invading to the serosa, through the entire thickness of the muscularis propria, which indicates a bad prognosis (**C**). Depth of invasion of the muscularis is a more important prognostic indicator than lymph node invasion when the patient has a colonic adenocarcinoma (**E**). Colonic adenocarcinoma commonly metastasizes to the liver (**D**).

161. Correct: Alveolar proteinosis (D)

Given that he is young and has no risk factors for cardiovascular disease, the diagnosis of congestive heart failure is unlikely (**A**). The image shows neither honeycomb change nor fibroblastic foci, the features of usual interstitial pneumonia (**B**). The clinical history is inconsistent with *Mycoplasma pneumoniae* in that it is recurrent and severe (as evidenced by the fungal infection) (**C**). With Goodpasture's syndrome, hemorrhage and hemosiderin deposition would be expected (**E**). Patients with alveolar proteinosis are at risk for recurrent lung infections, including with fungi. The histologic features and X-ray findings are characteristic of alveolar proteinosis (**D**).

162. Correct: Simple coal worker's pneumoconiosis (C)

The image illustrates a few scattered small collections of anthracotic pigment, which are consistent with either coal-dust macules or coal-dust nodules (**C**), with macules being nonpalpable, and nodules being palpable, features that cannot be appreciated in the image. Progressive massive fibrosis involves dense fibrosis of the lung in a lesion that is 2.0 cm or greater (**D**). Simple coal worker's pneumoconiosis has only small lesions, 1 to 5 mm in size, and it does not cause significant respiratory difficulties, while progressive massive fibrosis can (**C**). The lesions are not melanotic pigment or hemosiderin-laden macrophages (**A, B**), and the dilated airspaces are due to contraction associated with the pigment deposition, and not necessarily loss of parenchyma as would occur with emphysema (**E**).

163. Correct: Adenocarcinoma in situ (C)

The image illustrates tall mucus-producing cells lining essentially normal alveolar septa. This pattern is termed lepidic growth and is characteristic of adenocarcinoma in situ (formerly referred to as bronchioalveolar carcinoma) (**C**). As the lesion can be patchy in distribution, diagnosis as a pneumonia is possible (**A**). Type II pneumocyte hyperplasia can look similar; however, the underlying alveolar septa would be fibrotic, as the hyperplasia is a reaction to damage to the pulmonary parenchyma (**B**). There is no evidence of invasion (**D**). The image has no features to indicate *Legionella* or tuberculosis (**A, E**).

164. Correct: Blood vessel invasion (A)

The image illustrates caseating granulomas. Based on the gross inspection, these are scattered throughout the lung. The changes are consistent with miliary tuberculosis. Miliary tuberculosis occurs when a tuberculous infection erodes into a blood vessel, and the bacteria disseminate in that fashion (**A**). The other mechanisms listed are not the cause of this pathologic lesion (**B-E**).

165. Correct: Complete hydatidiform mole (C)

A complete hydatidiform mole results from fertilization of an ovum that lacks maternal chromosomes, whereas a partial hydatidiform mole results from two sperm fertilizing the same ovum, resulting in triploidy of the products of conception. In a complete mole, all villi are hydropic (**C**), whereas in a partial mole some are hydropic and others are not (**B**). Also, in a partial mole, the uterus is not large for gestational age, and the diagnosis is not often made grossly, but instead microscopically. While sarcoma botroides can present as a grape-like mass, the β-hCG would not be positive (**A**). An ectopic pregnancy and choriocarcinoma would not present with dilated villi being extruded from the uterus (**D, E**).

166. Correct: The karyotype is 46,XX. (C)

Given the clinical summary and pathologic condition illustrated, the diagnosis is a complete hydatidiform mole. The karyotype is 46,XX (**C**). In this condition, patients have a small risk of developing choriocarcinoma (**A**), an embryo is not present (**B**), the risk of persistence of the lesion after treatment is about 20% (**D**), and it is not associated with a granulosa cell tumor (**E**). Partial hydatidiform moles have no risk for future development of choriocarcinoma, an embryo is often present, the karyotype is 69,XXY or 69,XXX, and the rate of persistence is around 5%. Partial moles are also not characteristically associated with a granulosa cell tumor of the ovary.

167. Correct: Involvement of the optic nerves is common. (E)

The pathologic lesion illustrated in the image is a plaque, consistent with multiple sclerosis. Although the exact etiology of multiple sclerosis is unknown, possible underlying causes may include viral infections or an autoimmune disorder, but prion proteins are not implicated (**A**). The plaques in multiple sclerosis are due to the loss of oligodendroglial cells and subsequent loss of myelin (**B**). At first, the neurons remain viable; however, due to loss of myelin, nerve conduction is impaired. The diagnosis of multiple sclerosis requires lesions in different areas occurring at different times—it is temporally heterogenous (**D**). Patients with multiple sclerosis will often have involvement of the optic nerve (**E**). Involvement of the optic nerve can be the first presenting symptom of multiple sclerosis and sometimes the only episode. Microglial nodules and perivascular cuffing are typical histologic features of encephalitis (**C**).

168. Correct: The lesions in the slide will stain with β-amyloid precursor protein. (E)

The pathologic findings illustrated in the image are axonal spheroids, which are a finding in diffuse axonal injury. Diffuse axonal injury occurs due to head trauma, and grossly, punctate hemorrhages can be found in the corpus callosum and the brainstem. The lesion is due to tearing of axons, with subsequent pooling of amyloid precursor protein, a substance that is normally carried along the axon. As a result, axonal spheroids will stain with β-amyloid precursor protein but not Congo red (**C, E**). They do not represent a viral or fungal infection, and they do not follow a long bone fracture (**A-B, D**). The petechial hemorrhages that occur in the brain due to fatty emboli would be more widespread and not just concentrated in the corpus callosum and the brainstem.

169. Correct: Papillary necrosis (C)

Although commonly associated with phenacetin, papillary necrosis can occur in patients who routinely use a large amount of analgesics, including aspirin and acetaminophen (**C**). It is also associated with acute pyelonephritis. There are no stones or tumors present in the image (**A, B**). Xanthogranulomatous pyelonephritis results in a loss of architecture, and the renal parenchyma is more yellow in color, reflecting the accumulation of foamy macrophages in the parenchyma (**D**). The changes are not consistent with multiple myeloma (**E**).

170. Correct: Cysts of the liver are common (about 25% of patients). (D)

The gross pathologic features are consistent with autosomal dominant polycystic kidney disease (ADPKD) (**A**). The condition develops due to mutations in either the *PKD1* (polycystic kidney disease 1) or *PKD2* gene (**B**). Patients with ADPKD often have cysts in other organs, most commonly the liver, but also the spleen and pancreas (**D**). Although the kidney appears quite cystic, the cysts occur in only a small percentage of nephrons (**E**). As up to 20 to 25% of patients have berry aneurysms, a quite frequent cause of death is a subarachnoid hemorrhage (**C**).

171. Correct: Acute pyelonephritis (B)

The clinical history is consistent with acute pyelonephritis, and the kidney has features consistent with acute pyelonephritis, which are multiple small collections of pus (i.e., abscesses) within the cortex (**B**). Papillary necrosis can result from acute pyelonephritis, but it affects the renal papillae, not the cortex (**D**). Miliary tuberculosis would present a similar appearance to that in the image, and miliary tuberculosis commonly involves the kidney; however, in a young healthy female with no medical history, it would be very unlikely (**A**). Renomedullary interstitial cell tumors occur in the medulla, not the cortex, and a multifocal renal cell carcinoma would not appear in this way (i.e., innumerable small tumors) (**C, E**).

172. Correct: The patient may have endocarditis. (C)

Most cases of acute pyelonephritis develop secondary to a urinary tract infection. The most common bacterial cause is *Escherichia coli* (**A**). Although bilateral involvement of the kidneys can occur, it is not necessarily going to happen, as ascension of the bacteria from the bladder to the kidney often requires some dysfunction of the bladder-ureter junction, which may be present on only one side (**B**). Although most cases of acute pyelonephritis occur secondary to a urinary tract infection, hematogenous infection from another source such as endocarditis can occur (**C**). The condition is more common in females rather than males, as females are more at risk for urinary tract infections because of a shorter urethra and the fact that they lack the antibacterial activity of prostatic secretions (**E**). Acute pyelonephritis is a serious infection and can cause death. The white blood cell count will be elevated (**D**).

173. Correct: Renal cell carcinoma, clear cell type (A)

The histology is that of clear cells, with nuclei with little pleomorphism or mitotic figures. These changes are consistent with a clear cell renal cell carcinoma (**A**). In a papillary-type renal cell carcinoma, the tumor cells line papillary projections, and the cells are either basophilic or acidophilic (**B**). An angi-omyolipoma is a benign tumor that has blood vessel, smooth muscle, and fat components (**C**). A Wilms' tumor occurs in children and has immature tubules, loose stroma, and undifferentiated blastema in various amounts (**D**). A colonic adenocarcinoma would have neoplastic glands (**E**).

174. Correct: Some can produce a PTH-like hormone. (C)

Although most people with renal cell carcinoma do not have von Hippel–Lindau syndrome, almost all sporadic renal cell carcinomas have a loss of at least one *VHL* allele, and about 50% have mutations (**A**). Around 30% of renal cell carcinomas occur in individuals who have used tobacco products (**B**). Renal medullary carcinoma is almost always associated with sickle cell disease, but not clear cell renal cell carcinoma (**D**). The stage, and not the grade, of the tumor is the most significant prognostic indicator (**E**). Renal cell carcinomas can produce PTH and erythropoietin as paraneoplastic syndromes (**C**).

175. Correct: Clear cell renal cell carcinoma (A)

The image illustrates a mass in the upper pole, which is yellow in color, with focal red discoloration. The gross appearance of clear cell renal cell carcinoma is characteristic. The yellow discoloration is from the lipids and glycogen contained within the neoplastic cells (which also imparts the clear appearance under microscopic examination) (**A**). Based on the gross appearance, the other four tumor types listed can be excluded (**B-E**).

176. Correct: Uric acid calculi (C)

Calcium renal stones are the most common type of stone and can have either oxalate or phosphate. Calcium phosphate stones are pale (**A**). Staghorn calculi appear as the antlers of a deer, branching out into and through the renal pelvis. These types of stones can require nephrectomy for treatment (**B**). Uric acid stones are hard, yellow, and often smaller (**C**). Stones with calcium are radio dense, whereas stones with uric acid are radiolucent (**A, C**). Cystine stones are uncommon and occur only in individuals with hereditary cystinuria (**D**). Although urothelial polyps could calcify focally, this would be rare, and, the two lesions in the image are not pedunculated, nor apparently attached to the pelvis (**E**).

177. Correct: Emphysema (D)

Use of periodic acid–Schiff (PAS) stain followed by diastase digestion will highlight globules of α-1-antitrypsin protein and help to determine whether the patient's cirrhosis is due to this disease. Individuals with α-1-antitrypsin deficiency are also at risk for pulmonary emphysema because of the resultant uncontrolled activity of elastases (**D**). Kayser-Fleischer rings are associated with Wilson's disease (**A**), primary sclerosing cholangitis with ulcerative colitis (**B**), chronic pancreatitis with hereditary hemochromatosis (**C**), and cerebellar vermal atrophy with chronic alcoholism (**E**).

178. Correct: Adenomyosis (D)

Adenomyosis is a very common lesion identified in resected uteri, involving up to one-fourth. Although patients can be asymptomatic, adenomyosis can also cause dysfunctional uterine bleeding, dyspareunia, and pelvic pain. The pelvic pain occurs as during the menstrual cycle, hemorrhage into the glands occurs, with expansion of the tissue resulting and causing the pain (**D**). The glands in the myometrium have surrounding stroma, whereas an invasive endometrial adenocarcinoma would only be glands (**B**). Endometrial carcinoma can both arise within as well as extend into a focus of adenomyosis. An invasive mole would be placental villi (**A**). Both a leiomyoma and an endometrial stromal sarcoma would have a spindled architecture, albeit with other features, as the first is benign while the second is malignant (**C, E**).

179. Correct: Death in the neonatal period due to pulmonary hypoplasia is common. (D)

The image illustrates autosomal recessive polycystic kidney disease (ARPKD), which is due to dilated collecting ducts. The kidneys are large at birth and can impede delivery, and, because the kidneys are so large, lung development is inhibited and pulmonary hypoplasia is a cause of death in the neonatal period, affecting around 25% of infants born with this condition (**D**). ARPKD is due to a mutation of the *PKHD1* gene, which produces the protein fibrocystin (**C**). Berry aneurysms are associated with ADPKD (autosomal dominant PKD), and hepatic fibrosis is associated with ARPKD (**E**). The process is not neoplastic (**A**), and patients are not asymptomatic (**B**).

180. Correct: Wall of left atrium (A)

Given the age of the patient, and lack of risk factors for carotid artery atherosclerosis or an intracerebral hemorrhage, and with the mass identified within the heart, the most likely cause of his symptoms is an embolism. Without a patent foramen ovale, a lesion on the right side of the heart, either right atrium or tricuspid valve, could not produce a cerebral embolus (**D, E**). The image illustrates the histologic features of an atrial myxoma. It is not muscle (i.e., not a rhabdomyoma), papillary in architecture (i.e., not a papillary fibroelastoma), and not consistent with a carcinoma. Myxomas are the most primary tumor of the heart, and the majority arise in the left atrium (**A-C**).

181. Correct: At the least, frequent repeat biopsies would be recommended. (C)

The patient has intestinal-type glandular epithelium at the GE junction, which, in combination with the history, is consistent with Barrett's esophagus. In addition, there is dysplasia of the glandular epithe-

lium, putting the patient at higher risk for developing an invasive adenocarcinoma; thus, careful observation is necessary (**C**). Barrett's esophagus is due to acid reflux inducing metaplasia, which, in this case, progressed to dysplasia (**A**). There are no features of an HSV infection such as multinucleation or intranuclear inclusions (**B**). Achalasia is due to damage to the myenteric plexus (**D**). Mallory-Weiss tears are due to prolonged vomiting (**E**).

182. Correct: Basal cell carcinoma (A)

The histologic features illustrated in the image are consistent with a basal cell carcinoma (**A**). There are epithelial cells in nests invading the dermis. The nests of cells have peripheral palisading. There are no keratin pearls (**B**), dysplastic changes (**D**), epithelial hyperplasia (**E**), or changes consistent with a melanoma (**C**).

183. Correct: A similar disease can affect the vagina in older women. (E)

The image illustrates cervical intraepithelial neoplasia (CIN)II/CIN III. HPV 6 and 11 are low-risk, producing CIN I, whereas HPV 16, 18, 31, 33, 35 and others are high-risk, producing CIN II/III (**A**). As CIN II/III is a high-grade lesion, the Pap smear most likely showed HSIL (high-grade squamous intraepithelial lesion) (**B**). There is no perfect correlation (e.g., a person with LSIL on Pap smear can have CIN II/III on biopsy, and the reverse is true), but in general there is good correlation. The mechanism for low-grade dysplasia is accumulation of viral particles, producing the classic koilocyte; however, the mechanism for high-grade dysplasia is integration of viral genes *E6* and *E7* with the host genome, with the resultant proteins inactivating p53 (*E6*) and Rb (*E7*) (**C**). Although CIN II/III has a higher risk for progression to invasive cervical carcinoma, not all women experience this; in fact, only about 20% progress (**D**). VIN (vaginal intraepithelial neoplasia) is similar in appearance to CIN but affects the vagina and affects an older population. It may represent a field effect from viral infection of the cervix (**E**).

184. Correct: CIN III (C)

The patient has dysplasia of the cervix. By biopsy, the cervical dysplasia is graded, if there is dysplasia present, from CIN I-III. In CIN I, the dysplastic features are in the lower third of the thickness of the mucosa. In CIN II, the dysplastic features are involved in the lower half to two-thirds of the thickness of the mucosa. In CIN III, the dysplastic features involve the full thickness of the mucosa. The changes are a spectrum, and the actual division between the three grades is not always absolute. In the image, the dysplasia extends full thickness through the mucosa (**B, C**). The cervix is not normal (**A**). There is no evidence of invasion, as the basement membrane is intact, and the features are not consistent with a small-cell carcinoma (**D, E**).

185. Correct: Cytomegalovirus pneumonia (C)

The image illustrates scattered large cells (compared to the adjacent type I pneumocytes) that have intranuclear inclusions; the appearance is consistent with a cytomegalovirus infection (**C**). Influenza pneumonia, while caused by a virus, does not have inclusions that can be identified (**D**). There is no evidence of a neoplasm, and there are no hyaline membranes (**A**, **B**). The acute presentation alone would rule out a usual interstitial pneumonia (**E**).

186. Correct: High-grade ductal carcinoma in situ (C)

The image illustrates ducts expanded by dysplastic cells with central necrosis, referred to as comedo necrosis. There is no evidence of invasion of the basement membrane (**D**). Distinguishing low-grade from high-grade DCIS can be challenging; however, in general, the cells in low-grade DCIS have relatively uniform nuclei that are evenly spaced. Necrosis is not common, and usually smaller. The cells in high-grade DCIS have more atypical nuclei, and comedonecrosis is more common (**B, C**). Fibrocystic disease can have glands with hyperplasia. In general, in hyperplasia the cells appear more to be piled on top of each other, whereas in DCIS the cells appear to abut each other and form one layer (**A**). It is counterintuitive, but in DCIS the cells appear more organized, whereas in hyperplasia they appear more disorganized. The cellular features are not those of small-cell carcinoma (**E**).

187. Correct: Compound nevus (C)

The skin lesion has nevoid-type cells in the dermis and in clusters at the basal layer of the epidermis, which is consistent with a compound nevus (**C**). An intradermal nevus has nevoid cells in the dermis only (**A**), while in a junctional nevus, they are at the basal layer of the epidermis only (**B**). There is no evidence of dysplasia or migration of nevus cells upward in the epidermis, and there is no evidence of invasion into the dermis (**D, E**).

188. Correct: Physical examination could reveal erythema of the breast associated with this lesion. (C)

The image illustrates a low- or intermediate-grade DCIS. The cells are regular in size and form pseudolumens with a punched-out appearance. There is no comedonecrosis. Cells in DCIS stain positive for E-cadherin (**A**). Although lobular carcinoma in situ is often associated with invasive lobular carcinoma in the same breast as the in-situ lesion, women with lobular carcinoma in situ also, in general, have a higher risk for the development of invasive carcinoma, either lobular or ductal, and in either breast (**B**). Because of this fact, some women choose to have a bilateral mastectomy to reduce their risk. With DCIS, the resultant invasive carcinoma usually develops at the site of the DCIS. Paget's disease of the nipple, which is characterized by neoplastic cells in the epidermis, can appear as an erythematous region, and it is associated with underlying DCIS (**C**). Surgical excision can be curative, although adjuvant radiation may help prevent a recurrence (**D**). Although it is concerning, bloody nipple discharge most frequently indicates an underlying benign lesion, usually an intraductal papilloma (**E**).

189. Correct: Tubular adenoma (B)

The mass, on the lower right side of the image, has dysplasia, with the cells having a tubular and not villous architecture. These features are consistent with a tubular adenoma (**B**). A hyperplastic polyp has no dysplasia, and the lumen of the glands has a serrated appearance (**A**). There is no invasion (**C**). A juvenile polyp has dilated glands, of which none are present (**D**), and a lymphoid polyp has a prominent infiltrate of lymphoid cells forming germinal centers (**E**).

190. Correct: Cigarette use is a risk factor. (C)

The histologic features are characteristic of a tubular adenoma. Cigarette use, alcohol use, diets low in fruits and vegetables, obesity, and lack of physical exercise are risk factors for adenomas and resultant invasive colonic adenocarcinoma (**C**). When hundreds of tubular adenomas are present, the findings are consistent with familial adenomatous polyposis syndrome, which is caused by a mutation in the *APC* gene (**A**). Mutations of *hMSH2* or *hMLH1* are associated with Lynch's syndrome, which is a nonpolyposis hereditary colon cancer syndrome. Tubular adenomas, unless there is a hereditary cancer disorder, occur in older patients; hence the need for surveillance colonoscopies at age 50 years (**B**). The risk of a 1.0-cm polyp having an invasive carcinoma is only around 1% (**D**). Although polyps can develop in the small intestine, this is a rare occurrence (**E**).

191. Correct: Fibrocystic disease (A)

The mass consists of fibrous tissue and cysts. These changes are consistent with fibrocystic disease of the breast. Fibrocystic disease of the breast can be associated with proliferative lesions (i.e., epithelial hyperplasia, which can increase the risk of breast cancer very slightly; however, no such lesions are present in the biopsy) (**A**). Sclerosing adenosis has a disorderly proliferation of ducts and glands (**B**). Ductal carcinoma in situ has expansion of ducts by dysplastic cells, and invasive ductal carcinoma has invading elements, none of which are present in the image (**C, D**). Fat necrosis, which can mimic a neoplasm, is characterized by foamy macrophages (**E**).

192. Correct: Tophus (D)

The histologic findings are consistent with a tophus, being extracellular soft tissue composed of urate crystals that is surrounded by multinucleated giant cells (**D**). The lesion bears some resemblance to a granuloma. There is no cartilage, giant cells, or osteoid, and no evidence of neoplasia (**A-C**). A Charcot joint, usually occurring due to the peripheral neuropathy associated with diabetes mellitus, would be characterized by destruction of cartilage and bone, associated with cyst formation and sclerosis (**E**).

193.   Correct: Certain leukemias are a risk factor. (D)

The lesion is a tophus, which occurs in people with untreated gout. The tophus is uric acid deposition surrounded by a foreign body giant cell reaction. The source of uric acid is a breakdown of purines (**A**). As certain leukemias have a high turnover rate, most commonly the acute leukemias, an increased amount of uric acid can be produced, which leads to secondary gout (**D**). Uric acid is excreted only in the urine (**B**). Increased concentration of uric acid in the blood is due to increased production of purines, increased breakdown of nucleic acids, decreased turnover of purines, and decreased excretion of uric acid in the urine. Gout is not associated with Neimann-Pick disease (**C**); however, it is associated with Lesch-Nyhan syndrome, which has an increased production of purines due to a defect in hypoxanthine phosphoribosyl transferase. Gout quite frequently involves the big toe and is referred to as podagra (**E**).

194.   Correct: Graves' disease (B)

The symptoms are consistent with hyperthyroidism—weight loss, nervousness, intolerance to heat, and palpitations. The histologic image is consistent with Graves' disease, thyroid follicles with the follicular epithelium forming papillary projections into the colloid (**B**). An adenoma would be more cellular (**A**). Hashimoto's thyroiditis, which can cause hyperthyroidism early in its course, would have a lymphocytic infiltrate (**C**). A pheochromocytoma has clusters of neural-like cells (referred to as a zellballen pattern) (**D**). Papillary thyroid carcinoma has cleared-out cells, nuclear grooves, and psammoma bodies, and the amount of colloid would not be as abundant (**E**).

195.   Correct: Invasive lobular carcinoma (D)

The characteristic histologic feature of invasive lobular carcinoma is neoplastic cells organized in a single file, such as is exhibited in the image (**D**). Sclerosing adenosis is a disorganized collection of ducts and glands, but with a well-defined border (**A**). Ductal carcinoma in situ is a proliferation of dysplastic ductal cells filling a duct, and invasive ductal carcinoma quite frequently, unless very undifferentiated, has glandular elements (**B, C**). Neither cell-filled ducts nor glandular elements are present. Tubular carcinoma is a breast carcinoma with a better prognosis; however, as the name implies, the histologic features are infiltrative tubular structures (**E**).

196.   Correct: Ulcerative colitis (D)

The histology features are consistent with primary sclerosing cholangitis. Around the bile duct is a thick rim of fibrosis. Primary sclerosing cholangitis is most commonly associated with ulcerative colitis, but some patients with Crohn's disease also develop the disease (**D**). Riedel's thyroiditis and some forms of lymphoma are rarely associated with the condition (**B**). The other conditions listed are not normally associated with primary sclerosing cholangitis (**A, C, E**).

197.   Correct: Seminoma (A)

Seminomas are composed of a uniformly sized population of cells divided into clusters by fibrous septa. Within the fibrous septa can be lymphocytes and giant cells (**A**). Spermatocytic seminomas occur in an older age group than seminomas and are composed of a proliferation of three cell types—large, small, and intermediate (**B**). Yolk sac tumors occur most commonly in young boys, below the age of 4 years. Yolk sac tumors are composed of epithelial cells with a loose connective tissue stroma, which sometimes form glomerular-like structures, called Schiller-Duval bodies (**C**). Although the cells in the image may resemble a malignant lymphoma, lymphoma of the testicles is commonly bilateral and occurs in elderly men (**D**). Also, the CD117 positive is consistent with seminoma. A choriocarcinoma has syncytiotrophoblasts and cytotrophoblasts (**E**).

198.   Correct: Medullary thyroid carcinoma (C)

The histologic features are consistent with a medullary thyroid carcinoma. The eosinophilic material in the section is amyloid. Medullary thyroid carcinoma can produce a variety of hormones, including ACTH and serotonin (which could produce Cushing's syndrome and carcinoid syndrome, respectively). Watery diarrhea occurs in around 30 to 40% of patients with medullary thyroid carcinoma and is due mainly to the secretion of vasoactive intestinal peptide (**C**). The histologic features are not consistent with the remainder of the choices (**A-B, D-E**).

199.   Correct: The second polyp has a greater risk of harboring a neoplasm than the first polyp. (D)

The second polyp has villous architecture. The three types of adenomatous polyps are tubular, tubulovillous, and villous, depending upon the relative amount of each architectural type in the polyp. Polyps with villous architecture are more likely to harbor an invasive component (**A-E**). Also, as polyps increase in size, they are more likely to have an invasive component.

200. Correct: The tumor occurs as a part of Beckwith-Wiedemann syndrome (E)

The histology illustrates a Wilms' tumor. Blastema, immature tubules, and loose stroma are present. Almost all cases of Wilms' tumor occur in children under the age of 10 years (A). In sporadic Wilms' tumor, *WT1* mutations are less common (about one-fifth of patients) than in WAGR syndrome, where essentially all Wilms' tumors have *WT1* mutations. Loss of imprinting, or loss of heterozygosity on chromosome 11 (11p15.5), is found in around three-fourths of Wilms' tumors (B). With treatment, around 90% of children diagnosed with Wilms' tumor will have a long-term survival (C). Anaplasia, older age of presentation (i.e., greater than 2 years old), and extension outside the renal capsule have a worse prognosis (D). Wilms' tumor is a component of Beckwith-Wiedemann syndrome (E).

201. Correct: Eating poorly cooked pork (B)

The image illustrates encysted *Trichinella*. Hiking in the San Joaquin Valley can expose an individual to *Coccidioides immitis* (A). A tick bite can lead to a variety of bacterial and viral infections, including Lyme disease and Rocky Mountain spotted fever (C). The reduviid bug transmits *Trypanosoma cruzi*, which causes Chagas' disease (D). Drinking unfiltered lake or stream water is a risk factor for *Giardia lamblia* (E). The organism in the image is large and encysted in muscle. The other organisms described would be smaller. *Giardia lamblia* essentially infects only the colon, causing diarrhea (E). Trichinosis arises from eating poorly cooked pork (B).

202. Correct: Temporal arteritis (D)

Given the age of the patient and the symptoms, the diagnosis is temporal arteritis (also called giant cell arteritis) (D). The other vasculitides listed are not normally associated with involvement of the temporal artery. Takayasu's arterities, like giant cell arteritis, can involve the aorta and its branch vessels, but this condition occurs in patients who are under the age of 50 years (C). Polyarteritis nodosa and microscopic polyangiitis tend to have a more transmural inflammation, whereas the most prominent features in the image are intimal thickening, which is characteristic of temporal arteritis (A, B). In addition, the elastic laminae are fragmented, which is also characteristic for temporal arteritis. Granulomatosis with polyangiitis does not affect the temporal artery (E).

203. Correct: Low-grade papillary urothelial carcinoma (C)

The image illustrates a papillary neoplasm, which excludes an inverted papilloma, which appears more as a nodule and has growth downward into the lamina propria (A). The lack of invasion rules out an invasive urothelial carcinoma and squamous cell carcinoma (D, E). In addition, squamous cell carcinoma of the bladder is rare and, when it occurs, is commonly associated with a schistosomiasis infection. A urothelial papilloma would appear papillary; however, the lining epithelium would appear as normal transitional epithelium (B). In the image, there is increased cellularity and some atypia of the nuclei, which, of the choices, is most consistent with a low-grade papillary urothelial carcinoma (C).

204. Correct: Negri bodies (C)

The patient has symptoms that are characteristic of rabies. The characteristic histologic finding in rabies is the Negri body, which is a round eosinophilic inclusion in the cytoplasm of the neurons. Essentially every neuron in the image has a Negri body, and some neurons have two or more (C). HSV inclusions would be intranuclear and have a smudged appearance (B). Infection with a prion protein leads to vacuolation of the neuropil surrounding the neurons, and none exists in this image (D). *Naegleria fowleri* causes a meningoencephalitis and free amoebas would be identified (E). The neurons are not normal (A).

205. Correct: Aspirin use during recent chickenpox infection (B)

The image illustrates a microvesicular steatosis. In a young child, of the choices, the most likely diagnosis is Reye's syndrome, which occurs when aspirin is given to a child during an infection, most commonly chickenpox or influenza (B). Infection with hepatitis A, while capable of causing an acute illness, is very rarely lethal, and individuals recover (A). A recent blood transfusion could result in infection with hepatitis B or C; however, the histologic findings would not be diffuse microvesicular steatosis (C). A thrombus of the hepatic vein would cause severe congestion, and an accidental ingestion of alcohol would cause some macrovesicular steatosis of the liver (D, E). An acute alcohol ingestion can be lethal.

206. Correct: Complete hydatidiform mole (C)

The image illustrates swollen villi, and all of the villi are swollen. This appearance in combination with the history indicates a complete hydatidiform mole (C). With a partial hydatidiform mole, some villi are swollen while others are normal size. Also, the uterus is often not larger than the gestational age would predict (B). Choriocarcinoma has trophoblasts, cytotrophoblasts, and syncytiotrophoblasts, and not villi, and a placental site trophoblastic tumor has intermediate trophoblasts. (A, D) With HELLP syndrome (hemolysis, elevated liver enzymes, and low platelets), the fetus is not abnormal (E).

207.   Correct: Molluscum contagiosum (C)

The gross appearance and histologic appearance are characteristic of molluscum contagiosum, which is caused by poxvirus. The cells in the epidermis contain large intracytoplasmic inclusions, which are called molluscum bodies. The molluscum bodies are accumulations of viral particles (**C**). The histologic changes are not suggestive or consistent with the other conditions that are listed (**A-B, D-E**).

208.   Correct: Riedel's thyroiditis (D)

The image illustrates a thyroid gland that is replaced with fibrosis and has scattered clusters of inflammatory cells. This appearance is consistent with Riedel's thyroiditis (**D**). de Quervain's thyroiditis (i.e., subacute thyroiditis) is painful, and histologic examination would reveal granulomas and foreign body giant cells (**E**). Hashimoto's thyroiditis can have extensive fibrosis; however, some residual thyroid gland should be identifiable (**C**). There is no evidence of a neoplasm, and, with Graves' disease, thyroid follicles should be present throughout the gland (**A, B**).

209.   Correct: Encephalitis (C)

The image illustrates two of the three histologic features of a viral encephalitis: a microglial nodule and lymphocytic cuffing of the vessel in the Virchow-Robin space (**C**). There are many viral causes of encephalitis, and the symptoms can be variable. An acute cerebral infarct would have neuronal necrosis (i.e., red neurons) (**A**), multiple sclerosis would have evidence of myelin breakdown (**B**), and a low-grade astrocytoma would have a proliferation of astrocytes (**D**). Marchiafava-Bignami is a very rare demyelinating disorder associated with alcoholism (**E**).

210.   Correct: Brenner's tumor (B)

The image shows nests of transitional cell–like epithelium embedded in a fibrous background, which is the characteristic feature of a Brenner's tumor (**B**). A dysgerminoma would have a homogenous population of cells interspersed with fibrous septa containing lymphocytes (**A**). The tumor is histologically the same as seminoma. A granulosa cell tumor would have a homogeneous population of cells not arranged in nests and not with a prominent fibrous background (**C**). The cells are not atypical, do not have a papillary or glandular architecture, and there are no mitotic figures (**D**). There are no endometrial glands or stroma, and no hemosiderin (**E**).

211.   Correct: Apocrine metaplasia (D)

Apocrine metaplasia is a relatively common finding identified as a component of fibrocystic disease of the breast. It is benign. The cells appear enlarged and more eosinophilic (D). Both lobular carcinoma in situ and ductal carcinoma in situ involve hyperplasia and dysplasia of epithelial cells, filling lobular acini and ducts, respectively (A, B). Sclerosing adenosis appears as a scarred and disorganized area of breast tissue, with a well-defined border (C). The features are not normal glandular elements (E).

212.   Correct: Glandular epithelium (C)

The neoplasm is an adenocarcinoma. The image reveals a few rudimentary glandular structures, and some of the neoplastic cells contain large vacuoles, which represent mucus formation. Adenocarcinomas originate in the lung, gastrointestinal tract, pancreas, and prostate, predominantly (**C**). There are no histologic features of squamous cell carcinoma (e.g., keratin pearls or intercellular bridges), transitional epithelium, adipose tissue, or smooth muscle (**A-B, D-E**).

213.   Correct: Chronic pancreatitis (B)

The normal pancreatic parenchyma is divided into clusters of acini by variously sized bands of fibrosis. This appearance is consistent with chronic pancreatitis (**B**). Acute pancreatitis would not have the fibrous background, and the acini would be infiltrated by neutrophils (**A**). An adenocarcinoma would have infiltrating glandular elements (**C, D**). Nesidioblastosis is characterized by islet cell enlargement and dysplasia and causes a syndrome of hyperinsulinemia (**E**).

214.   Correct: Gallstones (C)

The image illustrates chronic pancreatitis. The two main causes of chronic pancreatitis are gallstones and alcohol (**B**). Both can cause acute pancreatitis, and, with recurring bouts, irreversible damage and subsequent fibrosis. Chronic pancreatitis can lead to malabsorption because of decreased production of digestive enzymes, and potentially to diabetes mellitus, although the endocrine portions of the pancreas are rather resilient. Hypertriglyceridemia is one cause of pancreatitis; however, compared to gallstones and alcohol, it is a much less common cause (**E**). Although a congenital malformation, a fungal infection, and an invasive neoplasm could damage the pancreas, and potentially, if the time course was long enough, lead to chronic pancreatitis, they would be a rare cause compared to alcohol or gallstones (**A-B, D**).

215.   Correct: Alzheimer's disease (A)

The neuron in the upper right corner has granulo-vacuolar degeneration, and the neuron in the lower left corner has a neurofibrillary tangle. These are histologic features characteristic of Alzheimer's disease. Also found in Alzheimer's disease are senile plaques and Hirano bodies (**A**). The diagnosis of Alzheimer's disease requires a correlation between autopsy findings and clinical history, as the histologic features of Alzheimer's disease are also found as a result of aging. Both Parkinson's disease, which can sometimes have dementia as a component, and diffuse Lewy body disease would have Lewy bodies (**C, E**), and Pick's disease would have Pick bodies (**B**). An acute hemorrhagic encephalitis would not cause dementia, and would instead cause a delirium (**D**).

216. Correct: Macrophages (D)

The image is an acid-fast stain, and within several cells in the field are *Mycobacterium tuberculosis* bacilli. In this stain, *M. tuberculosis* stains red. The type of inflammation associated with *M. tuberculosis* is granulomatous, which is composed of epithelioid histiocytes, which are macrophages (**D**). The other choices are incorrect (**A-C, E**).

217. Correct: Tuberous sclerosis (C)

The mass is an angiomyolipoma. The image illustrates histologic features of adipose tissue, blood vessels, and muscle tissue. Angiomyolipoma is a tumor type that is found in tuberous sclerosis (**C**). Other tumors associated with this condition are cardiac rhabdomyomas. Von Hippel–Lindau is associated with cerebellar hemangioblastomas and renal cell carcinoma (**A**). Hereditary hemochromatosis is not associated with tumors, unless the patient develops cirrhosis of the liver and subsequently has a hepatocellular carcinoma (**D**). Ollier's syndrome is associated with enchondromas (**E**). Cystic fibrosis is not associated with angiomyolipomas (**B**).

218. Correct: Spider angiomas (D)

The image illustrates cirrhosis of the liver. Cirrhosis of the liver is a cause of spider angiomas (**D**); however, it is not a cause of the remaining conditions listed (**A-C, E**). Patients with α-1-antitrypsin deficiency are at risk for both cirrhosis of the liver (due to buildup of abnormal protein damaging the liver) and emphysema (due to a lack of control of elastase); however, it is a relatively rare cause of cirrhosis of the liver.

219. Correct: Dysgerminoma (D)

The histology reveals large sheets of homogeneous cells interspersed with thin fibrous bands, which are vascular and contain a lymphocytic infiltrate. These histologic features are those of a dysgerminoma (**D**). Dysgerminomas have the same histologic appearance as seminomas, but the nomenclature used is different (**E**). Choriocarcinomas have cytotrophoblasts and syncytiotrophoblasts (**A**). A mucinous cyst adenoma would have mucus-producing cells lining cysts (**C**). The appearance is not consistent with a Sertoli-Leydig cell tumor (**B**).

220. Correct: Lisch nodules (C)

The decedent has neurofibromatosis. The diagnosis of neurofibromatosis 1 is based uon the presence of café au lait spots and cutaneous neurofibromas, both viewable in the image, and also Lisch nodules, which are iris hamartomas (**C**). Kayser-Fleischer rings are associated with Wilson's disease (**A**), Koplik spots with measles (**B**), and subependymal nodules are seen in tuberous sclerosis (**D**).

221. Correct: Malignant peripheral nerve sheath tumor (C)

The patient has features of neurofibromatosis, namely café au lait spots and neurofibromas. The lesions can be found in either neurofibromatosis 1 or 2, but are most consistent with NF1. Neurofibromatosis 1 is associated with a risk for development of peripheral nerve sheath tumors, with about 5% of patients with NF1 developing such a tumor, and with about 50% of peripheral nerve sheath tumors occurring in patients with NF1 (**C**). Other malignant tumors associated with NF1 are optic gliomas and glial tumors of other types. The other neoplasms listed do not occur with increased frequency in patients with neurofibromatosis (**A-B, D-E**).

222. Correct: Chronic pyelonephritis (B)

Her presenting symptoms and laboratory testing are consistent with renal failure that is not being due to dehydration or other form of pre-renal renal failure. Her clinical history indicates the possibility of past episodes of pyelonephritis. The image shows dilated tubules filled with an eosinophilic material, which is referred to as thyroidization of the tubules. Thyroidization of the tubules is a histologic feature that occurs in chronic pyelonephritis. Gross examination would reveal foci of cortical thinning associated with underlying blunting of the calyces (**B**). Acute pyelonephritis would have an interstitial infiltrate of neutrophils (**A**); renal cell carcinoma would, in the most common type, have clear cells on a delicate framework of vessels (**C**); acute tubular necrosis would have dilation of the tubules and coagulative necrosis of the renal tubular epithelial cells (**D**); and interstitial nephritis would have a lymphocytic infiltrate of the interstitium (**E**), none of which is present.

223. Correct: Synovial sarcoma (D)

The image illustrates a biphasic tumor—both epithelial cells and spindle cells. The epithelial cells have a gland-like architecture. This appearance is characteristic of a synovial sarcoma (**D**). Synovial sarcomas occur in young adults and commonly around the knees. A frequent genetic abnormality associated with the tumor is a t(X;18). A Baker's cyst occurs in the popliteal fossa; however, the image does not show a cyst (**A**). A rheumatoid nodule would have a necrotic core that is surrounded by histiocytes and giant cells (**B**). Nodular fasciitis is a benign, nonneoplastic proliferation that can be confused with a neoplasm. However, it is rapidly growing and would not have the epithelial component (**C**). An osteosarcoma has evidence of osteoid formation, none of which is present (**E**).

224. Correct: Myelofibrosis (E)

Myelofibrosis is a chronic myeloproliferative disorder that is characterized by fibrosis of the bone marrow. Myeloid metaplasia in the liver and spleen can lead to hepatosplenomegaly. The red blood cell morphology illustrated in the blood smear is dacryocytes (i.e., teardrop cells), which are characteristic of myelofibrosis (**E**). While megaloblastic anemia could present with fatigue and anemia, splenomegaly and the dacryocytes would not be normal. (**A**) Both hairy cell leukemia and infectious mononucleosis can have splenomegaly; however, dacryocytes are not characteristic (**C, D**). The white blood cell count is not as consistent with an acute lymphoblastic leukemia, and this form of leukemia is more common in a younger population (**B**).

225. Correct: 3p deletion (E)

The histology illustrates a neoplasm composed of cells with a small nuclear:cytoplasm ratio. There is no evidence of squamous (e.g., keratin pearls or intercellular bridges) or glandular differentiation. In the center of the figure is an example of nuclear molding, which is a histologic characteristic of small-cell carcinoma. A t(15;17) is associated with acute promyelocytic leukemia (**A**). *ALK* rearrangements, and *EGFR* and *KRAS* mutations are associated with lung cancer but are rare or absent in small-cell carcinoma (**B-D**). A 3p deletion is found in almost all small-cell carcinomas (**E**).

226. Correct: Coxsackievirus B (D)

The image illustrates a lymphocytic myocarditis. The most common cause of a lymphocytic myocarditis is an enterovirus infection, including coxsackievirus A and B (**D**). No organisms are identified in the figure, which would exclude *Aspergillus niger* and *Trypanosoma cruzi* (**B, C**). Also, in the United States, both would be extremely rare causes of myocarditis. *M. tuberculosis* would be a rare cause of myocarditis and the patient should have a granulomatous inflammation, and *S. aureus* would be a rare cause of myocarditis and the inflammation would be more likely neutrophilic.

227. Correct: Parkinson's disease (C)

The image illustrates Lewy bodies in a neuron in the substantia nigra. This finding is most characteristic of Parkinson's disease (**C**). About one-fifth of patients with Parkinson's disease can develop dementia. Amyotrophic lateral sclerosis is a disorder of motor neurons and does not cause dementia (**D**). Rabies encephalitis is associated with Negri bodies, which are eosinophilic inclusions in the cytoplasm of neurons, but are not necessarily as round as Lewy bodies and do not have the clearing around the inclusion (**E**). Infarcts would be associated with red neurons, foamy macrophages, or areas of gliosis (**B**). Alzheimer's disease has neurofibrillary tangles and senile plaques (**A**).

228. Correct: Pulmonary thromboembolus (C)

In a patient with a fractured ankle, immobility can lead to the development of deep venous thrombi, which can embolize the lung. Small emboli will reach the periphery of the lung, leading to infarction. The symptoms can include sharp chest pain and dyspnea. The infarct, due to the dual blood supply of the lung, is usually red and characteristically wedge-shaped. The image illustrates red infarcts of the lung, which developed from small pulmonary thromboemboli. His cause of death was most likely, based on the scenario and the findings in the image, a large pulmonary thromboembolus (**C**). The clinical scenario in combination with the autopsy findings do not support the remainder of the conditions listed (**A-B, D-E**).

229. Correct: Trauma (B)

The image illustrates foamy macrophages. The appearance is consistent with fat necrosis, which can occur as a result of trauma (**B**). Inheritance of *BRCA1* would predispose the patient to a neoplasm (**A**). Bacterial infections would have neutrophilic infiltrates (**E**), *M. tuberculosis* infection would have granulomatous inflammation (**D**), and an amoebic infection would be very rare. The cells in the image are foamy macrophages and not amoebas (**C**).

230. Correct: Incompetence of venous valves (B)

Dilated superficial vessels in the lower extremities are consistent with varicose veins. Varicose veins occur due to incompetence of the venous valves (**B**). Blood is propelled back to the heart from the lower extremities by action of the musculature on the veins, pushing blood along it; however, to prevent blood from backflowing, functioning venous valves are necessary. Given the history, heart failure is not likely (**D**). Hashimoto's thyroiditis and other autoimmune disorders are not commonly associated with varicose veins, and autoantibodies would not produce this effect (**E**). Although both obstruction of venous blood flow and neoplastic infiltration of lymphatic vessels could produce a similar appearance, given the time course of events, they are very unlikely (**A, C**).

231. Correct: Decubitus ulcer (C)

The lesion on the posterior surface of the thigh is a decubitus ulcer. Decubitus ulcers can occur in immobile patients due to constant pressure on skin surfaces. They commonly occur in areas that have overly bony prominences (e.g., the hips and the sacrum). Decubitus ulcers can extend deeply into the skin and to the bone. They can predispose to infection (**C**). The remainder of the choices are incorrect (**A-B, D-E**).

232. Correct: Coxsackievirus B infection (D)

The pericardial sac contains clear, watery, straw-colored fluid. These changes can be caused by a variety of conditions; however, Coxsackieviruses A and B, can produce a serous pericardial effusion (**D**). Given the history, the decedent most likely also has an underlying myocarditis. Metastatic tumor is associated with a hemorrhagic effusion (**A**), *Staphylococcus aureus* with a purulent effusion (**B**), and a recent myocardial infarct with a fibrinous pericarditis (note that the pericardial surface is smooth and glistening) (**C**). Chest trauma, if it caused an effusion, would produce hemorrhage (**E**).

233. Correct: Russell bodies (C)

The image illustrates cells containing a globule of acellular eosinophilic material. This material is immunoglobulin, and Russell bodies can be found in a variety of disorders (**C**). The appearance of the intracellular inclusions in the image is not consistent with the remainder of the lesions listed, nor is the clinical scenario (**A-B, D-E**).

234. Correct: Hyperplastic polyp (A)

The polyp has the typical features of a hyperplastic polyp, namely a serrated luminal border (**A**). There is no evidence of dysplasia, which would manifest as increase in nuclear size, hyperchromasia, and nuclear atypia (**B, C**). Also, in dysplastic glands, most frequently, mucus production is not evident. There is no evidence of invasion, and the cytologic features are not typical for an invasive adenocarcinoma of the colon (**D**). Barrett's metaplasia affects the esophagus (**E**).

235. Correct: Hypertension (C)

The image illustrates hyaline arteriolosclerosis, which is characterized by an acellular eosinophilic thickening of the vessel wall (**C**). A similar lesion can be identified in people with diabetes mellitus; however, although the histologic appearance is identical, the mechanism of formation in hypertension and diabetes mellitus is different. In hypertension it is due to damage to the vessel wall from pressure allowing plasma proteins to accumulate within the wall, whereas in diabetes mellitus it is due to the accumulation of advanced glycosylation end products. None of the other conditions produces a histologically similar lesion (**A-B, D-E**). Polyarteritis nodosa can have both a necrotizing transmural inflammation and scarring, as the disease has temporally heterogeneous lesions. Syphilis produces obliterative endarteritis.

236. Correct: Monospot test (C)

The clinical scenario is consistent with infectious mononucleosis. In infectious mononucleosis, patients can have atypical lymphocytes, such as that pictured in the image. Compared to normal lymphocytes, atypical lymphocytes have prominent cytoplasm (compared to a small rim around the nucleus) and more dispersed chromatin (compared to clumped chromatin). Atypical lymphocytes are found in infectious mononucleosis, and patients with infectious mononucleosis will have a positive monospot test (**C**). The other tests would not be expected to be positive (**A-B, D-E**).

237. Correct: *Streptococcus pneumoniae* (B)

The image illustrates meningitis. The surface of the brain has pus, which is unusual for *Neisseria meningitidis* because it usually develops so rapidly that the gross appearance of the brain is essentially normal (**A**). *Mycobacterium tuberculosis* is known for basilar involvement of the brain (**D**). *Aspergillus niger* and *Pseudomonas aeruginosa* would be rare causes of meningitis (**C, E**). The most common cause of meningitis in this age group would be *Streptococcus pneumoniae* (**B**).

238. Correct: Galactorrhea (A)

The image illustrates a pituitary adenoma. If the pituitary adenoma is functioning, the most commonly produced hormone is prolactin. Prolactin secretion can lead to galactorrhea and also amenorrhea and infertility (**A**). A TSH-secreting adenoma could lead to palpitations (**B**). TSH-secreting adenomas are rare. Oral hyperpigmentation can result from an ACTH-secreting adenoma, which is less common than those that secrete prolactin (**C**). Axillary and femoral hyperpigmentation is consistent with acanthosis nigricans, which is associated with diabetes mellitus and underlying malignancy (**D**). The pituitary adenoma is small and not as likely to produce mass effects, but mass effects are usually headache and visual field disturbances, and not commonly seizures (**E**).

239. Correct: Squamous cell carcinoma (D)

The image illustrates infiltrating nests of squamous cells. In the center of the image is a large keratin pearl, which is a characteristic feature of squamous cell carcinoma (**D**). The image does not contain malignant melanocytes (**E**), nests of cells with peripheral palisading (**C**), or adipose tissue (**B**). Seborrheic keratoses are pigmented, have a characteristic stuck-on appearance grossly, and would not have infiltrating nests or keratin pearls. The cells resemble the basal layer, and there is extensive accumulations of keratin (**A**).

240. Correct: Wilms' tumor (C)

The image illustrates two nephrogenic rests. Nephrogenic rests are a precursor for Wilms' tumor (**C**). When a Wilms' tumor is resected from a patient, identification of nephrogenic rests in the non-neoplastic kidney can predict the possible development of a Wilms' tumor in the remaining kidney. Although no glomeruli are present in the image, the presence of the tubules identifies the organ of origin. Nephrogenic rests are not characteristic of the remainder of the choices (**A-B, D-E**).

241.   Correct: Granulosa cell tumor (E)

The patient has an endometrial carcinoma. The tumor is filling the endometrial cavity and extending into the wall of the uterus. It is necrotic, which accounts for its friable appearance. Although there are other forms of uterine carcinoma, endometrial carcinoma is the most common. One condition that contributes to the development of an endometrial carcinoma is increased concentrations of estrogen. Granulosa cell tumors often secrete estrogen and, by doing so, serve as a risk factor for the development of endometrial and breast carcinoma (**E**). The other tumors listed do not contribute to the development of endometrial carcinoma (**A-D**).

242.   Correct: Colonic adenocarcinoma (B)

The image shows a cross-section of the liver with multiple tan-yellow nodules, consistent with metastatic tumor. Colonic adenocarcinoma is a common tumor type, and it most commonly metastasizes to the liver (**B**). The diagnosis of Crohn's disease for the first time at age 63 years would be unlikely, and it would be much less common than colonic adenocarcinoma, although Crohn's disease by itself is a risk factor for colonic adenocarcinoma (**A**). Brain tumors very rarely metastasize, and neither kidney stones nor granulomatosis with polyangiitis are associated with changes consistent with those seen in the liver (**C-D, E**).

243.   Correct: His hyperhomocysteinemia is a risk factor (D)

The image illustrates a coronary artery with a small atheromatous plaque. The plaque has a characteristic appearance, with a fibrous cap covering an atheromatous core. The plaque is small, causing less than 50% stenosis of the lumen of the vessel. To cause stable angina, the degree of stenosis would need to be around 75% (**A**). To cause unstable angina, the plaque would have to have some form of acute change, such as hemorrhage into the plaque (**B**). To cause his death, the plaque would have to have some form of acute change and, most likely, an occlusive thrombus (**C**). The main risk factors for atherosclerosis are family genetics, hypertension, diabetes mellitus, cigarette use, and hypercholesterolemia; however, there are other risk factors, including hyperhomocysteinemia (**D**). Cholesterol clefts are easily visible (**E**).

244.   Correct: Chronic obstructive pulmonary disease (D)

The image illustrates a dilated and hypertrophied right ventricle. The left ventricle is of normal thickness. The patient would have cor pulmonale, which can be due to four general categories of disease: diseases of the lung parenchyma, diseases of the pulmonary vasculature, diseases impairing normal chest movement, and conditions causing constriction of pulmonary arteries. Chronic obstructive pulmonary disease is a disease of the lung parenchyma that can

lead to right ventricular dilation and hypertrophy (**D**). The remainder of the conditions listed would not primarily affect the right ventricle (**A-C, E**).

245.   Correct: Subendocardial pallor and yellow discoloration in the anterior wall of the left ventricle (B)

The image illustrates an acute plaque change, with hemorrhage into the plaque, producing increased obstruction of the lumen of the vessel, but not occlusion, as a portion of the lumen still remains. With some lumen remaining, blood can reach the myocardium and prevent a transmural infarct (**A-B**). The left anterior descending supplies the anterior wall of the left ventricle (**D-E**). Circumferential subendocardial pallor would be due to decreased blood flow through all coronary arteries and could accompany shock (**A**).

246.   Correct: Hereditary spherocytosis (C)

The smear exhibits spherocytes, which are the small red blood cells with no central pallor (**C**). Hereditary spherocytosis is autosomal dominant, explaining its presence in three consecutive generations. Hereditary spherocytosis commonly is associated with splenomegaly. Sickle cell anemia is autosomal recessive, and no sickled red blood cells are present (**A**). Glucose-6-phosphate dehydrogenase deficiency is X-linked, and the characteristic cell is a bite cell (**B**). Iron deficiency is not hereditary, and the red blood cells characteristically have an increased central pallor (**E**). There is no evidence of malaria (**D**).

247.   Correct: Parvovirus B19 (C)

The history is consistent with hereditary spherocytosis. The blood smear illustrates spherocytes. Parvovirus B19 infects erythroblasts; their destruction can cause an acute lack of red blood cell production (**C**). Cytomegalovirus is a cause of infectious mononucleosis and can cause splenomegaly, but not the other features (**A**). Malaria can infect and lyse red blood cells, but the smear has no malarial organisms (**E**). Infection with Coxsackievirus A or hepatitis A virus would not produce the clinical scenario (**B, D**).

248.   Correct: AML (C)

The presenting symptoms are consistent with an acute leukemia, being rapid onset of symptoms related to deficiency of erythroid and myeloid lines. The bone marrow smear has blasts. The blasts have a large amount of cytoplasm, which is more characteristic of myeloblasts, and the CD33 confirms their origin. The morphology and the staining are inconsistent with the remainder of the choices (**A-B, D-E**).

249.   Correct: CLL (B)

The image illustrates an increased white blood cell count and resultant anemia. The white blood cells are predominantly of one type, which appear as mature lymphocytes, with clumped chromatin, giving the nucleus a cracked-earth or gingersnap appearance. There are also smudge cells. The morphology and the clinical scenario are consistent with CLL (**B**). ALL and AML would have blasts, with dispersed chromatin, and the presentation would be more acute (**A, C**). CML would have more mature myeloid cells (**D**). The morphology of the leukemic cells is not consistent with hairy cell leukemia (**E**).

250. Correct: CML (D)

The slide illustrates a chronic myelogenous leukemia, as there are myeloid precursors in various states of development, and there is a basophil in the image. There are no blasts; however, the final stage of CML is usually a blast crisis, which can be either myeloid or lymphoid in origin (**D**). The history is inconsistent with ALL or AML, which usually develop much more rapidly (**A, C**). The morphology is not consistent with hairy cell leukemia (**E**).

251. Correct: Iron deficiency anemia (C)

The image illustrates red blood cells that have an increased amount of central pallor. This appearance is characteristic for iron deficiency anemia. Another feature of iron deficiency anemia can be elongated, or pencil cells (**C**). The clinical scenario should suggest a neoplasm, such as colonic adenocarcinoma, with GI blood loss as the cause of the iron deficiency anemia. The morphologic changes are inconsistent with the remainder of the choices (**A-B, D-E**).

252. Correct: Bullous emphysema (D)

At the apex of the lung is a large bulla, which is an air-filled sac. Bullous emphysema can develop as a result of underlying emphysema. These air-filled sacs can rupture and can lead to the development of a pneumothorax (**D**). The other conditions would not produce the pathology illustrated in the image (**A-C, E**).

253. Correct: Desquamative interstitial pneumonitis (C)

The image shows accumulations of pigment-laden macrophages in essentially all of the alveolar airspaces. The pigment is anthracotic pigment. These histologic changes are consistent with desquamative interstitial pneumonitis, which is associated with cigarette use (**C**). Usual interstitial pneumonitis would not be diffuse and has fibroblastic foci and honeycomb change (**A**). Nonspecific interstitial pneumonitis would be diffuse but does not have the intra-alveolar macrophages (**B**). There are no neutrophils, and the alveolar airspaces are not increased in size due to loss of parenchyma (**D-E**).

254. Correct: Acute pyelonephritis (D)

The image illustrates a neutrophilic infiltrate in the interstitium. Given the clinical scenario, the patient most likely had a urinary tract infection that ascended to the kidneys, causing acute pyelonephritis (**D**). A drug-induced interstitial nephritis would also produce an interstitial infiltrate; however, it would be predominantly macrophages and lymphocytes, and some eosinophils would be visible (**A**). There is no evidence of vascular changes, a neoplasm, or microthrombi (**C, B, E**).

255. Correct: Clear cell renal cell carcinoma (D)

The histologic features illustrated in the image are consistent with clear cell renal cell carcinoma—clear cells with a fine vascular network. Although the nuclei appear bland, with little pleomorphism or mitotic figures, clear cell renal cell carcinoma can behave very aggressively (**D**). A papillary renal cell carcinoma has neoplastic cells arranged on papillae (**B**). A clear cell sarcoma would be very rare (**A**). Xanthogranulomatous pyelonephritis, with foamy macrophages, can mimic clear cell renal cell carcinoma, but it is most frequently associated with a staghorn calculus (**E**). There is no evidence of invasive glands (**C**).

256. Correct: Drug-induced interstitial nephritis (C)

The clinical scenario, hematuria and fever following 3 weeks after usage of a medication, is consistent with a drug-induced interstitial nephritis (**C**). Although eosinophils are often present, the main cell types are lymphocytes and macrophages. Given her young age and the clinical scenario, a follicular lymphoma is not likely (**B**). There are no neutrophils, viral inclusions, or neoplastic cells lining papillae (**A, E, D**).

257. Correct: Alcohol dehydrogenase (A)

The image illustrates oxalic acid crystals. While ethylene glycol as a compound is not injurious to the kidney, when it is broken down by alcohol dehydrogenase, it forms oxalic acid, which deposits in, and damages the kidney (**A**). The other choices are incorrect (**B-E**).

258. Correct: Retinal hemorrhage often occurs. (D)

The pathologic lesion is hyperplastic arteriolosclerosis, or onion-skinning, which is characteristic of severe hypertension. Clinically, severe hypertension can manifest as systolic blood pressure of greater than 200 mm Hg and diastolic blood pressure of greater than 120 mm Hg. Signs and symptoms can include retinal hemorrhage, renal failure, and papilledema (**D**). People with hypertension do not have c-ANCA or p-ANCA (**A**), most cases have a mixed etiology (both genetic and environmental) (**B**), and it is not associated with schistosomiasis (**C**). One of the most common causes of intracerebral hemorrhage is hypertension (**E**).

259. Correct: Patients can develop an acute cerebral infarct. (D)

The lesion is a papillary fibroelastoma. Papillary fibroelastomas are benign growths that occur on the cardiac valves (**A**). They are not malignant and do not predispose to malignancy (**B**). They are not the result of acute rheumatic carditis, and culture of the lesion should not grow any organisms (**C, E**). If the delicate papillary projections break loose, they can embolize, including to the brain (if the lesion is on the mitral and aortic valve), and would cause a cerebral infarct (**D**).

260. Correct: Pleomorphic adenoma (C)

Pleomorphic adenomas are the most common tumor of the parotid gland. They have both epithelial (ductal and myoepithelial) and mesenchymal components, with the epithelial cells being dispersed in the mesenchymal components. In this case, the background appears myxoid or cartilaginous. The tumors require a wide local resection, or they can recur, and malignant transformation can occur (**C**). Mucoepidermoid carcinomas have squamous, mucous, and intermediate cells (**D**). Warthin's tumor has a prominent lymphoid component (**E**). There is no malignant cartilage nor whorls with psammoma bodies. Meningiomas can, very rarely, involve the parotid gland (**A, B**).

261. Correct: Chronic gastritis (C)

The stomach has a prominent infiltrate of lymphoid cells in the mucosa, which are forming follicles. The histologic features are consistent with chronic gastritis (**C**). Further testing would most likely identify a *Helicobacter pylori* infection. Left untreated, these patients are at risk for developing a marginal zone lymphoma (or, MALToma), which can be cured by treating the underlying infection (**D**). There is no neutrophilic infiltrate, loss of mucosa, or evidence of neoplastic glands (**A-B, E**).

262. Correct: Cirrhosis (C)

The image illustrates a liver that is divided into variously sized nodules of hepatocytes by fibrous septa. There is a minimal amount of inflammation within the fibrous septa. These changes are consistent with cirrhosis (**C**). The lack of symptoms or a previous diagnosis of cirrhosis does not exclude the diagnosis, as many patients with cirrhosis can be asymptomatic for a period of time. The histologic changes are not consistent with the remainder of the conditions listed (**A-B, D-E**).

263. Correct: Alcohol (C)

The image illustrates a liver that is yellow-tan discolored, indicating steatosis, and also micronodular, indicating cirrhosis. Although most chronic alcoholics do not develop cirrhosis, chronic alcoholism is so common that in most cases, cirrhosis is due to underlying alcohol use (**C**). Alcohol use produces both fat accumulation in the liver and cirrhosis of the liver. Iron deposition can cause cirrhosis, but its incidence is much lower than that of chronic alcoholism (**A**). Hepatitis A does not cause chronic changes in the liver (**D**). Amyloidosis is not associated with cirrhosis, and *Clonorchis sinensis* would be very unlikely (**B, E**).

264. Correct: Coagulative necrosis (C)

The image illustrates coagulative necrosis (**C**)—hepatocytes with loss of nuclear and cytoplasmic basophilia, but with retention of architecture. Infarcts of the liver are uncommon, as the liver has a dual blood supply, and when they occur, hepatic infarcts are most often red infarcts, because of congestion. The infarct in the image is actually a white infarct, as there is no congestion. The image shows no changes consistent with any of the other conditions (**A-B, D-E**).

265. Correct: Mallory's hyaline (C)

The individual is most likely an alcoholic. Although not easily diagnosed from the image, the patient had alcoholic hepatitis, which can include a marked amount of Mallory's hyaline. In the image, multiple hepatocytes contain Mallory's hyaline, the ropy eosinophilic condensation of intermediate filaments that is occurring in the cytoplasm (**C**). Although there is also some steatosis, none of the other items listed are present (**A-B, D-E**). Given the circumstances, he most likely had a Mallory-Weiss tear, which in healthy individuals is not usually fatal; however, in individuals with cirrhosis and resultant clotting abnormalities, the condition can be fatal.

266. Correct: Chronic hepatitis C infection (C)

The image illustrates a marked portal tract lymphocytic infiltrate, which is characteristic of chronic hepatitis. Chronic hepatitis B often has ground-glass appearing hepatocytes, which are due to an accumulation of hepatitis B surface antigen in the hepatocyte (**B**), whereas chronic hepatitis C has lymphoid aggregates and bile duct epithelium proliferation (**C**). Hepatitis A does not have a chronic form (**A**). There is no fibrosis surrounding the bile ducts, and there is no evidence of a neoplasm (**D, E**).

267. Correct: Benign proliferation of cells (D)

The image illustrates a hemangioma. Hemangiomas are fairly common lesions of the liver and are usually of the cavernous form. They represent a benign proliferation of vascular cells (**D**). Although they are benign, and not capable of invasion or metastasis, the tumor can rupture and cause death through exsanguination. Many times, a person will have multiple hemangiomas. None of the other mechanisms explain the finding in the liver (**A-C, E**).

268. Correct: Prussian blue (D)

The patient has features of hereditary hemochromatosis—cirrhosis of the liver, diabetes mellitus, and increased skin pigmentation. The material in the liver is iron. A Prussian blue stain will highlight iron (**D**). A trichrome stain will highlight the fibrosis associated with cirrhosis; however, it would not add to the diagnosis of the underlying cause of the cirrhosis in this case (**E**). Oil Red O stains fat, Warthin-Starry stains bacteria, and a Congo red stain stains amyloid (**C, A, B**).

269. Correct: The disease causes some patients to develop arthritis. (D)

The clinical scenario is consistent with hereditary hemochromatosis, which is an autosomal recessive disease caused by a mutation in the *HFE* gene. The disease has a variable penetrance (**B**). Manifestations include those in the clinical scenario as well as arthritis and cardiomyopathy—with both dilated and restrictive forms being associated with the disease (**D**). The condition, in the primary form, develops due to excessive intestinal absorption of iron (**A**). It can easily be treated with routine phlebotomy; however, even with treatment, patients still have a high risk for developing hepatocellular carcinoma (**C**). The disease is not associated with dementia (**E**).

270. Correct: Cholesterolosis (B)

The mucosal surface of the gallbladder has many punctate yellow discolorations, which appear microscopically as accumulations of foamy cells. While many people who have their gallbladder resected have gallstones, some have only thick bile, and some have cholesterolosis (**B**). The gallbladder is not normal (**A**). In an acute infection, the wall would be thickened (**C**). There is no evidence of a stone or a neoplasm (**D, E**).

271. Correct: Acute cholangitis (C)

The clinical scenario is consistent with an individual who has cholecystitis, complicated by choledocholithiasis leading to acute cholangitis (**C**). The image illustrates an inflamed bile duct. Although *Clonorchis sinensis* is a common cause of cholangitis in Asia, in the United States the usual organisms are *Escherichia coli, Klebsiella, Clostridium,* and others (**D**). In the image, only the bile duct is involved, and the surrounding hepatocytes are essentially normal. There is no histologic evidence of the other conditions that are listed (**A, B, E**).

272. Correct: Reflux esophagitis (C)

The image illustrates a section of the esophagus with one eosinophil. In reflux esophagitis, the presence of eosinophils and basal zone hyperplasia help formulate the diagnosis (**C**). In eosinophilic esophagitis, the eosinophilic infiltrate would be much more extensive (**D**). There are no granulomas, evidence of a parasite, or intestinal metaplasia (**A-B, E**).

273. Correct: Pancreatic pseudocyst (C)

Given the clinical scenario, the patient, being a chronic alcoholic, is at risk for bouts of acute pancreatitis, which can lead to the development of a pseudocyst. The pseudocyst is normally lined with necrotic material, which causes the brown appearance (**C**). In a pseudocyst, however, there is no epithelial lining (**A, B**). Serous and mucinous tumors of the pancreas generally present at an older age and would present as a mass (**D, E**). In this case, there is just a gaping defect in the pancreatic parenchyma.

274. Correct: Acute pancreatitis (A)

The clinical scenario and laboratory testing are consistent with acute pancreatitis, and the image shows infiltration of neutrophils within the interstitium (**A**). Chronic pancreatitis would have lymphocytes, fibrosis, and loss of parenchyma as well as possible calcification (**B**). There are no neoplastic glands or lymphoid cells (**C, E**). The most common causes of acute pancreatitis are alcohol use and gallstones. The changes do not represent a type III hypersensitivity reaction (**D**).

275. Correct: Prostatic adenocarcinoma (D)

Between the ducts on the left and the acini on the right, there are small glands that are back-to-back in the intervening stroma. This low-power view is consistent with prostatic adenocarcinoma (**D**). The prostate is not normal (**A**), and there are no neutrophils, hyperplasia, or invasive colonic-type glands (**B, C, E**).

276. Correct: Endometrial polyps (B)

The endometrial surface of the uterus has two polypoid projections; however, the endometrium otherwise appears normal. The polyps are lined by endometrial glands that are similar to the basal layer of the endometrium (**B**). Endometrial polyps can rarely serve as the substrate for endometrial carcinoma; however, there is no evidence of a malignant neoplasm (**D**). The stromal cells of a polyp can be monoclonal. An intramural leiomyoma would be entirely within the wall of the uterus (**C**). Pelvic inflammatory disease affects the ovaries and fallopian tubes, but not the endometrial cavity (**E**). Dysfunctional uterine bleeding would not cause a mass lesion (**A**).

277. Correct: Phylloides tumor (B)

The tumor appears very similar to a fibroadenoma (**A**), however, it has some outward, leaf-like projections, which are consistent with a phylloides tumor (**B**). Most phylloides tumors are benign; some are malignant, but usually only locally aggressive. The histologic features are not consistent with a malignancy (**C-E**).

Index

A

Abdominal aortic aneurysm, 92, 93
Abscesses, 14, 287
Acanthosis nigricans, 48
ACA (anterior cerebral artery) stroke, 26
Accumulations, cellular, **4–5,** 8, 285
Acetaminophen toxicity, 74, 193, 194
Achalasia, 288
Acoustic schwannomas, 262
Acquired thrombocytopenia, 24
Acromegaly, 227
Acute appendicitis, 171
Acute bronchopneumonia, 138
Acute calculous cholecystitis, 192
Acute cerebral hemorrhage, 255
Acute infarct, 255
Acute inflammation, 13–14, 23, 284
Acute lymphangitis, 100
Acute lymphocytic leukemia, 121
Acute mastitis, 215
Acute myeloid leukemia, 121
Acute myocardial infarction, 26, 93, 94,
    97–98, 194, 283
Acute pancreatitis, 120, 198, 285
Acute primary adrenocortical insufficiency,
    232–233
Acute prostatitis, 212
Acute renal failure, 152
Acute respiratory distress, 65, 286, 287
Acute retroviral syndrome, 42
Acute tubular necrosis, 152
Adaption, cellular, **2–3,** 5–6
Adaptive immunity, 38
Addison's disease, 232, 233
Adenocarcinomas, 168, 173–175, 195,
    210–212, 289
Adenomas, 172, 174, 215, 227, 228, 230, 231
Adenomatous polyposis, 49, 174
Adenomyosis, 210
Adrenal glands, diseases of, 64, 94, **224–226,**
    228, 232–233
Adrenal hyperplasia, 64, 94, 232, 233
Aflatoxin, 73
Aging, cellular, **5,** 8
AIDS, 43
Air embolism, 26
Alcohol dehydrogenase, 152
Alcoholic liver disease, 188–190
Aldosterone-secreting tumors, 232
Alkaline phosphatase, 195
Allergic reactions, 284
Allergies, seasonal, 38
α-thalassemia, 118, 120
Alzheimer's disease, 259–260
Amniotic bands, 65
Amniotic fluid embolism, 25–26
Amyloidosis, 41
Amyloid protein, 260, 286
Amyotrophic lateral sclerosis, 261
Anaphylactic reaction, 38, 39, 284

Anemias
– autoimmune, 39, 117, 119, 122, 194
– dietary deficiencies and, 75, 116–119, 168,
    170, 174
– liver diseases and, 192–193, 194–195
– overview, **105–111,** 116–120
– red blood cell disorders and, 116–120
Aneurysms, **79–80,** 92–93, 95–96, 173, **247,**
    257
Angina, stable, 93
Angioedema, 42
Angiosarcomas, 73, 100
Anterior cerebral artery (ACA) stroke, 26
Antibiotic-induced diarrhea, 174–175
Antibodies, 194
Antiphospholipid antibody syndromes (APS),
    27
α-1-antitrypsin deficiency, 61, 190
Aortic dissection, 92, 93, 94, 95, 193
Aortic stenosis, 24
APC gene, 48–49
Aplastic anemia, 117, 122
Aplastic crises, 119
Apoplexy, pituitary, 228
Apoptosis, 7, 15, 285, 286
Appendicitis, 65, 171
Appendix, diseases of, 65, 171
APS (antiphospholipid antibody syndromes),
    27
Arachnoid cyst, 229
Arrhythmogenic right ventricular dysplasia-
    cardiomyopathy, 98
Arsenic poisoning, 73
Arteriolar nephrosclerosis, 94
Asbestos exposure, 73, 136, 137, 139
Ascites, 188
Ascitic fluid infection, 188
AST/ALT elevation, 190–191, 194
Asthma, 135–136
Atelectasis, 140
Atherosclerosis, **80–83,** 93–95, 97, 173, 283,
    285
Atherosclerotic coronary artery disease, 173
ATP7B gene, 191
Atrial septal defects, 96–97
Atrophy, 5, 6, 283, 285, 286
Autoimmune diseases, **32–35,** 39–41
Autoimmune gastritis, 170
Autoimmune hemolytic anemias, 39, 117,
    119, 122, 194
Autoimmune hepatitis, 193–194
Avascular necrosis, 239

B

Babesiosis, 119
Babinski's reflex, 260
Bacterial infections
– of CNS, 257–258
– of endocrine system, 233
– of genital tract, 209, 212

– of GI tract, 169–170, 171, 172, 174–175, 289
– pediatric, 60, 65, 287
– pulmonary, 15, 138, 286–287
Barrett's esophagus, 168
Basal cell carcinoma, 268
Basilar meningitis, 258
B-cell neoplasms, 121, 194–195
Benign prostatic hyperplasia (BPH), 211, 286
Benzocaine, 73
Bernard-Soulier's disease, 24
Berry aneurysms, 94, 257
Beryllium, 288
ß-carotene, 75
β-thalassemia, 116, 118, 120
Bile duct tumor, 195
Biliary tract diseases, **183–185,** 191–193
Birth defects, 65
Bitemporal hemianopia, 229
Blindness, 171
Blood pressure
– hypertension, **80–83,** 93–95, 189, 255, 285
– hypotension, 173
Boerhaave's syndrome, 168
Bone diseases, 235–240
– neoplastic, **238,** 239–240
– non-neoplastic, **236–237,** 238–239
Bone marrow, 121–122
Border zone infarct, 255
Bowel obstruction, 171, 172, 191
BPH (benign prostatic hyperplasia), 211, 286
Brain, diseases and disorders, **243–246,**
    254–257
Breast diseases, 213–216
Broca's aphasia, 254
Bronchiectasis, 286
Bronchitis, 135, 287
Bronchogenic carcinoma, 139–140
Bronchopneumonia, 138
Bruising, 23
Brunner's glands, 170
Budd-Chiari syndrome, 195
Bullous pemphigoid, 267
Burkitt lymphoma, 122

C

Cachexia, 15
CAH (congenital adrenal hyperplasia), 64, 94,
    232, 233
Calcifications, cellular, **5,** 8
Calcium pyrophosphate disease, 239
Calculi, renal, 153
Cancer, 48–49, 63, 74. *See also specific cancers*
Cannabis, 75
Carbon monoxide poisoning, 73
Carcinoid syndrome, 171
Carcinoid tumor, 171
Carcinomas
– adenocarcinomas, 168, 173–175, 195,
    210–212, 289
– breast, 215–216

Carcinomas (cont.)
– esophageal, 188, 289
– gastric, 169–170, 174, 289
– of genital tract, 208, 209, 212
– hepatic, 73, 188–189, 195
– neurodegenerative, 259
– pancreatic, 199
– pulmonary, 139–140, 228
– renal, 153
– of skin, 268
– of thyroid, 231
Cardiac myxomas, 100
Cardiogenic shock, 23–24
Cardiomyopathies, **88–89,** 98–99
Cardiovascular system, diseases of, 77–101
– aneurysms, **79–80,** 92–93, 95–96, 173, **247,** 257
– atherosclerosis and hypertension, **80–83,** 93–95, 97, 173, 283, 285
– cardiomyopathies, **88–89,** 98–99
– congenital heart disease, **84–85,** 96–97
– ischemic heart disease, **86–88,** 97–98
– miscellaneous, **89–92,** 99–101
– vasculitis, **84,** 95–96
ß-carotene, 75
Caseating granulomas, 15
Caseous necrosis, 6, 15
Catecholamine-secreting tumors, 232
Celiac disease, 169, 172, 290
Cells, 1–8
– accumulations, **4–5,** 8, 285
– adaption by, **2–3,** 5–6
– aging, **5,** 8
– calcifications, **5,** 8
– injury, **3–4,** 6–7
– red blood cell disorders, 116–120
– types of, 23, 38, 169, 174, 258
– white blood cell disorders, **111–115,** 120–123
Cellular casts, 150
Central diabetes insipidus, 229
Central nervous system, diseases of
– aneurysms, **247,** 257
– brain, **243–246,** 254–257
– infections, **247–248,** 257–258
– neoplasms, **253–254,** 261–262
Central pontine myelinolysis, 258–259
Centrilobular hepatic necrosis, 74
Cerebellar hemangioblastoma, 261
Cerebellar syndromes, 254
Cerebral edema, 24, 256
Cerebral hemorrhage, 255
Cerebral infarct, 94, 254–255
Cervical adenocarcinoma, 210
Cervical dysplasia, 209, 210
Cervical neoplasia, 210
Chediak-Higashi syndrome, 13, 41–42
Chemotherapeutic agents, 74
Chlamydia trachomatis, 209, 212
Cholangiocarcinoma, 195
Cholecystitis, 191–192
Choledocholithiasis, 192–193
Cholesterol embolization, 26
Cholesterol stones, 192–193
Choriocarcinoma, 208
Chromium toxicity, 74
Chromosomal disorders, **55–56,** 62–63
Chronic berylliosis, 288
Chronic bronchitis, 135, 287
Chronic cholecystitis, 191–192
Chronic gastritis, 170
Chronic granulomatous disease, 42
Chronic hypersensitivity pneumonitis, 137–138, 288

Chronic inflammation, 14
Chronic lymphocytic leukemia, 121, 123
Chronic myeloid leukemia, 121–122
Chronic obstructive pulmonary disease, 135, 136
Chronic pancreatitis, 171, 290
Chronic passive congestion, 24
Chronic renal failure, 152
Chronic venous insufficiency, 25
Chvostek's sign, 192
Cirrhosis, 168, **179–180,** 188–189, 191, 195
Claudication, 283
Clear cell adenocarcinoma, 210
Cleft lip, 65
Clostridium difficile, 65, 174–175
Coagulation, 24–25
Coagulative necrosis, 6, 7, 193
Coagulopathy, 26–27
Coarctation of the aorta, 63, 96
Cobalamin (vitamin B12) deficiency, 75, 76, 116, 170, 283
Cobalt toxicity, 74
Cocaine abuse, 74
Cold autoimmune hemolytic anemias, 117, 194
Colitis, 65
Colonic adenocarcinoma, 173, 174, 175
Communicating hydrocephalus, 260, 262
Community-acquired pneumonia, 42, 138
Compressive atelectasis, 140
Concentric hypertrophy, 100
Congenital adrenal hyperplasia (CAH), 64, 94, 232, 233
Congenital birth defects, 65
Congenital heart disease, **84–85,** 96–97
Congenital pyloric stenosis, 64, 65, 169, 289
Congestion, 23, 24, 284
Congestive heart failure, 23, 171
Conjugated bilirubin, 192
Contact dermatitis, 268
Contraction atelectasis, 140
Contusions, 23, 284–285
Conventional chondrosarcoma, 240
Copper deficiency, 76
Coronary arterial distribution, 98
Coronary artery atherosclerosis, 97
Coronary artery dissection, 97
Cortisol-secreting tumors, 232
Coumadin-induced skin necrosis, 74
Courvoisier's sign, 192, 198
Cowden's syndrome, 48
Craniopharyngioma, 228, 229, 262
Creutzfeldt-Jakob disease, 259, 261
Crohn's disease, 173–174, 175
Cryopyrin-associated periodic fever syndromes, 13
Crypt abscesses and ulcers, 174
Cryptococcal infections, 43
Curling's ulcers, 289
Cushing's disease, 94, 228, 232, 233
Cushing's syndrome, 94, 139
Cushing's ulcer, 289
Cyanotic congenital heart defects, 96
Cyclic vomiting, 75
Cystic fibrosis, 64–65, 290
Cytokines, 15

D

Dapsone, 73
DCIS (ductal carcinoma in situ), 216
DCS (decompression sickness), 25
D-dimer test, 141, 142
Decompression sickness (DCS), 25
Deep tendon reflexes, 260

Deep venous thrombi, 23, 99, 141
Delayed hemolytic transfusion reaction, 39
5p-deletion syndrome, 63
Dementia, 171, 259–260, 261
de Quervain's thyroiditis, 231
Dermatitis herpetiformis, 267, 269
Desquamative interstitial pneumonitis (DIP), 137
Diabetes, gestational, 64
Diabetes insipidus, 229
Diabetes mellitus, 190, 233
Diabetic ketoacidosis, 233, 234, 285
Dietary deficiencies, **71–73,** 75–76. See also specific dietary deficiencies
Diethylstilbestrol, 210
Diffuse-type gastric carcinoma, 289
DiGeorge's syndrome, 63
Digestive system diseases. See Gastrointestinal tract, diseases of
Dilated cardiomyopathy, 99
DIP (desquamative interstitial pneumonitis), 137
Disaccharidase deficiency, 172
Diseases
– adrenal gland, 64, 94, **224–226,** 228, 232–233
– autoimmune, **32–35,** 39–41
– biliary tract, **183–185,** 191–193
– bone, 235–240
– breast, 213–216
– cardiovascular system, 77–101. See also Cardiovascular system, diseases of
– endocrine, 217–234. See also Endocrine system, diseases of
– environmental, **68–69,** 73
– gastrointestinal tract, 155–175. See also Gastrointestinal tract, diseases of
– genital tract, 201–212. See also Genital tract, diseases of
– hematopoietic system, **105–111,** 116–120
– immune system, 29–43. See also Immune system, diseases of
– integumentary system, 263–269
– kidney and urinary tract, 143–153. See also Kidney and urinary tract, diseases of
– liver, 177–195. See also Liver, diseases of
– musculoskeletal system, 235–240
– nervous system, 241–262. See also Nervous system, diseases of
– pancreas, 197–199, **226–227,** 233–234, 285
– pediatric, **52–53, 56–60,** 60, 63–65
– respiratory system, 125–142. See also Respiratory system, diseases of
– structural proteins, **54,** 61–62
Disseminated intravascular coagulation, 25, 120
Diverticulosis, 173, 174
Down's syndrome, 62–63, 261
Drug-induced lupus, 40, 284
Drugs, therapeutic, **69–70,** 73–74
Drugs of abuse, **70–71,** 74–75
Dubin-Johnson syndrome, 189, 193
Duchenne's muscular dystrophy, 260
Ductal carcinoma in situ (DCIS), 216
Dysfunctional uterine bleeding, 209
Dysplasia, 209, 286, 289
Dystrophic calcification, 8

E

Eccentric hypertrophy, 100
Ecchymosis, 23
Ectasy (MDMA) abuse, 74
Ecthyma gangrenosum, 267
Ectopic pregnancy, 212

Edward's syndrome, 63
Effusions, 14, **134,** 141
Ehlers-Danlos syndrome, 61, 95
Eisenmenger's syndrome, 96
Embolic stroke, 25
Embolism
– hemodynamics of, 23, 25–26
– pulmonary, 26, 99–100, **133–135,** 140–142,
    199, 283
Embryonal carcinoma, 208
Emphysema, 101, 190, 287–288
Empyema, 138
Endocrine system, diseases of, 217–234
– adrenal glands, 64, 94, **224–226,** 228,
    232–233
– pancreas, **198,** 198–199, **226–227,** 233–234,
    285
– parathyroid gland, **223–224,** 231
– pituitary gland, **218–220,** 227–229, 230
– thyroid gland, **221–223,** 229–231
Endometrial carcinoma, 209
Endometrial hyperplasia, 209
Endometriosis, 210, 212
Entamoeba histolytica, 172, 174, 175
Environmental diseases and toxins, **68–69,** 73
Enzyme deficiencies, **52–53,** 60–61
Ependymoma, 262
Epidural hemorrhage, 256
Epstein-Barr virus, 121
Erythema multiforme, 267
Escherichia coli, 60
Esophageal adenocarcinoma, 168
Esophageal carcinoma, 188, 289
Esophageal varices, 168, 188, 189
Esophagus, diseases and disorders of, **157,**
    168, 173, 188, 189, 288, 289
Ethylene glycol, 152
Ewing's sarcoma, 239
Exogenous steroids, 233
Exophthalmos, 230
Extensive centrilobular necrosis, 194
Extrahepatic cholestasis, 192
Extravascular hemolysis, 119
Exudates, 13, 15, 285

F

Factor V Leiden mutations, 141, 283
Familial adenomatous polyposis, 49
Familial hypercholesterolemia, 93
Familial malignant melanoma, 48–49
Familial neoplasia syndromes, 48–49
Fanconi anemia, 119
Farmer's lung, 137
Fat accumulation (cellular), 8, 285
Fat embolism, 25
Fat necrosis, 7
Fat-soluble vitamin deficiency, 171
Fatty casts, 150, 152
Fatty streak, 93
Felty's syndrome, 40
Female reproductive system, diseases of
– ovaries, **205–206,** 210–211, 232
– pregnancy, **208,** 210, 212
– uterus, **202–205, 208,** 209–210, 212
Fetal alcohol syndrome, 63
Fibrillin, 93
Fibrinoid necrosis, 7
Fibroadenomas, 215
Fibrocystic disease, 215
Fibromuscular dysplasia, 283
Fibrous cap, 97
Fitz-Hugh-Curtis syndrome, 211
5p-deletion syndrome, 63
Focal segmental glomerulosclerosis (FSGS), 151

Folate (folic acid) deficiency, 75, 117, 118, 170
Foreign body in airway, **135,** 142
Fractures, pathological, 139
Fragile X syndrome, 63
Friedreich ataxia, 61
FSGS (focal segmental glomerulosclerosis),
    151

G

Galactosemia, 60
Gall bladder, **183–185,** 191–193, 198–199
Gall stones, 192–193
Gangrenous necrosis, 7
Gastric bleeding, 169–170, 188, 189
Gastric carcinoma, 169–170, 174
Gastric hemorrhage, 169–170
Gastric peptic ulcers, 169–170
Gastritis, autoimmune, 170
Gastroesophageal reflux, 173, 289
Gastrointestinal stromal tumor (GIST),
    289–290
Gastrointestinal tract, diseases of, 155–175
– esophagus, **157,** 168, 173, 188, 189, 288,
    289
– large intestine **163–168,** 173–175
– small intestine, **160–163,** 170–172
– stomach, **158–160,** 169–170, 289–290
Genetic disorders, **52–56,** 60–63. *See also*
    specific genetic disorders
Genital tract, diseases of, 201–212
– ovaries, **205–206,** 210–211, 232
– penis, **207,** 212
– pregnancy, **208,** 210, 212
– prostate, **206–207,** 211–212, 286
– testes, **202,** 208
– uterus, **202–205, 208,** 209–210, 212
Germ cell tumors, 208
Gestational diabetes, 64
GGT concentrations, 195
Ghon complex, 287
Giant cell arteritis, 95
Giant cell tumor, 240
Gilbert's syndrome, 189
GIST (gastrointestinal stromal tumor),
    289–290
Glioblastoma multiforme, 262
Glomerular diseases, **144–146,** 149–151, 152
Glomus tumor, 100
Glossitis, 168, 171
Glucose-6-phosphate dehydrogenase
    deficiency, 118
Gonococcal arthritis, 285
Goodpasture's syndrome, 287
Granulomas, 15, 174
Granulomatosis, 95
Granulomatous inflammation, 13, 15
Grave's disease, 230
Group B streptococcus (*Streptococcus
    agalactiae),* 287
Guillain-Barré syndrome, 259

H

HA (hereditary angioedema), 42
Hashimoto's thyroiditis, 229–230, 231
Heart. *See* Cardiovascular system, diseases of
Heartburn, 289
Heart-failure cells, 23
Heinz bodies, 118
Helicobacter pylori, 169–170, 172, 289
Hematopoietic system, diseases of, **105–111,**
    116–120
Hemiballismus, 254
Hemochromatosis, 190
Hemodynamics, 17–27

– coagulation, **19–20,** 24–25
– embolism, 23, 25–26, 99. *See also*
    Pulmonary embolism
– hereditary thrombophilia and coagulopathy,
    22–23, 26–27
– infarcts, 25–26, 92–94, 97–98, 194, 254–256,
    283, 285
– overview, **18–19,** 23–24
– thrombolysis, 24
– thrombosis, 25–26, 173, 285
Hemoglobin A1C, 232
Hemolytic anemias, 117, 119, 192–193,
    194–195
Hemorrhage
– of CNS, 255, 256, 257
– gastric, 169–170
– intraventricular, 172
– pituitary gland and, 228
– types of, 23, 284–285
Hemosiderin, 285
Hemostasis, **24,** 26
Henoch-Schonlein purpura, 150
Heparin-induced thrombocytopenia, 24
Hepatitis, alcoholic, 189
Hepatitis, autoimmune, 193–194
Hepatitis A, 190–191
Hepatitis B, 151, 189
Hepatitis D, 189
Hepatocellular carcinoma, 73, 188–189
Hereditary angioedema (HA), 42
Hereditary mixed hyperlipidemia, 234
Hereditary spherocytosis, 117, 118
Hereditary thrombophilia, 26–27
Herniation of brain, 256
Herpes simplex virus infection, 289
HHV-8, 100
Hiatal hernia, 289
Hirschsprung's disease, 173
Hirsutism, 232
Histamine, 13
HIV, 43, 48, 151, 258
Hodgkin's lymphoma, 74, 123
Homans' sign, 192
Homer-Wright pseudorosettes, 64
Homer-Wright rosettes, 233
Horner's syndrome, 259
Human papillomaviruses, 209–210
Huntington's chorea, 261
Hurler's syndrome, 62
Hyaline arteriolosclerosis, 95
Hyaline disease of the newborn, 65
Hyaline membrane disease, 172
Hydralazine-induced lupus, 40, 284
Hydrocephalus, 260, 262
Hyperadrenalism, 94, 228, 232, 233
Hypercalcemia, 139, 231
Hypercholesterolemia, 93
Hyperemia, 23
Hyperhomocysteinemia, 27
Hyper-IgM syndrome, 42
Hyperlipidemia, 234
Hyperparathyroidism, 231
Hyperplasia, 6, 209, 286
Hypersegmented neutrophils, 117
Hypersensitivity myocarditis, 99
Hypersensitivity pneumonitis, 137
Hypersensitivity reactions, **30–31,** 38–39, 284
Hypertension, **80–83,** 93–95, 189, 255, 285
Hypertensive neuropathy, 94
Hyperthermia, 74
Hyperthyroidism, 229, 230–231
Hypertonic hyponatremia, 232
Hypertrophic cardiomyopathy, 98, 99
Hypertrophy, 5, 6

Hypoadrenalism, 232–233
Hypocalcemia, 231
Hyponatremia, 74, 233
Hypoparathyroidism, 231
Hypophosphatemia, 75
Hypopituitarism, 228
Hypotension, 173
Hypothyroidism, 229, 230–231
Hypotonic hyponatremia, 232
Hypovolemic shock, 24

I

Idiopathic thrombocytopenic purpura (ITP), 119
Immediate transfusion reaction, 39, 284
Immune system, diseases of, 29–43
– autoimmune diseases, **32–35,** 39–41
– hypersensitivity reactions, **30–31,** 38–39, 284
– immunodeficiencies, **35–38,** 41–43
– overview, **30–31,** 38–39
Immunodeficiencies, **35–38,** 41–43
Inborn errors of metabolism, **52–53,** 60–61
Incomplete penetrance, 61
Infarcts, 25–26, 92–94, 97–98, 194, 254–256, 283, 285
Infections
– bacterial. *See* Bacterial infections
– CNS, **247–248,** 257–258
– liver, 188
– opportunist, 43
– parasitic, 153, 172, 174, 175
– pulmonary, 15, **129–130,** 138, 286–287
– renal, 150, 152, 153
– urinary tract, 212
– viral, 64, 119, 151, 189–191, 193–194, 257
– yeast, 269
Infectious mononucleosis, 120
Infertility, 211
Inflammation, **10–13,** 13–15, 23, 284, 285, 286
Inflammatory bowel disease, 174, 175
Inheritance, disorders of, **52–56,** 60–63. *See also specific genetic disorders*
Injury, cellular, **3–4,** 6–7
Innate immunity, 38
Integumentary system, diseases of, 263–269
Interstitial lung disease, 136, 137
Interstitial pneumonia, 138
Intestinal ischemia, 173
Intestinal obstruction, 171, 172, 191
Intracerebral hemorrhage, 255
Intradermal nevus, 268
Intraductal papillomas, 215–216
Intravascular hemolysis, 119
Intraventricular hemorrhage, 172
Intrinsic renal failure, 152
Intussusception, 63–64
Invasive ductal adenocarcinomas, 216
Iron deficiency anemia, 116–119, 168, 170, 174
Irreversible cellular injury, 6, 7, 14
Ischemic brain injuries, 254–256
Ischemic colitis, 173
Ischemic heart disease, **86–88,** 97–98
Isochromosome 12p, 208
Isotonic hyponatremia, 232
ITP (idiopathic thrombocytopenic purpura), 119

J

JAK2 mutation, 122
Jaundice, 191, 193
Juvenile rheumatoid arthritis (JRA), 239

K

Kaposi sarcoma, 42, 100
Kartagener's syndrome, 286
Kawasaki's disease, 95, 96
Kidney and urinary tract, diseases of, 143–153
– glomerular diseases, **144–146,** 149–151, 152
– renal tumors, cysts, and calculi, **148–149,** 153
– tubular and interstitial diseases, **146–148,** 151–152
Kidney failure, 151–152, 153
Kidney stones, 153
Klebsiella pneumoniae, 286–287
Klinefelter's syndrome, 63
Koilocyte, 209–210
Korsakoff's syndrome, 258

L

Laboratory testing reference ranges, 193
Lactase deficiency, 172
Lactose intolerance, 172
Lacunar infarct, 255
Lambert-Eaton syndrome, 259
Large intestine, diseases of, **163–168,** 173–175
Laryngeal tumors, 139
Lead poisoning, 73
Left-sided heart failure, 101
Left ventricular hypertrophy, 25
Leiomyomas, 174
Leukemias, 121–123, 153
Leukocyte adhesion deficiency, 13
Leukocyte rolling and adhesion, 13, 14, 15
Levamisole, 74
Lichen planus, 269
Li-Fraumeni syndrome, 48
Lines of Zahn, 141
Lipoprotein(a), 95
Liquefactive necrosis, 6, 24
Liver, diseases of, 177–195
– biliary tract, **183–185,** 191–193
– cirrhosis, 168, **179–180,** 188–189, 191, 195
– miscellaneous, **186–188,** 193–195
– viral, alcohol and metabolic, **180–183,** 189–191
Liver angiosarcoma, 73
Lividity, 23, 284
Lobar pneumonia, 138
Lower motor neuron disease, 260
Lung tumors, 100, 228, 240, 259
Lupus, 40, 284
Lyme disease, 239
Lymphangitis, 100
Lymphedema, 100
Lymphocytic leukemia, 121
Lymphoid system, diseases of, **111–115,** 120–123
Lymphomas, 48–49, 153, 208, 290
Lysosomal storage disorders, **54–55,** 62

M

Macrocytic anemia, 75, 117
Macrophages, 23
Malassezia, 269
Male reproductive system, diseases of
– penis, **207,** 212
– prostate, **206–207,** 211–212, 286
– testes, **202,** 208
Malignant melanoma, 48–49, 268
Mallory's hyaline, 188
Malnutrition and dietary deficiencies, **71–73,** 75–76. *See also specific dietary deficiencies*
MALT lymphomas, 289

Marfan's syndrome, 61–62, 93, 95, 284
Marginal zone lymphoma (MALTomas), 231
Massive hepatic necrosis, 193
Mastitis, 215
Maternal (gestational) diabetes, 64
McArdle's disease, 62
MCA (middle cerebral artery) stroke, 26
MDMA (ectasy) abuse, 74
Meckel's diverticulum, 64, 171, 172
Meconium ileus, 65
Medulloblastoma, 261
Megaloblastic anemia, 117, 170
Membranous glomerulonephropathy, 150, 151
Men. *See* Male reproductive system, diseases of
Meningiomas, 261, 262
Meningitis, 257
Mesenteric embolic infarction, 25
Mesenteric infarction, 25
Mesothelioma, 139
Metabolic liver disease, 190–191
Metaplasia, 5, 286
Metastases, 240
Metastatic calcification, 8
Metastatic colonic adenocarcinoma, 195
Metastatic prostatic adenocarcinoma, 211, 212
Methemoglobinemia, 73
Microcytic anemia, 116–120
Microglial cells, 258
Middle cerebral artery (MCA) stroke, 26
Migratory thrombophlebitis, 199
Minimal change disease, 151
Mitral insufficiency, 98
Monckeberg medial calcification, 95
Morbid obesity, 75
Morphogenesis abnormalities, 65
Motor neuron diseases, upper and lower, 260
Mouth, diseases of, **157,** 168
Mucopolysaccharidoses, 62
Multinucleated cells, 258
Multiple endocrine neoplasia type I, 172
Multiple myeloma, 122
Multiple sclerosis, 258, 259, 261
Mumps, 64
Mural thrombus, 98, 99
Murphy's sign, 192
Musculoskeletal system, diseases of, 235–240
Myasthenia gravis, 41, 260–261, 284
Mycobacterium tuberculosis, 15, 257–258, 287
Mycoplasma pneumoniae, 138
Mycotic aneurysm, 93
Myelofibrosis, 122
Myeloid leukemia, 121
Myocardial infarction, 26, 93, 94, 97–98, 194, 283
Myxomas, 100

N

Necrosis
– defined, 6
– inflammation and, 15
– types of, 6–7, 24, 74, 152, 193–194, 239, 289
Necrotizing enterocolitis, 65, 172
Neisseria gonorrheae, 209, 212
Neisseria meningitidis, 138, 233
Neonatal appendicitis, 65
Neonatal respiratory distress syndrome, 65
Neoplasia and neoplasms, 45–49. *See also specific neoplasms*
– bone, **238,** 239–240
– CNS, **253–254,** 261–262
– overview, **46–47,** 48–49
– pulmonary, **131–132,** 139–140
– skin, 48–49

Nephritic syndrome, 149–150, 287
Nephrogenic diabetes insipidus, 229
Nephrolithiasis, 153
Nephrotic syndrome, 149–150, 152
Nervous system, diseases of, 241–262
– brain and, **243–246,** 254–257
– demyelinating, alcohol-related, and
    miscellaneous, **248–250,** 258–259
– infections and aneurysms, **247–248,**
    257–258
– neoplasms, **253–254,** 261–262
– neurodegenerative, hydrocephalus, and
    motor neuron, **250–252,** 259–261, 262
Neuroblastomas, 64, 233
Neurofibrillary tangles, 259–260
Neurofibromatosis, 48, 60
Neutrophils, 117
Niacin deficiency, 171
Niemann-Pick disease, 62
Nitric oxide, 73
Nitrous oxide, 75
Noncaseating granulomas, 174
Noncommunicating hydrocephalus, 260, 262
Nondisjunction of chromosomes, 62
Non-neoplastic diseases of bone, **236–237,**
    238–239
Non–small cell carcinomas, 139
Nonspecific interstitial pneumonia (NSIP), 137
NSIP (nonspecific interstitial pneumonia), 137
Nutritional diseases, **71–73,** 75–76

O

Obstruction
– airway, **135,** 142
– bowel, 171, 172, 191
Obstructive atelectasis, 140
Obstructive lung disease, **126–127,** 135–136,
    190
Occipital lobe infarcts, 256
Occlusive thrombus, 97–98, 285
Oligodendroglioma, 262
Oncogenes, 48–49
Opportunist infections, 43
Opsonins, 13
Oral contraceptive pills (OCPs), 74
Organogenesis abnormalities, 65
Osteitis fibrosa cystica, 231
Osteoblastic metastatic adenocarcinoma,
    211, 212
Osteochondroma, 240
Osteogenesis imperfecta, 238
Osteoid osteoma, 240
Osteonecrosis, 239
Osteopetrosis, 238–239
Ovaries, diseases of, **205–206,** 210–211, 232

P

Paget's disease, 216
p-ANCA, 175, 191
Pancreas, diseases of, 197–199, **226–227,**
    233–234, 285
Pancreatic carcinoma, 199
Pancreatitis, 120, 171, 198, 285, 290
Papillary thyroid carcinoma, 231
Paradoxical embolus, 99
Paraesophageal hiatal hernia, 289
Parasitic infection, 153, 172, 174, 175
Parathyroid adenomas, 172, 231
Parathyroid gland, diseases of, 172, **223–224,**
    231
Paroxysmal nocturnal hemoglobinuria, 118
Parvovirus B19 infections, 119
Passive venous congestion, 24

Patau's syndrome, 63
Pathologic adaption, 5, 6
PCA (posterior cerebral artery) stroke, 26
Pediatric diseases, **52–53, 56–60,** 60, 63–65
– tumors, 48–49, 64, 208, 233
Pelvic inflammatory disease, 209, 210–211
Pemphigus foliaceous, 267
Pemphigus vulgaris, 267, 269
Pencil cells, 116, 117, 118
Penis, diseases of, **207,** 212
Perforated peptic ulcer, 169
Pericarditis, 40, 98, 285
Perihepatitis, 211
Peripheral neuropathy, 171
Peripheral vascular disease, 93–95
Peritonitis, 169–171
Peutz-Jeghers polyps, 174
Peyronie's disease, 290
Phenylketonuria, 61
Pheochromocytomas, 94, 232
Phosphorus, refeeding syndrome and, 75
Physiologic adaption, 5, 6
Pick's disease, 261
Pigmented granular casts, 150, 152
Pigment stones, 193
Pilocytic astrocytoma, 262
Pituitary adenomas, 230
Pituitary gland, diseases of, **218–220,**
    227–229, 230
Placental tissue, retained, 210
Pleura
– diseases of, **132–133,** 140
– effusions, **134,** 141
Plummer-Vinson syndrome, 168
Pneumonia, 42, 137, 138, 286–287, 288
Pneumonitis, 137–138, 288
Pneumothorax, **133, 134,** 140, 141
Poisoning, environmental, 73
Polyarteritis nodosa, 95
Polycystic ovarian syndrome, 232
Polycythemia vera, 122
Polymyalgia rheumatica, 40
Polyvinyl chloride exposure, 73
Pompe's disease, 62
Portal hypertension, 189
Posterior cerebral artery (PCA) stroke, 26
Postinfectious glomerulonephritis, 150
Post-renal azotemia, 152, 153
Precursor B-cell lymphoma, 122
Precursor T-cell lymphoma, 122
Pregnancy, **208,** 210, 212
Premature infants, conditions of, 172
Pre-renal azotemia, 152
Pre-renal failure, 151–152
Preterm (premature) infants, 65
Pretibial myxedema, 230
Primary biliary cirrhosis, 191
Primary hyperparathyroidism, 231
Primary hypoadrenalism, 232, 233
Primary hypothyroidism, 229
Primary pulmonary hypertension, 288
Primary sclerosing cholangitis, 174, 175,
    191, 192
Proliferative fibrocystic disease, 215
Prostate, diseases of, **206–207,** 211–212, 286
Prostatic adenocarcinoma, 211
Prostatic hyperplasia, benign (BPH), 211
Protein C deficiency, 74
Proteins
– cellular accumulation of, 8
– genetic diseases of, **54,** 61–62
Proximal jejunal peptic ulcer, 170
Pseudoaneurysm, 92

Pseudomembranes, 175
Pseudomonas aeruginosa, 233
Pseudomyxoma peritonei, 171
Pseudopolyps, 174
Psoriasis, 267, 268
Pulmonary asbestosis, 73, 136, 137, 139
Pulmonary embolism, 99–100, **133–135,**
    140–142, 199, 283
Pulmonary emphysema, 101, 190, 287–288
Pulmonary fibrosis, 101
Pulmonary function testing, 136
Pulmonary hypertension, 288
Pulmonary infections, **129–130,** 138
Pulmonary neoplasms, **131–132,** 139–140
Pulmonary tumors, 100, 228, 240, 259
Pure red cell aplasia, 116
Pyloric stenosis, 64, 65, 169, 289
Pyoderma gangrenosum, 174, 175

R

Radiotherapy agents, 74
Reactive arthritis, 239
Reactive oxygen species (ROS), 7, 14
Red blood cell casts, 150, 152
Red blood cell disorders, **105–111,** 116–120
Red infarcts, 25
Red neurons, 254
Refeeding syndrome, 75
Reference ranges for laboratory testing, 193
Reflux, gastroesophageal, 173, 289
Renal artery stenosis, 94, 232, 283, 285
Renal cell carcinomas, 153
Renal failure, 151–152, 153
Renal infarction, 25
Renal tumors, cysts, and calculi, **148–149,** 153
Reproductive system, diseases of, 201–212
– ovaries, **205–206,** 210–211, 232
– penis, **207,** 212
– pregnancy, **208,** 210, 212
– prostate, **206–207,** 211–212, 286
– testes, **202,** 208
– uterus, **202–205, 208,** 209–210, 212
Respiratory distress, 65, 286, 287
Respiratory system, diseases of, 125–142
– infections, 15, **129–130,** 138, 286–287
– neoplasms, **131–132,** 139–140
– obstructive lung disease, **126–127,** 135–136,
    190
– pleura, diseases of, **132–133,** 140
– pleural effusions, **134,** 141
– pneumothorax, **134,** 141
– restrictive lung disease, **127–129,** 136–138,
    288
– thromboembolism, 26, 99–100, **133–135,**
    140–142, 199, 283
Restrictive lung disease, **127–129,** 136–138,
    288
Retained placental tissue, 210
Reversible cellular injury, 6, 7, 285
Rhabdomyoma, 284
Rheumatoid arthritis, 39, 40
Riboflavin (vitamin B2) deficiency, 75
Right-sided colonic adenocarcinoma, 175
Right-sided heart failure, 101
Robertsonian translocations, 62
ROS (reactive oxygen species), 7, 14
Rosacea, 268
Rotor's syndrome, 189

S

Salicylate intoxication, 74
Sarcoidosis, 15, 137
Scarring, 14

Schistocytes, 120
Schistosoma haematobium infection, 153
Schwannoma, 262
SCID (severe combined immunodeficiency), 42, 43
Seasonal allergies, 38
Secondary aldosteronism, 232
Secondary hypertension, 94
Secondary hyperthyroidism, 230
Secondary hypothyroidism, 229
Secondary membranous glomerulonephropathy, 151
Selective IgA deficiency, 43
Seminoma, 208
Senile plaques, 259–260
Sepsis, 23, 24, 60
Septic arthritis, 239
Septic shock, 23–24
Serum sickness, 39
Severe combined immunodeficiency (SCID), 42, 43
Sheehan's syndrome, 227–228
Shock, 23–24
SIADH (syndrome of inappropriate antidiuretic hormone), 228
Sickle cell anemia, 117, 118
SIDS (sudden infant death syndrome), 64
Signet ring cells, 169, 174
Silica exposure, 137
Silicosis, 73
Sjögren's syndrome, 40–41
Skin, diseases of, **264–266,** 267–269
Skin necrosis, 74
SLE (systemic lupus erythematosus), 39–41, 229, 284
Small bowel obstruction, 191
Small cell carcinoma, 139, 228, 259
Small intestine, diseases of, **160–163,** 170–172
Sodium retention, 285
Spherocytes, 117, 118
Spina bifida, 64
Splenectomies, 138
Splenic flexure, 173
Spontaneous bacterial peritonitis, 188
Squamous cell carcinoma, 212, 289
Stable angina, 93
Stalk effect, 229
Steatorrhea, 172
Steroids, exogenous, 233
Stomach, diseases of, **158–160,** 169–170
Stool testing, 172
Storage disorders, lysosomal, 62
Streptococcus agalactiae (Group B streptococcus), 287
Streptococcus pneumoniae, 138, 257, 286
Strokes, 25, 26, 94, 254–255
Structural proteins, diseases of, **54,** 61–62
Struma ovarii, 231
Subacute thyroiditis, 231
Subarachnoid hemorrhage, 256, 257
Subdural hematoma, 285
Subdural hemorrhage, 256, 257
Subthalamic nucleus injuries, 254
Sudden infant death syndrome (SIDS), 64
Superficial thrombophlebitis, 25
Superior mesenteric artery, 173
Superior vena cava syndrome, 100, 139
Suppurative inflammation, 286
Syndrome of inappropriate antidiuretic hormone (SIADH), 228
Synovial cyst, 239
Systemic hypertension, 94, 285
Systemic lupus erythematosus (SLE), 39–41, 229, 284
Systemic sclerosis, 40, 41, 229

T

Takayasu's arteritis, 95
Target cells, 118
Tau protein, 260
Tay-Sachs disease, 62, 63
T-cell neoplasms, 121
Teardrop cells, 117
Telomerase, 8
Tendon reflexes, 260
Tension pneumothorax, **134,** 140, 141
Teratomas, 64, 208, 231, 233
Testes, diseases of, **202,** 208
Testicular torsion, 208
Tetralogy of Fallot, 96–97
Thalassemia, 116, 118, 120
Therapeutic drugs, **69–70,** 73–74
Thiamine (vitamin B1) deficiency, 75, 171, 258
Thoracic aortic aneurysms, 92, 93, 173
Thromboangiitis obliterans, 96
Thrombocytopenia, 24, 27
Thromboembolism, 26, 99–100, **133–135,** 140–142, 199, 283
Thrombolysis, 24
Thrombophilia, 26–27
Thrombosis, 25–26, 173, 285
Thrombotic thrombocytopenic purpura, 119
Thymomas, 284
Thyroid gland, diseases of, **221–223,** 229–231
Thyroid stimulating hormone (TSH), 229–230
Thyroid storm, 230
Thyrotoxicosis, 230
Tinea versicolor, 269
Toll-like receptors, 13
Tracheoesophageal fistula, 288
TRALI (transfusion-related acute lung injury), 120
Transfusion reactions, 39, 284
Transfusion-related acute lung injury (TRALI), 120
Transmigration of leukocytes, 13, 15
Transudates, 13, 15, 285
Tricuspid atresia, 96–97
Trisomy, 62–63
Tropheryma whipplei, 171
Trousseau's syndrome, 199
TSH (thyroid stimulating hormone), 229–230
Tuberculosis, 39, 287
Tuberous sclerosis (TS), 48–49, 60, 100, 284
Tubular adenomas, 174
Tumors. *See also* Neoplasia and neoplasms
– bile duct, 195
– bone, 239–240
– carcinoid, 171
– cardiovascular, 100
– endocrine, 228, 232
– esophageal, 168
– gastrointestinal, 289–290
– lung, 100, 228, 240, 259
– pancreas, 198
– pediatric, 48–49, 64, 208, 233
– renal, **148–149,** 153
– testicular, 208
– types of, 48–49
Tumor suppressor genes, 48–49
Turner's syndrome, 63
Type I-IV hypersensitivity reactions, **30–31,** 38–39, 284

U

UIP (usual interstitial pneumonia), 137, 288
Ulcerative colitis, 173–174, 175, 192, 195
Ulcers, 169–170, 172, 174, 289
Unconjugated hyperbilirubinemia, 192, 193, 194
Upper motor neuron disease, 260
Uric acid kidney stones, 153

Urinary calculi, 153
Urinary tract, diseases of. *See* Kidney and urinary tract, diseases of
Urinary tract infections (UTIs), 212
Usual interstitial pneumonia (UIP), 137, 288
Uterus, diseases of, **202–205, 208,** 209–210, 212

V

Valvular insufficiency, 283
Variable expressivity, 61
Varices, esophageal, 168, 188, 189
Varicose veins, 99
Vascular congestion, 24
Vasculitis, **84,** 95–96
Vasoconstriction, 14
Vasodilation, 14
Venous infarct, 255
Venous insufficiency, 25
Venous thromboembolism (VTE), 26
Ventricular septal defect, 96
Vertebral artery dissection, 256
Villous adenomas, 174
Vinyl chloride, 73
Viral infections, 64, 119, 151, 189–191, 193–194, 257
Vitamin A deficiency, 75
Vitamin B1 (thiamine) deficiency, 75, 171, 258
Vitamin B2 (riboflavin) deficiency, 75
Vitamin B6 deficiency, 171
Vitamin B12 (cobalamin) deficiency, 75, 76, 116, 170, 283
Vitamin K deficiency, 171
Vitiligo, 267
Vomiting, cyclic, 75
von Gierke's disease, 62
Von Hippel-Lindau (syndrome) disease, 60, 290
von Willebrand factor (VWF), 24
VTE (venous thromboembolism), 26
Vulnerable plaque, 97

W

WAGR syndrome, 64
Warfarin-induced skin necrosis, 74
Warm autoimmune hemolytic anemia, 117, 119, 194
Waterhouse-Friderichsen's syndrome, 232–233
Watershed infarct, 255
Wegener's granulomatosis, 95
Werdnig-Hoffman syndrome, 260
Wermer syndrome (MEN I), 228
Wernicke-Korsakoff syndrome, 75
Wernicke's aphasia, 254
Whipple's disease, 171
White blood cell casts, 150, 152
White blood cell disorders, **111–115,** 120–123
White infarcts, 25
Wilms tumor, 48, 49, 64
Wilson's disease, 191
Wiskott-Aldrich syndrome, 43
Women. *See* Breast diseases; Female reproductive system, diseases of

X

Xerophthalmia, 75
X-linked agammaglobulinemia, 43
X-linked lymphoproliferative disorder, 43

Y

Yeast infection, 269
Yolk sac tumors, 64, 208, 233

Z

Zollinger-Ellison syndrome, 171, 172